CUTANEOUS
NEUROIMMUNOMODULATION

THE PROOPIOMELANOCORTIN SYSTEM

ANNALS OF THE NEW YORK ACADEMY OF SCIENCES
Volume 885

CUTANEOUS NEUROIMMUNOMODULATION
THE PROOPIOMELANOCORTIN SYSTEM

*Edited by Thomas A. Luger, Ralf Paus,
James M. Lipton, and Andrzej T. Slominski*

The New York Academy of Sciences
New York, New York
1999

The cover of the paper-bound edition of this volume shows human dermal fibroblasts doubly immunostained for MC-1R (red fluorescence) and a marker for the endoplasmic reticulum (green fluorescence). Most of the MC-1R is distributed in vesicles in the cell periphery. (Photograph courtesy of Markus Böhm, Michael Raghunath, and Thomas A. Luger.)

**Library of Congress
Cataloging-in-Publication Data
is Available**

ISBN 1-57331-200-2 (cloth : alk. paper)
ISBN 1-57331-201-0 (pbk : alk. paper)

K-M Research/CCP
Printed in the United States of America
ISBN 1-57331-200-2 (cloth)
ISBN 1-57331-201-0 (paper)
ISSN 0077-8923

ANNALS OF THE NEW YORK ACADEMY OF SCIENCES

Volume 885

October 20, 1999

CUTANEOUS NEUROIMMUNOMODULATION
THE PROOPIOMELANOCORTIN SYSTEM

Editors and Conference Chairs
THOMAS A. LUGER, RALF PAUS, JAMES M. LIPTON, AND ANDRZEJ T. SLOMINSKI

Conference Organizers
THOMAS BRZOSKA, D.-HENNER KALDEN, RALF PAUS, AND CORD SUNDERKÖTTER

CONTENTS

The Proopiomelanocortin System in Cutaneous Neuroimmunomodulation:
An Introductory Overview. *By* THOMAS A. LUGER, RALF PAUS,
ANDRZEJ SLOMINSKI, AND JAMES LIPTON xi

Part I. Extracutaneous Proopiomelanocortin Biology

The Proopiomelanocortin System. *By* MAC E. HADLEY
AND CARRIE HASKELL-LUEVANO 1

POMC–Derived Peptides and Their Biological Action. *By* SAMUEL SOLOMON ... 22

The Pituitary–Skin Connection in Amphibians: Reciprocal Regulation of
Melanotrope Cells and Dermal Melanocytes. *By* H. VAUDRY,
N. CHARTREL, L. DESRUES, L. GALAS, S. KIKUYAMA, A. MOR,
P. NICOLAS, AND M.C. TONON 41

The Subtilisin/Kexin Family of Precursor Convertases: Emphasis on PC1, PC2/
7B2, POMC and the Novel Enzyme SKI-1. *By* NABIL G. SEIDAH,
SUZANNE BENJANNET, JOSÉE HAMELIN, AIDA M. MAMARBACHI,
AJOY BASAK, JADWIGA MARCINKIEWICZ, MAJAMBU MBIKAY,
MICHEL CHRÉTIEN, AND MIECZYSLAW MARCINKIEWICZ 57

The Role of Melanocortins in Adipocyte Function. *By* BRUCE A. BOSTON 75

An Immunocytochemical Approach to the Study of β-Endorphin Production in
Human Keratinocytes using Confocal Microscopy. *By* SUSANA B. ZANELLO,
DAVID M. JACKSON, AND MICHAEL F. HOLICK 85

Part II. The Melanocortin Receptors

UV Light and MSH Receptors. *By* ASHOK K. CHAKRABORTY, YOKO FUNASAKA,
ANDRZEJ SLOMINSKI, JEAN BOLOGNIA, STEFANO SODI,
MASAMITSU ICHIHASHI, AND JOHN M. PAWELEK 100

*a*This volume is the result of a conference entitled **Cutaneous Neuroimmunomodulation: The Proopiomelanocortin System** held by the New York Academy of Sciences on September 11–13, 1998 in Münster, Germany.

The Melanocortin-1 Receptor and Human Pigmentation. *By* ZALFA ABDEL-
MALEK, ITARU SUZUKI, AKIHIRO TADA, SUNGBIN IM, AND CAN AKCALI .. 117

Genetic Studies of the Human Melanocortin-1 Receptor. *By* JONATHAN L. REES,
MARK BIRCH-MACHIN, NIAMH FLANAGAN, EUGENE HEALY, SIÔN PHILLIPS,
AND CAROLE TODD 134

Molecular Pharmacology of Agouti Protein *in Vitro* and *in Vivo*.
By GREGORY S. BARSH, MICHAEL M. OLLMANN, BRENT D. WILSON,
KIMBERLY A. MILLER, AND TERESA M. GUNN 143

Synthetic Melanocortin Receptor Agonists and Antagonists.
By MICHAEL R. LERNER 153

Proopiomelanocortin and the Immune–Neuroendocrine Connection.
By J. EDWIN BLALOCK 161

**Part III. Proopiomelanocortin and the Skin Immune System:
Modulation of the Immune Response**

Mechanisms of Antiinflammatory Action of α-MSH Peptides: *In Vivo* and *in Vitro*
Evidence. *By* J.M. LIPTON, H. ZHAO, T. ICHIYAMA, G.S. BARSH,
AND A. CATANIA 173

α-MSH in Systemic Inflammation: Central and Peripheral Actions.
By ANNA CATANIA, RENÉ DELGADO, LORENA AIRAGHI,
MARIAGRAZIA CUTULI, LETIZIA GAROFALO, ANDREA CARLIN,
MARIA TERESA DEMITRI, AND JAMES M. LIPTON 183

Human Peripheral Blood-Derived Dendritic Cells Express Functional
Melanocortin Receptor MC-1R. *By* E. BECHER, K. MAHNKE,
T. BRZOSKA, D.-H. KALDEN, S. GRABBE, AND T.A. LUGER 188

Neural Influences on Induction of Contact Hypersensitivity.
By J. WAYNE STREILEIN, PASCALE ALARD, AND HIRONORI NIIZEKI 196

Role of Epidermal Cell-Derived α-Melanocyte Stimulating Hormone in
Ultraviolet Light Mediated Local Immunosuppression. *By* T.A. LUGER, T.
SCHWARZ, H. KALDEN, T. SCHOLZEN, A. SCHWARZ, AND T. BRZOSKA 209

Part IV. Modulation of Skin Physiology by Proopiomelanocortin Products

α-MSH and the Regulation of Melanocyte Function. *By* ANTHONY J. THODY. . . . 217

Molecular Basis of the α-MSH/IL-1 Antagonism. *By* T. BRZOSKA,
D.-H. KALDEN, T. SCHOLZEN, AND T.A. LUGER 230

Expression of Functional Melanocortin Receptors and Proopiomelanocortin
Peptides by Human Dermal Microvascular Endothelial Cells.
By THOMAS E. SCHOLZEN, THOMAS BRZOSKA, DIRK-HENNER KALDEN,
MECHTHILD HARTMEYER, MICHAELA FASTRICH, THOMAS A. LUGER,
CHERYL A. ARMSTRONG, AND JOHN C. ANSEL 239

Mechanisms of the Antiinflammatory Effects of α-MSH: Role of Transcription Factor NF-κB and Adhesion Molecule Expression. *By* D.-H. KALDEN, T. SCHOLZEN, T. BRZOSKA, AND T.A. LUGER 254

POMC and Fibroblast Biology. *By* TORELLO LOTTI, PATRIZIA TEOFOLI, BEATRICE BIANCHI, AND ALAIN MAUVIEL 262

The Role of Proopiomelanocortin-Derived Peptides in Skin Fibroblast and Mast Cell Functions. *By* PATRIZIA TEOFOLI, ALESSANDRA FREZZOLINI, PIETRO PUDDU, ORNELLA DE PITÀ, ALAIN MAUVIEL, AND TORELLO LOTTI . 268

Alpha-Melanocyte-Stimulating Hormone Modulates Activation of NF-κB and AP-1 and Secretion of Interleukin-8 in Human Dermal Fibroblasts. *By* MARKUS BÖHM, URSULA SCHULTE, HENNER KALDEN, AND T.A. LUGER . . . 277

Part V. Corticotropin-Releasing Hormone–Proopiomelanocortin Interactions

Cutaneous Expression of CRH and CRH-R: Is There a "Skin Stress Response System?" *By* ANDRZEJ T. SLOMINSKI, VLADIMIR BOTCHKAREV, MASHKOOR CHOUDHRY, NADEEM FAZAL, KLAUS FECHNER, JENS FURKERT, EBERHART KRAUSE, BIRGIT ROLOFF, MOHAMMAD SAYEED, EDWARD WEI, BLAZEJ ZBYTEK, JOSEF ZIPPER, JACOBO WORTSMAN, AND RALF PAUS 287

Corticotropin Releasing Factor Receptors and Their Ligand Family. *By* MARILYN H. PERRIN AND WYLIE W. VALE 312

Part VI. Proopiomelanocortin-Peptides—Clinical Relevance

α-MSH Can Control the Essential Cofactor 6-Tetrahydrobiopterin in Melanogenesis. *By* KARIN U. SCHALLREUTER, JEREMY MOORE, DESMOND J. TOBIN, NICHOLAS J.P. GIBBONS, HARRIET S. MARSHALL, TRACEY JENNER, WAYNE D. BEAZLEY, AND JOHN M. WOOD 329

Melanocortins and the Treatment of Nervous System Disease: Potential Relevance to the Skin? *By* WILLEM HENDRIK GISPEN AND ROGER A.H. ADAN 342

The Skin POMC System (SPS): Leads and Lessons from the Hair Follicle. *By* RALF PAUS, VLADIMIR A. BOTCHKAREV, NATALIA V. BOTCHKAREVA, LARS MECKLENBURG, THOMAS LUGER, AND ANDRZEJ SLOMINSKI 350

Part VII. Poster Papers

Expression of MC1- and MC5-Receptors on the Human Mast Cell Line HMC-1. *By* M. ARTUC, A. GRÜTZKAU, TH. LUGER, AND B.M. HENZ 364

Characterization of μ-Opiate Receptor in Human Epidermis and Keratinocytes. *By* M. BIGLIARDI-QI, P.L. BIGLIARDI, S. BÜCHNER, AND T. RUFLI 368

Characterization of a Polyclonal Antibody Raised Against the Human Melanocortin-1 Receptor. *By* MARKUS BÖHM, THOMAS BRZOSKA, URSULA SCHULTE, MEINHARD SCHILLER, ULRICH KUBITSCHECK, AND THOMAS A. LUGER 372

Effects of Ethanol Consumption on β-Endorphin Levels and Natural Killer Cell
Activity in Rats. *By* NADKA BOYADJIEVA, GARY MEADOWS,
AND DIPAK SARKAR 383

Murine Dendritic Cells Express Functional Delta-Type Opioid Receptors.
By CLEMENS ESCHE, VALERIA P. MAKARENKOVA, NATALIA V. KOST,
MICHAEL T. LOTZE, ANDREY A. ZOZULYA, AND MICHAEL R. SHURIN 387

Expression of Corticotropin Releasing Hormone in Malignant Melanoma.
By YOKO FUNASAKA, HIROFUMI SATO, AND MASAMITSU ICHIHASHI 391

Depression Modulates Pruritus Perception: A Study of Pruritus in Psoriasis,
Atopic Dermatitis and Chronic Idiopathic Urticaria.
By MADHULIKA A. GUPTA AND ADITYA K. GUPTA 394

α-MSH Immunomodulation Acts via Rel/NF-κB in Cutaneous and Ocular
Melanocytes and in Melanoma Cells. *By* J.W. HAYCOCK, M. WAGNER,
R. MORANDINI, G. GHANEM, I.G. RENNIE, AND S. MacNEIL 396

Microinjection of Alpha-MSH Followed by UV-Irradiation Blocks HSP 72 in
Human Keratinocytes. *By* BJÖRN HELD, SUSANNE AMATO, ERNST G. JUNG,
AND CHRISTIANE BAYERL 400

β-Endorphin Binding and Regulation of Cytokine Expression in Langerhans
Cells. *By* JUNICHI HOSOI, HIROAKI OZAWA, AND RICHARD D. GRANSTEIN .. 405

α-MSH Reduces Vasculitis in the Local Shwartzman Reaction.
By CORD SUNDERKÖTTER, H. KALDEN, T. BRZOSKA, CLEMENS SORG,
AND THOMAS A. LUGER 414

Implications of the Phenotype of POMC Deficiency for the Role of
POMC-Derived Peptides in Skin Physiology. *By* HEIKO KRUDE,
DIRK SCHNABEL, WERNER LUCK, AND ANNETTE GRÜTERS 419

Serotonin in Human Allergic Contact Dermatitis. *By* L. LUNDEBERG,
E. SUNDSTRÖM, K. NORDLIND, A. VERHOFSTAD, AND O. JOHANSSON 422

Differential Temporal and Spatial Expression of POMC mRNA and of the
Production of POMC Peptides During the Murine Hair Cycle.
By J.E. MAZURKIEWICZ, D. CORLISS, AND A. SLOMINSKI 427

Effective Treatment of Pruritus with Naltrexone, an Orally Active Opiate
Antagonist. *By* D. METZE, S. REIMANN, AND T.A. LUGER 430

Developmentally Regulated Expression of α-MSH and MC-1 Receptor in
C57BL/6 Mouse Skin Suggests Functions Beyond Pigmentation.
By V.A. BOTCHKAREV, N.V. BOTCHKAREVA, A. SLOMINSKI, B. ROLOFF,
T. LUGER, AND R. PAUS....................................... 433

Plasma β-Endorphin Concentrations During Natural and Artificially Induced
Winter Hair Growth in Mink (*Mustela vison*). *By* J. ROSE, K. WOOD,
J. BILLINGSLEY, J. OLBERTZ, A. LOVERING, AND J. CARR.............. 440

Expression of Proopiomelanocortin Peptides and Prohormone Convertases by Human Dermal Microvascular Endothelial Cells. *By* THOMAS E. SCHOLZEN, THOMAS BRZOSKA, DIRK-HENNER KALDEN, MECHTHILD HARTMEYER, THOMAS A. LUGER, CHERYL A. ARMSTRONG, AND JOHN C. ANSEL   444

ACTH Production in C57BL/6 Mouse Skin. *By* ANDRZEJ SLOMINSKI, NATALIA V. BOTCHKAREVA, VLADIMIR A. BOTCHKAREV, ASHOK CHAKRABORTY, THOMAS LUGER, MURAT UENALAN, AND RALF PAUS   448

Coexpression of Nitric Oxide Synthase and POMC Peptides in the Dystrophic C57BL/6J Mouse. *By* MARGARET E. SMITH AND RAVINDER K. PHUL   451

Ligand Binding Profile and Effects of Melanin-Concentrating Hormone on Fish and Mammalian Skin Cells. *By* T. SUPLY, B. CARDINAUD, S. KANAMORI, C. DAL FARRA, S. RICOIS, AND J.L. NAHON   455

Occurrence of Four MSHs in Dogfish POMC and Their Immunomodulating Effects. *By* AKIYOSHI TAKAHASHI, YUTAKA AMEMIYA, MASAHIRO SAKAI, AKIKAZU YASUDA, NOBUO SUZUKI, YUICHI SASAYAMA, AND HIROSHI KAWAUCHI   459

Specific Binding Sites for β-Endorphin on Keratinocytes. *By* K. EGELING, H. MÜLLER, B. KARSCHUNKE, M. TSCHISCHKA, V. SPENNEMANN, B. HAIN, AND H. TESCHEMACHER   464

Skin POMC Peptides: Their Binding Affinities and Activation of the Human MC1 Receptor. *By* MARINA TSATMALIA, KAZUMASA WAKAMATSU, ALISON J. GRAHAM, AND ANTHONY J. THODY   466

The Expression of α-MSH by Melanocytes Is Reduced in Vitiligo. *By* ALISON GRAHAM, WIETE WESTERHOF, AND ANTHONY J. THODY   470

α-MSH Inhibits Lipopolysaccharide Induced Nitric Oxide Production in B16 Mouse Melanoma Cells. *By* MARINA TSATMALI, PHILIP MANNING, CALUM J. MCNEIL, AND ANTHONY J. THODY   474

Index of Contributors   477

Financial assistance was received from:

Major Funders
- BUNDESMINISTERIUM FÜR BILDUNG UND FORSCHUNG
- DEUTSCHE FORSCHUNGSGESELLSCHAFT
- MINISTERIUM FÜR WISSENSCHAFT UND FORSCHUNG NORDRHEIN-WESTFALEN

Supporters
- CENTRE DE RECHERCHES ET D'INVESTIGATIONS EPIDERMIQUES ET SENSORIELLES
- ESSEX PHARMA GMBH
- HOFFMANN-LA ROCHE AG
- INTERDISZIPLINÄRES KLINISCHES FORSCHUNGSZENTRUM IN DER MEDIZINISCHEN FAKULTÄT DER UNIV. MÜNSTER
- LA ROCHE-POSAY
- SCHERING AG

Contributors
- CENTEON PHARMA GMBH
- CIRD GALDERMA SOPHIA ANTIPOLIS
- DPC BIERMANN GMBH
- DR. AUGUST WOLFF ARZNEIMITTEL
- GALDERMA FÖDERKREIS E.V.
- HERMAL
- LEO GMBH
- NOVARTIS PHARMA GMBH
- PHARMACIA & UPJOHN DIAGNOSTICS
- RENTSCHLER BIOTECHNOLOGY
- SYNTHÉLABO GMBH

The Proopiomelanocortin System in Cutaneous Neuroimmunomodulation

An Introductory Overview

THOMAS A. LUGER, RALF PAUS, ANDRZEJ SLOMINSKI, AND JAMES LIPTON

Proopiomelanocortin (POMC)-derived peptides have key roles in the coordination of complex neuroendocrine–immune interactions that maintain homeostasis and control stress-induced tissue damage. The POMC gene encoding that information is composed of three exons and two introns that are spliced from the primary transcripts to generate POMC mRNA, which is then translated into a single primary protein product. Subsequent tissue-specific processing by prohormone convertases and posttranslational modifications generate the regulatory neuropeptides adrenocorticotropin (ACTH), melanocyte stimulating hormones (α-, β-, γ-MSH), β-lipotropin (β-LP) and β-endorphin. The sequential steps from POMC gene transcription through the release of POMC-derived peptides are under multihormonal control. The process is also site-specific. In the pituitary it is lobe-specific, and in peripheral tissues it is organ-specific. In the pituitary, the predominant POMC producing organ, these steps are under hypothalamic control, in particular by the release of corticotropin releasing hormone (CRH).

Skin has long been recognized by pigment biologists, as well as by clinical and investigative dermatologists, to be the classical target organ for ACTH and MSH peptides. Due to its accessibility, and owing to the ease with which it can be manipulated experimentally, the skin lends itself as an ideal model system for exploring the role of POMC products in peripheral neuro-endocrine–immune interaction systems. Recent evidence indicates that, within the skin, keratinocytes, melanocytes, fibroblasts, and endothelial cells, as well as immunocytes, can produce POMC peptides and express the corresponding receptors. This suggests paracrine and autocrine modes of action for these neuropeptides. Thus, both the skin and its immune system (SIS) are not only targets for POMC peptide bioregulation, but are also sites of POMC expression and processing. The SIS is crucial for protecting the organism against infectious agents and it plays a critical role in the coordination of local and systemic immune responses. Together, the SIS, the pigmentary system, and locally produced neuropeptides can be viewed as forming a powerful early alarm network that reacts to noxious stimuli, such as solar radiation (ultraviolet light) and thermal, biological, and chemical insults.

The main goal of this New York Academy of Sciences Conference on Cutaneous Neuroimmunomodulation: The Proopiomelanocortin System, 1998, was to explore the role of POMC-derived peptides and their receptors in skin physiology and pathology. Particular emphasis was given to the regulation of immune functions, POMC participation in response to cutaneous stress, and to the pathogenesis of skin diseases that have significant neuroimmune components—such as psoriasis, atopic eczema, contact dermatitis, and urticaria. These problems were analyzed from a multidisciplinary approach involving the fields of neuroendocrinology, immunology, pharmacology, pigment and skin biology, and dermatology. A general assumption made during these presentations was that the skin has conserved the mechanisms known to regulate POMC gene expression and the production of POMC–derived peptides elsewhere. Since the discussions were focused on the mechanisms and functions of prohormone convertases, it was concluded that identification and characterization of the convertases, PC1 and PC2, in skin is crucial in order to obtain a proper understanding of cutaneous production of ACTH, α-MSH and β-endorphin.

The phenotypic effects of MSH- and ACTH-peptides are mediated by an interaction with G-protein linked melanocortin (MC) receptors, followed by a signal transduction pathway, coupled predominantly to the production of cAMP and the subsequent activation of cAMP dependent pathways. The presentations reminded us that the pigmentary system has provided the crucial model for defining the pharmacological and biochemical properties of MC receptors. This culminated in cloning the MC receptor family, which provided a better understanding of the function of these peptides. The newly developed molecular probes have been of great help in skin physiology, especially for the assignment of particular MC receptors to defined cell types. These discussions were extended by the analysis of endogenous MC receptor antagonists, including the product of the agouti locus, a natural antagonist of MC receptors. Finally, recent progress in the development of synthetic MC receptor agonists and antagonists was covered, since this opens new therapeutic possibilities for the treatment of various skin diseases.

The main topic of the conference, cutaneous neuroimmnomodulation via the skin POMC system, was preceded by an in-depth analysis of the role of POMC products in the immune-neuroendocrine connection. It appears that the immune system, in addition to protecting against infection, also acts as a diffuse sensory organ delivering to the brain information on biological insults different from that normally detected by sensory nerves. Moreover, the immune system also affects neuroendocrine functions via the production of neuropeptides, in particular of POMC-derived peptides, or directly by cytokine activation of the pituitary gland. Many of these neuroendocrine–immune interactions may be extrapolated to the skin, which also serves as a sensory, endocrine, and immune organ.　　　　•

One of the best-studied and, with respect to its immunomodulatory properties, an extremely potent POMC peptide, is α-MSH. The antinflammatory actions of α-MSH have been demonstrated pharmacologically, by central (brain) administration of inhibitory signals through descending nerve routes to target tissue, or by peripheral application. It appears that the antiflammatory actions of α-MSH are mediated via an antagonism of proinflammatory cytokines, such as interleukin (IL)-1, IL-6, and tumor necrosis factor α (TNFα). The α-MSH$_{11-13}$ sequence has been elucidated to represent the portion of the peptide responsible for its immunomodulatory properties.

In the skin, the effect of α-MSH on the local immune system is pleiotropic and includes, for example, modulation of the function of antigen-presenting cells, downregulation of adhesion molecules and MHC class-I antigen expression, IL-1 antagonism, and the stimulation of immunosuppressive factors (i.e., IL-10 production). Using animal models of systemic or topical application of α-MSH, this neuropeptide has been shown to inhibit the induction as well as the elicitation phase of contact hypersensitivity reactions, and to induce hapten-specific tolerance *in vivo.* In a skin model of septic shock, the Shwartzmann-Sanarelli reaction, α-MSH *in vivo* inhibits the associated vasculitis. There is also the intriguing possibility that α-MSH may inhibit the skin immune system via stimulation of melanogenesis in melanocytes. In this context, it is known that melanogenesis intermediate products such as L-DOPA can have immunosuppressive effects.

Not surprisingly, immunoregulatory properties of α-MSH may have a role in the therapy of inflammatory dermatoses. For example, one report covered the amelioration of contact dermatitis by topical application of α-MSH. Thus, it appears that we are on the verge of crossing the bridge between basic bench-research and clinical reality.

Recent evidence suggests that mast cells, neutrophils, and vascular endothelial cells can all express melanocortin receptors, especially MC-1R. Accordingly, it has been shown that some of the antinflammatory activities of α-MSH are due to its capacity to modulate adhesion molecule expression and cytokine production of these cells. Moreover, the detection of MC-1R expression on fibroblasts, and the finding that α-MSH is able to modulate collagen synthesis, raise the possibility that this neuropeptide is involved in the pathogenesis of fibrotic disorders such as scleroderma and keloids. However, these *in vitro* observations remain to be confirmed under *in vivo* conditions, and their clinical relevance is as yet obscure. Also, we are challenged to address the question: are there any skin cell populations that do *not* express MC-receptors, yet produce POMC-peptides; and are the functional effects mediated by the binding of MC receptor ligands the same in all these cells?

One of the most important cutaneous stressors is ultraviolet radiation (UVR). UVR stimulates, in a dose-dependent manner, the production of CRH peptide, expression of POMC mRNA, and release of ACTH and α-MSH. In addition, UVR upregulates expression of MC-1R mRNA, and increases α-MSH binding sites on keratinocytes and melanocytes. The latter phenomenon is connected with an increased melanogenic responsiveness to MSH peptides—as documented both in cell culture and *in vivo.* Thus, the stimulation of mammalian pigmentation by UV-light may be regulated by a stringently coordinated cascade of events in which stimulation of the local production of α-MSH, combined with increased expression of MSH receptors, would seem to play a central role. The implications of this model for other cutaneous systems should not be underestimated because of the pleiotropic effects of UVR, including inhibition of the skin immune system and increased epidermal thickness.

The size and functional diversity of skin requires a rapid, local, and efficient mode of responding to various environmental stressors in order to integrate the appropriate signals and to activate defense mechanisms that reestablish disturbed tissue homeostasis. Exciting recent evidence suggests that CRH, the most proximal element of the hypothalamo–pituitary–adrenal (HPA) axis and the neurochrome that coordinates systemic responses to stress in the mammalian organism, is indeed expressed in the skin along with CRH receptors. Furthermore, the cutaneous production of CRH is stimulated by UVR and by factors raising the intracellular cAMP concentration, whereas it is inhibited by dexamethasone. This raises the intriguing question, whether—in analogy to the systemic HPA response to stress—the skin has established an equivalent stress response system by means of which the local generation and release of CRH, and subsequently ACTH, initiates a signaling cascade that operates as a rapid, peripheral stress response system.

In summary, the combined efforts of all participants in this thought provoking conference has set the stage for further interdisciplinary studies on the mechanisms that regulate cutaneous POMC products and their bioregulatory role, as mediated by interaction with their corresponding receptors. A key challenge in this area will be to define how locally generated POMC products regulate the skin immune system under physiological and pathological conditions. Another key task is to develop novel therapeutic strategies for the management of inflammatory dermatoses by manipulating cutaneous POMC and/or MC receptor expression, as well as by topical and systemic administration of MC receptor agonists/antagonists. In this context the coordinated response of skin to stressors like UVR is also a most rewarding research subject. One of the most intriguing questions remains that of whether the skin does indeed contain a functional equivalent of the HPA axis as an evolutionary continuum of the general responses to stress developed by mammalian organisms. This would have far-reaching implications for cutaneous neuro-immunomodulation in health and disease.

The Proopiomelanocortin System

MAC E. HADLEY[a] AND CARRIE HASKELL-LUEVANO[b]

[a]Department of Cell Biology and Anatomy, College of Medicine,
The University of Arizona, Tucson, Arizona 85724-5044, USA

[b]Department of Medicinal Chemistry, University of Florida,
Gainesville, Florida 32610-0485, USA

ABSTRACT: POMC (31,000 MW) is localized to the pituitary, brain, skin, and other peripheral sites. The particular enzyme profile present within a cell dictates the nature of the hormonal ligand (melanocortin) synthesized and secreted: melanotropic peptides (α-MSH β-lipotropin, λ-MSH), corticotropin (ACTH), several endorphins (e.g., met-enkephalin). These POMC-derived peptides mediate their actions through typical seven-spanning membrane receptors (MCRs; MCR1, 2, 3, 4, and 5). A specific melanocortin acting on a specific MCR regulates a particular biological response; for example, α-MSH on MCR1 increases melanogenesis within melanocytes, ACTH on MCR2 increases cortisol production within adrenal zona fasciculata cells. Within the brain melanocortins regulate satiety (MCR4) and erectile activity (MCR?). MCRs have been localized by melanocortin macromolecular probes, for example, fluorescent to human epidermal melanocytes and also to keratinocytes, suggesting that systemic melanocortins or localized POMC products might regulate these integumental cellular elements in synchrony to enhance skin pigmentation and/or immunological responses. Superpotent, prolonged acting melanotropic peptides have been synthesized and their application in clinical medicine has been demonstrated. MCR antagonists have been used to discover and further delineate other roles of melanocortin ligands. For example, melanocortin–induced satiety can be antagonized by a melanocortin antagonist. Defects in melanocortin ligand biosynthesis, secretion, and melanocortin receptor function can lead to a diverse number of pathological states.

INTRODUCTION

This paper provides only a cursory overview of the proopiomelanocortin (POMC) system since other authors in this volume deal extensively with many of the topics surveyed. This review does, however, provide new information on more recent roles of the POMC system not discussed elsewhere in this volume. Clearly, very recent discoveries have broadened considerably our perspectives of the physiological roles of POMC ligands and receptors. In keeping with the general thrust of this volume, emphasis is placed on the melanocortins, and less so on the other class of POMC-derived ligands, the opioid peptides.

[a]Address for correspondence: 520-624-3093 (voice); 520-626-6354 (fax); seastman@u.arizona.edu (e-mail).

THE PROOPIOMELANOCORTIN SYSTEM

The proopiomelanocortin (POMC) system consists of POMC, a preprohormone, its numerous hormonal products, and the equally numerous receptors through which the POMC–derived chemical messengers mediate their actions to regulate a diverse number of physiological functions. Additionally, two naturally occurring MCR antagonists, agouti and agouti-related protein (AGRP), also play important roles in the regulation of the POMC system.

Proopiomelanocortin (POMC)

It was discovered by several investigative groups that some melanocortins were derived from a common precursor protein.[1,2] The nucleotide sequence of the cDNA for bovine POMC was first elucidated by Nakanishi *et al.*, by means of recombinant DNA technology.[3] POMC is a 31,000 molecular weight protein that possesses within its structure amino acid sequences common to a number of biologically important hormones. There is a single POMC gene per haploid nucleus located on chromosome 2p23. Depending on the regulated expression of cell-specific enzymes, POMC is proteolytically cleaved to yield a particular peptide species, for example melanocortin or corticotropin, from the melanotrophs or the corticotrophs, respectively, of the pituitary gland. Pairs of dibasic amino acids (arginine and lysine) within the POMC structure predict rather clearly the prospective cleavage sites and the possible peptides that can be derived from the parent protein (see FIGURE 1).

The sequences of POMC mRNAs have been determined in several species of mammals, amphibians, and teleosts. All POMC sequences from these jawed vertebrates (gnathostomes) reveal the same general structural organization. Although α-MSH, ACTH, and β-endorphin sequences are present, γ- and β-MSH sequences are absent or more likely nonfunctional.[4] The lamprey (an agnathan), most ancient of the vertebrates, pituitary contains recognizable POMC sequences with structural similarity to that of teleosts and higher vertebrates, suggesting that POMC was present in the common ancestor of lampreys and gnathostomes some 700 million or more years ago.[4]

With the discovery of Nature's own analgesics, the opiate-like peptides, it was determined that POMC was also the preprohormone for the generation of these neuropeptides. Proopiomelanocortin, therefore, is an epithet that signifies the hormonal nature of the three general classes of hormonal products to be derived from this preprohormone. The melanocortins (melanotropins and corticotropins) and opiate-like peptides (opioids) are biosynthesized in a variety of tissues; the specific expression and processing of the hormonal products is discussed in detail elsewhere in this volume.[5]

POMC Ligands (Agonists)

Melanocortins

The melanocortins comprise a family of peptides that possess structural similarity. The term melanocortin identifies two subgroups of peptides, the melanotropins and the corticotropins. Melanotropic activity refers to the action of these peptides on melanocytes present within the skin. Corticotropic activity refers to the action of

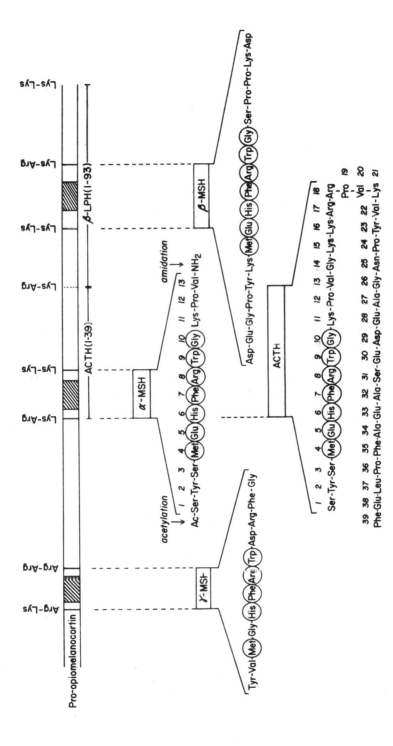

FIGURE 1. Processing of POMC to provide cell-specific opiomelanocortin peptides.

ACTH(1-39)	NH₂–SYSME	**HFRW**	GKPVGKKRRPVKVYPNGAEDESAEAFPLEF–OH
α-MSH	Ac–SYSME	**HFRW**	GKPV–NH₂
β-MSH	NH₂–AEKKDEGPYRME	**HFRW**	GSPPKD–OH
γ-MSH	NH₂–YVMG	**HFRW**	DRF–OH

Sequences of human MCs are provided

FIGURE 2. The melanocortin family of peptides. Note the invariant amino acid sequences in each peptide (*bold*).

these peptides on the adrenal cortex. Although these two classes of hormones regulate quite different functions, when secreted at abnormally high concentrations they may exhibit both melanotropic and corticotropic actions.

The melanotropic peptides were long ago shown to be derived from the pars intermedia of the pituitary gland. Melanocortins are also expressed in the brain, in the hypothalamic arcuate nucleus, and in the dorsal medullary nucleus of the solitary tract. The biosynthesis and release of these POMC-derived peptides is discussed elsewhere in this volume.[6] The melanotropins are characterized by an invariant heptapeptide sequence (see FIGURE 2). All of the melanotropins exhibit melanotropic activity, although at varying potencies. It is to be noted that α-MSH differs from the other melanocortins in that the peptide is N-terminally acetylated and C-terminally amidated (FIGS. 1–3). The shortest sequence that has been demonstrated to exhibit melanotropic activity is the 4–10 sequence, N-acetylated, C-amidated structure, Ac-His-Phe-Arg-Trp-NH$_2$.[7,8] Modifications of this minimal sequence has, however, resulted in a tripeptide analog with even greater potency.[9] Within the POMC structure are to be found two other peptides possessing the central heptapeptide sequence of α-MSH, γ-MSH, and β-MSH. There is no evidence that these peptides are secreted from the pituitary gland in order to play a systemic physiological role.

Corticotropin is 39 amino acids long, the first 13 being identical to α-MSH (but lacking N-terminal and C-terminal modifications (FIG. 2). Absence of the N-terminal acetyl group lowers the melanotropic potency of α-MSH (on melano-

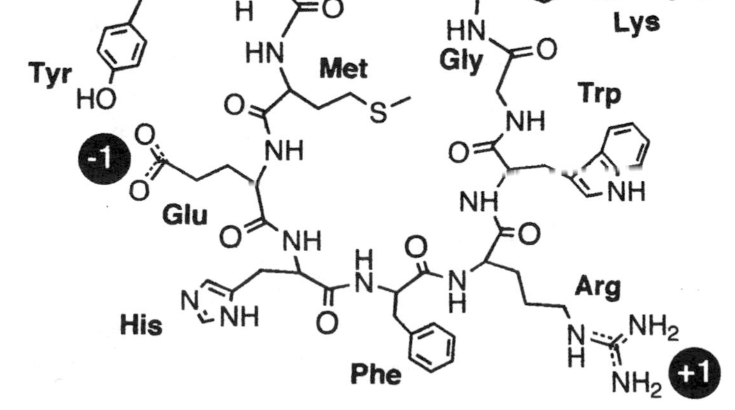

FIGURE 3. Primary structure of α-melanocortin (α-MSH).

cytes) considerably, whereas acetylation of ACTH 1–39 abolishes its corticotropic activity. It might be conjectured that these differences in the N-terminus provide an evolutionary mechanism for the restriction of the activities of α-MSH and ACTH to their appropriate receptors.

Corticotropin (adrenal cortical stimulating hormone, ACTH) is synthesized and secreted by corticotrophs of the anterior lobe of the pituitary gland. Synthesis and release of ACTH are subject to both positive regulation by corticotropin releasing hormone (CRH) and negative feedback by glucocorticoids (cortisol). The preferential expression of mRNA for ACTH in the pars distalis has been beautifully shown by hybridization studies.[10] mRNA for POMC is relatively unaffected by adrenalectomy in the pars intermedia, whereas anterior lobe levels of POMC mRNA are greatly increased. This increase in POMC production is abolished in adrenalectomized animals, however, if they are first treated with a synthetic glucocorticoid (dexamethasone). Intermediate lobe levels of POMC mRNA are unaffected by the glucocorticoid. These observations demonstrate the differential control of POMC mRNA synthesis by cells of the pars intermedia and pars distalis.

Superpotent Melanocortin Agonists

We have synthesized both natural melanotropins, α-MSH and β-MSH, as well as many α-MSH analogs.[11] We have systematically determined the essential features of α-MSH that are necessary for biological activity. We determined that the

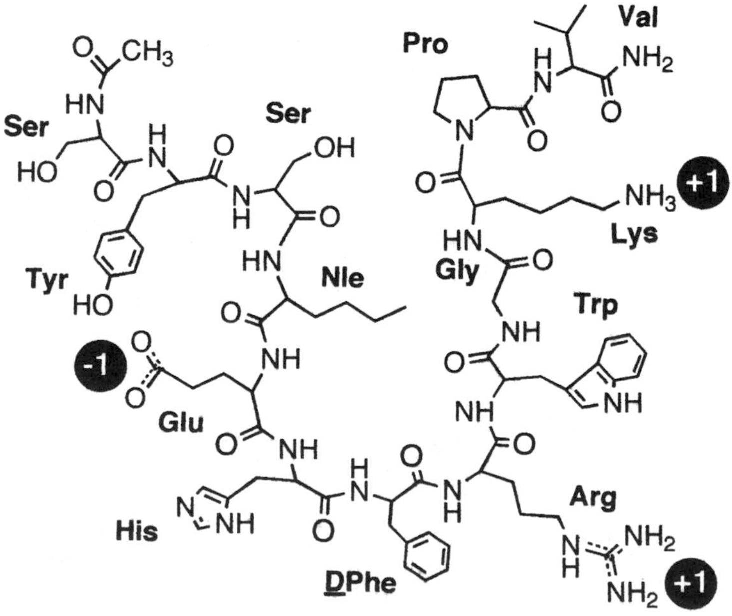

FIGURE 4. Primary structure of [Nle^4/DPhe^7]α-MSH.

N-terminal and C-terminal tripeptide sequences of α-MSH are not required for melanotropin action, and we have even prepared Ac-α-MSH$_{4-10}$-NH$_2$ analogs that are more potent than the tridecapeptide sequence of the native hormone. In an effort to develop α-MSH analogs that possess a variety of specific and desirable biological properties, we determined the structural, stereochemical, and conformational properties associated with biological properties. We have developed melanotropins that are superpotent, some of which, in addition, are nonbiodegradable, and exhibit ultraprolonged biological activity.[11]

We have synthesized a number of [Nle^4,DPhe^7]-substituted analogs of α-MSH. In most cases, these analogs are superpotent, exhibit prolonged activity (as discussed below), and are resistant to inactivation by proteolytic enzymes. The analog [Nle^4,DPhe^7]α-MSH (see FIGURE 4) was 10- to 1000-times more active than α-MSH depending upon the particular assay employed. We subsequently synthesized a number of [Nle^4,DPhe^7]-substituted fragment analogs of α-MSH. Ac-[Nle^4,DPhe^7]α-MSH$_{4-9}$NH$_2$, the smallest fragment that still contained the so-called active site of α-MSH, also proved to possess the qualities of superpotency, prolonged activity, and resistance to enzymic inactivation. On human MC receptors, stereochemical derivatives of the 6–9 and 7–9 core sequences identified subtype selective and specific agonists, albeit at μM concentrations.[12] These minimal fragment analogs may prove to be particularly useful for delivery across the skin or across a variety of mucosal epithelia.

Opiate Peptides

Opioid peptides are a family of endogenous neuromodulators. More than 20 peptides have been identified from brain, adrenals, and the pituitary gland. These peptides share a common N-terminal sequence (NH$_2$-Tyr-Gly-Gly-Phe-Met/Leu) and derive from cleavage of large precursor proteins that are translated from three different genes referred to as preproopiomelanocortin, preproenkephalen, and prodynorphin.[13] As shown in FIGURE 1, the β-LPH molecule, which contains the β-MSH and β-endorphin sequences is located at the C-terminal of POMC. Other shorter opiate fragments are enzymatically cleaved from β-endorphin, but all contain the 61–65 sequence necessary for opiate-like activity. Whether all these fragments actually play physiological roles is unclear. The late Thomas O'Donohue proposed that the differential regulation of acetylating enzymes within neurons could determine whether acetylated or nonacetylated forms of melanocortins or endorphins were released as neurotransmitters. These different forms of either class of peptide could act differentially on their respective receptors and possibly even antagonize the other receptor. Therefore, the cell-specific process of POMC degradation and subsequent differential enzymatic acetylation of POMC-products could produce a rather complex neural regulation. One might speculate that the relative contributions to the net response of α-MSH and β-endorphin release from the same neuron may be regulated by the activity of an opiomelanocortin acetylase.[14] It follows, therefore, that the expression of POMC in any particular tissue might lead to very cell-specific species of opiomelanocortin agonist ligands.

POMC Receptors

Like other peptide hormones, all POMC-derived hormones mediate their actions on membrane receptors, specifically the so-called seven-spanning membrane receptors. The N-terminus of the receptor is extracellular whereas the C-terminus is localized internally. Seven lipophilic, structurally related sequences transverse the plasma membrane as depicted in FIGURE 5. The extracellular C-terminus can vary considerably in length and degree of glycosylation. Opiomelanocortins (MCs) apparently interact with MC receptors (MCRs) within the helical channel formed by the seven-spanning membrane segments of the receptor, as determined by *in vitro* mutagenesis.

Presently five MCR subtypes are recognized; MCIR, MC2R, MC3R, MC4R, and MC5R. The detailed primary sequence of a MCR is shown[15] in FIGURE 6. Other aspects of the chemistry of these receptors are dealt with in greater detail in a subsequent paper in this volume.[16,17]

Cellular Mechanisms of Action of Opiomelanocortins

Opiomelanocortins, as noted above, mediate their actions through seven-spanning membrane receptors. The actions of these peptides are either to enhance or to decrease (inhibit) the basal activity of these receptors. Mutations in the structure of these receptors can result in constitutively active receptors, or in receptors that fail to respond to the ligand. Ligand-receptor interactions and signal transduction are quite complex and only a cursory discussion of these events is provided here.

Receptor Recognition. POMC-derived peptides interact (dock) with their receptors and apparently induce a conformational change in the receptor such that the active state of the protein can now transduce its signal to a second protein involved in

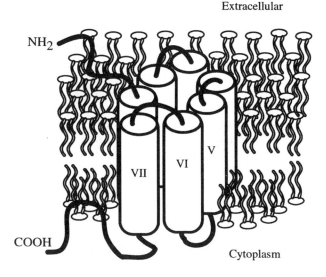

FIGURE 5. Depiction of a seven-spanning membrane receptor.

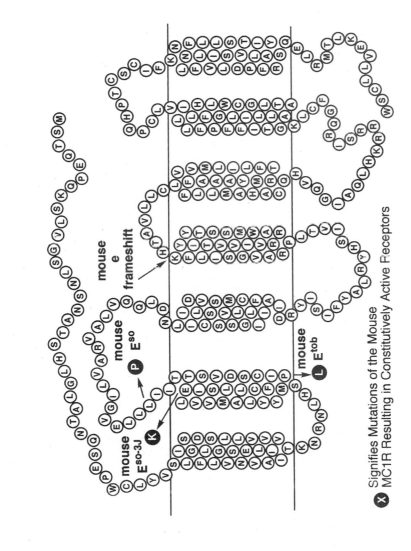

FIGURE 6. Primary structure of the mouse MC1R.[15]

receptor signal transduction (see below). We have designed and synthesized dozens of MCs to determine the structural features of those that enhance their efficacy and selectivity for receptor activation. By means of this process we have determined important clues to ligand-receptor interaction and activation.[12] Specificity of receptor recognition is a mechanism by which receptors are selectively activated although numerous other chemical messengers may also be present at the same time.

G-Protein Coupled Receptors and Second Messengers. Opiomelanocortins mediate their actions through G-protein coupled receptors (GPCRs). That is, following ligand-receptor interaction, the resulting conformational change in the receptor allows the active form of the receptor to interact with a second protein, a so-called G-protein. A stimulatory or inhibitory subunit of the trimeric G-protein is released and is now available to either stimulate or inhibit a third protein, adenylate cyclase, an enzyme that is able to convert ATP to cyclic adenosine monophosphate (cyclic AMR or cAMP)—a so-called "second messenger" of hormone action.

Melanocortin signal transduction pathways through any of the five MCRs involves the generation of cAMP. Elevated cAMP levels are then responsible for the various physiological responses engendered by each of the MCRs. Intracellular second messengers interact with proteins, usually enzymes, to activate a cellular response. Melanocortin-generated cAMP interacts with a protein kinase (PKA) which then phosphorylates CREB (cAMP response element-binding protein). Phosphorylation of CREB allows this transcription factor to interact with CRE (cDNA sequence) to activate transcription of a cell-specific mRNA for protein synthesis as shown in FIGURE 7.

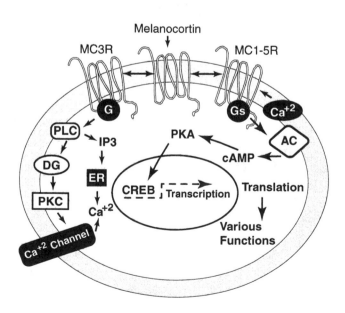

FIGURE 7. Melanocortin cellular mechanism of action.

The opioid receptor family has been characterized at the molecular level and consists of three homologous genes that encode for μ-, δ-, and κ-receptors. There exists heterogeneity within each receptor class. All three receptor classes have been shown to inhibit adenylate cyclase, decrease the conductance of voltage-gated Ca^{2+} channels or activate inwardly rectifying κ-channels depending on the particular species of cell. Depressed levels of intracellular cAMP are inhibitory to cellular activities. Further details on opioid mechanisms of action can be found elsewhere.[13]

Melanocortin Receptor Antagonists. The main way to understand the function of a particular hormonal ligand is to block the receptor through which it acts. Most interesting has been the discovery of natural ligands that can block MCRs, as will be discussed in a subsequent paper.[17] Synthetic antagonists of MCRs have also been designed that may prove to be clinically useful,[18–20] as will be discussed subsequently. An in-depth discussion of these MCR antagonists will be provided in a later paper.[19]

PHYSIOLOGICAL ROLES OF POMC PEPTIDES

Expression of the POMC gene is not restricted to the pituitary gland; it occurs normally in many other tissues including the brain. The diversity of POMC expression suggests, therefore, that the preprohormone regulates a great number of biological functions. POMC products can be delivered by the classical *endocrine* route, exemplified by the secretion of ACTH and α-MSH from the pituitary gland into the general circulation. POMC ligands are also released from neurons to act transsynaptically, a so-called *neurocrine* route of delivery. POMC peptides can also be released from neurons, and other cell types, to act on adjacent or nearby cells, a *paracrine* route of delivery. Some known and putative roles of POMC peptides are discussed in subsequent papers. Although POMC expression and secretion is regulated by a variety of stimuli, disregulated secretion of POMC peptides can lead to pathological physiological states (e.g., Cushing's disease; see below).

Melanocortins

Melanocortin-1 Receptor: Melanocortins and Cutaneous Pigmentation

α-Melanocyte stimulating hormone (α-MSH, α-melanocortin) of pituitary origin regulates rapid color changes (skin darkening) in many poikilothermic vertebrates (e.g., frogs and lizards). In humans and some mammals, melanocortins regulate skin and pelage (hair) coloration. α-MSH secreted by the pars intermedia of the pituitary gland probably regulates pelage coloration in some mammals (e.g., weasels and varying hares) where there is a change from a white winter pelage to a brown spring color.[21] Hair coloration in some strains of mice will change in response to injected melanotropins.[22] This change usually involves increased conversion to eumelanin (brown-black) synthesis over that of pheomelanin (yellow-red) synthesis in yellow mice.[23]

Melanocortins injected into humans also results in enhanced skin pigmentation due to increased melanogenesis.[24,25] The question therefore arises as to whether melanocortin ligands and receptors normally control skin pigmentation in man. The human pituitary gland lacks a recognizable pars intermedia, the source of α-MSH in most animals. Although α-MSH or a related melanocortin might be synthesized by cells of the pars distalis, there is at present no evidence to support this suggestion. It is interesting, therefore, that POMC expression in the skin has been demonstrated, as will be discussed in detail in this volume.[26,27] The control of integumental pigmentation has therefore evolved from a distant, systemic regulation, to a local regulatory mechanism. We have provided evidence that human epidermal melanocytes and keratinocytes (grown separately in culture) possess melanocortin receptors as demonstrated by direct visualization by fluorescence microscopy as well as by scanning electron microscopy.[20] Thus, these two cellular elements of the skin, which comprise the so-called "epidermal melanin unit",[28] provide a local mechanism for the control of cutaneous pigmentation by UVL, rather than by a pituitary melanotropin. This interesting hypothesis, first promulgated by Pawelek,[29] will be discussed at length in a subsequent paper.[26]

Melanotan-I: Hormone Analog for Tanning of the Skin. We have synthesized thousands of analogs of α-MSH, some of which have proven to be superpotent and prolonged acting. One analog, [Nle⁴,DPhe⁷]α-MSH (FIG. 4), referred to as melanotan-I (MT-I), has proved to be effective in FDA-sponsored clinical trials for tanning the human skin.[30] These studies are presently in progress. MT-I has been licensed to a biotechnology company in Australia for research and development, with the goal of providing a product for tanning the skin that might then prove to be photoprotective against light-induced skin cancer.

Melanocortin 2 Receptor: Corticotropin and Adrenal Steroidogenesis

Corticotropin (adrenal cortical stimulating hormone or ACTH) is produced by corticotrophs of the anterior lobe (pars distalis) of the pituitary gland. POMC expression is enhanced by corticotropin releasing hormone (CRH) of hypothalamic origin.[31] ACTH is released into the systemic circulation to act on MC2Rs possessed by adrenal cortical cells of the zona fasciculata. Negative feedback by cortisol to the hypothalamus leads to inhibition of CRH secretion, a subsequent decline of POMC expression, and, therefore, ACTH synthesis and secretion. Corticotropin is 39 amino acids in length, the first 24 residues from the N-terminus being invariant among the mammalian species studied. Apparently only one ACTH is expressed in any one species of animal.

Overexpression of pituitary POMC-derived melanocortins, as in Cushing's disease of secondary (pituitary) origin, can lead to a generalized hyperpigmentation of the skin, the so-called "cardinal symptom" of the disease. The enhanced circulating levels of ACTH, a peptide that shares some structural similarity to α-MSH (FIG. 2), stimulates melanogenesis by epidermal melanocytes. Extopic secretion of ACTH from a tumor (e.g., of the lung) can also result in cutaneous hyperpigmentation. In Addison's disease of primary origin, wherein there is a failure or lack of adrenal cortisol production, the resulting absence of a negative feedback to the hypothalamus leads to expression of pituitary ACTH secretion, resulting again in cutaneous hyperpigmentation. Null (inactivating) mutations in the adrenal cortical MC2R, such that it fails to recognize circulating ACTH, can be responsible for the above condition of excess ACTH secretion (due to failure of a negative feedback).

Melanocortin 3 Receptor: Unknown Function(s)

This receptor is expressed in several important tissue types including the brain, gut, and placenta. The MC3R recognizes all MCs having the heptapeptide central sequence of Met-Glu-His-Phe-Arg-Trp-Gly. λ-MSH peptides have a highly increased efficacy at the MC3R compared to α-MSH.[32] It is expressed in brain, placenta, and gut tissues, but not in melanoma cells or in the adrenal gland. The receptor has been implicated in cardiovascular control and natriuresis (see below).

Melanocortin 4 Receptor: Melanocortins and Ingestive Behavior

Extensive studies in rodents suggest that melanotropins acting within the brain control the desire for food intake; they cause satiety. For example, melanocortins injected into the third ventricle of the brain of rodents are inhibitory to food intake. The MC4R receptor is primarily expressed in the brain, and has been shown to be important for feeding behavior and weight homeostasis. Administration of the melanocortin agonist, MT-II (see FIGURE 8), or antagonist, SHU9119 (SEE FIGURE 9), result in decreased and increased food intake, respectively.[34] When the MC4R gene was deleted from the mouse genome, this resulted in an obese mouse.[35] Additionally, it is hypothesized that the obese phenotype of the agouti mouse is due to antagonism of MC4R by the agouti protein.[34] The naturally occurring antagonist, AGRP (see below), has been demonstrated to antagonize MC3R and MC4R, and when the protein is ubiquitously expressed, an obese mouse results, presumably due to antagonism of the MC4R.[36] Based on these experimental studies, the MC4R has become a drug target for the design of drugs for the treatment of obesity.

Melanocortin 5 Receptor: Melanocortins and Exocrine Secretions

The rather ubiquitous distribution of the MC5R suggested that systemically delivered and acting MSH/ACTH peptides might regulate these receptors. High levels

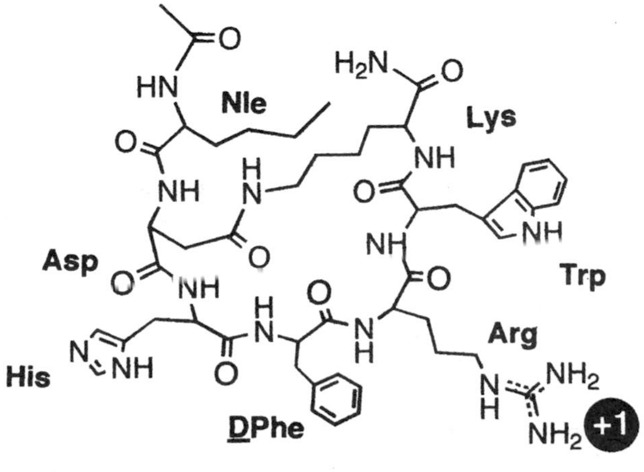

FIGURE 8. MT-II (Erectide), a superpotent MCR agonist. This MC differs considerably from α-MSH (FIG. 3).

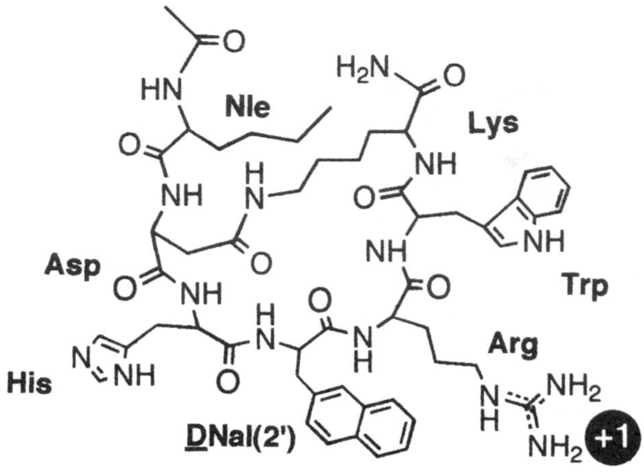

FIGURE 9. SHU919, an antagonist of MCR4 receptors. This analog differs from MT-II by the presence of a Dnapthalene moiety at position 9 rather than Dphenylalanine.

of MC5R expression are found in exocrine tissues, which include the Harderian, preputial, lacrimal, and sebaceous glands. A physiological role for the MC5R in the regulation of a wide variety of exocrine glands was determined by targeted disruption of the MC5R in the mouse. In such mice there was a severe defect in water repulsion and a decreased production of sebaceous lipids. Stress-induced synthesis of Harderian gland porphyrin production and lacrimal gland protein secretion were depressed. Elevated levels of ACTH/α-MSH may regulate stress-mediated exocrine gland function, including the release of odors (pheromones) from one or more exocrine glands.[23,37]

Melanocortins and other Putative Functions

Besides the functions listed above, melanocortins are claimed to regulate a large number of other functions.[14] The melanocortin ligands and receptors regulating these putative functions remain to be determined.

Erectile Function. Ac-Nle-c[Asp-His-DPhe-Arg-Trp-Lys]-NH$_2$ (MT-II) is a superpotent, prolonged acting, enzyme resistant, melanotropic peptide analog of α-MSH (FIG. 8). This cyclic lactam-bridged peptide is a superagonist of peripheral (melanocyte) MC1Rs, MT-II is also a potent agonist of melanocortin 3, 4, and 5 brain receptors. When injected intracerebroventricularly in the mouse, the peptide inhibited feeding, and mice lost weight (as discussed above). Most interestingly, MT-II also induced erections in human males, as discussed below.

Several normal white males were enrolled in a study after informed consent was obtained through protocol approval.[38] The starting dose of MT-II was 0.01 mg/kg, which was less than one-tenth the dose safely administered to rodents in unpublished preclinical toxicity tests. The trial was single-blinded; the placebo, 0.9% NaCl, was given on alternate days so that MT-II was never administered on successive days.

Each subject received a single daily subcutaneous injection for five days per week for two consecutive weeks. Thus, each subject received five injections of MT-II and five injections of saline over a two-week period. The MT-II dose was escalated by 0.005 mg/kg increments within the subjects. All three subjects developed an erection in response to MT-II for at least one of the concentrations administered. At a dose level of 0.025 mg/kg (three escalations from baseline), spontaneous penile erections were reported in all subjects. Satiety, flushing, yawning/stretching, gastrointestinal discomfort, and fatigue were transient side effects noted in the volunteers. None of the three subjects reported stretching and yawning or penile erections on any of the five days of saline injection.

Ten men with claimed erectile dysfunction of a psychogenic (nonorganic/physiological) nature were then enrolled in a double-blind crossover vehicle-controlled study.[39] Eight of the ten subjects developed erections to subcutaneous (non-penile) injections of MT-II (0.025–0.157 mg) as monitored objectively by Rigiscan (penile tumescence meter). This device measures rigidity of both the tip and the base of the penis. The erections were deemed satisfactory for intercourse.

Side effects were mild and no participants terminated participation because of toxicity associated with the test compound. Nevertheless, at high doses the peptide can cause gastrointestinal discomfort such as cramping and/or vomiting. The peptide does not appear to enhance libido, but rather, causes a transient erectile response (an erection on demand). The peptide may prove to be clinically effective for the differential diagnosis of erectile dysfunction and for the treatment of psychological (idiopathic) erectile dysfunction.

To our knowledge, these are the first studies to demonstrate that a melanotropic peptide administered by injection induces an erectile response in humans. Both α-MSH, β-MSH, as well as ACTH have been injected into humans.[24,25] Although other side effects were carefully documented, in no instance was induction of an erection reported. In fact, in the rat, it was reported that sexual responses such as penile erections can only be induced by direct intracerebro-ventricular injection of a melanotropic peptide.[40] Most interesting in the present study was the observation that, as in rodent studies, administration of a melanotropic peptide not only produced an erection but also induced a form of stretching-yawning response ("syndrome" SYS). Since these responses probably originate in the brain, then it suggests that subcutaneous injection of the peptide with delivery to the systemic circulation results, most likely, in the passage of the peptide across the blood-brain barrier into the central nervous system. MT-II therefore represents a model peptide for the development of peptides for delivery to the brain. The peptide and related analogs are patented and have been licensed for use in the diagnosis and treatment of impotency of psychogenic origin.

Cardiovascular Function. Melanocortins released by arcuate neurons (of the brain) activate MCRs (probably MC3R and MC4R) located in the dorsal-vagal complex (DVC) to elicit hypotension and bradycardia. Similar effects induced by β-endorphin (a peptide also derived from POMC) are mediated by opiate receptors at the same site. High concentrations of MC4R mRNA are found in the DVC, which suggests that this receptor may be involved in central cardiovascular control.[41] Microinjections of α-MSH into DVC causes a dose-dependent hypotension and bradycardia, and these effects are inhibited by an MC4R antagonist. The DVC is the site of the first synapse of the baroreceptor reflex, and it is the termination point of POMC–containing neurons descending from the arcuate nucleus. It was suggested that the release of α-MSH from arcuate neurons is mediated by neural MCRs (MC4/MC3) located in the DVC. The centrally mediated pressor and cardiac effects of γ-MSH do not appear to involve the MC3 and MC4Rs. The lack of involvement of any of the five MCRs in the pressor and tachycardiac effects γ-MSH suggests the existence of another, presently unknown, MCR in the brain or cerebral vasculatur.[41]

It is claimed that ACTH peptides cause a dose-dependent decrease in blood pressure along with a tachycardia. Again this action is not mediated through one of the presently recognized MCRs. Thus, two peptides, γ and ACTH, derived from a common precursor (POMC) and sharing a partial homology of primary structure have opposite effects on blood pressure (in rats). The antagonistic action of these two MCs appears to be mediated through an as yet to be determined MCR.[42] Other evidence suggests that the effects of γ-MSH are, at least in part, due to an increase in sympathetic outflow to the periphery possibly involving activation of vascular α_1-adrenoceptors and cardiac β_1-adrenoceptors.[43]

Neurotropic Role. There is evidence that repair of nerve damage can be effected by melanocortins.[44] It has been stated that melanocortins are able to accelerate the functional recovery of damaged (crushed) neurons, prevent the sensory neuropathy that occurs in patients as a side effect of certain anticancer drugs, and ameliorate diabetic neuropathy in certain animal models.[45] The following statements taken from journal references indicate some of the many views regarding the putative neurotropic actions of melanocortins.[14,46]

- Acceleration of recovery from sciatic nerve damage by $ACTH_{4-9}$ analog.
- α-MSH stimulates neurite outgrowth of chromaffin cells.
- Local control of neurite outgrowth of dorsal root ganglia and spinal cord neurons by an ACTH analog.
- ACTH accelerates recovery of neuromuscular function following crushing of peripheral nerve.[47]
- Recovery from peripheral nerve transection is accelerated by local application of α-MSH.
- Protective effects of α-MSH on canine brain stem ischemia.[48]
- Influences of fragments and analogs of ACTH/MSH upon recovery from nervous system injury.
- Effects of an analog of $ACTH_{4-10}$ on functional recovery after frontal cortex injury.
- Prevention of cisplatin neurotoxicity with an $ACTH_{4-9}$ analog.
- $ACTH_{4-10}$ accelerates ocular motor recovery in the guinea pig following vestibular deafferentation.
- ACTH/MSH analog stimulates microtubule formation in axons of central neurons of the snail.
- $[Nle^4,DPhe^7]\alpha$-MSH improves functional recovery in rats subjected to diencephalic hemisection.

- Analog of $ACTH_{4-9}$ protects against experimental allergic neuritis.[49]

- Reduction of amygdaloid kindled seizures by an analog of ACTH/MSH.

- Melanocortins stimulate proliferation and induce morphological changes in cultured rat astrocytes.

Adipocyte Function. Melanocortins possessing the core heptapeptide sequence possess lipolytic activity. This effect is apparently species specific since only the rabbit, but not human and rat adipocytes, are responsive. β-lipotropic hormone, in fact, was named by Dr. C.H. Li for its lipolytic actions on adipocytes. Since abnormally high concentrations of MCs are required to exert such an effect, it is unlikely that these peptides play a physiological role under normal circulating concentrations. The MCRs medicating such effects are discussed in a subsequent paper.[50]

Inflammation and Contact Hypersensitivity. There is substantial evidence that MCs modulate immune responses.[51] Some examples of manuscript titles supporting such a suggestion are as follows.

- Antiinflammatory effects of α-MSH on acute, chronic and systemic inflammation.

- α-MSH peptides inhibit acute inflammation and contact hypersensitivity.

- α-MSH inhibits immunostimulatory and inflammatory actions of interleukin-1.

- Modulation of host defense by α-MSH.

- α-MSH modulates contact hypersensitivity.

- α-MSH exhibits target selectivity in its capacity to affect interleukin-1–inducible responses *in vivo* and *in vitro*.

Antipyretic Role. Exogenous melanocortins are antipyretic when administered peripherally or centrally, and α-MSH administered peripherally or centrally antagonizes the proinflammatory actions of the cytokine, interleukin-1 (IL-1). The MCR antagonist, SHU-9119 (FIG. 9), significantly increased fever in the presence of a pyrogen. When co-injected with α-MSH, the antagonist prevented the antipyretic action of exogenous α-MSH.[52] It has been hypothesized, therefore, that endogenous central melanocortins exert an antipyretic effect during fever by acting on MCRs located within the brain.[51] Other evidence for an effect/role of MCs on thermoregulatory is suggested in the following information taken from journal references.[53]

- α-MSH suppresses fever and increases in plasma levels of prostaglandino.

- Antipyresis caused by stimulation of vasopressinergic neurons and intraseptal or systemic injections of γ-MSH.

- α-MSH conditioned suppression of a lipopolysaccharide-induced fever.

- α-MSH and $[Nle^4,DPhe^7]$α-MSH: effects on core temperature in rats.

- Central administration of α-MSH antiserum augments fever in the rabbit.

- Central and peripheral actions of α-MSH, the thermoregulation of rats.

- Central role of CRF on thermogenesis mediated by POMC products.

Cognitive Functions. A vast literature has accumulated on the putative actions/ roles of MCs on cognitive and related abilities. Only a sample can be provided here, but see Gispin[14,44] for more literature.

- ACTH and attention in humans.

- Injection of ACTH induces recovery from shuttle-box avoidance deficits in rats with amygdaloid lesions.

- Hormonal influences on motivation, learning, memory, and psychosis.

- The effects of neonatal injections of α-MSH on open-field behavior of juvenile and adult rats.

- Action of melanocortins on learning, performance, and retention.

- MSH/ACTH$_{4-10}$ influences on behavioral and physiological measures of attention.

- Neuropeptide MSH/ACTH enhances attention in the mentally retarded.

- MSH/ACTH$_{4-10}$ in men and women; effects upon performance of an attention an memory task.

Sexual Behavior. A large body of evidence suggests a role for MCs in sexual behavior in both male and female animals.[54] A sample of related references is provided.

- Sexual arousal in male animals: a central effect of ACTH-like peptides in mammals.

- Facilitation and inhibition of sexual receptivity in the female rat by α-MSH.

- Short- and long-term inhibitory action of α-MSH on lordosis in rats.

- α-MSH stimulates sexual behavior in the female rat.

- The role of melanotropins in sexual behavior.

- MSH and the pineals in the control of territorial aggression.

- Effects of α-MSH on social and exploratory behavior in the rat.

Opiate Peptides

POMC Expression and Pancreatic Islet Function

This introductory overview focusses mainly on the physiological roles of melanocortins. We give only a brief overview of POMC expression leading to opiate peptide production and function. Measurable POMC gene expression is present in pancreatic islets. Besides a truncated POMC-like mRNA, a full-length POMC mRNA is also transcribed. The function of POMC gene expression in the pancreatic islets is unknown. Opioid receptors (delta, kappa, but not mu) are present in islet tissue and opioid peptides bind to these receptors. Neoplastic expression of ACTH in islet tissue has been reported, and both β-endorphin and ACTH can lower or raise insulin and glucagon secretion by pancreatic islets depending on the species and other modifying factors.[55]

EVOLUTION OF THE POMC SYSTEM

Several decades of research on melanotropins and the control of skin pigmentation has led to a great deal of knowledge of the ligands and the structural features required for receptor activation. Most studies were done on frog skin melanophores.[56–58] Since human melanocytes possess MC1Rs, it could be assumed that these receptors are also the targets for melanotropic peptides, as in frogs. Generally, superpotent MC agonists of frog MC1Rs are also equally active on MC1Rs of other poikilothermic vertebrates as well as mammalian (mouse, human) melanocytes.[58] Several very potent antagonists of the frog MC1R have also been reported.[18,57,59] These antagonists are, in contrast, agonists of lizard melanocytes. More importantly, however, they are antagonists of hMC4Rs.[18] This raises the question of whether the MCR of one species is really closer, evolutionarily, to the equivalent MCR in the other species of concern. In other words, is the MC1R of humans evolved from the MC1R of frogs, or is the MC4R more closely related? Elucidation of the other MCRs (MC1-5R) of frogs and other species may provide an important view into receptor evolution.

Equally interesting is the evolution of opiomelanocortins from the primitive (primordial) POMC gene. What were the original receptors of the early secretory products of POMC expression? Are the receptors for the melanocortins and opiate peptides related? That is, do they contain overlapping sequences inherited from the evolutionary past? There are numerous reports, for example, that opioid agonists antagonize MCRs, and vice versa.[14] For example, dynorphin peptides can directly antagonize melanocortin MCRs. Dynorphins block the agonist actions of ACTH on MC2R. Antagonism of MCRs by dynorphin peptides is relatively selective since numerous other peptide receptors were not similarly blocked.[59] We have designed melanocortin agonists that also interact with somatostatin receptors, and it is known that the somatostatin receptors and opioid receptors have reciprocal actions on the other receptor.[57]

PERSPECTIVES

The roles of the melanocortins, α-MSH and ACTH, have been clearly recognized for many years. The discovery of at least five different MC receptors has revealed a diverse number of other functions also regulated by these peptides. The evidence is overwhelming that MCs also regulate: satiety (eating/feeding behavior), erectile and reproductive functions and behaviors, cognitive/learning skills, and immune responses. Most importantly in the context of this volume, there is overwhelming evidence for a role of the POMC system, its ligands, and receptors in the control of integumentary function. The role of MCs in skin pigmentation is rather well understood. It is also overwhelmingly documented by the papers to follow, that melanocortins also function in cutaneous neuroimmunomodulation.

ACKNOWLEDGMENTS

Carrie Haskell-Luevano was supported in part U.S. Public Health Service Grant DK09231 and is a recipient of a Burroughs Wellcome Fund Career Award in the Biomedical Sciences.

REFERENCES

1. MAINS, R.E. & B.A. EIPPER. 1976. J. Biol. Chem. **251:** 4115–4120.
2. EIPPER, B.A. & R.E. MAINS. 1978. J. Biol. Chem. **253:** 5732–5744.
3. NAKANISHI, S., A. INOUE, T. KITA, M. NARAMURA, A.C.Y. CHANG, S.N. COHEN & S. NUMA. 1979. Nature (Lond.) **278:** 423–427.
4. HEINIG, J.A., F.W. KEELEY, P. ROBSON, S.A. SOWER & J.H. YOUSON. 1995. Gen. Comp. Endocrinol. **99:** 136–144.
5. SEIDAH, N.A. 1999. Ann. N.Y. Acad. Sci. **885:** this volume.
6. VAUDRY, H. 1999. Ann. N.Y. Acad. Sci. **885:** this volume.
7. CASTRUCCI, A.M.L., M.E. HADLEY & V.J. HRUBY. 1984. Gen. Comp. Endocrinol. **55:** 104–111.
8. HRUBY, V.J., B.C. WILKES, M.E. HADLEY, F. AL-OBEIDI, T.K. SAWYER, D.J. STAPLES, E.D. DEVAUX, O. DYM, A.M.L. CASTRUCCI, M.E. HINTZ, J.P. RIEHM & K. RANGA RAO. 1987. J. Med. Chem. **30:** 2126–2130.
9. SAWYER, T.K., A.M. DE L. CASTRUCCI, D.J. STAPLES, J.A. AFFHOLTER, A.E. DEVOUT, V.J. HRUBY & M.E. HADLEY. 1993. Ann. N.Y. Acad. Sci. **680:** 597–599.
10. TONG, Y., J. COUET, J. SIMARD & G. PELLETIER. 1990. Mol. Cell. Neurosci. **1:** 78–83.
11. HRUBY, V.J., S.D. SHARMA, K. TOTH, J.Y. JAW, F. AL-OBEIDI, T.K. SAWYER & M.E. HADLEY. 1993. Ann. N.Y. Acad. Sci. **680:** 51–63.
12. HASKELL-LUEVANO, C., S. HENDRATA, C. NORTH, T.K. SAWYER, M.E. HADLEY, V.J. HRUBY, C. DICKINSON & I. GANTZ. 1997. J. Med. Chem. **40:** 2133–2139.
13. KIEFFER, B.L. 1995. Cellular Mol. Neurobiol. **15:** 615–635.
14. O'DONOHUE, T.L. & D.M. DORSA. 1982. Peptides. **3:** 353–395.
15. ROBBINS, L.S., J.H. MADEAU, K.R. JOHNSON, M.A. KELLY, L. ROSELLI-REHFUS, E. BAACK, K.G. MOUNTSOY & R.D. CONE. 1993. Cell **72:** 827–834.
16. EBERLE, A.N. 1999. Ann. N.Y. Acad. Sci. **885:** this volume.
17. BARSH, G. 1999. Ann. N.Y. Acad. Sci. **885:** this volume.
18. HRUBY, V.J., D. LU, S.D. SHARMA, A.M. DE L. CASTRUCCI, R.A. KESTERSON, F.A. AL-OBEIDI, M.E. HADLEY & R.D. CONE. 1995. J. Med. Chem. **38:** 3454–3461.
19. LERNER, M. 1999. Ann. N.Y. Acad. Sci. **885:** this volume.
20. HADLEY, M.E., V.J. HRUBY, J. JIANG, S.D. SHARMA, J.L. FINK, C. HASKELL-LUEVANO, D.L. BENTLEY, F. AL-OBEIDI & T.K. SAWYER. 1996. Pigment Cell Res. **9:** 213–234.
21. RUST, C.C. 1985. Gen. Comp. Endocrinol. **5:** 222–231.
22. GESCHWIND, I.I., R.A. HUSEBY & R. NISHIOKA. Rec. Prog. Horm. Res. **28:** 91.
23. THODY, A.J. 1999. Ann. N.Y. Acad. Sci. **885:** this volume.
24. LEMER, A.B. & J.S. MCGUIRE. 1961. Nature (Lond.) **189:** 176–179.
25. LERNER, A.B. & J.S. MCGUIRE. 1964. New Engl. J. Med. **270:** 539–546.
26. CHAKRABOTKY, A.K. & J.M. PAWELEK. 1999. Ann. N.Y. Acad. Sci. **885:** this volume.
27. SLOMINSKI, A.T. 1999. Ann. N.Y. Acad. Sci. **885:** this volume.
28. FITZPATRICK, T.B. & A.S. BREATHNACH. 1963. Dermatol. Wochenschr. **147:** 481–489
29. PAWELEK, J.M., M.P. CHAKRABORTY, M.P. OSBER, S.J. ORLOW & K.K. MIN. 1992. Pigment Cell Res. **5:** 348–356.

30. LEVINE, N., S.N. SHEFTEL, T. EYTAN, R.T. DORR, M.E. HADLEY, J.C. WEINRACH, G.A. ERTL, K. TOTH, D.L. MCGEE & V.J. HRUBY. 1991. J. Am. Med. Assoc. **266:** 2730–2736.
31. CHROUSOS, G.P. 1999. Ann. N.Y. Acad. Sci. **885:** this volume.
32. GANTZ, I., Y. KONDA, Y. TASHIRO, T. SHIMOTO, A. MIWA, G. MUNZERT, S.J. WATSON, J. DEVALLE & T. YAMADA. J. Biol. Chem. **268:** 8246–8250.
33. CHEN, W., M.A. KELLY, Y. OPITZ-ARAYA, R.E. THOMAS, M.J. LOW & R.D. CONE. 1997. Cell **91:** 789–798.
34. FAN, W., B.A. BOSTON, R.A. KESTERSON, V.J. HRUBY & R.D. CONE. 1997. Nature **385:** 165–168.
35. HUSZAR, D. *et al.* 1997. Cell **88:** 131–141.
36. OLLMANN, M.M., B.D. WILSON, Y.-K. YANG, J.A. KERNS, Y. CHEN, I. GANTZ & G.S. BARSH. 1997. Science **278:** 135–138.
37. LU, D., D. WILLARD, L.R. PATEL, S. KADWELL, L. OVERTON, T. KOSI, M. LUTHER, W. CHEN, R.P. WOYCHEK, W.O. WILKINSON & R.D. CONE. 1994. Nature **371:** 799 802.
38. DORR, R.T., R. LINES, N. LEVINE, C. BROOKS, L. YIANG, V.J. HRUBY & M.E. HADLEY. 1996. Life Sci. **58:** 1778–1784.
39. WESSELS, H., K. FUCIARELLI, J. HANSEN, M.E. HADLEY, V.J. HRUBY, R. DORR & N. LEVINE. 1998. J. Urology **160:** 389–393.
40. BERTOLINI, A. & G.L. GESSA. 1984. J. Endocrinol. Invest. **4:** 241–259.
41. LI, S.-J., K. VARGA, P. ARCHER, V.J. HRUBY, S.D. SHARMA, R.A. KESTERSON, R.D. CONE & G. KUNOS. 1996. J. Neurosci. **16:** 5182–5188.
42. VAN BERGEN, P., J.A. KLEIJNE, D.J. DEWILDT & D.H.G. VERSTEEG. 1996. Br. J. Pharmacol. **120:** 1561–1567.
43. VAN BERGEN, P., T.Y.C.E. DEWINTER, D.J. DEWILDT & D.H.G. VERSTEEG. 1997. Naunyn-Schmredeberg's Arch. Pharmacol. **355:** 720–726.
44. GISPIN, W. 1999. Ann. N.Y. Acad. Sci. **885:** this volume.
45. BÄR, P.R., E.M. HOL & W.H. GISPEN. 1993. Ann. N.Y. Acad. Sci. **692:** 284–286.
46. DEKKER, A.J.A.M., M.M. PRINCEN, H. DENIJS, L.G.J. DELEEDE, C.L.E. BROEKAMP. 1987. Peptides **8:** 1057–1059.
47. STRAND, F.L. & T.T. KUNG. 1980. Peptides **1:** 135–138.
48. HUH, S.-K., J.M. LIPTON & H.H. BATJER. 1997. Neurosurgery **40:** 132–140.
49. DUCKERS, H.J., J. VESHAAGEN & W.H. GISPEN. 1993. Brain **116:** 1059–1075.
50. BOSTON, B.A. 1999. Ann. N.Y. Acad. Sci. **885:** this volume.
51. CATANIA, A. & J.M. LIPTON. 1993. Endocr. Rev. **14:** 564–576.
52. HUANG, Q.-H., M.L. ENTWISTLE, J.D. ALVARO, R.S. DUMAN, V.J. HRUBY & J.B. TATRO. J. Neurosci. **17:** 3343–3351.
53. LIPTON, J.M., G. CERIANI, A. MACALUSO, D. MCCOY, K. CARNES, T. BILTZ & A. CATANIA. 1994. Ann. N.Y. Acad. Sci. **741:** 137–148.
54. GONZALES, M.I., S. VAZIRI & C.A. WILSON 1996. Peptides **17.** 171–177.
55. JAHN, R., U. PADEL, P.H. PORSCH & H.D. SOLING. 1982. Eur. J. Biochem. **126:** 623– 629.
56. Hadley, M.E. 1996. Endocrinology, 4th ed. Prentice-Hall, Englewood Cliffs.
57. HRUBY, V.J., G. HAN & M.E. HADLEY. Lett. Pept. Sci. **5:** 117–120.
58. HASKELL-LUEVANO, C., H. MEIVA, C. DICKINSON, M.E. HADLEY, V.J. HRUBY & T. YAMADA. 1996. J. Med. Chem. **39:** 432–435.
59. QUILLAN, J.M. & W. SADÉE. 1997. Pharmaceut. Res. **14:** 713–719.

POMC–Derived Peptides and Their Biological Action

SAMUEL SOLOMON[a]

Department of Medicine and Biochemistry,
McGill University and Royal Victoria Hospital, 687 Pine Avenue West,
M3.07 Montreal, Quebec H3A 1A1, Canada

ABSTRACT: It has long been known that a large number of POMC–related peptides are found in skin. In this introduction I describe the formation of POMC–derived peptides in various tissues to indicate that processing is largely tissue-dependent. I focus on the peptides from the N-terminal fragment, such as γ-MSH, ACTH and α-MSH, and β-lipopropin as well as β-endorphin. I touch on the factors that control the synthesis of the various peptides, which are now numerous and varied, and again are tissue specific. The biologic activity of the peptides generated from POMC are described in relation to their possible action in skin. In addition, I describe a new class of peptides induced in skin following injury and which are of great interest.

It is not possible in the space available to discuss all of the peptides derived from POMC and recently there have appeared excellent reviews on this subject.[1–4] Here I discuss the most recent advances with emphasis on the formation and biochemistry of the POMC-peptide in skin. The POMC gene and its peptides were first investigated in the pituitary gland of mammals.[5–7] However, it was soon discovered that the gene coding for POMC was also expressed in many peripheral and central nervous tissues, and that processing of the large precursor POMC molecule differs in different tissues. In lymphocytes and macrophages, depending on the nature of the stimulus, β-endorphin and $ACTH_{1–39}$ are formed and, in addition, $ACTH_{1–24}$, $ACTH_{1–25}$, and $ACTH_{1–26}$, as well as α- and γ-endorphin, have been found.[8,9] In the intestinal wall and in the duodenum POMC is processed to α-MSH, and in the small intestine β-endorphin is formed.[10] In the brain the POMC gene is expressed mostly in the arcuate nucleus of the hypothalamus where the POMC mRNA transcripts are the same size as those found in the pituitary except for a longer poly (A) tail.[11] POMC gene products have also been identified in several epidermal cells such as keratinocytes, melanocytes, Langerhans cells, thymocyte-1, and dendritic epidermal cells.[12–15] Keratinocytes normally produce low levels of α-MSH and ACTH but stimulation with the cytokine IL-1, UV light or tumor promoters induces POMC mRNA expression and α-MSH release.[12] POMC gene expression has also been found in skin and in melanomas.[16–18] As indicated in FIGURE 1, post-translational processing of POMC yields a large number of biologically active peptides. POMC is processed in the corticotropic cells of the anterior pituitary to form ACTH, β-LPH and pro-γ-MSH. Further processing occurs in the intermediate lobe to form α-MSH from ACTH and

[a]Address for correspondence: 514-842-1231 ext. 4358 (voice); 514-843-1695 (fax); ssolomon@rvhmed.lan.mcgill.ca (e-mail).

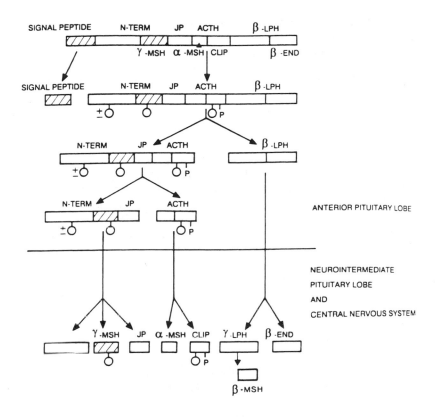

FIGURE 1. The structure of POMC and the products of posttranslational processing taken from Castro and Morrison.[2]

CLIP (Corticotrophin-like intermediate lobe peptide). β-MSH and pro γ- MSH are also cleaved to form a series of small peptides. All of the peptides formed in this manner also undergo amidation, mono- and diacetylation, phosphorylation, glycosylation, and methylation before POMC processing is complete.

POMC GENE EXPRESSION

There have been numerous reports in recent years detailing the interaction between POMC and leptin in the brain. Boston et al.[19] found that the mouse leptin weight–reducing effects are transmitted via POMC neurons. It was also shown that reduced central nervous leptin signalling due to fasting or to genetic defects in leptin or its receptor lowers POMC mRNA levels in the rostral arcuate nucleus. The stimulation of arcuate nucleus POMC gene expression was thought to proceed via a pathway involving leptin receptors, and that leptin signalling in the brain involves activation of the hypothalamic melanocortin system.[20] It was reasonable to suppose that because α-MSH reduction causes obesity and α-MSH infusion produces satiety, one should examine POMC gene expression following fasting in normal mice or in models of obesity characterized by leptin insufficiency (ob/ob) or leptin insensitivity (db/db). It was found that fasting in wild-type mice produces a fall in POMC mRNA which was positively correlated with leptin mRNA. POMC mRNA was decreased in both db/db and ob/ob mice. In ob/ob mice, treatment with leptin stimulated hypothalamic POMC mRNA. It was possible to deduce from these studies that impairment of α-MSH may be a common feature of obesity and that hypothalamic POMC neurons, stimulated by leptin, may constitute a link between leptin and the melanocortin system.[21] Cheung et al.[22] found that POMC neurons share a similar distribution with leptin receptor mRNA in the arcuate nucleus. They further showed that POMC neurons in the hypothalamus express leptin receptor mRNA and suggest that POMC neurons and the products of the POMC gene may be part of the signalling pathway mediating the action of leptin on feeding. In a separate study it was found that POMC mRNA levels were significantly reduced throughout the arcuate nucleus in leptin deficient ob/ob mice relative to wild-type controls but POMC mRNA levels in leptin-treated ob/ob mice were normal.[23] These observations suggest that products of POMC are a link between leptin and the central mechanism regulating body weight and reproduction. It was recently shown that decreased food intake in rats caused by the administration of leptin resulted in a decrease in hypothalamic galanin, melanin-concentrating hormone, POMC and neuropeptide Y gene expression, and an increase in neurotensin gene expression.[24]

Dietary sodium seems to influence POMC mRNA. Mayan et al.[25] found that after one week of high sodium intake in the rat, POMC mRNA was significantly increased and was further increased after two and three weeks. The increase was primarily in the neurointermediate lobe, and immunoreactive α-MSH was also increased in this lobe. It has long been established that glucocorticoids inhibit POMC gene transcription and peptide synthesis in the anterior pituitary,[26] but the effects of glucocorticoids on POMC gene expression in the hypothalamus is not fully understood. Recently the effects of adrenalectomy and glucorticoid replacement on POMC mRNA and β-EP plus α-MSH levels in medial basal hypothalamus (MBH) of the rat were examined.[27] It was found that POMC gene expression was significantly inhibited in the MBH after one and two weeks following adrenalectomy and that this effect was reversed by glucorticoid replacement. The role of 5-hydroxytryptamine (5-HT) neurons in mediating the effect of stress on POMC gene expression in the anterior and intermediate lobes of the pituitary gland has been studied.[28] It was found that stress increased POMC mRNA levels in the anterior and intermediate lobe of the pituitary. Depletion of 5-HT had no effect on basal POMC mRNA levels in the anterior pituitary of stressed rats and completely blocked POMC mRNA elevation in the intermediate lobe of stressed rats. It appears that 5-HT exerts a differential regulation of stress–induced activation of POMC gene expression in the anterior and intermediate lobes of the male rat pituitary.[28] Using AtT20PL cloned cells of the AtT20 line it was found that interleukin-1-beta (IL-1β) stimulated POMC promoter activity in a biphasic manner (weak short term effects followed by strong long term effects).[29] Tumor necrosis factor-α had a similar effect and IL-6 had a great stimulatory long term effect. IL-2 had no influence on POMC expression. Interferon and

INF-γ had acute stimulatory effects followed by a marked inhibitory effect. IL-1B, IL-6, and tumor necrosis factor-α significantly potentiated the stimulatory effect of CRH on POMC expression. The tyrosine phosphorylation cascade is needed for the effect of the cytokines on POMC gene expression.[29] Leukocytes themselves are capable of expressing the POMC gene. Evidence has been presented for the presence of full length POMC transcripts in splenic mononuclear cells (MNC) and that these MNC process POMC to form ACTH using the same pathway present in rat corticotrophs.[30]

The effect of various secretagogues on POMC gene expression in AtT-20 cells has been investigated[31] and it was found that CRH stimulated POMC promoter activity as well as cAMP generation and ACTH secretion. Epinephrine also was a stimulator and the effect was mimicked by beta- but not alpha-adrenergic agonists. The combined effect of epinephrine and CRH gave the highest results but both hormones were blocked by H89, an inhibitor of protein kinase A, indicating that the cAMP-PKA system is the intracellular signalling pathway for CRH and catecholamines.[31] In a separate study the role of pituitary adenylate cyclase-activating polypeptide (PACAP) and vasoactive intestinal polypeptide (VIP) on POMC gene expression was examined.[32] It was found that PACAP stimulated POMC 5′ promoter activity as well as cAMP generation and ACTH secretion. Similar effects were observed with VIP. PACAP and VIP enhanced the CRH stimulation of POMC gene, but there was no such effect between PACAP and VIP. The stimulatory effects of PACP and VIP on POMC gene expression use an intracellular signalling pathway distinct from that of protein kinase A.

POMC gene expression and peptide levels were examined in medial basal hypothalamus (MBH) of castrated rats after 10 days of treatment with subcutaneous morphine or placebo pellets and after pellet removal.[33] It was found that morphine suppresses POMC gene expression in the MBH and that this was accompanied by a fall in β-endorphin content. These effects were independent of the action of the sex steroids. In the rat median eminence (ME), gonadal hormone treatment decreased POMC mRNA expression. This suggests that POMC neurons directly innervated the ME and that POMC peptides could inhibit luteinizing hormone-releasing hormone following the preovulatory hormone surge.[34] N-terminal fragments of POMC act on the pituitary lactotrophs during early postnatal development. Lorsignol et al.[35] found that in immature pituitary cells POMC 1–76 induces an increase in $[Ca^{2+}]I$ through extracellular Ca^{2+} flux mediated in part by protein kinase A activation. In a separate study by the same group of investigators[36] it was found that human POMC (1–76) increased the number of DNA replicating lactotrophs. γ3-MSH (the C-terminal domain of hPOMC 1–76) mimicked the effect of h POMC (1–76) but to a lesser extent. α- and β-MSH were effective but less potent than γ3-MSH. Future consideration of the control of lactotrophs in the pituitary will change considerably now that Hinuma et al.[37] have isolated 31- and 20-membered peptides from the hypothalamus that only releases prolactin from the pituitary.

POMC peptides and gene expression in skin have been a subject of great interest recently. Ultraviolet B radiation stimulates POMC gene expression and the release of α-MSH and ACTH by normal and malignant human melanocytes and keratinocytes.[38] The synthesis and release of both peptides were stimulated by dbc-AMP and IL-α, but not by endothelin-1 (ET-1) or by TNF-α. Cultured dermal fibroblasts from normal skin and keloids express POMC.[39] TGF-B greatly reduced POMC gene expression which was counteracted by TNF-α, which stimulated POMC mRNA levels. POMC transcripts were reduced by TGF-B in keratinocytes but no effect was seen in keloid-derived fibroblasts.

POMC–PEPTIDES

POMC–derived peptides have varied biological activities and skin is one of their target tissues. α-MSH is the first 13 amino acid of ACTH which also has pigmentary action and is an agonist at the melanocortin-1 receptor (MC-1). Recently α-MSH was localized in keratinocytes, in melanocytes and in Langerhans cells. ACTH was also present. In cultured keratinocytes and in epidermis $ACTH_{1-39}$, $ACTH_{1-17}$, $ACTH_{1-10}$, acetylated $ACTH_{1-10}$, α-MSH, and desactyl α-MSH were isolated. All of the peptides could activate the human MC-1–receptor with an increase of adenylate cyclase.[40] Protein malnutrition in rats causes an increase in resting plasma ACTH and POMC mRNA in the anterior pituitary giving rise to increased plasma glucocorticoids.[41]

Gamma-MSH (γ-MSH) was found to be natriuretic[42] when it was infused intravenously into anesthetized rats. It was concluded that the natriuretic action of γ-MSH occurs primarily by an interaction with renal nerves. Atrial natriuretic peptides in plasma is also increased but it plays only a minor role in the natriuresis following γ-MSH infusion.[42] Fodor et al.,[43] using antisera against Lys-γ-2 MSH and γ-MSH found a wide distribution of the immunoreactive peptides in rat brain. Immunoreactive bodies were found in the intermediate and anterior lobes of the pituitary, in the hypothalamic arcuate nucleus, and in the commissural part of the nucleus of the solitary tract. Immunoreactivity was also found in the vascular system, the bronchi, and kidneys. The finding of immunoreactivity in regions involved in cardiovascular regulation suggests a role for the γ-MSH peptides in cardiac function. In addition to its opioid action, dynorphin-A (DynA) has a number of nonopioid effects such as inflammation and aggravation of traumatic nerve injury. Quillan and Godee[44] examined the interaction of DynA with the melanocortin system (MC) and found the DynA peptides (DynA 1–13 amide and related peptides) antagonize melanocortin receptors in vitro with potencies that parallel those reported for pharmacological nonopioid effects in vivo. Its des-Tyr derivatives such as DynA (2–17) lack opioid activity but antagonized each of the five MC receptors examined. Taylor et al.,[45] studied the action of dynorphin A 1–13 on fetal ACTH using the unanesthetized chronically catheterized fetal lamb model. They found that dynorphin A 1–13 in the ovine fetus may be acting via a mechanism different from that in the kappa-opioid system, and the dynorphins may act as direct secretagogues of ACTH at the anterior pituitary through nonopioid receptors. β-endorphin was measured in skin and found in increased amounts during anagen and declined during follicle evolution or in the resting phase. It was concluded that this neuropeptide had a regulatory role to play in the cyclic changes of hair growth.[46] There is good evidence for a hypothalamic role for endogenous opioids in the control gonadotropin secretion. Sanchez-Franco and Cacicedo[47] showed that β-endorphin blocks GnRH-stimulated LH release; and Kandeel and Swerdloff,[48] using individual pituitary cell assays, showed that β-endorphin modulated gonadal steroid effects on LH secretion by pituitary gonadotrophs.

α-MSH

In the papers that follow α-MSH and related melanocortins are discussed in detail as to their role in immunoregulation, their action in skin, and their action in neuroimmunoregulation. Here I want to highlight a few aspects that have recently been discovered but which are not related to the effects of α-MSH on skin. The structures of important melanocortins are shown in FIGURE 2. They all have the core sequence of α-MSH (Met-Glu-His-Ph-Arg-Trp) and there is substitution of a Gly for the Glu in the γ-melanocortins. Some time ago an interesting paper was published by Lis et al.,[49] on the corticotropin releasing activity of α-MSH. These authors used rat anterior pituitary cells and showed that arginine vasopressin and α-MSH together produced a greater amount of ACTH than the sum of that produced by the individual peptides. This has not been followed up and should be pursued. Another finding of great interest involves pituitary adenylate cyclase-activating polypeptide (PACAP). Rene et al.,[50] studied PACAP receptors and their function in mouse pituitary neurointermediate lobe explants. They showed that melanotropes express PACAP receptor type 1 isoforms that work via cAMP and the inositol phosphate pathways, PACAP 27 and PACAP 38, stimulate cAMP and PACAP 38, but not PACAP 27, stimulates inositol phosphate breakdown. Both ligands stimulate POMC gene transcription and peptide exocytosis. Recently, attempts have been made to identify the peptides responsible for the immunoreactivity observed in melanoma cells and in tumors. It was found that in tumor extracts the IR-α-MSH 4 was associated with a 16-kDa and a 5–9-kDa fraction,[51] This IR material promoted frog skin darkening, tryrosinase activity in Cloudman 591 melanoma cells, and could displace labelled α-MSH from its binding sites in human melanoma cells. In a further attempt to identify the IR material in melanoma cells using HPLC to purify these peptides, a peak corresponding to desacetyl α-MSH was found.[52] A high molecular form of IR material was also found but none of the peptides detected were identified.

ACTH	Ser-Tyr-Ser-**Met-Glu-His-Phe-Arg-Trp**-Gly-Lys-Pro-Val + 26 amino acids
α-MSH	Ac-Ser-Tyr-Ser-**Met-Glu-His-Phe-Arg-Trp**-Gly-Lys-Pro-Val-NH₂
γ-MSH (γ₂-MSH)	Tyr-Val-**Met-Gly-His-Phe-Arg-Trp**-Asp-Arg-Phe-Gly
γ₁-MSH[1]	Tyr-Val-**Met-Gly-His-Phe-Arg-Trp**-Asp-Arg-Phe-NH₂
γ₃-MSH[1]	Tyr-Val-**Met-Gly-His-Phe-Arg-Trp**-Asp-Arg-Phe-Gly + 15 amino acids
β-MSH[2]	Asp-Ser-Gly-Pro-Tyr-Lys-**Met-Glu-His-Phe-Arg-Trp**-Gly-Ser-Pro-Pro-Lys-Asp
NDP-MSH	Ac-Ser-Tyr-Ser-Nle-**Glu-His-D-Phe-Arg-Trp**-Gly-Lys-Pro-Val-NH₂

Conserved 'core' amino acids are shown in bold type. Ac = N-acetyl.
[1] Additional N-terminal Lys may be present.
[2] Bovine.

FIGURE 2. Primary structures of melanocortins, taken from Tatro.[3]

α-MSH has very recently been shown to have a biological action on intracellular adhesion molecule-1 (ICAM-1). It has been shown that α-MSH reduced TNF-α–stimulated upregulation of ICAM-1 in normal cutaneous melanocytes. In three human melanoma cell lines, α-MSH and forskolin reduced TNF-α–stimulated ICAM-1 expression.[53] In a follow-up publication it was reported that α-MSH inhibits ICAM-1 expression stimulated by TNF-α at the protein and gene expression level. Inhibition of ICAM-1 expression could only be observed in malignant melanocytes, where detectable MSH receptors were present.[54] Murate et al.,[55] used a Matrigel invasion assay to study the invasive ability of murine melanoma cells. They found that α-MSH readily blocked the invasion of B16-BL6 cells with high-metastatic potential, but that it was less effective in inhibiting the invasion of weakly metastatic B16-F1 cells.

It has been amply demonstrated in recent years that α-MSH is widely distributed in the brain and that it acts as a neurohormone. This aspect of α-MSH biology will be fully covered in subsequent papers but here I want to mention just a few recent findings. It has been shown that α-MSH stimulates axonal as well as dendrite outgrowth from both total and cholera toxin subunit B (CTB)-labelled neurons in cell culture of neonatal rat cortex.[56] It had been previously shown that α-MSH and ACTH stimulated outgrowth of neurites from peripheral and central nervous systems in vitro. The effect of melanocorticotropin-potentiating factor (MPF), a tetrapeptide, on neuronal regeneration in cell culture has been investigated.[57] It was found that MPF stimulates the growth of cultured astrocytes and neurite outgrowth from cultures of neocortical cholinergic and mesenchephalic dopaminergic neurons. The stimulatory action of α-MSH and MCH on monoaminergic levels in the preoptic area of the rat has been investigated by perfusing the hormones and quantifying the amount of amine formed.[58] In the medial preoptic area α-MSH raised the concentration of 5-HIAA and MCH reduced both 5-HT and 5-HIAA and neither had any effect on the ventromedial nucleus. The action of the two peptides in the medial preoptic area may be mediated by dopamine.

α-MSH modifies the action of proinflammatory cytokines and in particular TNF-α. When TNF-α was induced by injection of bacterial lipopolysaccharide locally and then α-MSH was given, it inhibited TNF-α production in brain tissue.[59] This was confirmed by showing an inhibition of TNF-α mRNA formation. After induction of inflammation, TNF-α plasma concentration was elevated and this increased level was inhibited by α-MSH treatment. This inhibition could also be shown in brain tissue in vitro indicating that α-MSH can act directly on brain cells to inhibit TNF-α formation. In human glioma cells (A-172, anaplastic astrocytoma cells) α-MSH and a C-terminal tripeptide were both effective in inhibiting TNF-α induced by bacterial endotoxin.[60]

α-MSH RECEPTORS

Melanocortins and melanocortin receptors are involved in the control of many physiological functions, including obesity, thermoregulation, inflammation, immunomodulation, and sexual behavior; all of which are part of the integration of central and peripheral actions of these hormones. FIGURE 3 shows the distribution of the five

MCR subtype	Agonist profile	Major tissue mRNA distribution
MC1	α-MSH > ACTH ≫ γ-MSH	melanoma, melanocytes
MC2	ACTH	adrenal cortex
		adipose tissue
MC3	γ-MSH = ACTH ≥ α-MSH	brain, gut, placenta
MC4	α-MSH = ACTH ≫ γ-MSH	brain
MC5	α-MSH ≥ ACTH > γ-MAH	brain and peripheral tissues (e.g. skeletal muscle, lung, gut, spleen, thymus, bone marrow, pituitary, adrenal, gonads, adipose tissue)

FIGURE 3. MCR subtypes and tissue distribution, taken from Tatro.[3]

MCR subtypes, their agonist profiles, and the tissue distribution of the mRNA for each. MC1 is mostly present in melanoma and melanocyte cells, MC2 is the ACTH receptor in the adrenal cortex and adipose tissue, whereas MC3 has been localized to brain, gut, and placenta. MC4 seems to be confined to brain. MC5 is present in brain and in many peripheral tissues. The papers that follow offer detailed discussion on the pharmacology and chemistry of the ligands that bind to the melanocortin receptors. In this section I highlight some recent findings concerning the role of melanocortin receptors in ACTH and α-MSH action. It should be pointed out at the start that, before the ACTH and α-MSH receptors were cloned, Tatro and colleagues in Reichlin's laboratory in Boston had established that melanocortin receptors were present in murine melanoma cells, in human melanoma tissue, and in human melanoma metastases.[61–63] In the laboratory of Dr. Victor Hruby the melanotropin peptide was conjugated with a fluorescent macromolecule and it was shown that this conjugated peptide binds to receptors of all melanoma cells examined,[64–66] including epidermal melanocytes and keratinocytes.

Very recently a lot of research has been done on the structure activity relationships of melanocortin receptors. Schioth and colleagues[67] found that MC1, MC3, MC4, and MC5 did not have a binding receptor for ACTH beyond the first 13 amino acids of α-MSH. If one deletes 27, 25, 28, and 20 amino acids from the N-terminal of human MC1, MC3, MC4, and MC5, respectively, there is no effect on ligand binding or expression levels.[68] These deletions include all potential N-terminal glycosylation sites on MC1 and MC4 receptors. Alterations of the C-terminal amino acids of α-MSH and γ-MSH have been studied to determine their effects on binding to MC1 and MC3 melanocortin receptors.[69] It was found that proline 12 of α-MSH was important for binding at the MC1 receptor. Alterations at the C-terminal end of the peptides have a much smaller effect on MC3-R binding and activity. Human melanocortin-5 receptor (hMC5R) has a low affinity toward α-MSH, and Frandberg *et al.*,[70] found that glutamine at position 235 and arginine at position 272 contribute to the low affinity of this receptor. When the glutamine was mutated to lysine and the arginine to cysteine the affinity of α-MSH for the hMC5R was increased 10-fold. The MC1R is a seven-transmembrane (TM) G-protein–coupled receptor whose natural ligands are the melanocortin peptides, ACTH and α-, β-, and γ-MSH. Using [Nle4, DPhe7] MSH (NDP-MSH) and human MC1R, Yang *et al.*,[71] examined the effects of site-directed mutagenesis on the binding affinity and potency of NDP-MSH. Mutagenesis of acidic receptor residues Glu 94 in TM2, and Asp 117 or Asp 121 in TM3, significantly altered the binding affinity and potency of NDP-MSH, α-MSH, γ-MSH and Ac-Nle 4-cyclic -[Asp 5, His 6, DPhe 7, Arg 8, Trp 9, Lys 10]NH$_2$. In addition, it was found that aromatic–aromatic ligand receptor interactions also participate in the binding of the melanocortins to MC1R. Schioth *et al.*,[72] found that the genomic DNA of the human melanocortin MC3 receptors had an unusually long N-terminus. They mutated two translation initiation sites, deleted the DNA between the two, and found that these changes did not alter ligand binding to the receptor. Therefore, the N-terminal of the human MC3 is not important for binding. These investigators[73] expressed the DNA encoding the human MC4 receptor in COS cells and tested its radio ligand binding properties using ^{125}I[Nle 4, DPhe 7] α-MSH. The order of potency in displacing the labelled ligand was [Nle 4, DPhe 7] α-MSH > Nle 4-α-MSH > β-MSH > desacetyl α-MSH 7 > α-MSH > ACTH $_{1-39}$ > ACTH$_{4-10}$ > gamma 1-MSH > gamma 2-MSH. The melanocortin receptor shows the highest affinity for β-MSH and a very low affinity for gamma MSH. In a separate study, a number of ACTH$_{4-10}$ analogues were tested for their ability to displace a radio labelled ligand from human melanocortin receptors MC1, MC3, MC4, and MC5, transiently expressed in COS cells.[74] It was found that [Phe-17] ACTH$_{4-10}$ had a higher affinity for the MC3, MC4, and MC5 receptors, but a lower affinity for the MC1 receptor. Ala 6 ACTH$_{4-10}$ did not bind the MC1 receptor but had the highest affinity for the MC4 receptor.

There is very little data on intracellular signalling resulting from the binding to the melanocortin receptors that are G-protein coupled. In a recent report[75] it was found that Ba/F3 pro-β-lymphocyte cells express the gene for the MC5 receptor that binds α-MSH. The binding of α-MSH stimulates Janus kinase 2 (JAK2) and signal transducers and activators of transcription (STAT1) tyrosine phosphorylation, in Ba/F3 cells and in human cultured IM-9 lymphocytes. α-MSH also activates JAK2 in mouse L-cells that stably express human MC5 receptor and α-MSH binding results in increased cellular proliferation.

It has recently been found that a cyclic analogue of MSH, HSO14, is a selective antagonist of the MC4 receptor.[76] HSO14 caused an increase in food intake in rats in the first hour after injection, and at four hours after injection. This effect was concentration dependent. This adds evidence to the hypothesis that activation of the MC4 receptor inhibits food intake. Recently Kistler-Heer and colleagues[77] studied the binding of ^{125}I-NDP, which binds to all five receptors including MC3-R and MC4-R, the predominant receptors in brain. They examined the mRNA of MC3-R and MC4-R in rats between gestational day 14 and postnatal day 27. MC4-R mRNA was the predominant species during the entire fetal period. It was localized in the sympathetic ganglia and epithalamus, the sensors trigeminal nuclei, the dorsal motor nucleus of vagus and cranial nerve ganglia, inferior olive and cerebellum, striated region, and entorhinal cortex. MC3-R mRNA was found only in the postnatal period. MC5-R mRNA has been also been found in a number of tissues of the rat.[78] It was found in exocrine glands, including lacromal, Harderian, preputial, prostate, pancreas, adrenals, esophagus, and thymus. In exocrine glands MC5-R mRNA expression was restricted to secretory epithelia. MC5-R is commonly and selectively expressed in exocrine glands and other peripheral organs. Zheng *et al.,*[79] studied pituitary cells from lactating rats and found that α-MSH binding was restricted to mammotropes and that a specific subpopulation of these express functional α-MSH receptors that are coupled to a Ca^{2+} signalling pathway.

LEUKEMIA-INHIBITORY FACTOR (LIF)

Melmed[80] has recently reviewed the status of LIF and related factors in the pituitary. It has recently been shown that IL-6, LIF, and oncostatin-M can regulate pituitary function. These cytokines act via their receptors, which share a common affinity converter subunit gp 130. This gp 130 may homodimerize with high affinity receptor units such as IL-6 or may heterodimerize with receptor molecules such as LIF or oncostatin-M. Following ligand induced activation of the receptor complexes, intracellular phosphorylation occurs as well as cytoplasmic-nuclear signal transduction. IL-6 stimulates hypothalamic CRH and thereby stimulates ACTH release.[81] LIF is a 4-helix bundle-cytokine capable of inhibiting embryonal stem cell differentiation, regulating neurotrophic development, inducing the proliferation of myeloid cells, and facilitating uterine blastocyst implantation.[82] In addition, LIF can stimulate bone reabsorption, inhibit lipoprotein lipase, and regulate the hypothalamic-pituitary-adrenal axis. LIF is expressed in human fetal pituitary, pituitary adenomas, and in normal and rodent pituitary tumors.[83,84] Human fetal pituitary tissue contains receptors for LIF, IL-4, and gp 130 subunit as early as 18 weeks gestation.[85]

In AtT 20 murine corticotroph tumor cells LIF stimulates ACTH secretion and POMC mRNA levels.[83] POMC expression seems to be regulated in an autocrine or paracrine fashion in the absence of LIF. In the corticotroph LIF seems to induce a JAK/STAT signalling pathway, which results in enhanced POMC transcription.[86] CRH and LIF both stimulate ACTH, but CRH acts through cAMP and LIF does not. Both interact at the (-173/-160) of the POMC promoter.[87] In the human fetal pituitary cells, gp 130 related cytokines such as oncostatin M and IL-6 induce basal levels of ACTH as well as CRH-stimulated ACTH secretion. Anti-gp 130 serum blocks ACTH induction by both LIF and IL-6, showing that LIF and CRH are very highly synergistic resulting in a very large stimulation of POMC transcription. CRH induces cell proliferation, and LIF inhibits cell number and attenuates entry of cells into the S phase. LIF and CRH potentiate POMC transcription at the level of gene expression. Cytokines gp 130 and their receptors are expressed in the pituitary where they induce POMC mRNA *in vivo* and *in vitro;* by acting alone or with CRH they greatly stimulate ACTH formation.

THE AGOUTI SIGNAL PROTEIN (ASP)

The mouse agouti gene was cloned in 1992 and it encoded a protein of 131 amino acids having a signal peptide, suggesting that it is a secreted protein.[88,89] The human agouti gene encoded 132 amino acids and was called the agouti signalling protein (ASP).[90] The agouti protein has a Cys rich C-terminal domain similar to that found in the conotoxins that are L-type Ca^{2+} channel blockers. All of the 10 cystine residues at the C-terminal end of the agouti proprotein are involved in disulphite linkages.[91] All of the MCR antagonist activity resides in the Cys-rich end of the molecule.[91] Shortly after cloning the agouti protein it was shown that it was a potent antagonist of MC1-R because inhibition of α-MSH induced cAMP content and binding of ^{125}I-NDP-MSH to B16 mouse melanoma cells.[92] The agouti protein also antagonized human MC4-R, but less so with the rat MC3-R and mouse MC5-R.[93] In addition to its antagonism of melanocortin receptors, the agouti protein has a wider role. Several strains of mice having the dominant mutant alleles of the agouti gene have been discovered and each has characteristic features of the yellow coat color, but also there is obesity, insulin resistance, and increased susceptibility to certain types of tumors.[94]

Recently a number of very interesting papers have appeared on the action of the agouti protein and which I will review briefly with the understanding that this subject will come up again in the papers that follow. α-MSH and ASP have antagonistic roles and possibly opposing mechanisms of action in the melanocyte. In the mouse, α-MSH promotes melanogenic enzyme function and elicits an increase in the amount of eumelanins formed, whereas ASP reduces total melanin and promotes the synthesis of pheomelanin.[95] It has recently been shown the ASP inhibits melanogenesis in B 16 FI melanomia cells in the presence and in the absence of α-MSH, and it also causes a dose-related decrease in the synthesis of both eumelanin and pheomelanin. These changes were not seen in B 16 G 4 F cells that lack the MC1 receptor, suggesting that even in the absence of α-MSH, ASP acts at the MC1 receptor.[96] Using cyclic analogues of those melanocortins that are potent agonists or antagonists of MC3 and MC4 receptors, it was possible to determine whether agouti causes obesity by antagonism of hypothalamic melanocortin receptors.[97] Intracerebroventricular administration of the agonist MT 11 inhibited feeding in four models of hyperphagia. Coadministration of the melanocortin antagonist and agouti-minetic SHV9119 completely blocked this inhibition. Administration of SHV9119 enhanced nocturnal feeding or feeding stimulated by a prior fast. Thus, melanocortinergic neurons exert a tonic inhibition on feeding behavior.[97] Inactivation of the MC4-R by gene targeting results in mice that develop a maturity onset obesity syndrome associated with hyperphasia, hyperinsulinemia, and hyperglycemia. It was found that the primary mechanism by which agouti induces obesity is chronic antagonism of the MC4 receptor in brain.[98] Agouti-related protein (AGRP) mRNA is normally expressed in the hypothalamus and its levels are increased eightfold in ob/ob mice. AGRP is a potent antagonist of MC3-R and MC4-R implicated in weight regulation. Human AGRP complementary DNA in transgenic mice caused obesity without altering pigmentation.[99] AGRP mRNA was found to be unregulated in the hypothalamus of ob/ob mice. Recombinant AGRP inhibits α-MSH from binding to MC3-R and MC4-R, but not to MC5-R. AGRP seems to be 100-fold more potent than the agouti in reference to MC3-R and MC4-R binding affinity. Thus AGRP may be a physiological regulator of feeding behavior.[100] In a separate study using a human homolog of agouti signalling protein (ASIP) it was found that it blocked the binding of α-MSH to the MC1-R and inhibited the effect α-MSH on human melanocytes. Recombinant mouse or human ASIP blocked the stimulatory effects of α-MSH on cAMP accumulation, tyrosinase activity, and cell proliferation. In the absence of α-MSH, ASIP inhibited basal levels of tyrosinase activity and cell proliferation, and it reduced the level of immunoreactive tyrosinase. ASIP also blocked the stimulatory effects of forskolin or dibutyryl cAMP on tyrosinase activity and cell proliferation. Thus, there is a potential role for ASIP in the regulation of human pigmentation.[101] To learn more about the effects of the orexigenic peptides, galanin and neuropeptide Y (NPY), as well as the anorexigenic POMC in the obesity syndrome, these peptides were studied in lethal yellow (A(Y)), MC4-R knockout (MC4-RKO), and leptin deficient (ob/ob) mice. No changes in galanin or POMC gene expression were observed. In obese A(Y) mice, arcuate nucleus NPY mRNA levels were the same as their C57BL/6J littermates. In the dorsal medial hypothalamic nucleus, NPY was expressed at high levels. This brain region is functionally altered by disruption of melanocortinergic signalling and suggests that it may have an etiological role in the melanocortinergic obesity syndrome.[102] It has recently been shown that a functional MC1-R is needed for the pigmentary effects of agouti protein to be observed. Agouti protein can act as an agonist for MC1-R in a way that differs from α-MSH action. It was shown that α-MSH and agouti protein or AGRP function as independent ligands that inhibit each other's binding and transduce opposite signals through a single receptor.[103] Intracellular free Ca^{2+} concentration is elevated in viable yellow mice. To study the mechanism of this increase, agouti protein was investigated in several cell types. Increases in $[Ca^{2+}]I$ were observed in AFr5 vascular smooth muscle cells and 3T3-L1 adipocytes. MC1-R and MC3-R are necessary to obtain the increased Ca^{2+} effect by the human agouti protein.[104] In order to determine which residues are important for melanocortin receptor binding inhibition of the agouti protein, carboxyl terminal, alanine-scanning mutagenesis was performed. When agouti residues Arg 116 and Phe 118 were changed to alanine, a large drop in agouti affinity for MCR1, MCR3, and MCR4 was observed. Mutation of Phe 117 to alanine causes a similar increase in agouti KIapp and MC4-R. When agouti residue Asp 108 was changed to alanine there was a large increase in KIapp for all three melanocortin receptors.[105]

PEPTIDES AND SKIN INJURY

In order to exert their effect, many effector molecules must bind to heparin sulfate chains found at the cell surface. The heparin sulfate is derived in great part from the four members of the syndecan family of transmembrane proteoglycans.[106] In a study of the mechanism by which cell surface syndecan is induced, the fluid accumulating in cutaneous wounds undergoing repair was analysed. From this fluid a peptide was isolated; it is called PR-39.[107] This peptide is proline– and arginine–rich and was previously isolated as an antibacterial peptide from pig intestine.[108] PR-39 can induce heparin sulfate at the wound surface and fight off bacteria to assist in the healing process. PR-39 is also a chemoattractant for neutrophils,[109] but not for mononuclear cells. The neutrophil chemoattractant domain is contained in the first 26 amino acids and is dependent on Ca^{2+}.

Mammalian mucosal epithelia contain several antimicrobial peptides, which include tracheal antimicrobial peptide (TAP) from bovine tracheal mucose, Paneth cell defensins from human and mouse, and a β-defensin called LAP (lingual antimicrobial peptide) expressed in bovine tongue epithelial cells. Recently, an antibacterial peptide has been isolated from granulocytes, and this is not a member of the defensin family. This peptide, called LL-37, is derived from the CAMP (cathelicidin antimicrobial peptide) gene coding for it—a peptide that is part of the cathelicidin family.[109] The human cathelicidin gene is upregulated in inflammatory skin disorders but no induction was found in normal skin. The transcript and peptide are found in keratinocytes of the epidermis of the inflammatory region. The peptide was also found in psoriatic scales. LL-37 is induced when the skin barrier is damaged and acts as an antibacterial agent in the first line of defence.

REFERENCES

1. OTTAVIANI, E., A. FRANCHINI & C. FRANCESCHI. 1997. Pro-opiomelanocortin-derived peptides, cytokines and nitric oxide in immune responses and stress: An evolutionary approach. Int. Rev. Cytology **170:** 79–141.
2. CASTRO, M.G. & E. MORISON. 1997. Post-translational processing of proopiomelanocortin in the pituitary and in the brain. Crit. Rev. Neurobiol. **11:** 35–57.
3. TATRO, J.B. 1996. Receptor biology of the melanocortins, a family of neuroimmunomodulatory peptides. Neuroimmunommodulation **3:** 259–284.
4. LUGER, T.A., R.S. BHARDIVAJ, S. GRABBE et al. 1996. Regulation of the immune response by epidermal cytokines and neurohormones. J. Dermatol. Sci. **13:** 5–10.
5. CHANG, A.C.Y., M. CHOCHET & S. COHEN. 1980. Structural organization of human genomic DNA encoding pro-opiomelanocortin peptide. Proc. Natl. Acad. Sci. USA **77:** 4890–4894.
6. DROUIN, J. & H.M. GOODMAN. 1980. Most of the coding region of rat ACTH, beta-LPH precursor gene lacks intervening sequences. Nature **288:** 610–613.
7. HAKANISHI, S., Y. TERANISHI, Y. WATANABI et al. 1981. Isolation and characterization of the bovine corticotropin/betalipotropin precursor gene. Eur. J. Biochem. **115:** 429–434.
8. HARBOUR-MCMENAMIN, D., E.M. SMITH & J.E. BLALOCK. 1985. Bacterial lipopolysaccharide induction of leukocyte-derived corticotropin and endorphins. Infec. Immunol. **48:** 813–817.
9. HARBOUR, D.V., E.M. SMITH & J.E. BLALOCK. 1987. A novel processing pathway for proopiomelanocortin in lymphocytes: Endotoxin induction of a new prohormone cleaving enzyme. J. Neurosci. Res. **18:** 95–101.
10. O'DONOHUE, T.L. & D.M. DORSA. 1982. The opiomelanotropinergic neuronal and endocrine system. Peptides (N.Y.) **3:** 353–395.
11. JEANNOTTE, L., J.P.H. BURBACH & J. DROUIN. 1987. Unusual proopiomelanocortin ribonucleic acids in extra pituitary tissues: intronless transcripts in testes and long poly A tails in hypothalamus. Mol. Endocrinol. **1:** 749–757.
12. SCHAUER, E., F. TRAUTINGER, A. KOCK et al. 1994. Proopiomelanocortin derived peptides are synthesized and released by human keratinocytes. J. Clin. Invest. **93:** 2258–2262.
13. LUNEC, J., J.C. PIERON, G.V. SHERBET et al. 1990. Alpha-melanocortin-stimulating hormone immunoreactivity in melanoma cell. Pathobiol. **58:** 193–197.
14. MORHENN, V.B. 1991. The physiology of scratching: Involvement of proopiomelanocortin gene-coded proteins in Langerhans cells. Prog. Neuro. Endo. Immun. **4:** 261–265.
15. FAROOQUI, J.Z., E.E. MEDRANO, R.E. BOISSY et al. 1995. Thy-1 + dendritic cells express a truncated form of POMC mRNA. Exp. Dermatol. **4:** 228–232.

16. SLOMINSKI, A. 1992. POMC gene expression in hamster and mouse melanoma cells. FEBS Lett. **291:** 165–168.

17. SLOMINSKI, A., R. PAUS & J. MAZURKIEWICZ. 1992. Proopiomelanocortin expression in the skin during induced hair growth in mice. Experientia **48:** 50–54.

18. SLOMINSKI, A., R. PAUS & J. WORTSMAN. 1993. On the potential role of proopiomelanocortin in skin physiology and pathology. Molec. Cell Endocrinol. **93:** C1–C6.

19. BOSTON, B.A., K.M. BLAYDON, J. VARNERIN et al. 1997. Independent and additive effects of central POMC and leptin pathways on murine obesity. Science **278:** 1641–1644.

20. SCHWARTZ, M.W., R.J. SEELY, S.C. WOODS et al. 1997. Leptin increased hypothalamic proopiomelanocortin mRNA expression in rostral arcuate nucleus. Diabetes **46:** 2119–2123.

21. MIZUNO, T.M., S.P. KLEOPOULOS, H.T. BERGEN et al. 1998. Hypothalamic proopiomelanocortin mRNA is reduced by fasting and (corrected) in ob/ob and db/db mice, but is stimulated by leptin. Diabetes **47:** 294–297.

22. CHEUNG, C.C., D.K. CLIFTON & R.A. STEINER. 1997. Proopiomelanocortin neurons are direct targets for leptin in the hypothalamus. Endocrinology **138:** 4489–4492.

23. THORTON, J.E., C.C. CHEUNG, D.K. CLIFTON et al. 1997. Regulation of hypothalamic proopiomelanocortin mRNA by leptin in ob/ob mice. Endocrinology **138:** 5063–5066.

24. SAHU, A. 1998. Evidence suggesting that galanin (GAL), melanin-concentrating hormone (MCH) neurotensin (NT), proopiomelanocortin (POMC) and neuropeptide Y(NPY) are targest of leptin signalling in the hypothalamus. Endocrinology **139:** 795–798.

25. MAYAN, H., K.T. LING, F.Y. LEE et al. 1996. Dietary sodium intake modulates pituitary proopiomelanocortin mRNA abundance. Hypertension **28:** 244–249.

26. LINDBLAD, J.R. & J.L. ROBERTS. 1988. Regulation of propiomelanocortin gene expression in pituitary. Endocr. Rev. **9:** 135–158.

27. WARDLAW, S.L., K.C. MCCARTHY & I.M. CONWELL. 1998. Glucocorticoid regulation of hypothalamic proopiomelanocortin. Neuroendocrinology **67:** 51–57.

28. GARCIA-GARCIA, L., J.A. FUENTES & J. MANZANARES. 1997. Differential 5-HT-mediated regulation of sites-induced activation of proopiomelanocortin (POMC) gene expression in the anterior and intermediate lobe of the pituitary in male rats. Brain Res. **772:** 115–120.

29. KATAHIRA, M., Y. IWASAKI, Y. AOKI et al. 1998. Cytokine regulation of the rat proopio- melanocortin gene expression in AtT-20 cells. Endocrinology **139:** 2414–2422.

30. LYONS, P.D. & J.E. BLALOCK. 1997. Proopiomelanocortin gene expession and protein processing in rat mononuclear leukocytes. J. Neuroimmunol. **78:** 47–56.

31. AOKI, Y., Y. IWASAKI, M. KATAHIRA et al. 1997. Regulation of the rat proopiomelanocortin gene expression in AtT-20 cells I: Effects of common secretogogues. Endocrinology **138:** 1923–1929.

32. AOKI, Y., Y. IWASAKI, M. KATAHIRA et al. 1997. Regulation of the rat proopiomelanocortin gene expression in AtT-20 cells II. Effects of the pituitary adenylate cyclase-activating polypeptide and vasoactive intestinal polypeptide. Endocrinology **138:** 1930–1934.

33. WARDLAW, S.L., J. KIM & S. SOBIESZCZYK. 1996. Effect of morphine on proopiomelanocortin gene expression and peptide levels in the hypothalamus. Brain Res. Mol. **41:** 140–147.

34. CHEUNG, S. & R.P. HAMMER, JR. 1997. Gonadal steroid hormone regulation of proopio- melanocortin gene expression in neurons that innervate the median eminence of the rat. Neurosci. Lett. **224:** 181–184.

35. LORSIGNOL, A., B. HIMPENS & C. DENEF. 1998. Stimulation of Ca^{2+} entry in lactotrophs and somatotrophs from immature rat pituitary by N-terminal fragments of proopiomelanocortin. J. Neuroendocrinol. **10:** 217–229.
36. TILEMANS, D., D. RAMECKERS, M. ANDRIES et al. 1997. Effect of POMC (1-76), its C-terminal fragment gamma 3-MSH and anti-POMC (1-76) antibodies on DNA replication in lactotrophs in aggregate cell cultures of immature rat pituitary. J. Neuroendocrinol. **9:** 627–637.
37. HINUMA, S., Y. HABATA, R. FIJII et al. 1998. A prolactin-releasing peptide in the brain. Nature **393:** 272–276.
38. CHAKRABORTY, A.K., Y. FUNASAKA, A. SLOMINSKI et al. 1996. Production and release of proopiomelanocortin (POMC) derived peptides by human melanocytes and keratinocytes in culture: regulation by ultraviolet B. Biochem. Biophys. Acta **1313:** 130–138.
39. TEOFOLI, P., K. MOTOKI, T.M. LOTTI et al. 1997. Proopiomelanocortin (POMC) gene expression by normal skin and keloid fibroblasts in culture: modulation by cytokines. Exp. Dermatol. **6:** 111–115.
40. WAKAMATSU, K., A. GRAHAM, D. COOK et al. 1997. Characterization of ACTH peptides in human skin and their activation of melanocortin-1 receptor. Pigment Cell Res. **10:** 288–297.
41. JACOBSON, L., D. ZURAKOWSKI & J.A. MAJZOUB. 1997. Protein malnutrition increases plasma adrenocorticotropin and anterior pituitary proopiomelanocortin messenger ribonucleic acid in the rat. Endocrinology **138:** 1048–1057.
42. CHEN, X.W., W.Z. YING, J.P. VALENTIN et al. 1997. Mechanism of the natriuretic action of gamma-melanocyte stimulating hormone. Am. J. Physiol. **272:** R1946–R1953.
43. FODOR, M., A. SLUITER, A. FRANKHUIZZEN-SIEREVOGEL et al. 1996. Distribution of Lys-gamma 2-melanocyte stimulating hormone (Lys-gamma 2-MSH)-like immunoreactivity in neuronal elements in the brain and peripheral tissues of the rat. Brain Res. **731:** 182–189.
44. QUILLAN, J.M. & W. SADEE. 1997. Dynorphin peptides: antagonists of melanocortin receptors Pharm. Res. **14:** 713–719.
45. CAYLOR, C.C., D. WU, Y. SOONG et al. 1997. Dynorphin A1-13 stimulates ovine fetal pituitary-adrenal function through a novel monopoid mechanism. J. Pharmacol. Exp. Ther. **280:** 416–421.
46. FURKERT, J., U. KLUG, A. SLOMINSKI et al. 1997. Identification and measurement of beta-endorphin levels in the skin during induced hair growth in mice. Biochem. Biophys. Acta **1336:** 315–322.
47. SANCHEZ-FRANCO, F. & L. CACICEDO. 1986. Inhibitory effect of β-endorphin on gonadotropin- releasing hormone and thyrotropin-releasing hormone releasing activity in cultured rat anterior pituitary cells. Horm. Res. **24:** 55–61.
48. KANDEEL, F.R. & R.S. SWERDLOFF. 1997. The interaction between beta-endorphin and gonadal steroids in regulation of luteinizing hormone (LH) secretion and sex steroid regulation of LH and proopiomelanocortin peptide secretion by individual pituitary cells. Endocrinology **138:** 649–656.
49. LIS, M., J. JULESZ, J. GUTKOWSKA et al. 1982. Corticotropin-releasing activity of alfamelanocortin. Science **215:** 675–677.
50. RENE, F., D. MONNIER, C. GAIDDON et al. 1996. Pituitry adenylate cyclase-activating polypeptide transduces through cAMP/PKA and PKC pathways and stimulates proopiomelanocortin gene transcription in mouse melanotropes. Neuroendocrinol. **64:** 2–13.
51. GHANEM, G., B. LOIR, M. HADLEY et al. 1992. Partial characterization of IR-alpha-MSH peptides found in melanoma tumors. Peptides **13:** 989–994.

52. LUNIEC, J., C. PIERON, G.V. SHERBET *et al.* 1990. Alpha-melanocyte-stimulating hormone immunoreactivity in melanoma cells. Pathobiol. **58:** 193–197.
53. HEDLEY, S.J., D.J. GAWKRODGER, A.P. WEETMAN *et al.* 1998. Alpha-melanocyte stimulating hormone inhibits tumor necrosis factor-alpha stimulated intercellular adhesion molecule-1 expression in normal cutaneous human melanocytes and in melanoma cell lines. Br. J. Dermatol. **138:** 536–543.
54. MORANDINI, R., J.M. BOEYMAEMS, S.J. HEDLEY *et al.* 1998. Modulation of ICAM-1 expression by α-MSH in human melanoma cells and melanocytes. J. Cell Physiol. **175:** 276–282.
55. MURATA, J., K. AYUKAWA, M. OGASAWARA *et al.* 1997. Alpha-melanocyte stimulating hormone blocks invasion of reconstituted basement membrane (Matrigel) by murine B16 melanoma cells. Invasion Metastasis **17:** 89–93.
56. JOOSTEN, E.A., S. VERHOOGH, D. MARTIN *et al.* 1996. Alpha-MSH stimulates neurite outgrowth of neonatal rat corticospinal neurons *in vitro.* Brain Res. **736:** 91–98.
57. OWEN, D.B., J.S. MORLEY, D.M. ENSOR *et al.* 1997. Trophic effects of melanocortin-potentiating factor (MPF) on cultures of cells of the central nervous system. Peptides **18:** 1015–1021.
58. GONZALEZ, M.I., V. KALEA, D.R. HOLE *et al.* 1997. Alpha-melanocyte-stimulating hormone (α-MSH) and melanin-concentrating hormone (MCH) modify monoaminergic levels in the preoptic area of the rat. Peptides **18:** 387–392.
59. Rajora, N., G. Boecoli, D. Burns, *et al.* 1997. Alpha-MSH modulates local and circulating tumor necrosis factor-alpha in experimental brain inflammation. J. Neurosci. **17:** 2181–2186.
60. WONG, K.Y., N. RAJORA, G. BOECOLI *et al.* 1997. A potential mechanism of local anti-inflammatory action of alpha-melanocyte-stimulating hormone within the brain: modulation of tumor necrosis factor-alpha production by human astrocytic cells. Neuroimmunomodulation **4:** 37–41.
61. TATRO, J.B., M.L. ENTWISTLE, B.R. LESTER *et al.* 1990. Melanotropin receptors of murine melanoma characterized in cultured cells and demonstrated in experimental tumors *in situ.* Cancer Res. **50:** 1237–1242.
62. TATRO, J.B., M. ATKINS, J.W. MIER *et al.* 1990. Melanotropin receptors demonstrated *in situ* in human melanoma. J. Clin. Invest. **85:** 1825–1832.
63. TATRO, J.B., Z. WEN, M.L. ENTWISTLE *et al.* 1992. Interaction of an alpha-melanocyte- stimulating hormone-diphtheria toxin fusion protein with melanotropin receptors in human melanoma metastases. Cancer Res. **52:** 2545–2548.
64. SHARMA, S.D., M.E. GRANBERRY, J. JIANG *et al.* 1994. Multivalent melanotropic peptide and fluorescent macromolecular conjugates: new reagents for characterization of melanotropin receptors. Bioconjug. Chem. **5:** 591–601.
65. SHARMA, S.D., J. JIANG, M.E. HADLEY *et al.* 1996. Melanotropic peptide-conjugated beads for microscopic and visualization and characterization of melanoma melanotropin receptors. Proc. Natl. Acad. Sci. USA **93:** 13715–13720.
66. JIANG, J., S.D. SHARMA, J.L. FINK *et al.* 1996. Melanotropic peptide receptors: membrane markers of human melanoma cells. Exp. Dermatol. **5:** 325–333.
67. SCHIOTH, H.B., R. MUCENIECE, M. LARSSON *et al.* 1997. The melanocortin 1,3,4 or 5 receptors do not have a binding epitope for ACTH beyond the sequence of α-MSH. J. Endocrinol. **155:** 73–78.
68. SCHIOTH, H.B., S. PETERSSON, R. MUCENIECE *et al.* 1997. Deletions of the N-terminal regions of the human melanocortin receoptors. FEBS Lett **410:** 223–228.
69. PENG, P.J., V.G. SAHM, R.V. DOHERTY *et al.* 1997. Binding and biological activity of C-terminally modified melanocortin peptides: a comparison between their actions at rodent MC1 and MC3 receptors. Peptides **18:** 1001–1008.

70. FRANDBERG, P.A., X. XU & V. CHHAJLANI. 1997. Glutamine 235 and arginine 272 in human melanocortin 5 receptor determines its low affinity for MSH. Biochem. Biophys. Res. Commun. **236:** 489–492.

71. YANG, Y.K., C. DICKINSON, C. HASKELL-LUEVANO et al. 1997. Molecular bases for the interaction of [Nle4,0-Phe 1] melanocyte stimulating hormone with the human melanocortin-1 receptor. J. Biol. Chem. **272:** 23000–23010.

72. SCHIOTH, H.B., R. MUCENIECE, J.E. WIKBERG et al. 1996. Alternative translation initiation codon for the human melanocortin MC3 receptor does not affect the ligand binding. Eur. J. Pharmacol. **314:** 381–384.

73. SCHIOTH, H.B., R. MUCENIECE & J.E. WIKBERG. 1996. Characterization of the melanocortin 4 receptor by radioligand binding. Pharmacol. Toxicol. **79:** 161–165.

74. SCHIOTH, H.B., R. MUCENIECE & J.E. WIKBERG. 1997. Selectivity of [Phe-17], [Al 6], and [D-ala 4, Glu 5, Tyr 6] substituted ACTH (4-10) analogues for the melanocortin receptors. Peptides **18:** 761–763.

75. BUGG, J.J. 1998. Binding of alpha-melanocyte-stimulating hormone to its G-protein-coupled receptor on β-lymophocytes activates the Jak/STAT pathway. Biochem. J. **331:** 211–216.

76. KASK, A., L. RAGO, F. MUTULIS et al. 1998. Selective antagonist for melanocortin 4 receptor (HS 014) increases food intake in free-feeding rats. Biochem. Biophys. Res. Commun. **245:** 90–93.

77. KISTLER-HEER, V., M.E. LAUBER & W. LICHTENSTEIGER. 1998. Different development patterns of melanocortin MC3 and MC4 receptor mRNA: predominance of MC4 in fetal rat nervous system. J. Neuroendocrinol. **10:** 133–146.

78. VAN DER KRAAN, M., R.A. ADAN, M.L. ENTWISTLE et al. 1998. Expression of melanocortin-5 receptor in secretory epithelia supports a functional role in exocrine and endocrine glands. Endocrinology **139:** 2348–2355.

79. ZHENG, T., C. VILLALOBOS, K.D. NUSSER et al. 1997. Phenotypic characterization and functional correlation of alpha-MSH binding to pituitary cells. Am. J. Physiol. **272:** E282–E287.

80. MALMED, S. 1998. gp 130-related cytokines and their receptors in the pituitary. Trends Endocrinol. Metab. **9:** 155–161.

81. MASTORAKOS, G., J.S. WEBER & M.-A. MAGIAKOU. 1994. Hypothalamic-pituitary adrenal axis activation and stimulation of systemic vasopressin secretion by recombinant interleukin-6 in humans: potential implication for the syndrome of inappropriate vasopressin secretion. J. Clin. Endocrinol. Metab. **79:** 934–939.

82. PATTERSON, P.H. 1994. LIF, a cytokine at the interface between neurology and immunology. Proc. Natl. Acad. Sci. USA **91:** 7833–7835.

83. AKITA, S., J. WEBSTER, S.G. REN et al. 1995. Human and murine pituitary expression of leukemia inhibitory factor-novel intrapituitary regulation of adrenocorticotropin hormone synthesis and secretion. J. Clin. Invest. **95:** 1288–1298.

84. WANG, Z., S.G. REN & S. MELMED. 1996. Hypothalamic and pituitary leukemia inhibitory factor gene expression in vivo: a novel endotoxin-inducible neuro-endocrine interface. Endocrinology **137:** 2947–2953.

85. SHIMON, I., X. YAN, D.W. RAY et al. 1996. Cytokine-dependent gp 130 receptor subunit regulates human fetal pituitary adrenocorticotropin hormone and growth hormone secretion. J. Clin. Invest. **100:** 357–363.

86. RAY, D., S.G. REN & S. MELMED. 1996. Leukemia inhibitory factor (LIF) stimulates proopiomelanocortin (POMC) expression in a corticotroph cell line: role of stat pathway. J. Clin. Invest. **97:** 1852–1859.

87. BOUSQUET, C., D. RAY & S. MELMED. 1997. A common proopiomelanocortin-binding element mediates leukemia inhibitory factor and corticotropin-releasing hormone transcriptional synergy. J. Biol. Chem. **272:** 10551–10557.

88. BULTMAN, S.J., E.J. MICHAUD & R.P. WOYCHIK. 1992. Molecular characterization of the mouse agouti locus. Cell **71:** 1195–1204.
89. MULLER, M.W., D.M.J. DUHL, H. VRIELING et al. 1993. Cloning of the mouse agouti gene predicts a secreted protein ubiquitously expressed in mice carrying the lethal yellow mutation. Gene Dev. **7:** 454–467.
90. WILSON, D.B., M.M. OLLMANN, L. KANG et al. 1994. Structure and function of ASP, the human homology of the mouse agouti gene. Hum. Mol. Genet. **4:** 223–230.
91. WILLARD, D.H., W. BODNAR, C. HARRIS et al. 1995. Agouti structure and function: Characterization of the potent α-melanocyte stimulating hormone receptor antagonist. Biochem. **34:** 12341–12346.
92. BLANCHARD, S.G., C.O. HARRIS, O.R.R. ITTOOP et al. 1995. Agouti antagonism of melanocortin-binding and action in the B16F10 murine melanoma cell line. Biochem. **34:** 10496–10411.
93. LU, D., D. WILLARD, I.R. PATEL et al. 1994. Agouti protein is an antagonist of the melano- cyte-stimulating-hormone receptor. Nature **371:** 799–804.
94. YEN, T.T., A.M. GILL, L.G. FRIGERI et al. 1994. Obesity, diabetes and neoplasia in yellow A^{vy/-} mice. Ectopic expression of the agouti gene. FASEB J. **8:** 479–488.
95. FURUMURA, M., C. SAKAI, Z. ABDEL-MALEK et al. 1996. The interaction of agouti signal protein and melanocyte stimulating hormone to regulate melanin formation in mammals. Pigment Cell Res. **9:** 191–203.
96. GRAHAM, A., K. WAKEMUTSU, G. HUNT et al. 1997. Agouti protein inhibits the production of eumelanin and phaeomelanin in the presence and absence of alpha-melanocyte stimulating hormone. Pigment Cell Res. **10:** 298–303.
97. FAN, W., B.A. BOSTON, R.A. KESTERSON et al. 1997. Role of melanocortinergic neurons in feeding and the agouti obesity syndrome. Nature **385:** 165–168.
98. HUSZAR, D., C.A. LYNCH, V. FAIRCHILD-HUNTRESS et al. 1997. Targeted disruption of the melanocortin-4 receptor results in obesity in mice. Cell **88:** 131–141.
99. OLLMANN, M.M., B.D. WILSON, Y.K. YANG et al. 1997. Antagonism of central melanocortin receptors in vitro and in vivo by agouti-related protein. Science **278:** 135–138.
100. FONG, T.M., C. MAO, T. MACNEIL et al. 1997. ART (protein product of agouti-related transcript) as an antagonist of MC-3 and MC-4 receptors. Biochem. Biophys. Acta **237:** 629–631.
101. SUZUKI, I., A. TADA, M.M. OLLMANN et al. 1997. Agouti signalling protein inhibits melanogenesis and the response of human melanocytes to alpha-melanotropin. J. Invest. Dermatol. **108:** 838–842.
102. KESTERSON, R.A., D. HUSZAR, C.A. LYNCH et al. 1997. Induction of neuropeptide Y gene expression is the dorsal medial hypothalamic nucleus in two models of the agouti obesity syndrome. Mol. Endocrinol. **11:** 630–637.
103. OLLMANN, M.M., M.L. LAMOREUX, B.D. WILSON et al. 1998. Interaction of agouti protein with the melanocortin 1 receptor in vitro and in vivo. Genes Dev. **12:** 316–330.
104. KIM, J.H., L.L. KIEFER, R.P. WOYCHEK et al. 1997. Agouti regulation of intracellular calcium: role of melanocortin receptors. Am. J. Physiol. **272:** E379–E384.
105. KIEFER, L.L., J.M. VEAL, K.G. MOUNTJOY et al. 1998. Melanocortin receptor binding determinants in the agouti protein. Biochem. **37:** 991–997.
106. DAVID, G., V. LORIES, B. DECOCK et al. 1990. Molecular cloning of a phosphatidyl inositol-anchored membrane heparan sulfate proteoglycan from human lung fibroblast. J. Cell Biol. **111:** 3165–3176.
107. GALLO, R.L., M. ONO, T. POOSIC et al. 1994. Syndecons, cell surface heparin sulfate proteoglycans, are induce by a proline-rich antimicrobial peptide from wounds. Proc. Natl. Acad. Sci. USA **91:** 11035–11039.
108. AGERBERTH, B., J.Y. LEE, T. BERGMAN et al. 1991. Amino acid sequence of PR-39. Isolation from pig intestine of a new member of the family of proline-arginine rich antibacterial peptides. Eur. J. Biochem. **202:** 849–854.

109. FROHM, M., B. AGERBERTH, G. AHANGARI *et al.* 1996. The expression of the gene coding for the antibacterial peptide LL-37 is induced in human keratinocytes during inflammatory disorders. J. Biol. Chem. **272:** 15258–15263.

The Pituitary–Skin Connection in Amphibians

Reciprocal Regulation of Melanotrope Cells and Dermal Melanocytes

H. VAUDRY,[a] N. CHARTREL,[a] L. DESRUES,[a] L. GALAS,[a] S. KIKUYAMA,[b]
A. MOR,[c] P. NICOLAS,[c] AND M.C. TONON[a]

[a]European Institute for Peptide Research (IFRMP n° 23),
Laboratory of Cellular and Molecular Neuroendocrinology,
INSERM U 413, UA CNRS,
University of Rouen, 76821 Mont-Saint-Aignan, France

[b]Department of Biology, School of Education,
Waseda University, Tokyo 169-50, Japan

[c]Institut Jacques Monod, Laboratoire de Bioactivation des Peptides,
CNRS UMR 9922, Université de Paris VII, 75251 Paris, France

ABSTRACT: In amphibians, α-MSH secreted by the pars intermedia of the pituitary plays a pivotal role in the process of skin color adaptation. Reciprocally, the skin of amphibians contains a number of regulatory peptides, some of which have been found to regulate the activity of pituitary melanotrope cells. In particular, the skin of certain species of amphibians harbours considerable amounts of thyrotropin–releasing hormone, a highly potent stimulator of α-MSH release. Recently, we have isolated and sequenced from the skin of the frog *Phyllomedusa bicolor*—a novel peptide named skin peptide tyrosine tyrosine (SPYY), which exhibits 94% similarity with PYY from the frog *Rana ridibunda*. For concentrations ranging from 5×10^{-10} to 10^{-7} M, SPYY induces a dose-related inhibition of α-MSH secretion. At a dose of 10^{-7} M, SPYY totally abolished α-MSH release. These data strongly suggest the existence of a regulatory loop between the pars intermedia of the pituitary and the skin in amphibians.

THE INTERMEDIATE LOBE OF THE FROG PITUITARY AS A MODEL OF NEUROENDOCRINE SYNAPSE

Experimental evidence that the pituitary gland produces melanotropic peptides was provided independently in 1916 by two American investigators, Philip E. Smith[1] and Bennet M. Allen,[2] who showed that hypophysectomy of frog tadpoles induces bleaching of their skin. An *in vitro* bioassay based on the reflectance of pieces of frog skin was set up by Kazuo Shizume to measure the melanotropic activity in pituitary fractions.[3] This sensitive and relatively specific assay was successfully applied by Aaron B. Lerner and Teh H. Lee to isolate melanocyte–stimulating hormone (MSH) from the porcine pituitary gland.[4–6] Subsequently, most investigations concerning the mechanism of regulation of MSH secretion by melanotrope cells have been conducted by using the pars intermedia of frogs[7–11] and toads.[12–14] Thus, our current

41

knowledge on the biochemistry and physiology of melanotropic hormones stems largely from studies in amphibians.

The pars intermedia of the frog pituitary presents several particular features that make it a very suitable model for investigating the process of neuroendocrine communication. In contrast to the intermediate lobe of mammals, which generally contains a certain proportion of corticotrope cells,[15,16] the frog pars intermedia is composed only of melanotrope cells.[17] Although two subpopulations of endocrine cells with distinct biochemical and functional characteristics coexist in the pars intermedia of the European green frog *Rana ridibunda*,[18,19] all endocrine cells of the intermediate lobe belong to the melanotrope phenotype. In this respect, the frog pars intermedia offers all the advantages of a cell line without the drawbacks of transformed tumor cells. In mammals, the intermediate lobe is directly innervated by aminergic nerve fibers originating from the hypothalamus. In the rat, catecholaminergic (mainly dopaminergic),[20,21] GABAergic,[22–24] and serotoninergic[25–27] nerve terminals innervate melanotrope cells. In amphibians, the fibers projecting to the pars intermedia contain, not only classical neurotransmitters,[28–31] but also a series of regulatory peptides.[30–36] *In vitro* studies have shown that, in frogs,[29,37–46] and toads,[47–55] most of these neurotransmitters and neuropeptides regulate the activity of melanotrope cells (see FIGURE 1). Because aminergic and peptidergic nerve terminals make close contacts with melanotrope cells, the intermediate lobe of amphibians appears to be an authentic model of neuro-endocrine synapse, where neuronal inputs are converted into endocrine signals.

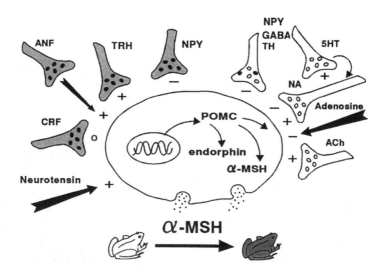

FIGURE 1. Schematic representation of the various neuroendocrine factors that may participate in the regulation of frog melanotrope cell activity.

THE AMPHIBIAN SKIN IS A RICH SOURCE OF BIOACTIVE PEPTIDES

The skin of a frog possesses a high density of acinuous glands embedded in the dermis and these glands communicate to the epidermal surface by means of secretory ducts.[56] Two categories of cutaneous glands can be distinguished according to their morphological features and biochemical content: the mucous glands and the granular glands—also called poison glands.[57] The poison glands are thought to arise from neuroendocrine-programmed cells derived from the neural crest and thus are part of the amine precursor uptake and decarboxylation (APUD) system.[58] These glands contain and release a large array of biologically active substances, including alkaloid toxins, classical neurotransmitters, and regulatory peptides.[56] Several of the peptides produced by the cutaneous glands exhibit a wide spectrum of antimicrobial activities and hence contribute to the defence mechanisms used by amphibians to protect themselves against invading pathogens.[59] Several dozens of antibacterial and antifungal peptides have now been isolated and characterized from the skin of various species of amphibians, including bombinin from the skin of the European toad *Bombina variegata*,[60] magainins from the South African clawed toad *Xenopus laevis*,[61] brevinin from the Japanese frog *Rana Brevipoda porsa*,[62] and dermaseptins from the South American tree frogs *Phyllomedusa sauvagei*[63] and *Phyllomedusa bicolor.*[59] Many other peptides produced by the poison glands of the amphibian skin are functionally related to various families of peptide hormones and/or neuropeptides such as the opioid peptides dermorphins[64] and deltorphins;[65] the tachykinins physalaemin,[66] hylambatin,[67] kassinin,[68] and phyllomedusin;[69] the cholecystokinin-related peptides caerulein[70] and phyllocaerulein;[71] the bradykinin-related peptides bradykinin,[66] phyllokinin,[72] and ranakinin;[72] and the bombesin-related peptides bombesin,[73] alytesin,[73] and ranatensin.[72] Interestingly, two other peptides purified from the skin of frogs exhibit potent hypophysiotropic activities: the tripeptide thyrotropin-releasing hormone (TRH),[74] which stimulates TSH release from pituitary thyrotrope cells, and the 41-amino acid residue peptide sauvagine,[75] which, like corticotropin–releasing hormone (CRF), urotensin I, and urocortin, stimulates ACTH release from pituitary corticotrope cells.

THYROTROPIN-RELEASING HORMONE

TRH was initially isolated from ovine[76] and porcine[77] hypothalamic extracts on the basis of its ability to stimulate TSH release, and its primary structure was established as P-Glu-His-Pro-NH$_2$. In mammals, TRH is widely distributed in the central nervous system[78,79] and in peripheral organs including the pancreas[80–82] and the gastrointestinal tract.[83,84] Consistent with its broad distribution, TRH exerts a large array of biological activities such as hyperthermia, hypertension, anorexia, and increase of colonic mobility.[85] In the pituitary of mammals, TRH stimulates not only TSH,[86] but also prolactin[87] and growth hormone secretion.[88] In the frog *Rana ridibunda*[37,38,89] and the toad *Xenopus laevis*,[51] TRH acts as an MSH-releasing hormone.

The skin of amphibians contains enormous amounts of TRH. In the leopard frog *Rana pipiens,* the concentration of TRH contained in the skin is twice that in the hypothalamus[90] and the amount of TRH in the skin of a single frog is approximately 85 μg.[91] Similarly, in a related species, the European green frog *Rana ridibunda,* high concentrations of TRH have been found in the dorsal skin (32 ng/mg protein).[92] In the toad *Xenopus laevis,* the level of TRH can reach 15 μg/g skin.[93] A high concentration of TRH has also been found in the skin of the Korean tree frog *Bombina orientalis,*[74] whereas a much lower level has been detected in the skin of the Mexican axolotl *Amblystoma mexicanum.*[94] Immunohistochemical studies have shown that, in the skin of *Rana ridibunda,* TRH is produced by a subpopulation of cells of the poison glands.[95] Interestingly, the dorsal skin of *Rana pipiens,*[95,96] *Rana ridibunda,*[95] and of *Xenopus laevis,*[93] which is more intensely pigmented than the ventral skin, contains the highest amount of TRH (see FIGURE 2).[91,92] The observation that the plasma concentrations of TRH in *Rana pipiens* are 1,000–10,000 times those measured in mammals[91] suggests that part of the TRH produced by the skin of amphibians can be released into the circulation. Thus, it appears that frog skin can be considered as an authentic endocrine organ that can release various regulatory peptides, including TRH, into the blood. In support of this concept, it has been reported that the secretion of TRH from the skin of amphibians is regulated by catecholamines. For instance, in *Rana pipiens,* TRH release is stimulated by noradrenaline (acting through α-adrenoreceptors) and inhibited by dopamine.[97,98] In *Xenopus laevis,* the secretion of TRH is also under catecholaminergic control.[93]

It has long been thought that, in amphibians, TRH was unable to stimulate TSH secretion.[99,100] Although it was subsequently demonstrated that this view is incorrect,[101] the reported lack of effect of TRH on amphibian thyrotrophs has prompted several groups to investigate other effects of TRH on pituitary cells in amphibians.

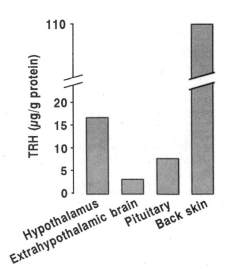

FIGURE 2. TRH concentration in different tissues of the frog *Rana pipiens* (adapted from Ref. 91).

These studies led to the discovery that, in *Rana catesbeiana,* TRH stimulates prolactin secretion.[102,103] They also revealed that, in *Rana ridibunda* and *Xenopus laevis,* TRH is a potent stimulator of α-MSH secretion.[37,38,51] The fact that, in amphibians, prolactin regulates water and ionic transport through the skin,[104] whereas α-MSH stimulates dermal melanocytes,[105] supports the existence of regulatory loops between skin TRH and pituitary hormones.

The transduction mechanisms associated with the activation of TRH receptors in amphibian melanotrope cells have been extensively studied. It has been found that, in *Rana ridibunda,* TRH induces a transient increase in inositol-1,4,5-triphosphate formation associated with a concomitant reduction of phosphatidylinositol bisphosphate indicating that, in frog melanotrope cells, TRH stimulates the phospholipase C pathway.[106] TRH also induces membrane depolarisation leading to an enhanced frequency of action potential discharge.[107] TRH causes a biphasic increase in cytosolic calcium concentrations ($[Ca^{2+}]i$), which can be accounted for by mobilization of intracellular calcium stores followed by the activation of membrane calcium channels.[89] The increase in $[Ca^{2+}]i$ is responsible for the stimulatory effect of TRH on α-MSH release.[89]

SKIN PEPTIDE TYROSINE TYROSINE

The pancreatic polypeptide (PP) family of regulatory peptides comprises three members in tetrapods: PP localized to endocrine cells in the pancreatic islets and in the intestine,[108] peptide tyrosine tyrosine (PYY) localized primarily to endocrine cells in the lower intestinal tract,[109] and neuropeptide tyrosine (NPY) synthesized in neurons of the central and peripheral nervous systems and in chromaffin cells of the adrenal medulla.[110,111] All three peptides exhibit structural similarities, suggesting that the PP family has arisen from successive duplications of an ancestral gene.[112–114] The primary structure of the different members of the PP family has now been determined in a number of vertebrate species (see Refs. 41, 115, and 116 for reviews): it appears that the sequence of PP and PYY has been moderately well conserved during evolution whereas the sequence of NPY has been very strongly preserved. For example, in the frog *Rana ridibunda,* the sequences of PP and PYY exhibit only 61% and 75% identity with their human counterparts, respectively,[115,116] whereas frog NPY differs from human NPY by a single, conservative amino acid substitution.[41] PP-related peptides exert a large array of biological effects in the central nervous system[117–120] and in peripheral organs.[121–124] In the frog *Rana ridibunda*[34,125,126] and in the toad *Xenopus laevis,*[55] NPY acts as an MSH-release inhibiting factor.

A peptide belonging to the PP family has been recently isolated in pure form from the skin of the South American arboreal frog *Phyllomedusa bicolor* on the basis of its antifungal activity. The primary structure of the peptide was determined (see TABLE 1) and it became apparent that this regulatory peptide is homologous to *Rana ridibunda* PYY. Therefore, this novel peptide was named skin peptide tyrosine tyrosine (SPYY).[127] Comparison of the sequence of *Phyllomedusa bicolor* SPYY with that of *Rana ridibunda* PYY indicates that these peptides differ only by two amino acid substitutions ($Ser^7 \rightarrow Asn$ and $Asn^{18} \rightarrow Thr$) suggesting that SPYY may simply

TABLE 1. A comparison of the primary structure of frog pancreatic polypeptide–related peptides

Peptide (origin)	Sequence	Similarity score (%)	Ref.
SPYY (*P. bicolor*)	Y P P K P E S P G E D A S P E E M N K Y L T A L R H Y I N L V T R Q R Y - NH$_2$		127
PYY (*R. ridibunda*)	Y P P K P E S P G E D A S P E E M T K Y L T A L R H Y I N L V T R Q R Y - NH$_2$	94	116
NPY (*R. ridibunda*)	Y P S K P D S P G E D A P A E D M A K Y Y S A L R H Y I N L I T R Q R Y - NH$_2$	72	41
PP (*R. ridibunda*)	A P S E P H H P G D Q A T P D Q L A Q Y Y S D L Y Q Y I T F I T R P R F - NH$_2$	39	115

correspond to the expression product of the PYY gene in the skin of *Phyllomedusa bicolor.* Alternatively, two closely related genes encoding PYY and SPYY may exist in the genome of *Phyllomedusa bicolor* as previously demonstrated for brain and skin proTRH.[128,129]

The skin of *Phyllomedusa bicolor* contains considerable amounts of SPYY (100 μg/g tissue) as compared to the concentration of NPY in the brain (5.5 μg/g tissue) or PYY in the gut (0.5 μg/g tissue) in *Rana ridibunda.* This suggests that SPYY, in very much the same way as TRH, may be released into the general circulation and, thus, may act as a hormone. As a matter of fact, it was found that SPYY is a potent inhibitor of α-MSH release by perifused frog neurointermediate lobes[127] (see FIGURE 3). Comparison of the dose-response curves revealed that SPYY is 15 times more potent than NPY in inhibiting α-MSH release.[41,127] The C-terminal fragment SPYY$_{14-36}$ is also capable of inhibiting α-MSH release (although this short-chain analog was a less potent inhibitor than SPYY) indicating that the action of SPYY is mediated through a Y$_2$ receptor subtype[127] (see FIGURE 3). Consistent with this observation, we have recently observed that the inhibitory effect of NPY on the electrophysiological activity of frog melanotrope cells[43] is mimicked by the Y$_2$ receptor agonist NPY$_{16-36}$ whereas the selective Y$_1$ receptor agonist [Leu^{31}, Pro^{34}]NPY is much less active (unpublished data). Interestingly, it has been found that the stimulatory effect of TRH on α-MSH secretion is dose-dependently inhibit

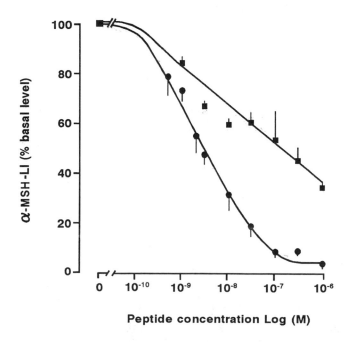

FIGURE 3. Effects of graded doses of SPYY (●) and SPYY-(14–36) (■) on α-MSH secretion by perifused frog neurointermediate lobes.

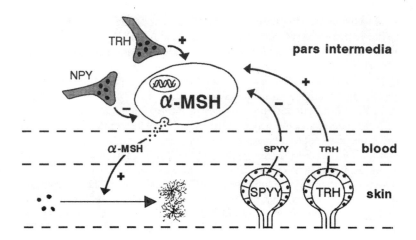

FIGURE 4. Schematic representation of putative regulatory loops between skin TRH and SPYY, and pituitary melanotrope cells. +, stimulatory effect; −, inhibitory effect.

ed by NPY[126] suggesting that the two skin peptides TRH and SPYY may interact on their common target melanotrope cells (see FIGURE 4).

CONCLUSION

The skin of amphibians is a rich source of regulatory peptides. Two biologically active peptides, TRH and SPYY, produced in large amounts by frog skin, are capable of regulating the secretion of α-MSH from the intermediate lobe. The fact that, in amphibians, dermal melanocytes are the main target cells for α-MSH, together with the occurrence of TRH and SPYY in frog skin, suggests the existence of a regulatory loop between the pars intermedia of the pituitary and the skin in amphibians.

ACKNOWLEDGMENTS

This work was supported by grants from INSERM (U 413), CNRS (UMR 9922), and the Conseil Régional de Haute-Normandie.

REFERENCES

1. SMITH, P.E. 1916. Experimental ablation of the hypophysis in the frog embryo. Sciences **44:** 230–282.
2. ALLEN, B.M. 1916. Extirpation of the hypophysis and thyroid gland of *Rana pipiens.* Science **44:** 755–757.
3. SHIZUME, K., A.B. LERNER & T.B. FITZPATRICK. 1954. *In vitro* bioassay for melanocyte stimulating hormone. Endocrinology **54:** 553–560.

4. LEE, T.H. & A.B. LERNER. 1956. Isolation of melanocyte-stimulating hormone from hog pituitary gland. J. Biol. Chem. **221:** 943–959.

5. LERNER A.B. & T.H. LEE. 1955. Isolation of a homogeneous melanocyte-stimulating hormone from hog pituitary gland. J. Am. Chem. Soc. **77:** 1066–1067.

6. LERNER, A. 1993. The discovery of the melanotropins. *In* The Melanotropic Peptides. H. Vaudry & A.N. Eberle, Eds. Ann. N.Y. Acad. Sci. **680:** 1–12.

7. BOWER, A., M.E. HADLEY & V.J. HRUBY. 1974. Biogenic amines and control of melanophore stimulating hormone release. Science **184:** 70–72.

8. DAVIS, M.D. & M.E. HADLEY. 1978. Pars intermedia electrical potentials changes in spike frequency induced by regulatory factors of melanocyte stimulating hormone (MSH) secretion. Neuroendocrinology **26:** 277–282.

9. TONON, M.C., J.M. DANGER, M. LAMACZ, P. LEROUX, S. ADJEROUD, A.C. ANDERSEN, B.M.L. VERBURG-VAN KEMENADE, B.G. JENKS, G. PELLETIER, M.E. STOECKEL, A. BURLET, G. KUPRYSZEWSKI & H. VAUDRY. 1988. Multihormonal control of melanotropin secretion in cold blooded vertebrates. *In* The Melanotropic Peptides. M.E. Hadley, Ed. **1:** 127–171. CRC Press. New York.

10. TONON, M.C., L. DESRUES, M. LAMACZ, N. CHARTREL, B.G. JENKS & H. VAUDRY. 1993. Multihormonal regulation of pituitary melanotrophs. *In* The Melanotropic Peptides, H. Vaudry & A.N. Eberle, Eds. Ann. N.Y. Acad. Sci. **680:** 175–187.

11. VAUDRY, H., M. LAMACZ, L. DESRUES, E. LOUISET, J. VALENTIJN, Y.A. MEI, N. CHARTREL, J.M. CONLON, L. CAZIN & M.C. TONON. 1994. The melanotrope cell of the frog pituitary as a model of neuroendocrine integration. *In* Perspectives in Comparative Endocrinology. K.G. Davey, R.E. Peter & S.S. Tobe, Eds.: 5–11, Nat. Res. Council Canada.

12. ITURRIZA, F.C. 1966 Monoamines and control of the pars intermedia of the toad pituitary. Gen. Comp. Endocrinol. **6:** 19–25.

13. ROUBOS, E.W. 1997. Background adaptation by *Xenopus laevis:* a model for studying neuronal information processing in the pituitary pars intermedia. Comp. Biochem. Physiol. **3:** 533–550.

14. JENKS, B., M. BUZZI, C. DOTMAN, H. DE KONING, W. SCHEENEN, J. LIESTE, H. LEENDERS, P. CRUIJSEN & E. ROUBOS. 1998. The significance of multiple inhibitory mechanisms converging on the melanotrope cell of *Xenopus laevis*. *In* Trends in Comprartive Endocrinology and Neurobiology, H. Vaudry, M.C. Tonon, E.W. Roubos & A. De Loof, Eds. Ann. N.Y. Acad. Sci. **839:** 229–234.

15. STOECKEL, M.E., H.D. DELLMANN, A. PORTE & C. GERTNER. 1971. The rostral zone of the intermediate lobe of the mouse hypophysis, a zone of particular concentration of corticotropic cells. A light and electron microscopic study. Z. Zellforsch. Mikrosk. Anat. **122:** 310–322.

16. STOECKEL, M.E., G. SCHMITT & A. PORTE. 1981. Fine structure and cytochemistry of the mammalian pars intermedia. Ciba Found. Symp. **81:** 101–122.

17. BENYAMINA, M., C. DELBENDE, S. JEGOU, P. LEROUX, F. LEBOULENGER, M.C. TONON, J. GUY, G. PELLETIER & H. VAUDRY. 1986. Localization and identification of α-melanocyte-stimulating hormone (α-MSH) in the frog brain. Brain Res. **366:** 230–237.

18. GONZALEZ DE AGUILAR, J.L., M.C. TONON, H. VAUDRY & F. GRACIA-NAVARRO. 1994. Morphological and functional heterogeneity of frog melanotrope cells. Neuroendocrinology **59:** 176–182.

19. GONZALEZ DE AGUILAR, J.L., M. MALAGON, R.M. VAZQUEZ-MARTINEZ, I. LIHRMANN, M.C. TONON, H. VAUDRY & F. GRACIA-NAVARRO. 1997. Two frog melanotrope cell subpopulations exhibiting distinct biochemical and physiological patterns in basal conditions and under thyrotropin-releasing hormone stimulation. Endocrinology **138:** 970–977.

20. BAUMGARTEN, H.G., A. BJORKLUND, A.F. HOLSTEIN & A. NOBIN. 1972. Organisation and ultrastructural identification of the catecholamine nerve terminals in the neural lobe and pars intermedia of the rat pituitary. Z. Zellforsch. Mikrosk. Anat. **126:** 483–517.

21. BJORKLUND, A. & A. NOBIN. 1973. Organization of tuberohypophyseal and reticulo-infundibular catecholamine neuron systems in the rat brain. Brain Res. **51:** 171–191.

22. OERTEL, W.H., E. MUGNAINI, M.C. TAPPAZ, V.K. WEISE, A.L. DAHL, D.E. SCHMECHEL & I.J. KOPIN. 1982. Central GABAergic innervation of neurointermediate pituitary lobe: biochemical and immunocytochemical study in the rat. Proc. Natl. Acad. Sci. USA **79:** 675–679.

23. VINCENT, S.R., T. HÖKFELT & J.Y. WU. 1982. GABA neuron system in hypothalamus and the pituitary gland. Neuroendocrinology **34:** 117–125.

24. VUILLEZ, P., S. CARBAJO-PEREZ & M.E. STOECKEL. 1987. Colocalization of GABA and tyrosine hydroxylase immunoreactivities in the axons innervating the neurointermediate lobe of the rat pituitary: An ultrastructural immunogold study. Neurosci. Lett. **79:** 53–58.

25. WESTLUND, K.N. & G.V. CHILDS. 1982. Localization of serotonin fibers in the rat adenohypophysis. Endocrinology **111:** 1761–1769.

26. FRIEDMAN, E., D.T. KRIEGER, E. MEZEY, C. LERANTH, M.J. BROWSTEIN & M. PALKOVITS. 1983. Serotonin innervation of the pituitary intermediate lobe decreases after stalk section. Endocrinology **112:** 1943–1947.

27. SALAND, L.C., J.A. WALLACE & F. COMUNAS. 1986. Serotonin-immunoreactive nerve fibers of the rat pituitary: effects of anticatecholamine and antiserotonin drugs on staining patterns. Brain Res. **368:** 310–318.

28. KONDO, Y., I. NAGATSU, M. YOSHIDA, N. KARASAWA & T. NAGATSU. 1983. Existence of noradrenaline cells and serotonin cells in the pituitary gland of *Rana catesbeiana.* Cell Tissue Res. **228:** 405–408.

29. LAMACZ, M., M.C. TONON, F. LEBOULENGER, F. HERY, A.J. VERHOFSTAD, G. PELLETIER & H. VAUDRY. 1989. Effect of serotonin on alpha-melanocyte-stimulating hormone (α-MSH) secretion from perifused frog neurointermediate lobe. Evidence for the presence of serotonin-containing cells in the frog pars intermedia. J. Endocrinol. **122:** 135–146.

30. DE RIJK, E.P.C.T., F.J.C. VAN STRIEN & E.W. ROUBOS. 1992. Demonstration of coexisting catecholamine (dopamine), amino acid (GABA), and peptide (NPY) involved in inhibition of melanotrope cell activity in *Xenopus laevis:* a quantitative ultrastructural, freeze-substitution immunocytochemical study. J. Neurosci. **12:** 864–871.

31. TONON, M.C., O. BOSLER, M.E. STOECKEL, G. PELLETIER, M. TAPPAZ & H. VAUDRY. 1992. Colocalization of tyrosine hydroxylase, GABA and neuropeptide Y within axon terminals innervating the intermediate lobe of the frog *Rana ridibunda.* J. Comp. Neurol. **319:** 599–605.

32. SEKI, T., Y. NAKAI, S. SHIODA, T. MITSUMA & S. KIKUYAMA. 1983. Distribution of immunoreactive thyrotropin-releasing hormone in the forebrain and hypophysis of the bullfrog, *Rana catesbeiana.* Cell Tissue Res. **233:** 507–516.

33. TONON, M.C., A. BURLET, M. LAUBER, P. CUET, S. JEGOU, L. GOUTEUX, N. LING & H. VAUDRY. 1985. Immunohistological localization and radioimmunoassay of corticotropin-releasing factor in the forebrain and hypophysis of the frog *Rana ridibunda.* Neuroendocrinology **40:** 109–119.

34. DANGER, J.M., F. LEBOULENGER, J. GUY, M.C. TONON, M. BENYAMINA, J.C. MARTEL, S. SAINT-PIERRE, G. PELLETIER & H. VAUDRY. 1986. Neuropeptide Y in the intermediate lobe of the frog pituitary acts as an α-MSH-release inhibiting factor. Life Sci. **39:** 1183–1192.

35. VERBURG-VAN KEMENADE, B.M.L., B.G. JENKS, J.M. DANGER, H. VAUDRY, G. PELLE-
TIER & S. SAINT-PIERRE. 1987. A NPY-like peptide may function as MSH-release
inhibiting factor in *Xenopus laevis*. Peptides **8:** 61–67.

36. LAMACZ, M., C. HINDELANG, M.C. TONON, H. VAUDRY & M.E. STOECKEL. 1989.
Three distinct TRH-immunoreactive axonal systems project in the median eminence-
pituitary complex of the frog *Rana ridibunda*. Immunocytochemical evidence for colocalization of TRH and mesotocin in fibers innervating pars intermedia cells. Neuroscience **32:** 451–462.

37. TONON, M.C., P. LEROUX, F. LEBOULENGER, C. DELARUE, S. JEGOU, J. FRESEL &
H. VAUDRY. 1980. Thyrotropin-releasing hormone stimulates the release of melanotropin from frog neurointermediate lobe *in vitro*. Life Sci. **26:** 869–875.

38. TONON, M.C., P. LEROUX, M.E. STOECKEL, S. JEGOU, G. PELLETIER & H. VAUDRY.
1983. Catecholaminergic control of α-melanocyte-stimulating hormone (α-MSH)
release by frog neurointermediate lobe *in vitro:* evidence for direct stimulation of
α-MSH release by thyrotropin-releasing hormone. Endocrinology **112:** 133–141.

39. LAMACZ, M., M.C. TONON, E. LOUISET, L. CAZIN & H. VAUDRY. 1989. Acetylcholine
stimulates melanocyte-stimulating hormone release from frog pituitary melanotrophs
through activation of muscarinic and nicotinic receptors. Endocrinology **125:** 707–
714.

40. TONON, M.C., S. ADJEROUD, M. LAMACZ, E. LOUISET, J.M. DANGER, L. DESRUES,
L. CAZIN, P. NICOLAS & H. VAUDRY. 1989. Central-type benzodiazepines and the
octadecaneuropeptide (ODN) modulate the effects of γ-aminobutyric acid on the
release of α-melanocyte-stimulating hormone from frog neurointermediate lobe *in
vitro*. Neuroscience **31:** 485–493.

41. CHARTREL, N., J.M. CONLON, J.M. DANGER, A. FOURNIER, M.C. TONON & H.
VAUDRY. 1991. Characterization of melanotropin-release-inhibiting factor (mel-
anostatin) from frog brain: Homology with human neuropeptide Y. Proc. Natl. Acad.
Sci. **88:** 3862–3866.

42. VALENTIJN, J.A., E. LOUISET, H. VAUDRY & L. CAZIN. 1991. Dopamine-induced inhibition of action potentials in cultured frog pituitary melanotrophs is mediated
through activation of potassium channels and inhibition of calcium and sodium
channels. Neuroscience **42:** 29–39.

43. VALENTIJN, J.A., H. VAUDRY, W. KLOAS & L. CAZIN. 1994. Melanostatin (NPY)
inhibited electrical activity in frog melanotrophs through modulation of K^+, Na^+ and
Ca^{2+} currents. J. Physiol. (Lond) **475:** 185–195.

44. LAMACZ, M., M. GARNIER, F. HERY, M.C. TONON & H. VAUDRY. 1995. The adrener-
gic control of α-MSH release in frog pituitary is mediated by both β- and a non conventional $α_2$ subtype of adrenoreceptor. Neuroendocrinology **61:** 430–436.

45. DESRUES, L., M.C. TONON, J. LEPRINCE, H. VAUDRY & J.M. CONLON. 1998. Isolation,
primary structure and effects on α-MSH release of frog neurotensin. Endocrinology.
139: 4140–4146.

46. GARNIER, M., M. LAMACZ, L. GALAS, S. LENGLET, M.C. TONON & H. VAUDRY. 1998
Pharmacological and functional characterization of muscarinic receptors in the frog
pars intermedia. Endocrinology. **139:** 3525–3533.

47. VERBURG-VAN KEMENADE, B.M.L., M. TAPPAZ, L. PAUT & B.G. JENKS. 1986. GABA-
ergic regulation of melanocyte-stimulating hormone secretion from the pars intermedia of *Xenopus laevis:* immunocytochemical and physiological evidence. Endocrinology **118:** 260–267.

48. VERBURG-VAN KEMENADE, B.M.L., M.C. TONON, B.G. JENKS & H. VAUDRY. 1986.
Characterization of dopamine receptors in the pars intermedia of the amphibian
Xenopus laevis. Neuroendocrinology **44:** 446–456.

49. VERBURG-VAN KEMENADE, B.M.L., B.G. JENKS, P.M.J.M. CRUIJSEN, A. DINGS, M.C. TONON & H. VAUDRY. 1987. Regulation of MSH release from the neurointermediate lobe of *Xenopus laevis* by CRF-like peptides. Peptides **8:** 1093–1100.

50. VERBURG-VAN KEMENADE, B.M.L., B.G. JENKS & R.J.M. SMITS. 1987. N-terminal acetylation of MSH in the pars intermedia of *Xenopus laevis* is a physiologically regulated process. Neuroendocrinology **46:** 289–296.

51. VERBURG-VAN KEMENADE, B.M.L., B.G. JENKS, T. VISSER, M.C. TONON & H. VAUDRY. 1987. Assessment of TRH as a potential MSH release stimulating factor in *Xenopus laevis*. Peptides **8:** 69–76.

52. DE KONING, H.P., B.G. JENKS & E.W. ROUBOS. 1993. Analysis of $GABA_A$ receptor function in the *in vitro* and *in vivo* regulation of α-MSH secretion from melanotrope cells of *Xenopus laevis*. Endocrinology **132:** 674–681.

53. SHIBUYA, I. & W.W. DOUGLAS. 1993. Spontaneous cytosolic calcium pulsing detected in *Xenopus* melanotrophs: modulation by secreto-inhibitory and stimulant ligands. Endocrinology **132:** 2166–2175.

54. SCHEENEN, W.J.J.M., H.G. YNTEMA, P.H.G.M. WILLEMS, E.W. ROUBOS, J.R. LIESTE & B.G. JENKS. 1995. Neuropeptide Y inhibits Ca^{2+} oscillations, cyclic AMP, and secretion in melanotrope cells of *Xenopus laevis* via a Y_1 receptor. Peptides **16:** 889–895.

55. VAN STRIEN, F., E.W. ROUBOS, H. VAUDRY & B.G. JENKS. 1996. Acetylcholine autoexcites release of proopiomelanocortin-derived peptides from melanotrope cells of *Xenopus laevis* via a M_1 muscarinic receptor. Endocrinology **137:** 4298–4307.

56. LAZARUS, L.H. & M. ATTILA. 1993. The toad, ugly and venomous, wears yet a precious jewel in his skin. Prog. Neurobiol. **41:** 473–507.

57. NEUWIRTH, M., J.W. DAILY, C.W. MYERS & L.W. TICE. 1979. Morphology of the granular secretory glands in skin of poison-dart frogs (*Dendrobatidae*). Tissue Cell **11:** 755–771.

58. PEARSE, A.G.E. 1976. Peptides in brain and intestin. Nature **262:** 92–94.

59. MOR, A., M. AMICHE & P. NICOLAS. 1994. Structure, synthesis and activity of dermaseptin b, a novel vertebrate defensive peptide from frog skin: relationship with adenoregulin. Biochemistry **33:** 6642–6650.

60. CSORDAS, A. & H. MICHL. 1970. Isolierung und Strukturaufklärung eines hämolytisch wirkenden polypeptides aus abwehrsekret europäischer unken. Monatsh. Chem. **101:** 182–189.

61. ZASLOFF, M. 1987. Magainins, a class of antimicrobial peptides from *Xenopus* skin: isolation, characterization of two active forms, and partial cDNA sequence of a precursor. Proc. Natl. Acad. Sci. USA **84:** 5449–5453.

62. MORIKAWA, H., K. HAGIWARA & P. NICOLAS. 1992. Brevinin-1 and -2, unique antimicrobial peptides from the skin of the frog, *Rana brevipoda porsa*. Biochem. Biophys. Res. Commun. **189:** 184–190.

63. MOR, A., N. VAN HUONG, A. DELFOUR, D. MIGLIORE-SAMOUR & P. NICOLAS. 1991. Isolation, amino acid sequence, and synthesis of dermaseptin, a novel antimicrobial peptide of amphibian skin. Biochemistry **30:** 8824–8830.

64. MONTECUCCHI, P.C., R. DE CASTIGLIONE, R.S. PIANI, L. GOZZINI & V. ERSPAMER. 1981. Amino acid composition and sequence of dermophin. A novel opiate-like peptide from the skin of *Phyllomedusa sauvagei*. Int. J. Pept. Prot. Res. **17:** 275–283.

65. RICHTER, K., R. EGGER & G. KREIL. 1987. D-Alanine in the frog skin peptide dermorphin is derived from L-alanine in the precursor. Science **238:** 200–202.

66. ERSPAMER, V., G. BERTACCINI & J.M. CEI. 1962. Occurrence of an eledoisin-like polypeptide (physalaemin) in skin extracts of *Physalaemus fuscumaculatus*. Experientia **18:** 526–563.

67. YASUHARA, T., T. NAKAJIMA, G. FALCONIERI-ERSPAMER & V. ERSPAMER. 1981. New tachykinins, Glu^2,Pro^5-kassinin (hylambates-kassinin) and hylambatin, in the skin of the African rhacophorid frog *Hylambates maculatus*. Biomed. Res. **2**: 613–617.

68. ANASTASI, A., P. MONTECUCCHI, V. ERSPAMER & J. VISSER. 1977. Amino acid composition and sequences of kassinin, a tachykinin dodecapeptide from the skin of the African frog *Kassina senegalensis*. Experientia **33**: 857–858.

69. ERSPAMER, V., G. FALCONIERI-ERSPAMER, P. MELCHIORRI & R. ENDEAN. 1985. A potent factor in extracts of the skin of the Australian frog, *Pseudophryne coriacea*. Apparent facilitation of transmitter release in isolated smooth muscle preparations. Neuropharmacology **24**: 783–792.

70. ANASTASI, A., V. ERSPAMER, & R. ENDEAN. 1968. Isolation and amino sequence of caerulein, the active decapeptide of the skin *Hyla caerulea*. Arch. Biochem. Biophys. **125**: 57–68.

71. ERSPAMER, V. & P. MELCHIORRI. 1973. Active polypeptides of the amphibian skin and their synthetic analogs. Pure Appl. Chem. **35**: 463–494.

72. NAKAJIMA, T. 1974. New vasoactive peptides of nonmammalian origin. *In* The Chemistry and Biology of the Kallikrein-Kinin System in Health and Disease. J.J. Pisano & K.F. Austen, Eds.: 165–168, Fogarty International Center Proceeding n° 27 DHEW n° 76–791, Bethesda.

73. ANASTASI, A., V. ERSPAMER & M. BUCCI. 1971. Isolation and structure of bombesin and alytesin, 2 analogous active peptides from the skin of the European amphibians *Bombina* and *Alytes*. Experientia **27**: 166–167.

74. YASUHARA, T. & T. NAKAJIMA. 1975. Occurrence of $Pyr-His-Pro-NH_2$ in the frog skin. Chem. Pharmacol. Bull. **23**: 3301–3303.

75. MONTECUCCHI, P.C., A. ANASTASI, R. DECASTIGLIONE & V. ERSPAMER. 1980. Isolation and amino acid composition of sauvagine. An active polypeptide from ethanol extracts of the skin of the South American frog *Phyllomedusa sauvagei*. Int. J. Pept. Prot. Res. **16**: 191–199.

76. BURGUS, R., T.F. DUNN, D. DESIDERIO, D.N. WARD, W. VALE & R. GUILLEMIN. 1970. Characterization of ovine hypothalamic hypophysiotropic TSH-releasing factor. Nature **226**: 321–325.

77. NAIR, R.M.G., T. BARRET, C.Y. BOWERS & A.V. SCHALLY. 1970. Structure of porcine thyrotropin-releasing hormone. Biochemistry **9**: 1103–1106.

78. BROWNSTEIN, M.J., M. PALKOVITS, J.M. SAAVEDRA, R.M. BASSIRI & R.T UTIGER. 1974. Thyrotropin-releasing hormone in specific nuclei of rat brain. Science **185**: 267–269.

79. OLIVER, C., R.L. ESKAY, N. BEN-JONATHAN & J.C. PORTER. 1974. Distribution and concentration of TRH in the rat brain. Endocrinology **95**: 540–546.

80. MARTINO, E., A. LEMMARK, H. SEO, D.F. STEINER & S. REFETOFF. 1978. High concentration of thyrotropin-releasing hormone in pancreatic islets. Proc. Natl. Acad. Sci. USA **75**: 4265–4267.

81. KOIVUSALO, F. & J. LEPPÄLUOTO. 1979. High TRF immunoreactivity in purified pancreatic extracts of fetal and newborn rats. Life Sci. **24**: 1655–1659.

82. DUTOUR, A., L. L'OUAFIK, E. CASTANAS, F. BOUDOURESQUE & C. OLIVER. 1985. TRH and TRH-OH in the pancreas of adult and newborn rats. Life Sci. **37**: 177–183.

83. MORLEY, J.E., J.J. GARVIN, A.E. PEKARY & J.H. HERSHMANN. 1977. Thyrotropin-releasing hormone in the gastrointestinal tract. Biochem. Biophys. Res. Commun. **79**: 314–317.

84. LEPPALUOTO, J., F. KOIVUSALO & R. KRAAMA. 1978. Thyrotropin-releasing factor: Distribution in neural and gastrointestinal tissues. Acta Physiol. Scand. **104**: 175–179.

85. Griffiths, E.C. 1985. Thyrotropin-releasing hormone: endocrine and central effects. Psychoneuroendocrinology **10:** 225–235.

86. BOWERS, C.Y., A.V. SCHALLY, F. ENZMANN, J. BØHLER & K. FOLKERS. 1970. Porcine thyrotropin releasing hormone is (Pyro)-Glu-His-Pro-(NH_2). Endocrinology **86:** 1143–1153.

87. VALE, W., R. BLACKWELL, G. GRANT & R. GUILLEMIN. 1973. TRF and thyroid hormones on prolactin secretion by rat anterior pituitary cells *in vitro*. Endocrinology **93:** 26–33.

88. SZABO, M., M.E. STACHURA, N. PALEOLOGOS, D.E. BYBEE & L.A. FROHMAN. 1984. Thyrotropin-releasing hormone stimulates growth hormone release from the anterior pituitary of hypothyroid rats *in vitro*. Endocrinology **114:** 1344–1351.

89. GALAS, L., M. LAMACZ, M. GARNIER, E.W. ROUBOS, M.C. TONON & H. VAUDRY. 1998. Involvement of extracellular and intracellular calcium sources in TRH-induced α-MSH secretion in frog melanotrope cells. Mol. Cell. Endocrinol. **138:** 25–39.

90. JACKSON, I.M.D. & S. REICHLIN. 1977. Thyrotropin-releasing hormone: abundance in the skin of the frog *Rana pipiens*. Science **198:** 414–415.

91. JACKSON, I.M.D. & S. REICHLIN. 1979. Thyrotropin-releasing hormone in the blood of the frog, *Rana pipiens*: its nature and possible derivation from regional locations in the skin. Endocrinology **104:** 1814–1820.

92. GIRAUD, P.G., P. GILLIOZ, B. CONTE-DEVOIX & C. OLIVER. 1979. Distribution de thyrolibérine (TRH), α-melanocyte-stimulating hormone (α-MSH) et somatostatine dans les tissus de la grenouille verte (*Rana esculenta*). C.R. Acad. Sci. Paris **288:** 118–124.

93. BENNETT, G.W., M. BALLS, R.H. CLOTHIER, C.A. MARSDEN, G. ROBINSON, & G.D. WEMYSS-HOLDEN. 1981. Location and release of TRH and 5HT from amphibian skin. Cell Biol. Internat. Reports. **5:** 151–158.

94. SAWIN, C.T., J.L. BOLAFFI, I.P. CALLARD, P. BACHARACH, & I.M.D. JACKSON. 1978. Induced metamorphosis in *Amblystoma mexicanum*: lack of effect of triodothyronine on tissue or blood levels of TRH. Gen. Comp. Endocrinol. **36:** 427–432.

95. RAVAZZOLA, M., D. BROWN, J. LEPPÄLUOTO & L. ORCI. 1979. Localisation by immunofluorescence of thyrotropin-releasing hormone in the cutaneous glands of the frogs, *Rana ridibunda*. Life Sci. **25:** 1331–1334.

96. BOLAFFI, J.L. & I.M.D. JACKSON. 1979. Immunohistochemical localization of TRH in skin of *Rana pipiens*. Cell Tissue Res. **202:** 505–508.

97. MUELLER, G.P., L. ALPERT, S. REICHLIN, & I.M.D. JACKSON. 1980. Thyrotropin-releasing hormone and serotonin secretion from frog skin are stimulated by norepinephrine. Endocrinology **106:** 1–4.

98. BOLAFFI, J.L. & I.M. JACKSON. 1982. Regulation of thyrotropin-releasing hormone secretion from frog skin. Endocrinology **110:** 842–846.

99. ETKIN, W. & A.G. GONA. 1968. Failure of mammalian thyrotropin-releasing factor preparation to elicit metamorphic responses in tadpoles. Endocrinology **82:** 1067–1068.

100. TAUROG, A., C. OLIVER, R.L. ESKAY, J.C. PORTER, & J.M. MCKENZIE. 1974. The role of TRH in the neoteny of the Mexican axolotl (*Amblystoma mexicanum*). Gen. Comp. Endocrinol. **24:** 267–279.

101. DARRAS, V.M. & E.R. KÜHN. 1982. Increased plasma levels of thyroid hormones in a frog *Rana ridibunda* following intravenous administration of TRH. Gen. Comp. Endocrinol. **48:** 469–475.

102. CLEMONS, G.K., S.M. RUSSELS & C.S. NICOLL. 1979. Effect of mammalian thyrotropin-releasing hormone on prolactin secretion by bullfrog adenohypophysis *in vitro*. Gen. Comp. Endocrinol. **38:** 62–67.

103. SEKI, T. & S. KIKUYAMA. 1986. Effect of thyrotropin-releasing hormone and dopamine on the *in vitro* secretion of prolactin by the bullfrog pituitary gland. Gen. Comp. Endocrinol. **61:** 197–202.

104. BOLE-FEYSOT, C., V. GOFFIN, M. EDERY, N. BINART & P.A. KELLY. 1998. Prolactin (PRL) and its receptor: actions, signal transduction pathways and phenotypes observed in PRL receptor knockout mice. Endocr. Rev. **19:** 225–268.
105. BAGNARA, J.T. & M.E. HADLEY. 1973. Chromatophores and color change; the comparative physiology of animal pigmentation. Prentice Hall Inc. Engelwood Cliffs.
106. DESRUES, L., M.C. TONON & H. VAUDRY. 1990. Thyrotropin-releasing hormone (TRH) stimulates polyphosphoinositide metabolism in frog neurointermediate lobes. J. Mol. Endocrinol. **5:** 129–136.
107. LOUISET, E., L. CAZIN, M. LAMACZ, M.C TONON & H. VAUDRY. 1989. Dual effect of thyrotrophin-releasing hormone (TRH) on K$^+$ conductance in frog pituitary melanotrophs. TRH-induced α-melanocyte-stimulating hormone release is not mediated through voltage-sensitive K$^+$ channels. J. Mol. Endocrinol. **3:** 207–218.
108. KIMMEL, J.R., L. HAYDEN & H.G. POLLOCK. 1975. Isolation and characterization of a new pancreatic polypeptide hormone. J. Biol. Chem. **250:** 9369–9376.
109. TATEMOTO, K. 1982. Isolation and characterization of peptide YY (PYY), a candidate gut hormone that inhibits pancreatic exocrine secretion. Proc. Natl. Acad. Sci. USA **79:** 2514–2518.
110. TATEMOTO, K., V. CARLQUIST & V. MUTT. 1982. Neuropeptide Y—A novel brain peptide with structural similarities to peptide YY and pancreatic polypeptide. Nature **296:** 659–660.
111. TATEMOTO, K. 1982. Neuropeptide Y: Complete amino acid sequence of the brain peptide. Proc. Natl. Acad. Sci. USA **79:** 5485–5489.
112. SCHWARTZ, T.W., J. FUHLENDORFF, N. LANGELAND, H. THOGERSEN, J.C. JORGENSEN & S.P. SHEIKH. 1989. *In* Neuropeptide Y.V. Mutt, T. Hökfelt, K. Fuxe & J.M. Lundberg, Eds.: 143–157, Raven Press, New York.
113. LARHAMMAR, D., A.G. BLOMQVIST & C. SODERBERG. 1993. Evolution of neuropeptide Y and its related peptides. Comp. Biochem. Physiol. **106C:** 743–752.
114. LARHAMMAR, D. 1996. Evolution of neuroepeitde Y, peptide YY and pancreatic polypeptide. Regul. Pept. **62:** 1–11.
115. CONLON, J.M., J.E. PLATZ, N. CHARTREL, H. VAUDRY & P.F. NIELSEN. 1998. Amino acid sequence diversity of pancreatic polypeptide among the amphibia. Gen Comp. Endocrinol. **112:** 146–152.
116. CONLON, J.M., N. CHARTREL & H. VAUDRY. 1992. Primary structure of frog PYY: Implications for the molecular evolution of the pancreatic polypeptide family. Peptides **13:** 145–149.
117. DUMONT, Y., A. FOURNIER, S. ST-PIERRE, T.W. SCHWARTZ & R. QUIRION. 1992. Neuropeptide Y and neuropeptide Y receptor subtypes in brain and peripheral tissues. Prog. Neurobiol. **38:** 125–167.
118. WAHLESTEDT, C. & D.J. REIS. 1993. Neuropeptide Y-related peptides and their receptors: Are the receptors potential therapeutic drug targets? Annu. Rev. Pharmacol. Toxiol. **32:** 309–352.
119. HEILIG M. & E. WIDERLOV. 1995. Neurobiology and clinical aspects of neuropeptide Y. Crit. Rev. Neurobiol. **9:** 115–136.
120. MUNGLANI, R., M.J. HUDSPITH & S.P. HUNT. 1996. The therapeutic potential of neuropeptide Y: analgesic, anxiolytic, and antihypertensive. Drug **52:** 371–389.
121. DANGER, J.M., M.C TONON, B.G. JENKS, S. SAINT-PIERRE, J.C. MARTEL, A. FASOLO, B. BRETON, R. QUIRION, G. PELLETIER & H. VAUDRY. 1990. Neuropeptide Y: localization in the central nervous system and neuroendocrine functions. Fundamental Clin. Pharmacol. **4:** 307–340.
122. KARLA, S.P. & W.R. CROWLEY. 1992. Neuropeptide Y: a novel neuroendocrine peptide in the control of pituitary hormone secretion, and its relation to luteinizing hormones. Front. Neuroendocrinol. **13:** 1–46.

123. LUNDBERG, J.M., K. TATEMOTO, L. TERENIUS P.M. HELLSTROM, V. MUTT, T. HOKFELT & B. HAMBERGER. 1982. Localization of peptide YY (PYY) in gastrointestinal endocrine cells and effects on intestinal blood and motility. Proc. Natl. Acad. Sci. USA **79:** 4471–4475.
124. SHEIKH, S. 1991. Neuropeptide Y and peptide YY: major modulators of gastrointestinal blood flow and function. Am. J. Physiol. **261:** 6701–6715.
125. DANGER, J.M., M.C. TONON, M. LAMACZ, J.C. MARTEL, S. SAINT-PIERRE, G. PELLETIER & H. VAUDRY. 1987. Melanotropin-release inhibiting action of neuropeptide Y: structure activity relationships. Life Sci. **40:** 1875–1880.
126. DANGER, J.M., M. LAMACZ, F. MAUVIARD, S. SAINT-PIERRE, B.G. JENKS, M.C. TONON & H. VAUDRY. 1990: Neuropeptide Y inhibits thyrotropin-releasing hormone-induced stimulation of melanotropin release from the intermediate lobe of the frog pituitary. Gen. Comp. Endocrinol. **77:** 143–149.
127. MOR, A., N. CHARTREL, H. VAUDRY & P. NICOLAS. 1994. Skin peptide tyrosine-tyrosine, a member of the pancreatic polypeptide family: isolation, structure, synthesis, and endocrine activity. Proc. Natl. Acad. Sci. USA **91:** 10295–10299.
128. KUCHLER, K., K. RICHTER, J. TRNOVSKY, R. EGGER & G. KREIL. 1990. Two precursors of thyrotropin-releasing hormone from skin of *Xenopus laevis*. Each contains seven copies of the end product. J. Biol. Chem. **265:** 11731–11733.
129. BULANT, M., K. RICHTER, K. KUCHLER & G. KREIL. 1992. A cDNA from brain of *Xenopus laevis* coding for a new precursor of thyrotropin-releasing hormone. FEBS Lett. **300:** 197.

The Subtilisin/Kexin Family of Precursor Convertases

Emphasis on PC1, PC2/7B2, POMC and the Novel Enzyme SKI-1

NABIL G. SEIDAH,[a] SUZANNE BENJANNET,[b] JOSÉE HAMELIN,[a]
AIDA M. MAMARBACHI,[a] AJOY BASAK,[a,c] JADWIGA MARCINKIEWICZ,[b]
MAJAMBU MBIKAY,[b] MICHEL CHRÉTIEN,[b,c]
AND MIECZYSLAW MARCINKIEWICZ[b]

[a]Laboratory of Biochemical Neuroendocrinology,
Clinical Research Institute of Montreal,
110 Pine Ave. West, Montreal, QC, Canada H2W 1R7

[b]Laboratory of Molecular Neuroendocrinology,
Clinical Research Institute of Montreal,
110 Pine Ave. West, Montreal, QC, Canada H2W 1R7

ABSTRACT: Proopiomelanocortin (POMC) is a precursor to various, bioactive peptides Including ACTH, βLPH, αMSH, and βendorphin (βEND). Processing of POMC at dibasic residues is tissue-specific and is performed by either PC1 alone (resulting in ACTH and βLPH, anterior pituitary corticotrophes) or by a combination of PC1 and PC2 (yielding αMSH and βEND, pituitary neurointermediate lobe and hypothalamus). The PC2-specific binding protein 7B2 is intimately involved in the zymogen activation of proPC2 into PC2. Structure–function studies of these enzymes demonstrated the presence of N- and C-terminal domains, as well as specific amino acids within the catalytic segment that influence the degree of activity of each enzyme and the interaction of PC2 with 7B2. The tissue distribution, plasticity of expression, and the multiple precursors that are differentially cleaved by PC1 and/or PC2, predict a wide array of combinatorial activities of these convertases within the endocrine and neuroendocrine system. The phenotypic consequences of the absence of genetic expression of either PC1 or PC2 are now explored using knockout mice and in human patients suffering from obesity and diabetes.

INTRODUCTION

Biologically active proteins and peptides are often generated by intracellular limited proteolysis of inactive precursors. This evolutionary ancient mechanism resulted in the elaboration of specific secretory enzymes and a tight regulation of their activities. These processing enzymes usually cleave proproteins at selected sites, composed of single or paired basic amino acids. The latter are found in precursors

[c]Present address: Loeb Health Research Institute at the Ottawa Hospital, 725 Parkdale Avenue, Ottawa, Ontario, Canada K1Y 4K9.

of most neural and peptide hormones, proteolytic enzymes, growth factors, numerous type-I membrane–bound proteins (including receptors, cell adhesion molecules, and cell surface glycoproteins of pathogenic species such as viruses and bacteria), and even cell signaling molecules. Thus, the generation of biologically active peptides and proteins requires two major components—the polypeptide precursor substrate and the proteolytic enzyme(s) responsible for the conversion of the precursor into its final bioactive protein/peptide product(s). A debate has raged about whether biologically active peptides/proteins are generated by unique enzymes that process each precursor, or by relatively few enzymes with general and possibly redundant functions. Recently, these questions have been brought to sharp focus and answered.

The secretory enzymes responsible for this intracellular cleavage have now been molecularly and functionally characterized, and are shown to belong to an evolutionary conserved family of serine proteinases of the subtilisin/kexin-type. The seven known mammalian *precursor convertases* (PCs) cleaving at single and/or pairs of basic residues have been named PC1 (also called PC3), PC2, furin (also called PACE), PACE4, PC4, PC5 (also called PC6), and PC7 (also called SPC7, LPC, or PC8).[1–5] These enzymes specialize in the cleavage of basic residues within the general motif Arg-$(X)_n$-Arg$\downarrow$ where $n = 0, 2, 4,$ or 6 and X is any amino acid except Cys or, rarely, Pro. However, a number of precursors are also cleaved at nonbasic sites, such as the C-terminal to Ala, Ser, Thr, Val, and Leu.[5] In this context, an evolutionary conserved new *subtilisin-kexin-isozyme* has been very recently characterized, and named SKI-1, since it cleaves some precursors at single (and possible pairs of) hydroxylated amino acids, such as Thr.[6] The detailed study of the tissue expression, regulation, ontogeny, gene silencing, and biological functions of these "convertases" and their mutants, suggests that they exhibit both complementary and specific functions.[1–9] The data demonstrate that PCs exhibit a remarkable temporal and spatial specificity of expression patterns, making them available in various proportions and combinations in different loci. This raises questions about the redundancy of the convertases *versus* their specialization. Since the PC family actually counts eight paralogs, with some exhibiting additional protein-isoforms (PACE4,[10,11] PC4,[12] PC5,[13] PC7,[9] and SKI-1[6]) produced by alternative splicing of their precursor RNA, the distribution picture remains open to future exploration.

The conservation of the catalytic domains and the variability around these domains suggests that PC genes evolved from a common ancestral gene through duplications, translocations, insertions, or deletions. Except for furin and PACE4, which are closely linked, all the other PCs genes are dispersed on various chromosomes. The synteny between mouse and human for all the chromosomal regions carrying PC loci suggests that their multiplication and divergence occurred before the human and murine evolutionary lines branched—about 80 million years ago. The multiplicity of PC genes suggests both redundancy and differentiation of functions among their products. Redundancy serves the survival of a biological system, whereas differentiation affords complexity to it. The challenge in such cases is in delimiting the degree of overlap and distinctiveness. Cellular coexpression of substrates and convertases provides invaluable insights into the substrate and cleavage site preferences of many convertases, as well as their trafficking pathways within the cells.

What is emerging is that, although many PCs could cleave the same precursor *in vitro,* it is the regulation of the level of their individual cellular expression and their activities, as well as their dynamic intraorganellar localization, that are critical for each *in vivo* processing reaction.

THE NEURAL AND ENDOCRINE CONVERTASES PC1 AND PC2

Analysis of the tissue-expression and cellular localization of the convertases revealed that only PC1[14] and PC2,[14] and in some cases PC5-A[15] (the short soluble isoform of PC5), can be found within dense core secretory granules. Cellular coexpression studies and gene knockout results confirmed the key role of PC1 and PC2 in processing most neuropeptide and endocrine precursors for which products are stored in granules.[1,2,4,5,8,14] All the other enzymes, including furin, PC7, PACE4, PC4, as well as PC5, seem to concentrate and act at the level of the *trans*-Golgi Network (TGN), en route to the cell surface or at the level of the plasma membrane.[1-9] Thus, the latter enzymes seem to be primarily responsible for processing precursors for which products reach the cell surface and/or are secreted constitutively. In this part of the report we summarize and add new data concerning the cellular biology of PC1 and PC2; and we present an updated version of the proposed models of action for these enzymes, as well as for the regulation of their enzymatic activities.

Cellular Biology of PC1

The PCs exhibit an N-terminal signal peptide, followed by a pro-segment, a catalytic-domain, a P-domain, and an enzyme-specific C-terminal segment.[1-9] The most conserved catalytic domain of eukaryotic precursor convertases exhibits the closest similarity to bacterial subtilisins and contains the catalytic triad Asp, His, and Ser, as well as the oxyanion hole, Asn.[1-9] As is shown in FIGURE 1, PC1 first autocatalytically cleaves its N-terminal inhibitory pro-segment within the endoplasmic reticulum (ER).[16-18] The resulting 84-kDa PC1 is then transported to the TGN and immature secretory granules (ISGs) where it undergoes a second autocatalytic cleavage reaction to produce a very active 66-kDa form and this is subsequently stored in mature secretory granules.[17,19-21] Although the 84-kDa[16,17,23] and 66-kDa[21,23] forms of PC1 are enzymatically active, both *ex vivo* coexpression studies[21-23] and *in vitro* data[24] reveal that the 66-kDa form is much more active than the longer form. This led to the suggestion that the C-terminally excised segment might somehow dampen the activity of the 84-kDa PC1. Formal confirmation of this hypothesis was recently achieved using human prorenin as a substrate.[23] Mouse PC1 (mPC1) had previously been shown to cleave human prorenin in GH4 cells (which contain secretory granules) but are unable to cleave prorenin in CHO or BSC40 cells (which are devoid of secretory granules.)[16] In contrast, a recent study showed that removal of the C-terminal tail of mPC1 allows the efficient cleavage of prorenin in the constitutive secretory pathway of CHO cells.[23] The C-terminal tail thus appears to act as an inhibitor to PC1 activity against certain substrates. Its autocatalytic removal and further processing within ISGs (see FIGURE 1), may explain the observed granule-

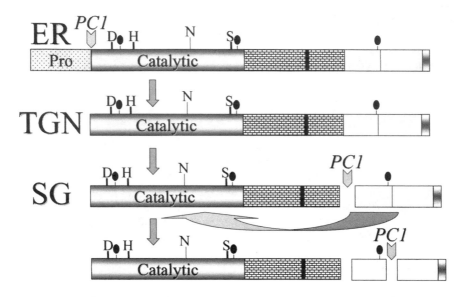

FIGURE 1. Schematic representation of the autocatalytic activation of PC1. The zymogen proPC1 is autocatalytically converted into PC1 in the ER. The cleaved products PC1 and the inhibitory pro-segment are presumably transported as a complex to the TGN where PC1 may further cleave the pro-segment at a secondary site (not shown) and be free to act on substrates. However, the C-terminal segment is still inhibitory. Only when PC1 (84-kDa) reaches the ISG, autocatalytically converts itself to the very active 66-kDa form, and further cleaves the C-terminal peptide, can this convertase be finally free to act *in trans* on the majority of its substrates.

specific processing of some proproteins. However, since PC1 can cleave POMC into β-LPH at the level of the TGN, it is also evident that it is present in a partially active state prior to reaching the secretory granules, where it is then processed to a maximally active state. Thus, regulation of the activity of PC1 occurs from both ends of the molecule—that is, from the pro-segment in the ER and Golgi, and from the C-terminal segment in the TGN/ISGs. This ensures a tight control of the intracellular activity of PC1 until it reaches its major conversion compartment, which is the ISG in many cases; for example, in pancreatic β-cells and pituitary corticotrophes. Very recent data from our laboratory revealed that the C-terminal segment of PC1 is also critical for its entry within secretory granules, since the cellular expression of a truncated 66-kDa version of PC1 results in the constitutive release of the enzyme. In addition, coexpression of the 66-kDa mPC1, together with a plasmid carrying only the C-terminal segment. redirects the 66-kDda mPC1 back toward the granules (C. Rovère, T. Reudelhuber, and N.G. Seidah, manuscript in preparation). This is somewhat analogous to the effect of the C-terminal 38-amino-acid segment of the luminal convertase PC5-A, which was shown to be important for the entry of this PC5–isoform within the regulated secretory pathway.[15] Finally, recent data also demonstrate that the conserved R*RGD*L sequence found in the P-domain of six out of the seven mammalian PCs[4,5] (FIG. 1) is critical for PC1 trafficking and its entry within secretory granules.[25]

Cellular Biology of PC2 and its Binding Protein 7B2

All PCs are first synthesized as zymogens (proPCs) that undergo autocatalytic processing of their prosegment within the ER, with the exception of proPC2, which is processed to PC2 within the TGN/ISG compartments.[2-5,17] Of all the PCs, only PC2 requires a specific binding protein, known as 7B2,[26] and such binding improves the efficiency of zymogen activation of proPC2 to PC2.[1,27-29] The PC2–specific binding protein 7B2 is itself first synthesized as a 186-amino acid (aa) precursor,[30] pro7B2$_{1-186}$, which is cleaved within the TGN by a furin-like enzyme into the 150-aa 7B2$_{1-150}$. It has been proposed that at least two PC2-binding sites exist in pro7B2$_{1-186}$. The first resides in the C-terminal (CT) 31-aa peptide, which is also a potent PC2-specific inhibitor containing a critical LysLys sequence,[31,32] whereas the second[28] may encompass a poly-proline-containing segment.[33] The oxyanion hole Asp$_{309}$, which is an Asn in all other PCs as well as in subtilases,[1-9] has been reported to be important in the initial binding of proPC2 to pro7B2$_{1-186}$ within the ER.[29]

To delineate the amino acids that play a key role in the zymogen activation of PC2 and in its binding to 7B2, we began to investigate the critical importance of six amino acids within the catalytic segment. The latter are unique to PC2 since they are different and conserved in all other PCs. These include[5] Ser$_{189}$ in PC2, which is an Asn in all other PCs (*Ser*189Asn), *Tyr*194Asp, *Ala*219Asn, *Gln*242Gly, *Asn*273Asp, and the oxyanion hole *Asp*309Asn. Thus we first isolated vaccinia virus recombinants (VV) of mouse PC2-mutants generated by site-directed mutagenesis of Tyr$_{194}$ and Asp$_{309}$.[34] These allowed us to demonstrate that the Y194D mutation markedly increases the *ex vivo* ability of PC2 to process POMC into β-endorphin in cells devoid of 7B2; for example, BSC40 cells.[34] In these cells, expression of native PC2 does not result in the secretion of measurable *in vitro* activity against a pentapeptide fluorogenic substrate. In contrast, secreted Y194D-PC2 exhibited significant enzymatic activity, even in the absence of 7B2. To further test the fate of PC2 and its mutants we used Western blots to analyze the molecular forms of PC2 obtained from BSC40 cells infected with the corresponding vaccinia virus recombinants. The media and cell extracts were first immunoprecipitated with a 7B2-antibody and then analyzed by Western blot using a C-terminal PC2-antibody (see FIGURE 2). Examination of the media provided evidence that only native PC2 that contains Tyr$_{194}$ can bind 7B2$_{1-150}$. None of the mutants of this residue bind it, indicating that Tyr$_{194}$ participates in the interaction of PC2 with 7B2 (see FIGURE 3), in agreement with pulse–chase analysis and coimmunoprecipitation data.[34] The data shown in FIGURE 2 also indicate that the oxyanion hole Asp$_{309}$ is critical for binding proPC2 with pro7B2$_{1-186}$ since both intracellularly, and in the media, insignificant amounts of pro7B2$_{1-186}$ associate with the D309N mutant. These and previous[34] data indicate that Tyr$_{194}$ is crucial for binding PC2 to 7B2 and less so to pro7B2, whereas the oxyanion hole Asn$_{309}$ is critical for binding proPC2 to pro7B2 but less so to 7B2 (FIG. 3).

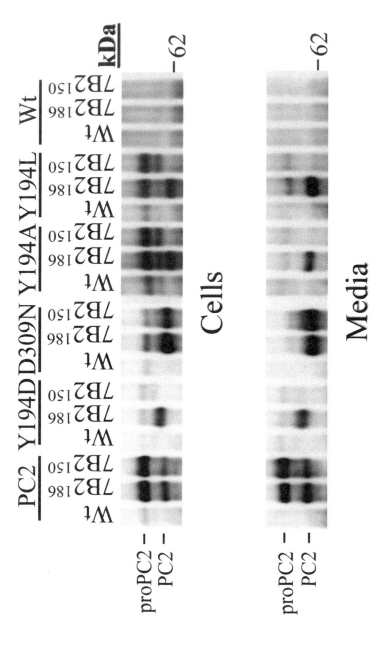

FIGURE 2. Western blot of PC2 and its Tyr$_{194}$ and Asp$_{309}$ mutants expressed in BSC40 cells. 2×10^6 cells were infected with VV:recombinants of either native PC2, or its mutants Y194A, Y194D, Y194L, and D309N, at a multiplicity of 1 pfu/cell. Following overnight culture, the cells were washed and then further incubated for 6 h in 0.01% fetal bovine serum. One sixth of the total media and cell extracts were immunoprecipitated with a 7B2 antibody and the precipitates separated on SDS-PAGE, (8% T, 2.7% C), and fluorographed as described.[17] The gels were then blotted onto a PVDF membrane and incubated with a C-terminal PC2-antibody at a 1/4000 dilution. The immunoreactive bands were visualized with a donkey anti-rabbit horse radish peroxidase conjugate according to instructions from the manufacturer (Amersham, Little Chalfont, Buckinghamshire, U.K.).

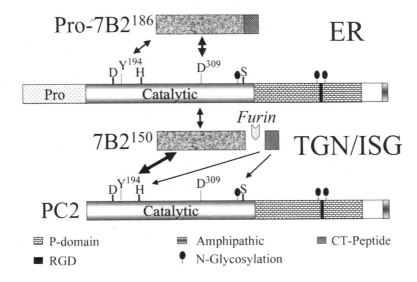

FIGURE 3. Schematic representation of the interactions of proPC1 and PC2 with either pro7B2$_{1-186}$ (pro7B2^{186}) or 7B2$_{1-150}$ (7B2^{150}). The *heavy arrows* denote major interactions and the *lighter arrows* depict less critical interactions. Thus, Asp$_{309}$ and Tyr$_{194}$ are critical for binding proPC2 with pro7B2$_{1-186}$ (pro7B2^{186}) in the ER, and PC2 with 7B2$_{1-150}$ (7B2^{150}) in the TGN/ISG, respectively. The inhibitory CT-peptide presumably interacts with the active site residues via its critical LysLys sequence.[32]

In conclusion, we propose that the highly conserved structure of PC2 evolved to retain specific amino acids and these, together with the participation of 7B2, ensure the proper spatial and temporal autocatalytic activation,[35] and enzymatic functioning of PC2.

POMC Processing by PC1 and PC2 and other PCs

When PC1 and PC2 were discovered in 1989–1990, one of the first potential substrates tested was proopiomelanocortin (POMC), the precursor of ACTH, αMSH, and β-endorphin.[22] This choice was guided by the high level of expression of these enzymes in the pituitary POMC–producing cells.[36,37] The data clearly showed that PC1 generated ACTH and β-LPH, whereas PC2 was critical for the production of both αMSH and β-endorphin (see FIGURE 4).[22] This was the first evidence that tissue-specific processing of POMC could be explained by the relative levels of its convertases. Thus, in the corticotrophes where PC1 predominates, ACTH and β-LPH are the final POMC-processing products. In contrast, the high expression of PC2 in the pituitary pars intermedia provided a rationale for the long known production of αMSH and β-endorphin in this tissue. Both regulation[38] and ontogeny[39] data corroborated this model. More detailed analysis of POMC processing further showed that

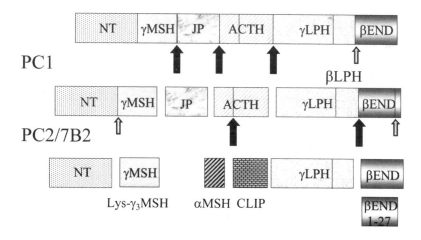

FIGURE 4. Schematic representation of POMC processing by PC1 and PC2. Major cleavage sites afforded by either enzymes are represented as *large dark arrows*. Minor sites are depicted as *small light arrows*. The importance of 7B2 for the maximal activity of PC2 is emphasized.

PC2 was critical for the formation of Lys-γ_3MSH and β-endorphin[1–27] (FIG. 4), implicating late cleavages at the less favored ArgLys and LysLys sites, respectively.[40]

Very recently, an obese and diabetic female patient was found to have both PC1 alleles mutated at residues which, based on *ex vivo* data, suggest that they would result in the synthesis of an inactive enzyme.[41] Interestingly, this patient had some ACTH circulating in the bloodstream and, hence, one wonders if the allelic mutations really caused the complete disappearance of PC1 activity, as suggested by overexpression studies in the non-endocrine CHO cells.[41] Alternatively, the small amount of circulating ACTH may be produced by yet another PC present in corticotrophes.[1,5,9] Accordingly, we tested the ability of all the other PCs to process POMC. As shown in FIGURE 5, PC1 cleaves POMC into ACTH and β-LPH. PC2 is critical for the generation of αMSH (as assessed by radioimmunassay, data not shown) and β-endorphin. Coexpression of POMC with each of the other PCs revealed that furin and PACE4 can generate ACTH, β-LPH, and β-endorphin; whereas PC7 produces little β-LPH and no β-endorphin. In contrast, overexpressed PC5-A and SKI-1 (not shown) do not seem to be able to cleave POMC. Interestingly, yeast kexin very efficiently processes POMC into β-endorphin as a final product (not shown). Therefore, we suggest, it is likely that PACE4, which is expressed in pituitary corticotrophes and highly regulated by the thyroid status,[42] may be in part responsible for processing POMC into ACTH.

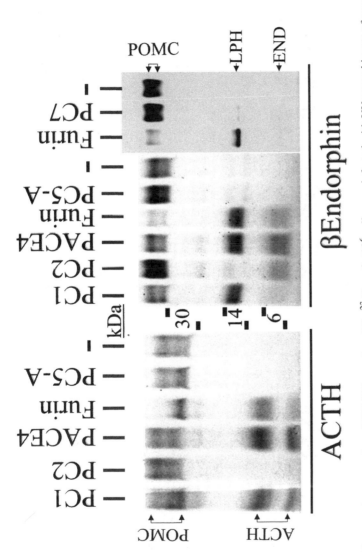

FIGURE 5. Comparative processing of POMC by various PCs.[22] Here, 2×10^6 cells were infected with VV:recombinants of mouse POMC together with recombinants of either mPC1, mPC2, hPACE4, hFurin, mPC5-A, rPC7, or the wild-type virus as control (−), each using a multiplicity of 1 pfu/cell. After overnight culture, the cells (BSC40 for the *two left panels*, and GH4C1 for the *right panel*) were washed and then pulse labeled for either 2 h (BSC40 cells) or 4 h (for GH4C1 cells) with [^{35}S]Met. The production of ACTH (13-kDa glycosylated form and 4.5-kDa nonglycosylated form) was measured by SDS-PAGE analysis (14% T, 3% C, Tricine gels) of media proteins immunoprecipitated by using either an ACTH-specific antibody that does not recognize αMSH, or a β-endorphin antibody that recognizes both β-LPH and β-endorphin. Notice that unprocessed heterogeneously glycosylated POMC migrates as multiple bands.[22] Data from cellular extracts confirm the conclusions reached from analysis of the media (not shown).

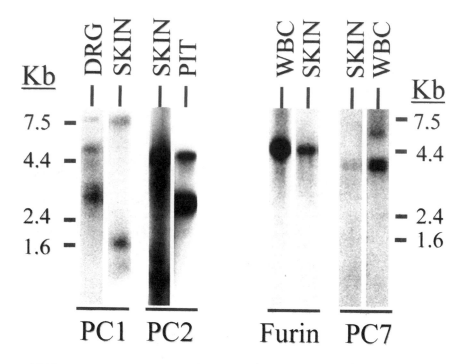

FIGURE 6. Northern blot analysis of total RNAs coding for PC1, PC2, Furin, and PC7 in the skin of adult rat and, for comparison, in some other tissues and cells, such as the dorsal root ganglion (DRG), pituitary gland (PIT), and white blood cells (WBC). The sizes of standard RNA are in kilobases (Kb).

Expression of PCs in Skin

Recently, it became evident that POMC, PC1, and PC2 are likely to be coexpressed in extra-pituitary tissues including the immune system[43] and skin-melanocytes.[44] In the latter, the expression of these proteins is upregulated by exposure to UV-radiation.[44,45] It was, therefore, of interest to compare the mRNA transcripts of the PCs in skin and other tissues and cells. As is shown in FIGURE 6, Northern blot analysis of the expression of PC1 and PC2 revealed that, even though these enzymes are expressed in skin, their mRNA transcripts are much longer. For example, although PC1[36,37,46] and PC2[37,47] are known to have multiple mRNA transcripts that only differ by virtue of the size of their noncoding 3′ ends, the major forms are 2.8 to 3.0 Kb long in most endocrine and neural tissues. In contrast, the major mRNA transcripts in skin are of size 8 Kb for PC1 and 5 Kb for PC2. Although these longer transcripts are expected to code for the same proteins, no advantage gained from such alternative splicing of the *PC1* and *PC2* genes is known.[46] In contrast, in both skin and white blood cells, furin,[3] and PC7[9] mRNA transcripts have the expected sizes of about 4.4 and 3.8 Kb, respectively (FIG. 6).

THE NEW ENZYME SKI-1 AND ITS EXPRESSION IN
ADULT PITUITARY AND IN THE SKIN OF NEWBORN RATS

Very recently, we identified cDNAs from rat, mouse, and human sources corresponding to a *subtilisin-kexin-isozyme* named SKI-1, for the first member of a possible new family of convertases related to subtilisins and to yeast kexin.[6] The schematic representation of the molecular architecture of the 1052-aa SKI-1 is shown in FIGURE 7. The catalytic domain of human SKI-1 is 35% identical to bacterial subtilisin BPN´, and is remarkably conserved between species. It exhibits complete identity between mouse and rat SKI-1, and 99% identity between the human and rat enzymes. This very high degree of sequence identity, even higher than that observed for the PCs,[48] suggests considerable evolutionary pressure for retaining this structure. We have recently confirmed that SKI-1 is a type-I membrane-anchored protein, as was predicted from its primary sequence.[6] The significance of the presence of a cytokine receptor/growth factor motif within the C-terminal half of the structure has not yet been elucidated.

Cellular expression studies demonstrated that, unlike the PCs, SKI-1 does not cleave postsingle or pairs of basic residues. Rather, we found that SKI-1 can cleave postsingle and possibly pairs of Thr residues in certain precursors. This unexpected cleavage specificity of SKI-1 will have to be investigated further in order to define the minimal motif surrounding this recognition sequence. Phylogenetic analysis based on the alignment of the amino acid sequence in the catalytic subunits, revealed that this evolutionary ancient Thr-cleaving enzyme seems to have emerged before the appearance of the PCs since it is the closest paralog to subtilisin BPN´ (see FIGURE 8).

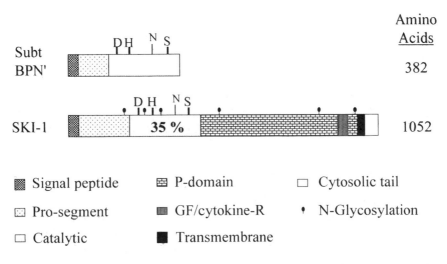

FIGURE 7. Schematic representation of the molecular architecture of SKI-1 as compared to that of bacterial subtilisin BPN´.

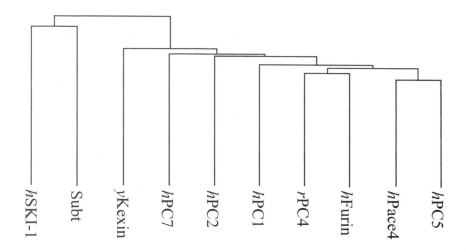

FIGURE 8. Dendogram representing the phylogenetic tree of the seven known human (rat for PC4) convertases, as compared to yeast Kexin, bacterial subtilisin BPN′ and human SKI-1. The data were obtained from the GCG Wisconsin package using the program Pileup applied to the catalytic subunits of each enzyme and Phylogenetic tree.

In an effort to identify some of the physiological substrates of SKI-1, we embarked on a detailed analysis of its mRNA and protein expression in tissues during ontogeny and in the adult. Accordingly, SKI-1 mRNA was found to be very widely (if not ubiquitously) distributed, showing high expression in the thymus, adrenal, submaxillary gland, and pituitary.[6] In FIGURE 9, we present an *in situ* hybridization (ISH) analysis of the mRNA expression of SKI-1 in an adult rat pituitary. SKI-1 mRNA is highly expressed in the anterior lobe (AL), less so in the intermediate lobe (IL), and lower expression is also observed in pituicytes of the posterior lobe (PL). Although the endogenous substrates of SKI-1 in the pituitary have not yet been defined, our preliminary overexpression studies indicate that POMC is not likely to be one of them.

Since SKI-1 mRNA was found to be abundant in rat newborn skin,[6] we undertook a more detailed analysis of its expression by ISH in the skin of a 2-day old rat (p2) (see FIGURE 10). In this tissue, SKI-1 mRNA is present at high levels in germinal cells and in the hypodermis, especially in the inner (and less so in the outer) hair sheath. These data strongly suggest that SKI-1 may play an important role in skin and/or hair development by virtue of processing as yet unknown endogenous substrates within germinal cells. It would also seem that some SKI-1 mRNA could be found within skin melanocytes, and the function therein will need further exploration.

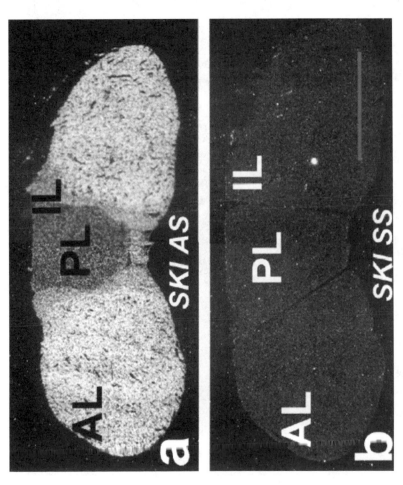

FIGURE 9. *In situ* hybridization showing SKI-1 mRNA expression in the pituitary gland of an adult rat using specific [^{35}S]radiolabeled antisense (*SKI AS*) and control sense (*SKI SS*) riboprobes. The hybridization signal was detected in the anterior (*AL*), intermediate (*IL*) and posterior pituitary lobe (*PL*). Most of the labeling was confined to endocrine cells in AL and IL and to some pituicytes in the PL. Magnification ×5; *bar* (in **b**), length 1 mm.

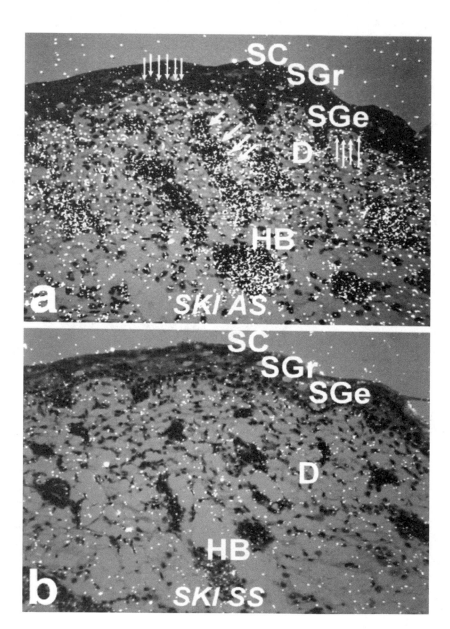

FIGURE 10. *In situ* hybridization showing SKI-1 mRNA sites in the skin of a newborn two-days-old (p2) rat using antisense (*SKI AS*) and control sense (*SKI SS*) riboprobes. The hybridization signal was detected in the stratum germinativum (*small vertical arrows* in SGe), in both outer and inner hair sheath (*medium arrows*) and in some cells within the dermis (*D*). Other abbreviations: HB, hair bulb; SC, stratum corneum; SGr, stratum granulosum. Magnification ×80.

CONCLUSIONS

The data presented in this paper and the cumulative knowledge acquired over the last eight years has revealed that a wide array of secretory precursors are processed intracellularly by a limited set of convertases. The choice of processing sites made by the seven known PCs, namely, PC1, PC2, furin, PACE4, PC4, PC5, and PC7, suggest that, within the context of single or dibasic residues, they prefer to cleave precursors at Arg residues, and less so following Lys residues. Very recently, analysis of SKI-1 cleavage specificity—the first member of a possibly new family of subtilisin-kexin-isozymes—revealed that cleavage post basic residues is not the only motif recognized by mammalian subtilases. Therefore, a new set of rules must exist and these will have to be defined from the study of the cleavage specificity of such enzymes. The observed cleavage at a single, and possibly pairs of Thr residues, is only the beginning of our quest for the minimal motif recognized by SKI-1. Are there other subtilisin/kexin-like convertases to be found? Only the future can tell. However, with what we know, it is clear that these convertases exert a variety of functions from neuroendocrine to immune response regulation. The recent discovery of the expression of these enzymes in skin suggests that exciting new functions will be discovered, which could find applications in the therapeutic treatment of certain pathologies.

ACKNOWLEDGMENTS

We wish to thank Sylvie Emond for her secretarial help and Dr. Annik Prat for critically reading this manuscript. The expert technical assistance of Jim Rochemont, Andrew Chen, and Annie Lemieux are very much appreciated. This work was supported by MRC group Grant #11474.

REFERENCES

1. SEIDAH, N.G., M. CHRÉTIEN & R. DAY. 1994. The family of subtilisin/kexin like proprotein and prohormone convertases: divergent or shared functions. Biochimie **76:** 197–209.
2. ROUILLÉ, Y., S.J. DUGUAY, K. LUND, M. FURUTA, Q. GONG, G. LIPKIND, A.A. OLIVA, JR., S.J. CHAN & D.F. STEINER. 1995. Proteolytic processing mechanisms in the biosynthesis of neuroendocrine peptides—The subtilisin-like proprotein convertases. Front. Neuroendocrinol. **16:** 322–361.
3. VAN DE VEN, W.J.M. & A. ROEBROEK. 1993. Structure and function of eukaryotic proprotein processing enzymes of the subtilisin family of serine proteases. Crit. Rev. Oncog. **4:** 115–136.
4. SEIDAH, N.G., R. DAY, M. MARCINKIEWICZ & M. CHRÉTIEN. 1998. Precursor convertases: an evolutionary ancient, cell-specific, combinatorial mechanism yielding diverse bioactive peptides and proteins. Ann. N.Y. Acad. Sci. **839:** 9–24.
5. SEIDAH, N.G., M. MBIKAY, M. MARCINKIEWICZ & M. CHRÉTIEN. 1998. The mammalian precursor convertases: paralogs of the subtilisin/kexin family of calcium-dependent serine proteinases. *In* Proteolytic and Cellular Mechanisms in Prohormone and Neuropeptide Precursor Processing. V.Y.H. Hook, Ed.: 49–76. R.G. Landes Company, Austin.

6. SEIDAH, N.G., S.J. MOWLA, J. HAMELIN, A.M. MAMARBACHI, S. BENJANNET, B.B. TOURÉ, A. BASAK, J.S. MUNZER, J. MARCINKIEWICZ, M. ZHONG, J.-C. BARALE, C. LAZURE, R.A. MURPHY, M. CHRÉTIEN & M. MARCINKIEWICZ. 1999. Mammalian subtilisin/kexin isozyme SKI-1: a widely expressed proprotein convertase with a unique cleavage specificity and cellular localization. Proc. Natl. Acad. Sci. USA **96:** 1321–1326.

7. MBIKAY, M., H. TADROS, N. ISHIDA, C.P. LERNER, E. DE LAMIRANDE, A. CHEN, M. EL-ALFY, Y. CLERMONT, N.G. SEIDAH, M. CHRÉTIEN, C. GAGNON & E.M. SIMPSON. 1997. Impaired fertility in mice deficient for the testicular germ-cell protease PC4. Proc. Natl. Acad. Sci. USA **94:** 6842–6846.

8. FURUTA, M., H. YANO, A. ZHOU, Y. ROUILLÉ, J. HOLST, J. CARROLL, M. RAVAZZOLA, L. ORCI, H. FURUTA & D.F. STEINER. 1997. Defective prohormone processing and altered pancreatic islet morphology in mice lacking active SPC2. Proc. Natl. Acad. Sci. USA **94:** 6646–6651.

9. SEIDAH, N.G., J. HAMELIN, A.M. MAMARBACHI, W. DONG, H. TADROS, M. MBIKAY, M. CHRÉTIEN & R. DAY. 1996. cDNA structure, tissue distribution and chromosomal localization of rat PC7: a novel mammalian proprotein convertase closest to yeast kexin-like proteinases. Proc. Natl. Acad. Sci. USA **93:** 3388–3393.

10. MORI, K., S. KII, A. TSUJI, M. NAGAHAMA, A. IMAMAKI, K. HAYASHI, T. AKAMATSU, H. NAGAMUNE & Y. MATSUDA. 1997. A novel human pace4 isoform, PACE4-E is an active processing protease containing a hydrophobic cluster at the carboxy terminus. J. Biochem. **121:** 941–948.

11. ZHONG, M., S. BENJANNET, C. LAZURE, S. MUNZER & N.G. SEIDAH. 1996. Functional analysis of human PACE4-A and PACE4-C isoforms: identification of a new PACE4-CS isoform. FEBS Lett. **396:** 31–36.

12. SEIDAH, N.G., R. DAY, J. HAMELIN, L. GASPAR, M.W. COLLARD & M. CHRÉTIEN. 1992. Testicular expression of PC4 in the rat: molecular diversity of a novel germ cell-specific Kex2/subtilisin-like proprotein convertase. Mol. Endocrinol. **6:** 1559–1570.

13. NAKAGAWA, T., M. HOSAKA & K. NAKAYAMA. 1993. Identification of an isoform with an extremely large Cys-rich region of PC6, a kex2-like processing endoprotease. FEBS Lett. **327:** 165–171.

14. MALIDE, D., N.G. SEIDAH, M. CHRÉTIEN & M. BENDAYAN. 1995. Electron microscopy immunocytochemical evidence for the involvement of the convertases PC1 and PC2 in the processing of proinsulin in pancreatic β-cells. J. Histochem. Cytochem. **43:** 11–19.

15. DE BIE, I., M. MARCINKIEWICZ, D. MALIDE, C. LAZURE, K. NAKAYAMA, M. BENDAYAN & N.G. SEIDAH. 1996. The isoforms of the proprotein convertase 5 are sorted to different subcellular compartments. J. Cell Biol. **135:** 1261–1275.

16. BENJANNET, S., T. REUDELHUBER, C. MERCURE, N. RONDEAU, M. CHRÉTIEN & N.G. SEIDAH. 1992. Pro-protein conversion is determined by a multiplicity of factors including convertase processing, substrate specificity and intracellular environment. J. Biol. Chem. **267:** 11417–11423.

17. BENJANNET, S., N. RONDEAU, L. PAQUET, A. BOUDREAULT, C. LAZURE, M. CHRÉTIEN & N.G. SEIDAH. 1993. Comparative biosynthesis, post-translational modifications and efficiency of prosegment cleavage of the pro-hormone convertases PC1 and PC2: Glycosylation, sulfation and identification of the intracellular site of prosegment cleavage of PC1 and PC2. Biochem. J. **294:** 735–743.

18. GOODMAN, L.J. & C.M. GORMAN. 1994. Autoproteolytic activation of the mouse prohormone convertase mPC1. Biochem. Biophys. Res. Commun. **201:** 795–804.

19. VINDROLA, O. & I. LINDBERG. 1992. Biosynthesis of the prohormone convertase-mPC1 in AtT-20 cells. Mol. Endocrinol. **6:** 1088–1094.

20. ZHOU, A., L. PAQUET & R.E. MAINS. 1995. Structural elements that direct specific processing of different mammalian subtilisin-like prohormone convertases. J. Biol. Chem. **270:** 21509–21516.

21. ZHOU, Y., C. ROVÈRE, P. KITABGI & I. LINDBERG. 1995. Mutational analysis of PC1 (SPC3) in PC12 cells. 66-kDa PC1 is fully functional. J. Biol. Chem. **270:** 24702–24706.

22. BENJANNET, S., N. RONDEAU, R. DAY, M. CHRÉTIEN & N.G. SEIDAH. 1991. PC1 and PC2 are pro-protein convertases capable of cleaving POMC at distinct pairs of basic residues. Proc. Natl. Acad. Sci. USA **88:** 3564–3568.

23. JUTRAS, I., N.G. SEIDAH, T.L. REUDELHUBER & V. BRECHLER. 1997. Two activation states of the prohormone convertase PC1 in the secretory pathway. J. Biol. Chem. **272:** 15184–15188.

24. ZHOU, Y. & I. LINDBERG. 1994. Enzymatic properties of carboxyl-terminally truncated prohormone convertase 1 (PC1/SPC3) and evidence for autocatalytic conversion. J. Biol. Chem. **269:** 18408–18413.

25. LUSSON, J., S. BENJANNET, J. HAMELIN, D. SAVARIA, M. CHRÉTIEN & N.G. SEIDAH. 1997. The integrity of the RRGDL sequence of the proprotein convertase PC1 is critical for its zymogen and C-terminal processing, and for its cellular trafficking. Biochem. J. **326:** 737–744.

26. SEIDAH, N.G., K.L. HSI, G. DE SERRES, J. ROCHEMONT, J. HAMELIN, T. ANTAKLY, M. CANTIN & M. CHRÉTIEN. 1983. Isolation and NH$_2$-terminal sequence of a highly conserved human and porcine pituitary protein belonging to a new superfamily: Immunocytochemical localization in pars distalis and pars nervosa of the pituitary and in the supraoptic nucleus of the hypothalamus. Arch. Biochem. Biophys. **225:** 525–534.

27. BRAKS, J.A. & G.J.M. MARTENS. 1994. 7B2 is a neuroendocrine chaperone that transiently interacts with prohormone convertase PC2 in the secretory pathway. Cell **78:** 263–273.

28. BENJANNET, S., D. SAVARIA, M. CHRÉTIEN & N.G. SEIDAH. 1995. 7B2 is a specific intracellular binding protein of the prohormone convertase PC2. J. Neurochem. **64:** 2303–2311.

29. BENJANNET, S., J. LUSSON, J. HAMELIN, D. SAVARIA, M. CHRÉTIEN & N.G. SEIDAH. 1995. Structure-function studies on the biosynthesis and bioactivity of the precursor convertase PC2 and the formation of the PC2/7B2 complex. FEBS Lett **362:** 151–155.

30. PAQUET, L., F. BERGERON, N.G. SEIDAH, M. CHRÉTIEN, M. MBIKAY & C. LAZURE. 1994. The neuroendocrine precursor 7B2 is a sulfated protein proteolytically processed by a ubiquitous furin-like convertase. J. Biol. Chem. **269:** 19279–19285.

31. MARTENS, G.J.M., J.A.M. BRAKS, D.W. EIB, Y. ZHOU & I. LINDBERG. 1994. The neuroendocrine polypeptide 7B2 is an endogenous inhibitor of prohormone convertase PC2. Proc. Natl. Acad. Sci. USA **91:** 5784–5787.

32. ZHU, X., Y. ROUILLE, N.S. LAMANGO, D.F. STEINER & I. LINDBERG. 1996. Internal cleavage of the inhibitory 7B2 carboxyl-terminal peptide by PC2: a potential mechanism for its inactivation. Proc. Nat. Acad. Sci. USA **93:** 4919–4924.

33. ZHU, X.R., N.S. LAMANGO & I. LINDBERG. 1996. Involvement of a polyproline helix-like structure in the interaction of 7B2 with prohormone convertase 2. J. Biol. Chem. **271:** 23582–23587.

34. BENJANNET, S., M. MAMARBACHI, J. HAMELIN, D. SAVARIA, J.S. MUNZER, M. CHRÉTIEN & N.G. SEIDAH. 1998. Residues unique to the prohormone convertase PC2 modulate its autoactivation, binding to 7B2 and enzymatic activity. FEBS Lett. **428:** 37–42.

35. MATTHEWS, G., K.I.J. SHENNAN, A.J. SEAL, N.A. TAYLOR, A. COLMAN & K. DOCHERTY. 1994. Autocatalytic maturation of the prohormone convertase PC2. J. Biol. Chem. **269:** 588–592.

36. SEIDAH, N.G., M. MARCINKIEWICZ, S. BENJANNET, L. GASPAR, G. BEAUBIEN, M.G. MATTEI, C. LAZURE, M. MBIKAY & M. CHRÉTIEN. 1991. Cloning and primary sequence of a mouse candidate pro-hormone convertase PC1 homologous to PC2, furin and Kex2: Distinct chromosomal localization and mRNA distribution in brain and pituitary as compared to PC2. Mol. Endocrinol. **5:** 111–122.

37. SEIDAH, N.G., L. GASPAR, P. MION, M. MARCINKIEWICZ, M. MBIKAY & M. CHRÉTIEN. 1990. cDNA sequence of two distinct pituitary proteins homologous to Kex2 and furin gene products: tissue-specific mRNAs encoding candidates for pro-hormone processing proteinases. DNA **9:** 415–424.

38. DAY, R., M.K.H. SCHÄFER, S.J. WATSON, M. CHRÉTIEN & N.G. SEIDAH. 1992. Distribution and regulation of the prohormone convertases PC1 and PC2 in the rat pituitary. Mol. Endocrinol. **6:** 485–497.

39. MARCINKIEWICZ, M., R. DAY, N.G. SEIDAH & M. CHRÉTIEN. 1993. Ontogeny of the prohormone convertases PC1 and PC2 in the mouse hypophysis and their colocalization with corticotropin and α-melanotropin. Proc. Natl. Acad. Sci. USA **90:** 4922–4926.

40. ZHOU, A. & R.E. MAINS. 1994. Endoproteolytic processing of proopiomelanocortin and prohormone convertases 1 and 2 in neuroendocrine cells overexpressing prohormone convertases 1 or 2. J. Biol. Chem. **269:** 17440–17447.

41. JACKSON, R.S., J.W.M. CREEMERS, S. OHAGI, M-L. RAFFIN-SANSON, L. SANDERS, C.T. MONTAGUE, J.C. HUTTON & S. O'RAHILLY. 1997. Obesity and impaired prohormone processing associated with mutations in the human prohormone convertase 1 gene. Nature Genetics **16:** 303–306.

42. JOHNSON, R.C., D.N. DARLINGTON, T.A. HAND, B.T. BLOOMQUIST & R.E. MAINS. 1994. PACE4: A subtilisin-like endoprotease prevalent in the anterior pituitary and regulated by thyroid status. Endocrinology **135:** 1178–1185.

43. BLALOCK, J.E. 1985. Proopiomelanocortin-derived peptides in the immune system. Clin. Endocrinol. **22:** 823–827.

44. WAKAMATSU, K., A. GRAHAM, D. COOK & A.J. THODY. 1997. Characterisation of ACTH peptides in human skin and their activation of the melanocortin-1 receptor. Pigment Cell Res. **10:** 288–297.

45. SLOMINSKI, A. & J. PAWELEK. 1998. Animals under the sun: effects of ultraviolet radiation on mammalian skin. Clin. Dermatol. **16:** 503–515.

46. FTOUHI N., R. DAY, M. MBIKAY, M. CHRÉTIEN & N.G. SEIDAH. 1994. Gene organization of the mouse pro-hormone and pro-protein convertase PC1. DNA Cell Biol. **13:** 395–407.

47. OHAGI S., J. LAMENDOLA, M.M. LEBEAU, R. ESPINOSA, J. TAKEDA, S.P. SMEEKENS, S.J. CHAN & D.F. STEINER. 1992. Identification and analysis of the gene encoding human PC2, a prohormone convertase expressed in neuroendocrine tissues. Proc. Natl. Acad. Sci. USA **89:** 4977–4981.

48. SEIDAH, N.G. 1995. The mammalian family of subtilisin/kexin-like pro-protein convertases. *In* Intramolecular Chaperones and Protein Folding. U. Shinde & M. Inouye, Eds.: 181–203. R.G. Landes Company, Austin.

The Role of Melanocortins in Adipocyte Function

BRUCE A. BOSTON[a]

Department of Pediatrics, Oregon Health Sciences University, Mail Code HRC 5,
3181 SW Sam Jackson Park Road, Portland, Oregon 97201, USA

ABSTRACT: It has been demonstrated that adipocytes express high affinity ACTH and α-MSH binding sites, and that ACTH, α-MSH, and β-LPH are potent lipolytic hormones. Considerable species variability exists in the lipolytic response to melanocortins, however. Recently, MC2 and MC5 receptor-mRNA was found in both murine adipocytes and in the 3T3-L1 murine embryonic fibroblast cell line, but only after the 3T3-L1 cells had differentiated into adipocytes. The 3T3-L1 cell line was used to characterize the pharmacological properties of both MC2 and MC5 receptors *in situ*. Both murine MC2 and MC5 receptors are functional in the adipocyte, although the MC5 receptor required high doses of α-MSH to activate cylase. ACTH potently stimulates cyclase with EC_{50} values that are consistent with the hypothesis that the murine MC2 receptor, not the MC5 receptor, mediates stress-induced lipolysis via release of ACTH from the pituitary.

INTRODUCTION

The adipocyte is a complex cell that has multiple important metabolic functions. Excess carbohydrates are converted to lipids and are stored in the adipocyte for future use. However, the cell does not simply serve as an energy storage depot. The adipocyte also plays an important role in secreting leptin, a hormone that completes a nutritional feedback loop to the hypothalamus.[1] Therefore, the adipocyte is emerging as a major player in metabolic regulation, rather than simply acting as a caloric reservoir. The metabolic balance between lipogenesis and lipolysis in the adipocyte is determined by multiple different peptide and steroid hormones and their respective receptors. Very early in the study of the adipocyte, it was discovered that derivatives of proopiomelanocortin participated in this balance by stimulating lipolysis.[2–6] This review will focus on the role of melanocortins and their receptors on the metabolic regulation of the adipocyte.

POMC AND THE MELANOCORTIN RECEPTORS

Proopiomelanocortin (POMC) peptides have been implicated in a wide variety of biological functions since the discovery of POMC in 1977,[7,8] and the cloning of the POMC gene in 1979.[9] Many of the peptides derived from proteolytic cleavage of

[a]Address for correspondence: 503-494-1926 (voice); 503-494-1933 (fax); bostonbr@ohsu.edu (e-mail).

POMC are classified as melanocortins, because of their ability to stimulate steroid production in the adrenocortical cell, or to stimulate eumelanogenesis in the melanocyte. The two most thoroughly studied of the melanocortin biological functions are adrenocorticotropic hormone (ACTH)-stimulation of adrenal steroidogenesis, and melanocyte stimulating hormone (MSH)-stimulation of eumelanin production. However, numerous other effects of these peptides have been reported. In addition to stimulating lipolysis in the adipocyte, melanocortins have been implicated in the regulation of feeding and grooming behavior, learning and memory, thermogenesis, neural regeneration, metabolism, inflammation, exocrine gland function, and natriuresis.

Investigators have recently identified a family of five distinct G-protein coupled receptors, all with the ability to bind ACTH. Each of these receptors stimulates adenylyl cyclase via the $G_s\alpha$ subunit to increase intracellular cAMP levels.[10–21] The MC1 receptor was the first to be cloned and it is the classic "MSH receptor" responsible for cAMP induced eumelanin formation in melanocytes.[11,12,22] This receptor exhibits an approximate fivefold specificity for α-MSH, when compared to ACTH. A second receptor, the MC2 receptor, was found to correspond to the adrenal cortex ACTH receptor, and binds only ACTH. The MC3 and MC4 receptors are primarily neural melanocortin receptors.[13–15,20] The MC3 receptor is unique in that it has the highest affinity for γ-MSH among all the melanocortin receptors. The MC4 receptor has recently been shown to regulate feeding behavior and weight homeostasis.[23,24] Finally, the MC5 gene encodes a melanocortin receptor with a very wide tissue distribution. Northern hybridization[16] and RNase protection analysis[19] have detected the MC5-R mRNA at high levels in skin and muscle as well as in lung, liver, spleen, and adrenal tissue.

MELANOCORTIN STIMULATION OF LIPOLYSIS

Multiple different POMC peptides, including ACTH, α-MSH, and β-lipotropin (β-LPH), have been shown to stimulate lipolysis in the adipocyte.[2–6,25] One of the earliest studies by White and Engel, in 1958, demonstrated that purified ACTH caused a loss of extractable lipid from adipose tissue in mice.[25] These investigators followed up on these *in vivo* experiments by demonstrating that ACTH-induced lipolysis is a direct effect of the melanocortin peptide on the rat adipocyte.[5] They were, however, unable to demonstrate any significant effect of either α-MSH or β-MSH on the same rat adipocyte preparations. Using adipose cells isolated from rabbits, Richter and colleagues demonstrated a significant lipolytic response to both α-MSH and β-MSH.[26] Minimal effective concentrations of both α-MSH and β-MSH were 1×10^{-9} M, similar to the minimal concentration of ACTH required to induce lipolysis in these experiments. Furthermore, they were able to demonstrate a requirement for the Met-Glu-His-Phe-Arg-Trp-Gly peptide sequence in the induction of lipolysis *in vitro*.[26] The core His-Phe-Arg-Trp sequence has subsequently been shown to be necessary for activation of all the melanocortin receptors, and therefore indicates that melanocortin receptors are directly involved in the stimulation of lipolysis in these experiments. Furthermore, since the MC2 (ACTH) receptor does not bind α-MSH,[27] the observation that α-MSH stimulates lipolysis indicates

Table 1. Lipolytic potency of ACTH and α-MSH in different mammalian species

Species	ACTH	α-MSH
Rabbit[a]	EC_{50} = 16.4 nM	EC_{50} = 3.7 nM
Guinea Pig[b]		
Rat, Mouse[a]	EC_{50} = 1.34 nM	EC_{50} = 1530 nM
Hamster[b]		
Primates[c]	EC_{50} > 1000 nM	EC_{50} > 1000 nM

[a]Refs. 3 and 4
[b]Ref. 28
[c]Ref. 29

the presence of a functional melanocortin receptor other than the MC2 receptor on the rabbit adipocyte cell surface.

Significant species differences have been noted with regard to the relative lipolytic activity of the melanocortins (see TABLE 1). Both α-MSH (EC_{50} = 3.7 nM) and ACTH (EC_{50} = 16.4 nM) are potent lipolytic agents for the rabbit adipocyte, whereas in the rat, only ACTH (EC_{50} = 1.34 nM) has potent lipolytic activity.[3,4] α-MSH does stimulate lipolysis in the rat but is much less potent (EC_{50} = 1530 nM) than ACTH. Guinea pig adipocytes are also responsive to both α-MSH and ACTH, but hamster adipocytes only respond to ACTH.[28] Despite lipolytic activity in rodents and in rabbits, ACTH has very little effect on lipolysis in isolated human and nonhuman primate adipocytes, even at concentrations as high as 1 μM.[29] With this high degree of variability in the lipolytic response to melanocortins, there may be major species differences in the expression of the receptor subtypes on the cell surface. Alternatively, subtle structural differences in the specific receptor subtypes between species may change the affinity of the adipocyte receptors for the various melanocortin peptides.

MELANOCORTIN BINDING

Tatro and Reichlin reported a comprehensive investigation of α-MSH binding sites in both mice and rats using the radioiodinated superpotent α-MSH analogue Nle[4], D-Phe[7]-α-MSH (NDP-α-MSH).[30] Binding studies using this radiolabeled peptide revealed potential sites of expression of MC1, MC3, MC4, and MC5 receptors but not MC2, since the MC2 (ACTH) receptor has little affinity for MSH or its analogs. In addition to multiple other melanocortin binding sites, Tatro and Reichlin found significant binding of NDP-α-MSH in white adipose tissue. Later studies by Oelofsen demonstrated specific binding in isolated rat adipocytes using radiolabeled ACTH.[6] These studies indicate that ACTH binds to a single high affinity site on the rat adipocyte with an apparent K_d of 0.15 to 0.18 nM.[6] Although ACTH binds to all of the known melanocortin receptors, the high affinity ACTH binding site demonstrated in this experiment probably represents the MC2 receptor, since ACTH is the most potent lipolytic melanocortin peptide in rats. α-MSH does not bind the MC2 receptor and has little lipolytic activity in rats. Taken together, this evidence suggests that the NDP-α-MSH binding demonstrated by Tatro and Reichlin in rodents, likely represents a lower affinity melanocortin receptor subtype, and not the MC2 receptor.

MELANOCORTIN RECEPTOR SUBTYPES IN ADIPOCYTES

Although initial observations reported only a single class of ACTH binding sites on the adipocyte, the responsiveness of the adipocyte to α-MSH and β-LPH indicated, at least in some species, expression of a melanocortin receptor other than the MC2 receptor. The recent cloning and characterization of the five known melanocortin receptors made it possible to determine the specific melanocortin receptor subtypes present on the mouse adipocyte. Using RT/PCR and Northern blot hybridization, high levels of MC2 receptor mRNA were found in mouse adipose tissues isolated from multiple sites.[31] Furthermore, MC5 receptor-mRNA was found in a subset of these sites, although this mRNA was considerably less abundant. RT/PCR using melanocortin receptor subtype-specific primer pairs failed to demonstrate the presence of mRNA coding for MC1, MC3, or MC4 in mouse adipose tissues.

Both the MC2 and MC5 receptor-mRNAs were also found in the 3T3-L1 cell line, a murine embryonic fibroblast cell line that could be induced to differentiate into adipocytes.[32] This cell line has been demonstrated to be good model system for studying the adipocyte *in vitro*. Prior to differentiation, no melanocortin receptors were detected on the preadipocyte. However, after the cells had differentiated into adipocytes, both the MC2 and the MC5 receptors were detected by Northern blot.[31] This observation is consistent with data from Grunfeld and Ramachandran that demonstrates specific binding of labeled ACTH to the differentiated 3T3-L1 adipocytes, but lack of binding to undifferentiated cells.[33]

MELANOCORTIN PHARMACOLOGY IN THE ADIPOCYTE

Cell surface expression of the melanocortin receptor subtypes in the mouse adipocyte has been characterized by both binding experiments and measurements of melanocortin–stimulated intracellular cAMP. Binding experiments using labeled NDP-α-MSH demonstrate a high affinity MSH binding site on the differentiated 3T3-L1 cell surface (see FIGURE 1).[31] This indicates the presence of a melanocortin receptor other than the MC2 receptor, since the MC2 receptor does not bind NDP-α-MSH with high affinity.[27] The IC_{50} value observed using cold NDP-α-MSH as a competing ligand (0.99 ± 0.02 nM) is similar to the IC_{50} reported for the murine MC5 receptor (1.1 ± 0.2 nM) in transfected CHO-K1 cells.[19] The IC_{50} value observed using cold $ACTH_{1-39}$ as a competing ligand (60 ± 2 nM) is also consistent with previously reported values (236 ± 41 nM) in that it indicates a lower affinity of the murine MC5 receptor for ACTH.[19] These data support expression of a functional MC5 receptor in the 3T3-L1 adipocyte and also support the MC5 receptor as the source of the specific NDP-α-MSH binding in mouse and rat adipose tissue in the Tatro and Reichlin experiments.[30] Grunfeld and Ramachandran report specific ACTH binding to 3T3-L1 cells with an IC_{50} value of 4.3 nM using cold ACTH as a

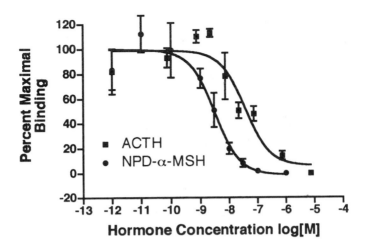

FIGURE 1. Characterization of a high affinity NDP-MSH binding site in differentiated 3T3-L1 cells. Confluent 3T3-L1 cells were differentiated into adipocytes in 12-well plates. Cells were washed once with DMEM containing 1% bovine serum albumin and 0.1% bacitracin. Incubation media, consisting of DMEM with 1% bovine serum albumin and 0.1% bacitracin, was added to each well. 400,000 cpm of ^{125}I NDP-MSH (specific activity 2000 cpm/fmol) per ml of media was added to each well together with varying concentrations of NDP-MSH and ACTH$_{1-39}$. Wells were incubated for 60 minutes at room temperature then washed three times with phosphate buffered saline. The cells were solubilized with 0.1 M NaOH and counted in a gamma counter. Competition binding curves were graphed and statistics calculated using the PRISM software program (Graph Pad, San Diego, CA). Each point is the mean of triplicate values. The IC$_{50}$ values for displayed curves are 0.99 ± 0.02 nM for NDP-MSH and 60 ± 2 nM for ACTH$_{1-39}$. (Reproduced, with permission, from Ref. 31. ©The Endocrine Society.)

competing ligand.[33] Although this is most likely binding to the MC2 receptor, since ACTH can also bind to the murine MC5 receptor, the possibility remains that this ligand is detecting cell surface expression of the MC5 receptor rather than, or in addition to, the MC2 receptor. Therefore, binding studies alone do not confirm the expression of the MC2 receptor on the 3T3-L1 murine adipocyte surface.

Although binding experiments confirm a cell surface site consistent with the MC5 receptor, functional coupling studies were required to demonstrate functional expression of the MC2 receptor in the murine adipocyte. ACTH potently stimulates cAMP production in 3T3-L1 adipocytes with an EC$_{50}$ value of 1.4 ± 0.6 nM (see FIGURE 2).[31] This EC$_{50}$ value is similar to the IC$_{50}$ value observed in Grunfeld's labeled ACTH binding experiments.[33] Since both the murine MC2 and MC5 receptors bind ACTH avidly, ACTH stimulation of adenylyl cyclase alone does not distinguish the receptor subtypes.

α-MSH also stimulates adenylyl cyclase in 3T3-L1 cells (FIG. 2), although at a lower than expected EC$_{50}$ for the murine MC5 receptor (EC$_{50}$ of 130 ± 10 nM).[31]

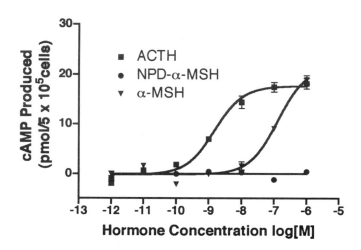

FIGURE 2. Melanocortin stimulation of adenylyl cyclase in differentiated 3T3-L1 cells by ACTH, α-MSH, and NDP-MSH. Confluent 3T3-L1 cells were differentiated into adipocytes in 12-well plates. The differentiated cells were washed with DMEM containing 1% bovine serum albumin and 0.1% bacitracin. Incubation media consisting of DMEM with 1% bovine serum albumin, 0.1% bacitracin, 0.1 mM IBMX, and varying concentrations of $ACTH_{1-39}$, α-MSH, or NDP-MSH, were added to the wells and incubated at room temperature for 30 minutes. The media were removed and the cells rinsed twice with phosphate buffered saline. Sixty-percent ethanol was added to wells and the cell monolayer was transferred into eppendorf tubes to be dried under vacuum. cAMP content in each tube was determined by RIA. Dose response curves were graphed and statistics calculated using the PRISM software program (Graph Pad, San Diego, CA). Each point is the mean of triplicate values. The EC_{50} values for displayed curves are 130 ± 10 nM for α-MSH and 1.4 ± 0.6 nM for $ACTH_{1-39}$. (Reproduced, with permission, from Ref. 31. ©The Endocrine Society.)

Experiments measuring intracellular cAMP in the Chinese hamster ovary (CHO) cell line, transfected with the murine MC5 receptor and incubated with α-MSH, reveal an EC_{50} of 1.07 ± 0.13 nM.[19] The low EC_{50} for cyclase activation observed in the adipocyte, however, is consistent with *in vivo* observations, that only very high α-MSH concentrations (EC_{50} 1.53 μM) stimulate lipolysis in rodents.[4,6,28] Surprisingly, the potent α-MSH analogue, NDP-α-MSH, does not stimulate adenylyl cyclase, despite high affinity binding in the 3T3-L1 adipocyte (FIG. 2).[31] Since NDP-α-MSH binds but does not activate the murine MC5 receptor site, it can be used as an antagonist to block the MC5 receptor and allow the MC2 receptor site to be studied in isolation. When NDP-α-MSH is used to antagonize the murine MC5 receptor, α-MSH stimulated cyclase activity disappears in the 3T3-L1 cells confirming antagonism of the MC5 receptor site (see FIGURE 3). As expected, however, ACTH-mediated cAMP production was unaffected by preincubation with NDP-α-MSH (FIG. 3), confirming functional expression of the MC2 receptor in the mouse adipo-

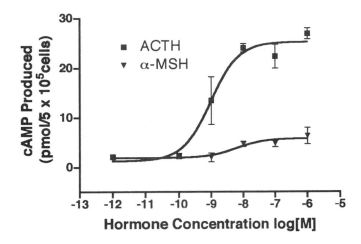

FIGURE 3. Stimulation of adenylyl cyclase in differentiated 3T3-L1 cells by ACTH and α-MSH in the presence of 1 mM NDP-αMSH. Methods as described in FIGURE 2 except that 1 µM NDP-MSH was added to incubation media. The EC_{50} value for $ACTH_{1-39}$ is 0.98 ± 0.02 nM. (Reproduced, with permission, from Ref. 31. ©The Endocrine Society.)

cyte.[31] Although release of free fatty acids into the medium was not measured in these experiments, previous investigators have shown that lipolysis is mediated by an increase in adenylyl cyclase activity.[3] Therefore, melanocortins stimulate lipolysis in the adipocyte by increasing adenylyl cyclase activity in either the MC2 and/or the MC5 receptor. The pharmacology, however, is most consistent with the MC2 receptor as the major contributor to ACTH-mediated cAMP production, and the MC5 receptor as responsible for the minimal lipolysis seen with α-MSH in murine adipocytes.

The observation, that NDP-α-MSH binds to the MC5 receptor with high affinity but does not activate adenylyl cyclase, is an intriguing one. The pharmacology of the murine MC5 receptor has primarily been studied in heterologous cell expression systems.[16,19,34,35] In these systems, NDP-α-MSH binds to the receptor and stimulates adenylyl cyclase with very high affinity (EC_{50} of 0.051 to 1.8 nM).[19,35] The discrepancy between experiments demonstrating NDP-α-MSH as a potent agonist of the transfected MC5 receptor and those that show it as a potent antagonist of the MC5 receptor in the 3T3-L1 cells, is difficult to explain. The unique pharmacological properties of the murine MC5 receptor described here may be the normal response of the MC5 receptor in murine cells such as 3T3-L1 adipocytes that naturally express this receptor. Since the cells that have been used to express the murine MC5 receptor, human 293 cells and Chinese hamster ovary, do not normally express melanocortin receptors, the natural biology of the MC5 receptor may have been altered. These cells may lack cofactor(s) necessary for the normal function of these receptors. Alternatively, although MC5 is detected by Northern blot in 3T3-L1 and primary mouse adipocytes, this receptor may not be expressed on the cell surface and the binding and cyclase studies may be pharmacologically characterizing another, as yet undescribed, melanocortin receptor. Regardless of the mechanism, the antagonistic properties of NDP-α-MSH seen here are important to note since many biological activities have been reported using this compound under the assumption that it is a potent melanocortin agonist.

SUMMARY

Melanocortin receptors, including both the MC2 and MC5 receptors, have been demonstrated and characterized in the adipocyte. The physiologic importance of these receptors, however, has yet to be clearly defined and may vary from species to species. Although both the MC2 and MC5 receptors can stimulate lipolysis in the rodent, it is more likely that the MC2 receptor plays a physiological role in lipid metabolism. For example, only ACTH has significant lipolytic activity in the rat adipocyte with reported EC_{50} values between 0.15 nM and 1.34 nM, whereas α-MSH has relatively little lipolytic activity (EC50 of 1.53 μM).[4,6] These concentrations of ACTH in experiments using 3T3-L1 adipocytes would stimulate approximately 20% of maximal cAMP production. Previous experiments have shown that small increases in cAMP over basal levels may maximally activate lipolysis in rat adipocytes.[3] Since the concentrations of ACTH that promote lipolysis approximate the levels seen in the rat during stress (up to 0.43 nM),[36] ACTH stimulation of the adipocyte MC2 receptor may serve to augment release of energy stored into the circulation during times of increased energy demand.

The physiological relevance of the MC5 receptor in the adipocyte remains uncertain. Lipolysis and cAMP production in response to α-MSH in the 3T3-L1 occur at α-MSH levels much higher than those found in serum. Although ACTH also stimulates the murine MC5 receptor, blocking this receptor with NDP-α-MSH caused no change in ACTH mediated intracellular cAMP production.[31] Therefore, in the mouse adipocyte, the MC5 receptor is unlikely to have a physiologic role in ACTH mediated lipolysis. The MC5 receptor, however, may play a significant role in rabbit and hamster adipocytes since both of these animals are responsive to α-MSH administration. The mechanism behind the species differences in melanocortin response is unclear. It is possible that the different responsiveness to α-MSH and ACTH in rabbit and rat adipocytes is due to different levels of expression of the MC2 and MC5 receptors in these animals. This hypothesis remains to be tested.

Although the melanocortins appear to play a role in adipocyte regulation in most mammals, it is unlikely that melanocortins regulate lipolysis in humans. Even high concentrations of ACTH have no effect on the human adipocyte. At the present time, it is unclear whether primates even express melanocortin receptors on the adipocyte cell surface. Despite the apparent lack of importance in human physiology, the mere presence of these receptors on the adipocyte in other mammals argues for a physiologic role—even if it is only a small one. The melanocortin receptors may therefore play a role along with other hormone receptors in regulating the adipocyte, and allowing it to function as an efficient energy storage depot.

REFERENCES

1. ZHANG, Y., R. PROENCA, M. MAFFEI *et al.* 1994. Positional cloning of the mouse obese gene and its human homologue. Nature **372:** 425–432.

2. RAMACHANDRAN, J., S.W. FARMER, S. LILES *et al.* 1976. Comparison of the steroidogenic and melanotropic activities of corticotropin, alpha-melanotropin, and analogs with their lipolytic activities in rat and rabbit adipocytes. Biochim. Biophys. Acta **428:** 347–354.

3. RAMACHANDRAN, J. & V. LEE. 1976. Divergent effects of adrenocorticotropin and melanotropin on isolated rat and rabbit adipocytes. Biochim. Biophys. Acta **428:** 339–346.

4. RICHTER, W.O. & P. SCHWANDT. 1987. Lipolytic potency of proopiomelanocorticotropin peptides *in vitro*. Neuropeptides **9:** 59–74.

5. WHITE, J.E. & F.L. ENGEL. 1958. Lipolytic action of corticotropin on rat adipose tissue *in vitro*. J. Clin. Invest. **37:** 1556–1563.

6. OELOFSEN, W. & J. RAMACHANDRAN. 1983. Studies of corticotropin receptors on rat adipocytes. Arch. Biochem. and Biophys. **225:** 414–421.

7. MAINS, R.E., B.A. EIPPER & N. LING. 1977. Common precursor to corticotropins and endorphins. Proc. Natl. Acad. Sci. USA **74:** 3014–3018.

8. ROBERTS, J.L. & E. HERBERT. 1977. Characterization of a common precursor to corticotropin and beta-lipotropin: cell-free synthesis of the precursor and identification of corticotropin peptides in the molecule. Proc. Natl. Acad. Sci. USA **74:** 4826–4830.

9. NAKANISHI, S., A. INOUE, K. KITA *et al.* 1979. Nucleotide sequence of cloned cDNA for bovine corticotropin-B lipotropin precursor. Nature **278:** 423–427.

10. BARRET, P., A. MACDONALD, R. HELLIWELL *et al.* 1994. Cloning and expression of a new member of the melanocyte-stimulating hormone receptor family. J. Mol. Endocrinol. **12:** 203–213.

11. MOUNTJOY, K.G., L.S. ROBBINS, M.T. MORTRUD *et al.* 1992. The cloning of a family of genes that encode the melanocortin receptors. Science **257:** 543–546.

12. CHHAJLANI, V. & J.E.S. WIKBERG. 1992. Molecular cloning and expression of the human melanocyte stimulating hormone receptor cDNA. FEBS Lett. **309:** 417–420.

13. ROSELLI-REHFUSS, L., K.G. MOUNTJOY, L.S. ROBBINS *et al.* 1993. Identification of a receptor for γ-MSH and other proopiomelanocortin peptides in the hypothalamus and limbic system. Proc. Natl. Acad. Sci. USA **90:** 8856–8860.

14. GANTZ, I., Y. KONDA, T. TASHIRO *et al.* 1993. Molecular cloning of a novel melanocortin receptor. J. Biol. Chem. **268:** 8246–8250.

15. GANTZ, I., H. MIWA, Y. KONDA *et al.* 1993. Molecular cloning, expression, and gene localization of a fourth melanocortin receptor. J. Biol. Chem. **268:** 15174–15179.

16. GANTZ, I., Y. SHIMOTO, Y. KONDA *et al.* 1994. Molecular cloning, expression, and characterization of a fifth melanocortin receptor. Biochem. Biophys. Res. Comm. **200:** 1214–1220.

17. CHHAJLANI, V., R. MUCENIECE & J.E.S. WIKBERG. 1993. Molecular cloning of a novel human melanocortin receptor. Biochem. Biophys. Res. Comm. **195:** 866–873.

18. DESARNAUD, F., O. LABBE, D. EGGERICKX *et al.* 1994. Molecular cloning, functional expression and pharmacological characterization of a mouse melanocortin receptor gene. Biochem. J. **299:** 367–373.

19. LABBE, O., F. DESARNAUD, D. EGGERICKX *et al.* 1994. Molecular cloning of a mouse melanocortin 5 receptor gene widely expressed in peripheral tissues. Biochem. **33:** 4543–4549.

20. MOUNTJOY, K.G., M.T. MORTRUD, M.J. LOW *et al.* 1994. Localization of the melanocortin-4 receptor (MC4-R) in neuroendocrine and autonomic control circuits in the brain. Mol. Endo. **8:** 1298–1308.

21. GRIFFON, N., V. MIGNON, P. FACCHINETTI et al. 1994. Molecular cloning and characterization of the rat fifth melanocortin receptor. Biochem. Biophys. Res. Comm. **200:** 1007–1014.

22. ROBBINS, L.S., J.H. NADEAU, K.R. JOHNSON et al. 1993. Pigmentation phenotypes of variant extension locus alleles result from point mutations that alter MSH receptor function. Cell **72:** 827–834.

23. FAN, W., B.A. BOSTON, R.A. KESTERSON et al. 1997. Role of melanocortinergic neurons in feeding and the agouti obesity syndrome. Nature **384:** 165–168.

24. HUSZAR, D., C.A. LYNCH, V. FAIRCHILD-HUNTRESS et al. 1997. Targeted disruption of the melanocortin-4 receptor results in obesity in mice. Cell **88:** 131–141.

25. WHITE, J.E. & F.L. ENGLE. 1958. A direct effect of purified ACTH on depot fat in the mouse. Amer. J. Med **25:** 136–142.

26. RICHTER, W.O. & P. SCHWANDT. 1983. *In vitro* lipolysis of proopiocortin peptides. Life Sciences **33:** 747–750.

27. BAUMANN, J.B., A.N. EBERLE, E. CHRISTEN et al. 1986. Steroidogenic activity of highly potent melanotropic peptides in the adrenal cortex of the rat. Acta Endocrin. **113:** 396–402.

28. NG, T.B. 1990. Studies on hormonal regulation of lipolysis and lipogenesis in fat cells of various mammalian species. Comparative Biochemistry & Physiology-B: Comparative Biochemistry **97:** 441–446.

29. BOUSQUET-MELOU, A., J. GALITZKY, M. LAFONTAN et al. 1995. Control of lipolysis in intra-abdominal fat cells of nonhuman primates: comparison with humans. J. Lipid Res. **36:** 451–61.

30. TATRO, J.B. & S. REICHLIN. 1987. Specific receptors for α-melanocyte-stimulating hormone are widely distributed in tissues of rodents. Endocrinology **121:** 1900–1907.

31. BOSTON, B.A. & R.D. CONE. 1996. Characterization of melanocortin receptor subtype expression in murine adipose tissues and in the 3T3-L1 cell line. Endocrinology **137:** 2043–2050.

32. CORNELIUS, P., O.A. MACDOUGALD & M.D. LANE. 1994. Regulation of adipocyte development. Annu. Rev. Nutr. **14:** 99–129.

33. GRUNFELD, C., J. HAGMAN, E.A. SABIN et al. 1985. Characterization of adrenocorticotropin receptors that appear when 3T3-L1 cells differentiate into adipocytes. Endocrinology **116:** 113–117.

34. CHEN, W., T.S. SHIELDS, P.J.S. STORK et al. 1995. A colorimetric assay for measuring activation of Gs and Gq coupled signaling pathways. Anal. Biochem. **226:** 349–354.

35. FATHI, Z., G.I. LAWERENCE & E.M. PARKER. 1995. Cloning, expression, and tissue distribution of a fifth melanocortin receptor subtype. Neurochem. Res. **20:** 107–113.

36. REES, L.H., D.M. COOK, J.W. KENDELL et al. 1971. A radioimmunoassay for rat plasma ACTH. Endocrinology **89:** 254–261.

An Immunocytochemical Approach to the Study of β-Endorphin Production in Human Keratinocytes using Confocal Microscopy

SUSANA B. ZANELLO,[a] DAVID M. JACKSON, AND MICHAEL F. HOLICK

Vitamin D, Skin and Bone Research Laboratory,
Departments of Physiology and Medicine,
Boston University School of Medicine,
715 Albany Street, M-1013, Boston, Massachusetts 02118, USA

ABSTRACT: Proopiomelanocortin (POMC) is a protein that is posttranslationally processed to yield POMC peptides. The main site of POMC expression is the anterior pituitary lobe but many other sources have been identified. There is evidence that the skin produces POMC peptides, although their roles have not yet been defined. In the skin, regulation of POMC gene expression is known to be hair-cycle dependent, and it is localized to the sebaceous gland. In particular, β-endorphin, a POMC peptide, has been shown to be modulated by TPA, IL-1α, and ultraviolet radiation in keratinocytes. These results were obtained by examination of POMC mRNA levels using the Northern blot method; β-endorphin protein production by the Western blot method on cultured cells; and immunocytochemistry for tissue preparations. This report represents an approach to use immunocytochemistry to quantify β-endorphin production in cultured human keratinocytes. Additionally, we examined whether exposure to 20 mJ ultraviolet B radiation (UVB) and/or UVA could influence β-endorphin production in these cells. Keratinocytes were grown in monolayers, in serum-free medium, fixed, and incubated with antiserum to whole synthetic β-endorphin. Fluorescence microscopy was performed with a confocal laser scanning microscope. The integrated level of fluorescence was evaluated in $n = 18 \pm 8$ individual cells, and this was assumed to be proportional to β-endorphin content. High variability was observed in the fluorescence intensity among cells. No significant differences between control and UVB- or UVA+UVB-treated cells was found. Similar results were produced by using brefeldin A, a compound that disrupts the secretory pathway, eliminating the possibility that the absence of a difference between β-endorphin content in the treated and control cells was due to secretion of the peptide into the medium. We conclude that: (1) β-endorphin or β-endorphin-like peptides are produced in human keratinocytes and are readily detected by immunocytochemistry; (2) under the conditions tested, UVA and/or UVB did not increase β-endorphin-like immunoreactivity in these cells.

INTRODUCTION

The skin is a large organ that, in addition to functioning as a protective barrier, possesses a diversity of cells and a complex hormonal environment. Research has ex-

[a]Address for correspondence: 617-638-8882 (fax); szanello@br.edu

tended into how stimuli of different origins provoke skin responses to reestablish tissue homeostasis.[1] In this field, several opioid peptides (endogenous substances involved in antinociception, or the suppression of pain[2]) have been shown to be produced in the skin.[3,4]

Proopiomelanocortin (POMC) is a protein synthesized mainly in the anterior and neurointermediate lobes of the pituitary gland[5,6] and is the precursor of the neuropeptides adrenocorticotropic hormone (ACTH), melanocyte-stimulating-hormone (MSH), β-lipotropin, and β-endorphin, among others, that are derived after further posttranslational processing.[7] The regulation of the POMC gene has been extensively studied,[8–12] and its gene and 5´-regulatory sequences have been cloned.[13,14] In the pituitary gland, its expression is mainly downregulated by glucocorticoids,[15,16] stimulated by corticotropin-releasing hormone (CRH),[17,18] and directed by transcriptional activating factors for pituitary-specific gene expression.[19]

In the skin, regulation of POMC gene expression is known to be hair-cycle dependent. It is localized in the sebaceous gland[20] and modulated in keratinocytes by TPA, IL-1a, and ultraviolet radiation.[21] It has been shown that exposure to UV-radiation increases plasma levels of β-endorphin,[22] suggesting that the skin may be a significant source for β-endorphin released into the circulation. To further characterize the potential induction of β-endorphin in human keratinocytes after UV-radiation exposure, we employed an immunocytochemical approach to evaluate this stimulation.

METHODS

Antibodies

Rabbit antiserum to whole synthetic human β-endorphin was kindly provided by Dr. A.F. Parlow, Harbor-UCLA Medical Center, CA. Biotinylated secondary antibodies and streptavidin-Oregon Green were purchased from Molecular Probes, Eugene, OR.

Cell Culture

Human keratinocytes were cultured under serum-free conditions using a modification of methods previously reported.[23,24] Briefly, the dermis and epidermis of neonatal foreskins were separated by trypsin treatment. Subsequent trypsinization of the epidermis-separated basal cells was performed by plating them onto a feeder layer of γ-irradiated NIH 3T3 cells in nutrient medium MCDB 153 supplemented with 50 mg/ml histidine, 99 mg/ml isoleucine, 14 mg/ml methionine, 15 mg/ml phenylalanine, 10 mg/ml tryptophan, 14 mg/ml tyrosine, 20 ng/ml epidermal growth factor (EGF), 5 mg/ml insulin, 0.1 mM ethanolamine, 50 ng/ml prostaglandin E_1, 0.15 mM $CaCl_2$, and 3 mg/ml bovine pituitary extract. First passage cells used for all experiments were obtained by trypsinization of the cells grown on the feeder layer, followed by replating in MCDB 153 together with the above additives, 0.5 mM hydrocortisone, and 100 nM cholera toxin. The medium was replaced two days after plating with MCDB 153, without additives.

3T3 NIH fibroblasts and murine pituitary AtT20 were maintained in Dulbecco's Modified Eagle Medium (DMEM) supplemented with 5% fetal bovine serum (FBS). Cells used for all experiments were obtained by trypsinization followed by replating in DMEM supplemented with 5% FBS, with a change into medium without serum for 24 h prior to treatment.

Ultraviolet Irradiation

The source was a solar simulator (Kratos, Ramsey, NJ) using a 1-KW Xenon arc lamp and optical filters to provide the spectral simulation of Air Mass 0 (AM0), or extraterrestrial solar spectrum and Air Mass 2 (AM2), or terrestrial solar spectrum at 60° elevation. Cells were irradiated in phosphate-buffered saline (PBS) through the plastic Petri dish cover at a perpendicular distance of 6.25 cm from the source for 13 min. This yielded an incident UVB energy of 20 mJ/cm^2 when AM0 was used. Irradiance was measured with a spectroradiometer (Optronics, Orlando, FL). After deciding upon a dose (20 mJ/cm^2), the above irradiation parameters were calculated as follows: The spectral values were plotted on a semilog scale. Integration of the regressed linear graph furnished the total 280 nm–320 nm irradiance per unit area at 27.5 cm distance from the light source. The time of exposure at 6.25 cm necessary to attain 20 mJ/cm^2 was then calculated from the relationship $E = I_{tot}\int dt$. Sham irradiated cells or controls were treated in the same way, but were covered with aluminum foil. The transmission spectrum of AM0 plus PBS and Petri dish plastic cover included portions of both UVB and UVA wavelengths. Therefore, the cells were receiving both UVB and UVA under this treatment. AM2 almost precluded the penetration of all UVB radiation but not UVA. Hence, the exposure of the cells at the same distance and during the same period of time, ensured that they were dosed with UVA in both treatments, retaining the addition of UVB and a surplus of UVA as the sole difference.

Immunocytochemistry

Cells were seeded on plastic multiwell slides (Labtek, Nunc) and subsequently fixed and permeabilized in formaldehyde/glutaraldehyde/Triton X-100 in stabilization buffer, as previously described.[25] A wash with 0.5 mg/ml sodium borohydride in PBS was included to eliminate autofluorescence due to the glutaraldehyde. The preparations were blocked in 5% goat serum/1% BSA in PBS 30 min. All incuba tions were performed at room temperature. Rabbit antiserum against human synthetic whole human β-endorphin (dilution 1:500) was a generous gift from Dr. Parlow. Goat secondary-biotinylated-antibodies to rabbit (Molecular Probes, Eugene, OR) IgGs were used at a dilution of 1:400. Finally, streptavidin coupled to Oregon Green 514 (Molecular Probes) was added at a final concentration 10 mg/ml in PBS, and 5 mg/ml propidium iodide (Molecular Probes) was used to stain the nuclei. The specimens were mounted with Prolong Antifade (Molecular Probes) to preserve fluorescence, and visualized under a Meridian Insight Plus (Genomic Solutions, Inc., Ann Harbor, MI) confocal microscope with the 488 nm Argon laser line.

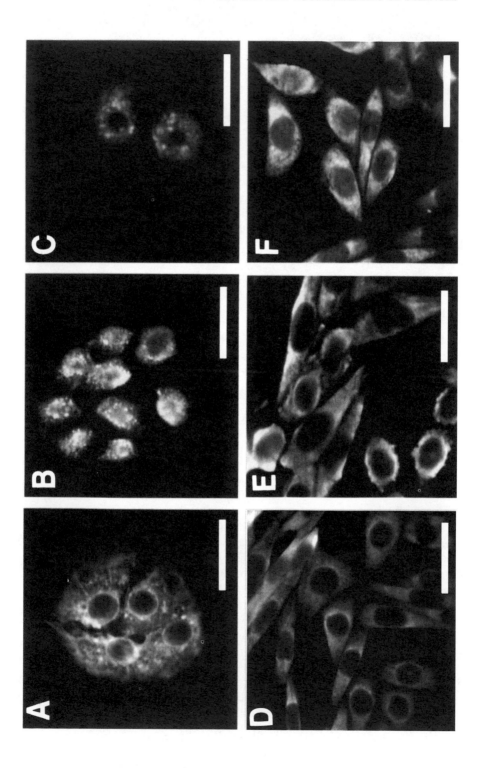

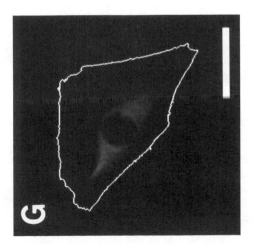

FIGURE 1. Confocal micrograph showing the typical appearance and β-endorphin immunoreactivity levels in human keratinocytes (**A**, **B**, and **C**), rat pituitary AtT20 cells (**D**, **E**, and **F**), and 3T3 NIH fibroblasts (**G**). Samples were prepared as described in the text. Control cells (**A**, **D**, and **G**), UVA treated cells (**B** and **E**), and UVB treated cells (**C** and **F**) are shown. *Scale bars*, 50 μm.

Computerized Image Analysis

Relative fluorescence measurements were performed by using the Meridian Image Analysis program (Genomic Solutions, Inc., Ann Harbor, MI) in randomly chosen fields to gather numerous cells—the only criteria for elimination being a cell surface value very different from the mean. Boundaries of nonoverlapping cells were traced with a computer cursor to determine a polygon within which the measurements were made. The parameters measured were integrated pixel intensity, in arbitrary units, and area of the cells (except in AtT20 cells, for which only integrated pixel intensity was measured, due to the consistent cell size).

Statistical Analysis

Statistical comparison between treatments in each experiment was made by using an independent t-test. To incorporate data from the five separate experiments, the average pixel intensity of each treatment, in each experiment, was taken as a single observation, normalized to the value for the control treatment. Thus, an analysis with $n = 5$ was performed by unpaired and paired t-tests. The unpaired t-test was computed using the SigmaPlot program, and the standard deviation (SD) was calculated as the sum of the SD values for each experiment and treatment. To reduce the variability in the observations due to differences among the experimental sets, a paired t-test was used to test the hypothesis that the average difference (D_{av}) in pixel intensity (i.e. β-endorphin content) was null. The t-values, computed from $t = D_{av}/SD$, where SD is the standard deviation of the D values, were compared with the critical value for $n - 1$ degrees of freedom ($n = 5$, number of experiments) in the t-table.

RESULTS

Detection of β-Endorphin in Human Keratinocytes by Immunocytochemistry

In order to test whether β-endorphin could be detected by immunofluorescence in cultured human keratinocytes, we used specific antibodies for the peptide on fixed cell specimens. FIGURE 1 shows a typical result. β-Endorphin immunoreactivity appeared in the cytoplasm, with a distribution that resembled the endoplasmic reticulum, and possibly secretory vesicles (FIG. 1A, B, and C). The pituitary cell line AtT20 was used a positive control (FIG. 1D, E, and F). The fluorescence was markedly lower in NIH 3T3 fibroblasts (FIG. 1G), which have been shown not to react to β-endorphin antibodies.[26]

Quantitative Immunofluorescence Revealed no Differences of β-Endorphin Production in Human Keratinocytes after UV-Stimulation

We examined control and UV-irradiated human keratinocytes by immunofluorescence using a specific antiserum to human β-endorphin. To evaluate the results quantitatively, the cells were examined with a confocal microscope and the digital images were computer analyzed in order to obtain measurements of fluorescence in arbitrary units (AU). The measurements were assumed to be proportional to the β-endorphin content under the imaging conditions used (see below). The results varied with the

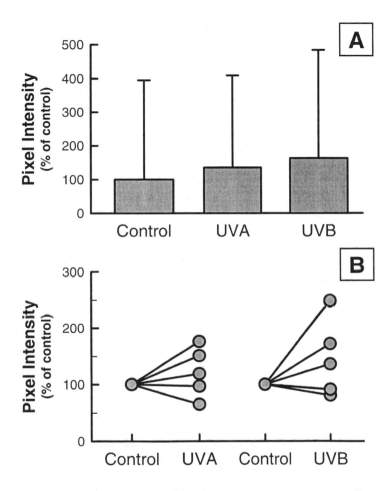

FIGURE 2. Statistical analysis summary of quantitative immunocytochemical results for β-endorphin-like peptides in cultured human keratinocytes. Pixel intensity in arbitrary units is expressed as percentage of control for five different experiments. In **panel A,** each averaged value was obtained as the mean of *n* observations (*n* = 115, 100, and 101 for control, UVA-, and UVB-treated cells, respectively) and the SD is expressed as the sum of the SD values for each of the five experiments in each treatment. **Panel B** shows the same results with the actual values from the averages of the five experiments; a paired *t*-test was used to compare controls and each UV treatment. No significant differences were detected ($t_{c/UVA}$ = 0.49; $t_{c/uvB}$ = 0.85) *t*-values did not exceed the critical values in the 1% and 5% *t*-distribution.

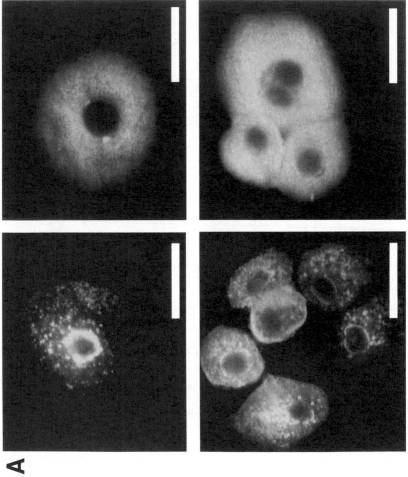

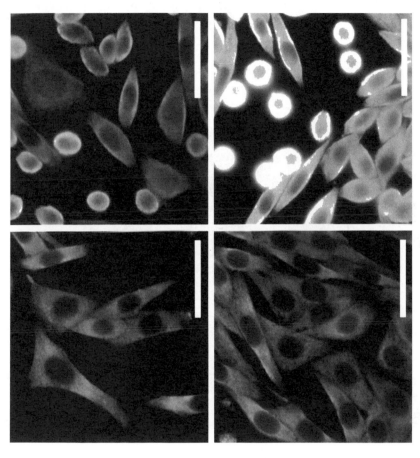

FIGURE 3. Effect of brefeldin A on the intracellular distribution of β-endorphin-immunoreactivity. Human keratinocytes (**A**) and AtT20 cells (**B**) were treated with brefeldin A for 16 h and then fixed samples were immunostained for β-endorphin (*right*). Control cells are shown on the *left*. The *upper, right panel* in (**B**) was generated from an exposure that was half that used in the *lower, right panel*, so as to avoid the saturation notable in the latter. *Scale bars*, 50 μm.

different cell lots; no consistency was found to support the induction of β-endorphin production after UV-irradiation.[21] FIGURE 2 summarizes the statistical analysis of 115 control cells, 100 UVA exposed cells, and 101 UVB exposed cells. FIGURE 1A, B, and C, respectively, show a typical average set of micrographs corresponding to control, UVA, and UVB treated keratinocytes. For the statistical analysis, 115 control cells, 100 UVA exposed cells, and 101 UVB exposed cells were examined.

To test the possibility that UV-radiation could stimulate the secretion of β-endorphin as well as its production, we treated the cells with brefeldin A, a compound that interrupts the secretory pathway by disrupting the endoplasmic reticu-

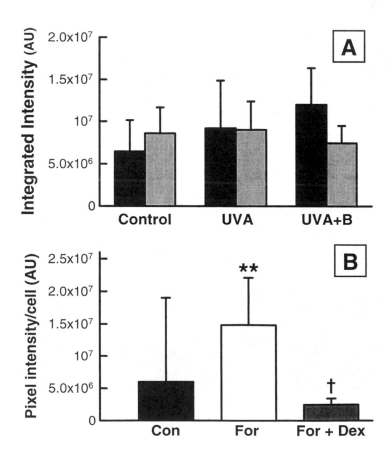

FIGURE 4. β-endorphin immunostaining in AtT20 cells. (A) Cells were exposed to 20 mJ/cm² UVB-light plus UVA, UVA, or sham irradiated, and their relative β-endorphin immunoreactivity was quantified as described in the text. (B) Cells were treated with 10 mM forskolin and 10 nM dexamethasone, and the relative β-endorphin immunoreactivity was quantified as described in the text. The results are expressed as the percentage of control of integrated pixel intensity ± SD. The experiment was repeated with or without brefeldin A treatment (*grey* and *black bars*, respectively).

lum/Golgi continuity.[27] In this case, secretory proteins accumulate in the cell, augmenting immunofluorescence signals[28] and, therefore, giving a more accurate value of the amount of protein actually produced but not released into the medium. An undetectable difference in β-endorphin production due to its secretion into the medium would be, thus, be rendered detectable. FIGURE 3 shows micrographs of keratinocytes treated and untreated with brefeldin A, and where immunocytochemistry for β-endorphin was performed. The effect of the drug was manifested by the disappearance of the typical secretory vesicles, and β-endorphin immunoreactivity spread throughout the endoplasmic reticulum. The same results concerning differences in β-endorphin content were observed in UV-treated keratinocytes with respect to controls, when the cells were exposed to brefeldin A in the medium after irradiation for 18 h (data not shown). The cells examined displayed a uniform surface area distribution. To provide a control, the average pixel intensity per unit area—in AU/mm^2— and its statistical variation were similar in all cases (data not shown).

AtT20 pituitary cells also did not alter β-endorphin production after UV-exposure (see FIGURE 4A, and also FIG. 1D, E, and F), even though the fluorescence level was in general higher, in agreement with the fact that this cell type represents the paradigm for POMC peptide production. The same results were also observed after brefeldin A treatment, in this case the alterations in shape caused by the drug were dramatic (FIG. 3B). AtT20 cells treated with 10 mM forskolin provoked an approximately threefold increase in β-endorphin immunoreactivity. This effect was suppressed to below control levels when the cells were simultaneously treated with 10 nM dexamethasone (FIG. 4B).

DISCUSSION

Since the first observations of an increase in β-endorphin and β-lipotropin in human plasma after exposure to UV radiation,[22] substantial attention has been directed to the skin as a probable source of these POMC peptides, because it is exposed to solar radiation. The presence of both messenger RNA for POMC, and several of its final processed peptides, was demonstrated by various techniques in whole skin, hair follicles, cultured human keratinocytes, and melanocytes.[3,20,21,29] However, less additional evidence of β-endorphin expression in skin cells has been provided by immunocytochemistry. POMC products—ACTH, β-MSH, and β-endorphin—have been detected in areas of skin affected by diseases like psoriasis, basal cell carcinoma, and melanoma,[30] as well as in hair follicles.[20] Cells infiltrating the inflamed subcutaneous tissue; including T- and B-lymphocytes, monocytes, and macrophages; have been stained with antibodies to β-endorphin.[31] To the best of our knowledge, the work presented here represents the first immunocytochemical demonstration of β-endorphin immunoreactivity in cultured human keratinocytes. By using AtT20 pituitary cells and NIH fibroblasts as positive and negative controls, respectively, we were able to ascertain that the fluorescence observed was due to presence of β-endorphin or β-endorphin-like peptides in keratinocytes that are reactive to the cognate antibodies, with a minor component of nonspecific binding to other components of the antiserum, as seen in the 3T3 NIH fibroblast preparations.

The immunostaining pattern with the β-endorphin antiserum followed the typical granular arrangement of secretory vesicles, as has been observed previously for other neuropeptides.[32] We cannot exclude the possibility that the antiserum crossreacts with other β-endorphin precursors like β-lipotropin. The immunoreactivity switched to a more diffused distribution when the cells were treated with brefeldin A, suggesting that the secretory pathway was indeed disrupted and the peptides accumulated throughout the endoplasmic reticulum.

One of our objectives was to determine whether quantitative immunocytochemical analysis could be used to study the induction of β-endorphin by UV-radiation exposure in cultured human keratinocytes. We chose an extensive digital image analysis to pursue this aim, and a stringent statistical analysis to express the results. Similar quantitative approaches have been reported in the literature.[33,34] The reproducibility of previous results on β-endorphin expression in the pituitary cell line, AtT20, validated this technique as a feasible way to estimate β-endorphin-like immunoreactivity levels in human keratinocytes. It had been demonstrated previously that 10 mM forskolin, during a 5 h treatment, provoked a fivefold increase of POMC promoter activity compared to the basal level.[12] Our observation, of a threefold increase in β-endorphin immunoreactivity after a 18 h treatment with the same forskolin concentration, has the same order of magnitude. The slightly smaller increase we obtained may be due to the fact that the treatment was prolonged to 18 h, since a decrease in the effect had been observed after 6 h treatment in previous experiments by other groups.[12] Similarly, 10 nM dexamethasone inhibited forskolin stimulation of POMC product formation, as previously reported.[35] Thus, we conclude that our immunocytochemical quantitative assessment of β-endorphin levels was an adequate means for similar studies in human keratinocytes.

The preparation of the samples seems to be critical for the correct fixation and exposure of the antigen-epitopes in quantitative immunocytochemistry, especially when compartmentalization is an issue—that is, in secretory vesicles. Particular care was taken to choose the right fixation and staining procedures and to process all samples in the same way, so that comparison between the preparations was meaningful.

The results of the experiments involving treatments of human keratinocytes with UV-radiation and its effect on β-endorphin-immunoreactivity were highly variable. Although earlier publications had shown an induction of β-endorphin in irradiated cells,[21] these results proved to be erratic as well: the conditions of growth being a critical parameter influencing the consistency of the results (Wintzen, personal communication). The average of fluorescence intensity values of various experiments allowed us to conclude that differences in β-endorphin production were not UV-radiation dependent, even though a slight increase in β-endorphin-like immunoreactivity was observed in UVB-treated keratinocytes. Individual experiments were analyzed with a standard t-test in order to uncover any significant differences among the treatments. We have observed similar frequency of occurrence of experiments in which an increment in β-endorphin content occurred after UV-irradiation of the cells, and of experiments in which no difference, or even a decrease, was observed.

The integration of all results from six independent experiments analyzed by an unpaired t-test did not show significant differences in the β-endorphin content between control and UV-exposed cells. In order to explore the possibility that the cell population of each experiment exhibited any proclivity to respond, or not, to

UV-irradiation, a paired *t*-test was performed. This showed no relevant differences either.

In conclusion, this work documents the expression of β-endorphin-like peptides in cultured human keratinocytes by immunocytochemistry. These peptides appear to be localized mainly in endoplasmic reticulum and secretory vesicles. The analysis of the modulation of their expression was performed by a conscientious quantitative application of confocal microscopy, and no significant differences were found between control samples and those that were UV-irradiated. Apart from a certain common crossreactivity of the antiserum used with other POMC derivatives, which could affect the results, adequate controls were included to validate the technique.

ACKNOWLEDGEMENTS

We are especially thankful to Dr. A.F. Parlow (Pituitary Hormones & Antisera Center, Harbor-UCLA Medical Center), who provided the antiserum to β-endorphin. We also thank Dr. Ray Stephens for invaluable discussions on microscopy and statistical techniques and K. Persons for the cell cultures. This work was supported by the Heliotherapy, Light and Skin Research Center at Boston University School of Medicine and the generous support by California Tan, Los Angeles, CA.

REFERENCES

1. SLOMINSKI, A., R. PAUS & J. WORTSMAN. 1993. On the potential role of proopiomelanocortin in skin physiology and pathology. Mol. Cell. Endoc. **93:** C1–C6.

2. TERENIUS, L. 1992. Opioid peptides, pain and stress. Prog. Brain Res. **92:** 375–383.

3. SCHAUER, E., F. TRAUTINGER, A. KÖCK, A. SCHWARZ, R. BHARDWAJ, M. SIMON, J.C. ANSEL, T. SCHWARZ & T.A. LUGER. 1994. Proopiomelanocortin-derived peptides are synthesized and released by human keratinocytes. J. Clin. Invest. **93:** 2258–2262.

4. WINTZEN, M. & B.A. GILCHREST. 1996. Proopiomelanocortin, its derived peptides and the skin. J. Invest. Dermatol. **106:** 3-10.

5. CIVELLI, O., N. BIRNBER & E. HERBERT. 1982. Detection and quantitation of proopiomelanocortin mRNA in pituitary and brain tissues from different species. J. Biol. Chem. **257**(12): 6783–6787.

6. SMITH, A.I. & J.W. FUNDER. 1988. Proopiomelanocortin processing in the pituitary, central nervous system, and peripheral tissues. Endocrine Rev. **9**(1): 159–179.

7. KRIEGER, D.T., A. LIOTTA & M.J. BROWNSTEIN. 1977. Presence of corticotropin in brain of normal and hypophysectomized rats. Proc. Natl. Acad. Sci. USA **74**(2): 648–652.

8. PELLETIER, G. 1993. Regulation of proopiomelanocortin gene expression in rat brain and pituitary as studied by in situ hybridization. Ann. N.Y. Acad. Sci. **680:** 246–259.

9. AUTELITANO, D.J., J.R. LUNDBLAD, M. BLUM & J.L. ROBERTS. 1989. Hormonal regulation of POMC expression. Annu. Rev. Physiol. **51:** 715–726.

10. LUNDBLAD, J.R. & J.M. ROBERTS. 1988. Regulation of proopiomelanocortin gene expression in pituitary. Endoc. Rev. **9:** 135–158.

11. AOKI, Y., Y. IWASAKI, M. KATHIRA, Y. OISO & H. SAITO. 1997. Regulation of the rat proopiomelanocortin gene expression in AtT-20 cells. I: Effects of common secretagogues. Endocrinology **138**(5): 1923–1929.

12. AOKI, Y., Y. IWASAKI, M. KATHIRA, Y. OISO & H. SAITO. 1997. Regulation of the rat proopiomelanocortin gene expression in AtT-20 cells. II: Effects of the pituitary adenylate cyclase-activating polypeptide and vasoactive intestinal polypeptide. Endocrinology 138(5): 1930–1934.

13. COCHET, M., A.C.Y. CHANG & S. COHEN. 1982. Characterization of the structural gene and putative 5´-regulatory sequences for human proopiomelanocortin. Nature 297: 335–339.

14. TAKAHASHI, H., Y. TERANISHI, S. NAKANISHI & S. NUMA. 1981. Isolation and structural organization of the human corticotropin-beta-lipotropin precursor gene. FEBS Lett. 135(1): 97–102.

15. EBERWINE, J.H. & J.L. ROBERTS. 1984. Glucocorticoid regulation of proopiomelanocortin gene transcription in the rat pituitary. J. Biol. Chem. 259: 2166–2170.

16. NAKAI, Y., T. USUI, T. TSUKADA, H. TAKAHASHI, J. FUKATA, M. FUKUSHIMA, K. SENOO & H. IMURA. 1991. Molecular mechanisms of glucocorticoid inhibition of human POMC gene transcription. J. Steroid Biochem. Mol. Biol. 40: 301–306.

17. JIN, W.D., A.-L. BOUTILLIER, M.J. GLUCKSMAN, S.R.J. SALTON, J.P. LOEFFLER & J.L. ROBERTS. 1994. Characterization of a corticotropin-releasing hormone-responsive element in the rat proopiomelanocortin gene promoter and molecular cloning of its binding protein. Mol. Endoc. 8: 1377–1388.

18. BOUTILLIER, A.-L., D. MONNIER, D. LORANG, J.R. LUNDBLAD, J.L. ROBERTS & J.P. LOEFFLER. 1995. Corticotropin-releasing hormone stimulates proopiomelanocortin transcription by cFos-dependent and -independent pathways: characterization of an AP1 site in exon 1. Mol. Endoc. 9: 745–755.

19. LIU, B., M. MORTRUD & M.J. LOW. 1995. DNA elements with AT rich core sequences direct pituitary cell-specific expression of the pro-opiomelanocortin gene in transgenic mice. Biochem. J. 312: 827–832.

20. SLOMINSKI, A., R. PAUS & J. MAZURKIEWICZ. 1992. Proopiomelanocortin expression in the skin during induced hair growth in mice. Experientia 48: 50–54.

21. WINTZEN, M., Y. YAAR, P.H. BURBACH & B.A. GILCHREST. 1996. Proopiomelanocortin gene product regulation in keratinocytes. J. Invest. Dermatol. 106: 673–678.

22. LEVINS, P.C., D.B. CARR, J.E. FISHER, K. MOMTAZ & J.A. PARRISH. 1983. Plasma β-endorphin and β–lipotropin response to ultraviolet radiation. Lancet 2: 166.

23. RHEINWALD, J.G. & H. GREEN. 1977. Epidermal growth factor and the multiplication of cultured human epidermal keratinocytes. Nature 265: 421–424.

24. CHEN, T.C., K. PERSONS, W.-W. LIU, M.L. CHEN & M.F. HOLICK. 1995. The antiproliferative and differentiative activities of 1,25-dihydroxyvitamin D_3 are potentiated by epidermal growth factor and attenuated by insulin in cultured human keratinocytes. J. Invest. Dermatol. 104: 113–117.

25. HOLLERAN, E.A., M.K. TOKITO, S. KARKI & E.L.F. HOLZBAUR. 1996. Centractin (ARP1) associates with spectrin revealing a potential mechanism to link dynactin to intracellular organelles. J. Cell. Biol. 135(6): 1815–1829.

26. BEUTLER, A.S., M. BANCK, F.W. BACH, F.H. GAGE, F. PORRECA, E.J. BILSKY & T.L. YAKSH. 1995. Retrovirus-mediated expression of an artificial β-endorphin precursor in primary fibroblasts. J. Neurochem. 64: 475–481.

27. FUJIWARA, T., K. ODA, S. YOKOTA, A. TAKATSUKI & Y. IKEHARA. 1988. Brefeldin A causes disassembly of the Golgi complex and accumulation of secretory proteins in the endoplasmic reticulum. J. Biol. Chem. 263(34): 18545–18552.

28. PICKER, L.J., M.K. SINGH, Z. ZDRAVESKI, J.R. TREER, S.L. WALDROP, P.R. BERGSTRESSER & V.C. MAINO. 1995. Direct demonstration of cytokine synthesis heterogeneity among human memory/effector T cells by flow cytometry. Blood 86(4): 1408–1419.

29. LUNEC, J., C. FISHEER, C. PARKER, G.V. SHERBET & A.J. THODY. 1988. Pigment cells are able to synthesize MSH peptides. (Abstract). J. Invest. Dermatol. **91:** 407.
30. SLOMINSKI, A., J. WORTSMAN, J.E. MAZURKIEWICZ, L. MATSUOKA, J. DIETRICH, K. LAWRENCE, A. GORBANI & R. PAUS. 1993. Detection of proopiomelanocortin-derived antigens in normal and pathologic human skin. J. Lab. Clin. Med. **122:** 658–666.
31. PRZEWLOCKI, R., A.H.S. HASSAN, W. LASON, C. EPPLEN, A. HERZ & C. STEIN. 1992. Gene expression and localization of opioid peptides in immune cells of inflamed tissue: functional role in antinoception. Neuroscience **48**(2): 491–500.
32. FISHER, J.M., W. SOSSIN, R. NEWCOMB & R.H. SCHELLER. 1988. Multiple neuropeptides derived from a common precursor are differentially packaged and transported. Cell **54:** 813–822.
33. FOUSER, L., H.E. SAGE, J. CLARK & P. BORNSTEIN. 1991. Feedback regulation of collagen gene expression: a Trojan horse approach. PNAS **88:** 10158–10162.
34. EL-SALHY, M., O. SANDSTRÖM, M. NÄSSTRÖM, M. MUSTAJBASIC & S. ZACHRISSON. 1997. Application of computer image analysis in endocrine cell quantification. Histochem. J. **29:** 249–256.
35. RAY, D.W., S.-G. REN & S. MELMED. 1996. Leukemia inhibitory factor (LIF) stimulates proopiomelanocortin (POMC) expression in a corticotroph cell line. J. Clin. Invest. **97:** 1852–1859.

UV Light and MSH Receptors

ASHOK K. CHAKRABORTY,[a,b] YOKO FUNASAKA,[c] ANDRZEJ SLOMINSKI,[d] JEAN BOLOGNIA,[b] STEFANO SODI,[b] MASAMITSU ICHIHASHI,[c] AND JOHN M. PAWELEK[b]

[b]Department of Dermatology, Yale University School of Medicine, New Haven, Connecticut 06520, USA

[c]Department of Dermatology, Kobe University School of Medicine, Kobe 650, Japan

[d]Department of Pathology, Loyola University Medical Center, 2160 South First Avenue, Maywood, Illinois 60153, USA

ABSTRACT: Ultraviolet B (UVB) radiation in the skin induces pigmentation that protects cells from further UVB damage and reduces photocarcinogenesis. Although the mechanisms are not well understood, our laboratory has shown that UVB radiation causes increased MSH receptor activity by redistributing MSH receptors from internal pools to the external surface, with a resultant increase in cellular responsiveness to MSH. By this means, UVB and MSH act synergistically to increase melanin content in the skin of mice and guinea pigs. In humans, MSH causes increased skin pigmentation, predominantly in sun-exposed areas. We have shown recently that UVB irradiation and exposure to MSH or to dbcAMP, stimulates production of mRNAs for both αMSH receptors and POMC in human melanocytes and keratinocytes. This indicates that at least one action of UVB on the pigmentary system is mediated through increased MSH receptor production, as well as through the production of the signal peptides, MSH and ACTH, that can further activate MSH receptors. The results add support to the hypothesis that the effects of UVB on cutaneous melanogenesis are mediated through a series of coordinated events in which MSH receptors and POMC-derived peptides play a central role.

INTRODUCTION

It is ironic that the cutaneous pigmentary system, which protects skin from solar radiation, as evidenced by an inverse relationship between the melanin content of human skin and the incidence of skin carcinomas induced by solar radiation,[1,2] is also the system from which melanomas are generated. Epidemiological studies agree that the incidence of malignant melanomas and other forms of skin cancer are increasing in humans, and there is considerable evidence that UV light is a major causative factor.[3–5]

We do not yet fully understand the mechanism by which UV transduces its signal to exert its effect. For some years our laboratories, and those of others, have focused on the mechanisms of action of UV on skin, and specifically on the transduction of UV energy into organized biological responses at both cellular and tissue levels.[6–12]

[a]Address for correspondence: Ashok K. Chakraborty, Ph.D., Department of Dermatology, Yale University School of Medicine, 333 Cedar Street, New Haven, CT 06520, USA. 203-785-4963 (voice); 203-785-7637 (fax); sodi@biomed.med.yale.edu (e-mail).

UV-induced damage as a signaling mechanism has been suggested by Gilchrest *et al.*,[13] who showed that UV-induced thymine dimers stimulate pigmentation. Evidence for specific UV-receptors has also been documented in both vertebrates and invertebrates.[14–22] In addition, our laboratories have produced results supporting the hypothesis that the effects of UVB on cutaneous pigmentation are mediated through a series of coordinated events in which MSH receptors and proopiomelanocortin–derived peptides play a central role.[6–12]

UV AND PIGMENTARY SYSTEM

In mammals, exposure to UV light results in an increase in the number of active melanocytes, the rate of melanin synthesis, and in the transfer of pigment granules to surrounding keratinocytes.[23–28] Similar effects were also documented for cyclic AMP or agents that increase the level of cyclic AMP, particularly in rodents.[29] The melanotropins (MSH)—proopiomelanocortin derived peptides—are known to stimulate the cyclic AMP system in rodents[30,31] through an interaction with high affinity of receptors, and can induce melanin content in melanocytes (see Ref. 32 for a review).

Several years ago, it was shown that exposure to sunlight causes increased levels of circulating melanocyte-stimulating hormone (MSH) and adrenocorticotropic hormone (ACTH) in both horses and humans.[33,34] In fact, Lerner and McGuire,[35] and subsequently Levine *et al.*[36] showed MSH and ACTH caused increased skin darkening in humans, but predominantly in sun-exposed areas. Individuals with Addison's disease, characterized by an overproduction of ACTH, show generalized skin darkening, which is enhanced in sun-exposed areas.[37] Similar effects were also reported with both injected and topically applied MSH in mice.[38–41] This information prompted us to study the relationship of UVB and MSH in inducing skin pigmentation.

UVB Acts Synergistically with MSH

We observed that UVB and MSH act synergistically to increase melanin content in the skin of mice and guinea pigs.[6] In the areas of guinea pig skin that received both UVB and MSH, there was a significant increase in melanin formation when compared to that in the areas receiving either MSH or UVB separately (see FIGURE 1). Shave biopsies were performed in each of the four areas shown in Figure 1. The epidermis was isolated and incubated with LDOPA to assess DOPA oxidase activity, a key product of active differentiated melanocytes. Suboptimal MSH treatments alone had no effect on the number of active melanocytes seen in control area of skin, whereas suboptimal UVB caused a fivefold increase in active melanocytes. However, combined suboptimal UVB/MSH treatment show a significant increase over the sum of active melanocytes observed with the separate treatments.[6] Similar results were also obtained with cultured Cloudman S91 melanoma cells, where UVB and MSH potentiate each other to induce tyrosinase activity and melanin content (see FIGURE 2).[7] This indicated that at least one action of UVB may be mediated through MSH receptors.

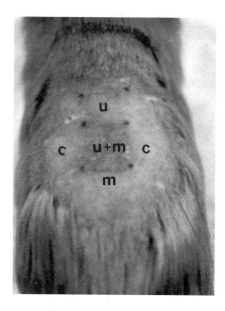

FIGURE 1. An experimental demonstration of the interactions between UVB, MSH, and the mammalian pigmentary system. Shown is a red-haired guinea pig that was treated in separate areas of its shaved back for 7 days with vehicle alone (control); suboptimal concentrations of either UVB alone or MSH alone; or MSH plus UVB. Marked pigmentation was seen with MSH and UVB in contrast to either of the single treatments. (Reprinted, with permission, from Bolognia et al.[6])

UV, MSH RECEPTORS, AND MELANOGENESIS

The melanotropins (MSH), proopiomelanocortin-derived peptides, bind to high affinity receptors, stimulate cyclic AMP level, and induce melanin content in melanocytes (see Ref. 32 for review). Thus far, five different melanocortin receptors (MC1-R to MC5-R) have been cloned and they are found to differ in their tissue distribution, relative affinities for different melanotropic peptides, and, perhaps, to exhibit different physiological roles.[42–47] However, MC1-R is the key MSH receptor of pigmentation,[32,48–50] and has binding affinities with αMSH = ACTH > βMSH > γMSH in order of potency.[42,43,51]

Numerous studies on regulation of the MSH receptor system have been carried out in cultured mouse and hamster melanoma cells, resulting in the following observations: (1) MSH receptors are linked through G-proteins to the adenylate cyclase system.[30,31,42,52–54] (2) In Cloudman melanoma cells, MSH receptors are cell-cycle specific, being expressed predominantly in the late S-G2/M phases of the cell cycle; the phase when cells are most responsive to MSH in terms of increased cyclic AMP levels, tyrosinase activity, and melanin production.[55–57] (3) MSH receptors on synchronized cells exhibit positive cooperativity in late S-G2/M.[57] (4) MSH receptor expression is stimulated by various compounds that influence melanogenesis.[6,7,12,58–62] (5) There are internal binding sites for MSH, associated with coated

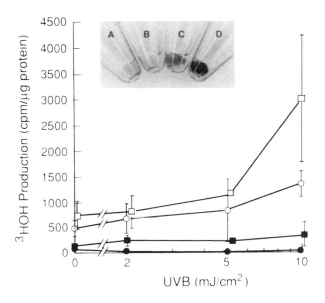

FIGURE 2. UVB acts synergistically with MSH to induce tyrosinase activity and melanin content of Cloudman S91 melanoma cells. Results represent averages ± SD for quadruplicate culture flasks. (●, no MSH; ■, MSH 1×10^{-9} M; ○, MSH 3×10^{-9} M; □, MSII 1×10^{-8} M). The experiments were repeated several times with similar results. **Inset:** *A*, untreated cell pellets; and cell pellets from treatment with; *B*, UUB 10mJ/cm²; *C*, MSH 1×10^{-8} M; *D*, MSH + UVB. (Reprinted, with permission, from Chakraborty *et al.*[7])

vesicles, and they share structural and antigenic characteristics with external receptors.[7,63] (6) The expression of internal MSH receptors is also essential for cellular responsiveness to MSH, in that mutant cell lines that are unable to express internal receptors are nonresponsive to MSH.[63]

Upregulation of MSH Receptors by MSH and UVB

Incubation of cultured Cloudman melanoma cells with MSH elevates expression of both internal and external pools of MSH receptors.[64] Similar homologous upregulation was also observed with human melanoma cells, by others.[65] Under identical culture conditions and with the same Cloudman cell line, UVB also causes increased binding of ¹²⁵I-MSH to cells within 24 h,[7,8] but possibly through a different mechanism. Preceding the rise in tyrosinase activity in cultured cells, UVB elicited a decrease in internal MSH binding sites and a concomitant increase in external sites (see FIGURE 3).[7] Furthermore, a comparison made with the effects of UVB and MSH, alone and in combination on cultured Cloudman melanoma cells, revealed that their effects were additive,[64] suggesting that UVB and MSH act through separate pathways on the MSH receptor system.

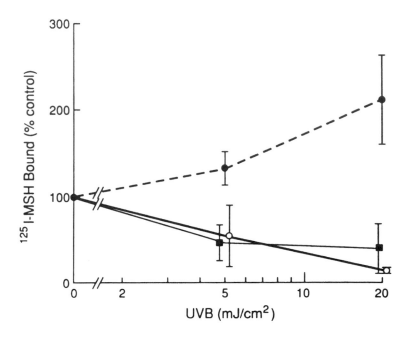

FIGURE 3. Effects of UVB induced on external and internal MSH binding sites from Cloudman melanoma cells. Results are expressed as the mean ± SE for four independent experiments. All experimental data points were statistically significant with $p \leq 0.001$. For each individual experiment, the binding of ^{125}I-MSH to control (nonirradiated) cells was placed at 100%. ●, outer cell surface; ■, binding sites sedimenting to a 47% sucrose region; ○, binding sites sedimenting to a 50% sucrose region. (Reprinted, with permission, from Chakraborty *et al.*[7])

From the data shown in FIGURE 3, it is tempting to speculate that one action of UVB is to enhance redistribution of MSH receptor from internal vesicles to cell surface, or conversely, to prevent internalization of cell surface receptors. However we have not ruled out other explanations, such as nonspecific toxicity of UVB toward the internal MSH binding sites (e.g., proteolysis and denaturation). Another possibility is that UVB promotes autocrine production of MSH or MSH–like peptides, and that the internal binding sites are occupied and thus less available to bind the ^{125}I-MSH following irradiation. No attempt was made in our studies to measure the protein production of MSH receptors. However, since Scatchard analysis of MSH binding shows positive cooperativity, assessment of change in receptor affinity, and/ or number, was not possible, but could represent a mechanism for biological amplification of the MSH signal.

Northern blot analysis, however, showed that Cloudman murine melanoma cells responds to both UVB and MSH in culture, with increased production of mRNAs for MC1-R (see FIGURE 4). The MC1-R transcript migrated as 4-Kb species, as reported previously.[42] With regard to normal human melanocytes, similar results were obtained in that UVB irradiation stimulates specific binding activity of MSH-R in a dose- and time-dependent manner[12] that correlates with increased expression of mRNA for MC1-R (see FIGURE 5).

Together, the above observations provide compelling evidence for an interaction between the UVB and MSH receptor systems. However, the initial effect of UV irradiation may not be directly on MC1-R, but through such mechanisms as direct activation of melanocytes by active oxygen species, via DNA damage, or due to

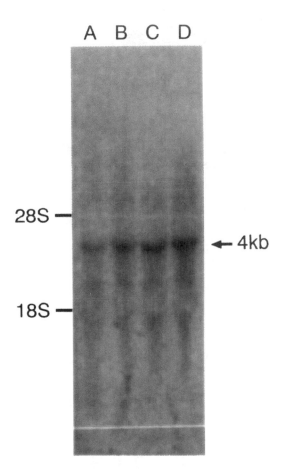

FIGURE 4. Northern blot analysis of hybridizable RNAs for the αMSH receptor in Cloudman S91 melanoma cells. Pretreatment of the cells in culture was: *A*, none (control); *B*, MSH (2×10^{-7} M) plus IBMX (10^{-4}) M, a cyclic nucleotide phosphodiesterase inhibitor that potentiates the action of MSH; *C*, dibutyryl cyclic AMP (1 mM); *D*, UVB (20 mJ/cm^2). Shown is an autoradiogram marking the positions of labeled RNAs. Molecular size markers are 18S and 28S RNA. *Arrow* denotes the position of authentic αMSH receptor mRNA. (Reprinted, with permission, from Chakraborty *et al.*[9])

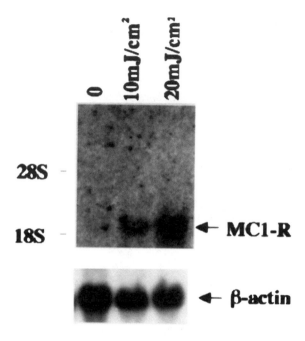

FIGURE 5. UVB induces expression of mRNA for MC1-R in normal human melanocytes. Northern blot of RNA (50 μg/lane) extracted from human melanocytes 24 h after UVB irradiation at the dosages 0, 10, and 20 mJ/cm^2. The sample described as 0 mJ/cm^2 was sham-irradiated with PBS(−) and cultured for 24 h in keratinocyte serum free medium, containing 1 mM of dbcAMP and 10 ng/ml of bFGF. Positions of the 18S and 28S ribosomal bands are shown on the *left*. ^{32}P-labeled coding region of human MC1-R and β-actin were used as probes.

indirect, paracrine activation of melanocytes by a variety of factors, including cytokines, growth factors, and POMC peptides produced in and released from epidermal keratinocytes (see Ref. 66 for a review).

UVB AND POMC PEPTIDES

POMC is a 31-kDa prohormone protein that is processed to various bioactive peptides including adrenocorticotropin (ACTH), melanotropins (α-, β-, and γ-MSH), lipotropins, and endorphins.[67] Historically, POMC was considered to be produced solely by pituitary cells.[68–70] However, it has become apparent that POMC mRNA or POMC-derived peptides, are expressed in extrapituitary tissues including skin.[71–78] For example, Slominski *et al.*[79,80] reported the expression of POMC gene expression in mouse and human skin *in vivo*. They also have shown the existence of POMC-derived peptides in 24 of 39 human skin biopsy specimens examined,[76, 77] suggesting that local production of POMC peptides, following the activation of its own corticotropic releasing hormone (CRH), similar to hypothalamic/pituitary system,[11] might play a role in both cutaneous melanogenesis as well as in regulation of the skin immune system.[76] Melanocytes and keratinocytes are included as members of the neuroendocrine and immune systems of the skin,[81,82] and there is evidence that all these cells produce POMC-derived peptides.[74–79,81–86] In this respect, we have demonstrated that UVB markedly enhances production of POMC peptides, MSH and ACTH by epidermal cells.[9,10]

UVB Stimulates POMC Expression by Melanocytes and Keratinocytes

UVB stimulates production and release αMSH and ACTH in both mouse melanoma cells and transformed keratinocytes.[9] Northern blot experiments demonstrate markedly stimulated production of POMC mRNA in UVB-irradiated cells. The detected POMC mRNAs migrated on electrophoretic gels with approximate sizes of 6.5 Kb, 3.5 Kb, and 1.1 Kb, representing nonspliced primary transcription product, alternatively spliced product, and mature POMC transcript coding for full-length protein, respectively. cAMP, or its inducers, also has some stimulatory effect (see

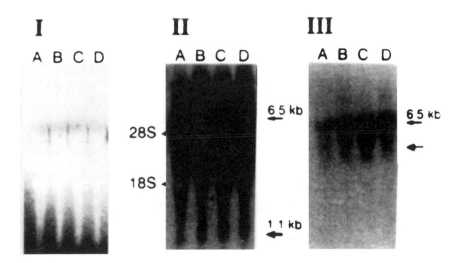

FIGURE 6. Northern blot analysis of hybridizable RNAs for POMC in Cloudman S91 mouse melanoma cells. Pretreatment of the cells in culture was: *A*, none (control); *B*, MSH (2×10^{-7} M) plus IBMX (10^{-4} M); *C*, dibutyryl cyclic AMP (1 mM); *D*, UVB, (20 mJ/cm^2). **I,** ethidium bromide staining of RNA samples showing relative concentration of ribosomal RNA, added as an internal loading control for each lane. Patterns of hybridized mRNA for POMC after prolonged (**II**) and short (**III**) autoradiography. Molecular size markers are 18S and 28S ribosomal RNA. *Arrows* denote positions of POMC transcripts, 6.5 Kb and 1.1 Kb, representing non-spliced primary product and mature POMC transcript, respectively. *Arrowhead* (**III**) corresponds to a 3.5-Kb, alternatively spliced POMC product. (Reprinted, with permission, from Chakraborty *et al.*[9]).

FIGURE 6). Extending this study with normal human melanocytes and keratinocytes revealed similar increases in the production and release of POMC peptides after UVB irradiation, in a dose dependent manner.[10] The RT-PCR assay showed that UVB stimulated the expression of a 260-bp product of POMC-transcript[80] that migrated identically with a POMC transcript run as a positive control (see upper panel of FIGURE 7); the concentration of the amplified fragment of the GAPDH transcript, used as an internal control, remained unchanged during the treatment (see lower panel of FIGURE 7).

This observations suggest a system involving positive feedback regulatory steps, as a mechanism for UVB-induced pigmentation. That is, factors that stimulate melanogenesis also upregulate cellular responsiveness to the MSH/MSH receptor sys-

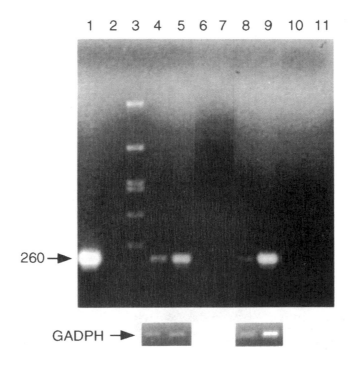

FIGURE 7. Detection of POMC mRNA by semiquantitative RT-PCR in normal human melanocytes and keratinocytes treated with UVB. **Upper panel:** 260-bp POMC mRNA from exon 3 (*arrow*) was amplified (30 cycles) using primers described in Slominski *et al.*[80] **Lower panel:** amplification of the glycerol phosphate dehydrogenase gene (GAPDH, *arrow*). Human pituitary (positive control, *lane 1*); buffer (*lane 2*); DNA size markers of 1000-, 700-, 525-, 400-, 300-, and 100-bp (*lane 3*); normal human keratinocytes (*lanes 4 and 5*) and melanocytes (*lanes 8 and 9*) with no treatment (*lanes 4 and 8*); or exposed to UVB, 25 mJ/cm^2 (*lanes 5 and 9*). Negative control for keratinocytes (*lanes 6 and 7*) and melanocytes (*lanes 10 and 11*) represents PCR amplifications of RNA corresponding to samples in *lanes 4, 5,* and *lanes 8, 9,* respectively, without prior reverse transcription. (Reprinted, with permission, from Chakraborty *et al.*[10])

tem, through increased MSH receptor production as well as through production of the signal peptides, MSH and ACTH, which in turn can further activate MSH receptors.

UVB and Oxidative Stress

UV irradiation causes lipid peroxidation followed by generation of free radicals[87] and depletion of the intracellular pool of reduced glutathione (GSH), resulting in oxidative stress.[88] There is evidence that the active oxygen species (AOS) produced by UVB irradiation may play a role in melanogenesis.[89] In this context, UV-induced AOS could regulate the epidermal melanin unit by increased expression of melanogenic αMSH and ACTH peptides. To test this, we used N-acetylcysteine (NAC), which is readily taken up by cells, and is rapidly converted to GSH that acts as an intracellular free radical scavenger.[90] We observed that UVB-induced α-MSH and ACTH production were suppressed to the nonirradiated control level by NAC (500 μM) treatment, suggesting the involvement of UVB-mediated oxidative stress in POMC production.[10]

Gilchrest *et al.* have reported that dipyrimidine dithymidylic acid (pTpT), which is generated during DNA damage by UV radiation, can directly activate the tyrosinase gene, and upregulate MSH-receptor signaling systems in both cultured mouse melanoma cells and in guinea pig skin.[13,91]

UVB Arrest of the Cell Cycle

We observed that UVB irradiation on Cloudman melanoma cells causes prolongation of the G2 phase of their cell cycle, where expression of MSH receptors, as well as increased responsiveness to MSH, were maximal.[55–57,92,93] The results raise the possibility that an increase in the number of cells in G2 phase of the cell cycle is a generalized cellular response to injury, such as that caused by UV radiation. In the case of pigment cells, this might be a generalized mechanism for increasing other G2/M injury responses. For example, it has been suggested that in addition to its direct effects on pigmentation, MSH may play a crucial role in the downregulation of inflammatory reactions in the skin through antagonisms of the proinflammatory cytokines.[61,84,94]

UVB AND MELANOCYTE/KERATINOCYTE INTERACTIONS

The epidermal melanin unit is composed of melanocytes and keratinocytes, and the activity of this unit is observed, for example, when melanin is donated from the melanocytes to surrounding keratinocytes in response to ultraviolet light. The close relationship between melanocytes and keratinocytes in this intricate process suggests that there are communication mechanisms between them. Experimental results are consistent with at least four categories of UV-regulated communication: (1) unidirectional from keratinocytes to melanocytes,[95–97] (2) unidirectional from melanocytes to keratinocytes,[61,98,99] (3) bidirectional between the two cell types,[61,99] and (4) peripheral regulation from a source other than keratinocytes and melanocytes.[33,34,79,100] Such forms of communication between keratinocytes and melanocytes have not yet been demonstrated to be functional *in vivo*. Considering that several cytokines that might be involved in melanocyte/keratinocyte interactions, the question is quite complex as to *how* the communication systems are regulated. With this in mind, we studied the MSH responsive system (MSH/MSH receptor) on keratinocytes, since keratinocytes express POMC peptides and are regulated by UVB, analogous to that described above for melanocytes.

Keratinocytes Express UVB-Regulated MSH Receptors

Employing cultured human squamous carcinoma cells as a model, we found that MSH-receptor proteins are expressed on the surface of keratinocytes, and that these proteins are quite similar to, if not identical to, those expressed on mouse melanocytes.[101] We also found that interleukin-1, MSH, and UVB upregulated keratinocyte MSH receptors in a manner similar to that observed in mouse melanoma cells.[61,101] The striking similarities between receptors suggested that they may be functional in keratinocyte *in vivo* in the response to UV light. Functional MSH receptors were recently reported in normal human epidermal keratinocytes,[102–104] although Suzuki *et al.*[51] do not confirm these findings. In this respect, our immunohistochemical observations of stronger expression of POMC peptides near the suprabasal layer of the

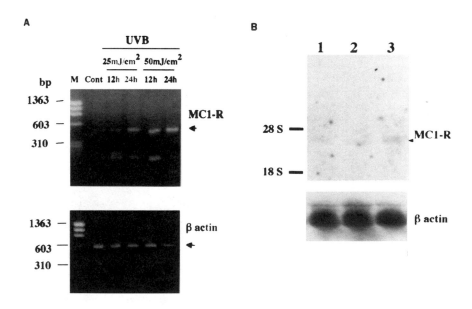

FIGURE 8. A. Detection of MC1-R mRNA by semiquantitative RT-PCR in normal human keratinocytes treated with UVB. **Upper panel:** 580-bp MC1-R mRNA (*arrow*) was amplified (30 cycles) using primers as described in Bhardwaj *et al.*[105] **Lower panel:** shows amplification of β-actin gene. DNA size marker, *M*. **B.** Northern blot of MC1-R (**upper panel**) and β-actin (**lower panel**). Untreated human keratinocytes (*lane 1*); human keratinocytes exposed to UVB, 25 mJ/cm^2 after 12 h (*lane 2*) and 24 h (*lane 3*).

epidermis, where the keratinocytes are mostly differentiated, indicates that increased production and/or increased receptor–mediated binding may be induced during differentiation of keratinocytes.[106] By using both Northern blot analysis and RT-PCR, we confirmed that normal human keratinocytes, indeed, express MC1-R, and that this is enhanced during differentiation induced by exogenous agents like Ca^{2+} or UVB (see FIGURE 8).

These observations are consistent with a model in which ultraviolet mediated release of POMC peptides, and ultraviolet mediated increase in MSH receptor activity could initiate ultraviolet responses in both keratinocytes and melanocytes in a coordinated fashion.[8–10]

CONCLUSION

The existence of POMC peptides, their receptors in melanocytes and keratinocytes, and their stimulation by UVB, implies an existence of autoregulatory loops as well as crosstalk between epidermal cells. In conclusion, we propose the following: (1) the melanogenic response to UVB may include increased expression of MSH receptors and production of their ligand peptides, ACTH, MSH, by cells of cutaneous origin; (2) the system is regulated in a positive feed-back manner, resulting in a biological amplification of the UV signal; and (3) DNA damage—resulting in a prolonged G2 phase of the cycle—could be an initiating mechanism for this process.

ACKNOWLEDGMENTS

We thank Dr. J. Roberts for mouse and human POMC cDNA, and Dr. R. Cone for mouse αMSH receptor cDNA. The work was supported by grants from Vion, Inc., to Dr. John Pawelek, NSF Grant # IBM-9405242 to Dr. Andrzej Slominski; Grant-in-Aid for Cancer Research and ICMR (Japan) to Dr. Masamitsu Ichihashi; and grants from the basic Science Foundation, Shinryokukai, the Research Foundation from the Japanese Society of Women Doctors, and the basic Medical Science Foundation, to Dr. Yoko Funasaka.

REFERENCES

1. KAIDBEY, K.H., P.P. AGIN, R.M. SAYRE *et al.* 1979. Photoprotection by melanin a comparison of black and Caucasian skin. J. Am. Acad. Dermatol. **1**: 249–260.
2. LUANDEE, J., C.I. HENSCHKE & N. MOHAMMED. 1985. The Tanzanian human albino skin: natural history. Cancer **55**: 1823–1828.
3. BALCH, C.M. & G.W. MILTON. 1985. Cutaneous melanoma. J.B. Lippincott and Company, New York.
4. MAGNUS, K. 1987. Epidemiology of malignant melanoma: Status of knowledge and future prospectives. U. Veronessi, N. Cascinelli & M. Santinami, Eds.: 1–13. Academic Press, New York.
5. ARMSTRONG, B.K. 1988. Epidemiology of malignant melanoma: intermittent or total accumulated exposure to the skin. J. Dermatol. Surg. Oncol. **14**: 835–849.
6. BOLOGNIA, J.L., M. MURPHY & J. PAWELEK. 1989. UVB induced melanogenesis may be mediated through the MSH-receptor system. J. Invest. Dermatol. **92**: 651–656.

7. CHAKRABORTY, A.K., S.J. ORLOW & J.L. BOLOGNIA. 1991. Structural/functional relationship between internal and external MSH receptors: Modulation of expression in Cloudman melanoma cells by UVB radiation. J. Cell Physiol. **147:** 1–6.

8. PAWELEK, J., A.K. CHAKRABORTY, M.P. OSBER *et al.* 1992. Molecular cascade in UV-induced melanogenesis: A central role for melanotropins? Pigment Cell Res. **5:** 348–356.

9. CHAKRABORTY, A.K., A. SLOMINSKI, G. ERMAK *et al.* 1995. Ultraviolet B and melanocyte-stimulating hormone (MSH) stimulate mRNA production of αMSH receptors and pro-opiomelanocortin-derived peptides in mouse melanoma cells and transformed keratinocytes. J. Invest. Dermatol. **105:** 655–659.

10. CHAKRABORTY, A.K., Y. FUNASAKA, A. SLOMINSKI *et al.* 1996. Production and release of proopiomelanocortin (POMC) derived peptides by human melanocytes and keratinocytes in culture: regulation by ultraviolet B. Biochem. Biophys. Acta **1313:** 130–138.

11. SLOMINSKI, A., J. BAKER, G. ERMAK *et al.* 1996. UVB stimulates production of corticotrophin releasing factor (CRF) by human melanocytes. FEBS Lett. **399:** 175–176.

12. FUNASAKA, Y., A.K. CHAKRABORTY, Y. HAYASHI *et al.* 1998. Modulation of melanocyte stimulating hormone receptor expression on normal human melanocytes: Evidence for a regulatory role of UVB, IL-1α, IL-1β, ET-1, and TNF-α. Br. J. Dermatol. **139:** 216–224.

13. GILCHREST, B.A., H.Y. PARK., M.S. ELLER *et al.* 1996. Mechanism of ultraviolet light-induced pigmentation. Photochem. Photobiol. **63:** 1–10.

14. ROBINSON J., E.A. SCHMITT, F.I. HAROSI *et al.* 1993. Zebrafish ultraviolet visual pigment: Absorption spectrum, sequence and localization. Proc. Natl. Acad. Sci. USA **90:** 6009–6012.

15. LOEW, E.R., V.I. GOVARDOVSKII, P. ROHLICH *et al.* 1996. Microspectro- photometric and immunocytochemical identification of ultraviolet photoreceptors in geckos. Visual Neurosci. **13:** 247–256.

16. PLACIOS, A.G., T.H. GOLDSMITH & G.D. BERNARD. 1996. Sensitivity of cones from cyprinid fish (Danio aequipinnatus) to ultraviolet and visible light. Visual Neurosci. **13:** 411–421.

17. RAYMOND, P.A., L.K. BARTHEL & D.L. STENKAMP. 1996. The zebra fish ultraviolet cone opsin reported previously is expressed in rods. Invest. Opthalmol. Visual Sci. **37:** 411–421.

18. TOWNER, P., P. HARRIS, A.J. WOLSTENHOLME *et al.* 1997. Primary structure of locust opsin: A speculative model which may account for ultraviolet wavelength light detection. Vision Res. **37:** 495–503.

19. SILLMAN A.J., V.I. VOVARDOVSKII, P. ROHLICH *et al.* 1997. The photoreceptors and visual pigments of the garter snake (Thamnophis sirtalis): A microspectrophotmetric, scanning electron microscopic and immunocytochemical study. J. Comp. Physiol. **181:** 89–101.

20. BENNET, A.T., I.C. CUTHIL, J.C. PATRIDGE *et al.* 1997. Ultraviolet plumage colors predict mate preferences in starlings. Proc. Natl. Acad. Sci. USA **94:** 8618–8621.

21. KAWAMURA, S. & S. YOKOYAMA. 1997. Functional characterization of visual and non visual pigments of american chameleon (*Anolis carolinensis*). Vision Res. **770:** 131–138.

22. VONSCHANTZ, M., S.M. ARGAMASOHERMAN, A. SZEL *et al.* 1997. Photopigments and photoentrainment in the Syrian golden hamsters. Brain Res. **770:** 131–138.

23. SZABO, G. 1967. Photobiology of melanogenesis. *In* The Pigmentary system. Advances in Biology of Skin, vol. 8. W. Montangna & F. Hu, Eds.: 379–391. Pergamon Press, Oxford.

24. QUEVEDO, W.C., G. SZABO & J. VIRKS. 1969. Influence of age and UV on the population of dopa-positive melanocytes in human skin. J. Invest. Dermatol. **52:** 287–290.

25. ROSDAHL, I.K. 1979. Local and systemic effects on the epidermal melanocyte population in UV-irradiated mouse skin. J. Invest. Dermatol. **73:** 306–309.

26. PATHAK, M.A. 1985. Activation of the melanocyte system by ultraviolet radiation and cell transformation. Ann. N.Y. Acad. Sci. **453:** 328–339.

27. STIERNER, U., I. ROSDAHL, A. AUGUSTSSON *et al.* 1989. UVB irradiation induces melanocyte increase in both exposed and shielded human skin. J. Invest. Dermatol. **92:** 561–564.

28. GOLDSMITH, L.A. 1991. Physiology, Biochemistry, and Molecular Biology of the Skin. Oxford University Press, New York.

29. WIKSOW, M.A. 1973. Action of cyclic AMP on pigment donation between mammalian melanocytes and keratinocytes. Yale J. Biol. Med. **46:** 592–601.

30. KREINER, P.W., C.J. GOLD, J.J. KEIRNS *et al.* 1973. MSH-sensitive adenenyl cyclase in the Cloudman melanoma. Yale J. Biol. Med. **46:** 583–591.

31. WONG G., & J. PAWELEK. 1973. Control of phenotypic expression of cultured melanoma cells by melanocyte stimulating hormones. Nature New Biol. **241:** 213–215.

32. LU, D., W. CHEN & R. CONE. 1998. Regulation of melanogenesis by the MSH receptor. *In* Pigmentary System, Physiology and Pathophysiology. J.J. Nordlund, R. Boissy, V.J. Hearing, R.A. King & J.P. Ortonne, Eds.: 183–196. Oxford University Press, Oxford and New York.

33. HOLZMANN, H., P. ALTMEYER & W. SCHULTZ-AMLING. 1982. Der Einfluss ultravioletter Strtahlen auf die Hypothalamus-Hypophysenachse des Menschen. Act. Dermatol. **8:** 119–123.

34. HOLZMANN, H., P. ALTMEYER, L. STOHR *et al.* 1983. Die Beeinfussung des alpha-MSH durch UVA-Bestrahlunger der Hautein funktionstest. Hautarzt. **34:** 294–297.

35. LERNER, A.B. & J.S McGUIRE. 1961. Effect of alpha-and beta-melanocyte stimulating hormone on the skin color of man. Nature **189:** 176–179.

36. LEVINE, N., S.N. SHEFTEL, T. EYTAN *et al.* 1991. Induction of skin tanning by subcutaneous administration of a potent synthetic melanotropin. JAMA **266:** 2730–2736.

37. FRIENKEL, R.K. & N. FRIENKEL. 1987. Cutaneous manifestation of endocrine disorders. *In* Dermatology in General Medicine. T.B. Fitzpatrick, A.Z. Eisen, K. Wolff, I.M. Freedberg & K.F. Austen, Eds.: 2063–2081. McGraw-Hill, New York.

38. GESCHWIND H., R.A. HUSBY & R. NISHIOKA. 1972. The effect of melanocyte stimulating hormone on coat color in the mice. Recent Prog. Hormone Res. **28:** 91–120.

39. HIROBA, T. & T. TAKEUCHI. 1977. Induction of melanogenesis in the epidermal melanoblasts of newborn mouse skin by MSH. J. Embryol. Exp. Morphol. **37:** 79–90.

40. BURCHILL S.A. & A.J. THODY. 1986. Melanocyte–stimulating hormone and the regulation of tyrosinase activity in hair follicular melanocytes of the mouse. J. Endocrinol. **111:** 225–232.

41. LEVINE N., A. LEMUS-WILSON, S.H. WOOD *et al.* 1987. Stimulation of follicular melanogenesis in the mouse by topical and injected melanotropins. J. Invest. Dermatol. **89:** 269–273.

42. MOUNTJOI, K.G., L.S. ROBBINS, M.T. MOTRUD *et al.* 1992. The cloning of a family of genes that encode the melanocortin receptors. Science **257:** 1248–1251.

43. CHHAJLANI, V. & J.E.S. WIKBERG. 1992. Molecular cloning and expression of the human melanocyte stimulating hormone receptor cDNA. FEBS Lett. **309:** 417–420.

44. GANTZ, I., Y. KONDA, T. TASHIRO *et al.* 1993. Molecular cloning of a novel melanocortin receptor. J. Biol. Chem. **268:** 8246–8250.

45. GANTZ, I., H. MIWA, Y. KONDA *et al.* 1993. Molecular cloning, expression, and gene localization of a fourth melanocortin receptor. J. Biol. Chem. **268:** 15174–15179.

46. ROSELLI-REHFUSS, L., K.G. MOUNTJOY, R.S. ROBBINS *et al.* 1993. Identification of a receptor for gamma-melanotropin and other proopiomelanocortin peptides in the hypothalamus and limbic system. Proc. Natl. Acad. Sci. USA **90:** 8856–8860.

47. LABBE, O., F. DESARNAUD, D. EGGERICKX et al. 1994. Molecular cloning of a mouse melanocortin 5 receptor gene widely expressed in peripheral tissues. Biochem. **33:** 4543–4549.
48. REES, J. & E. HEALY. 1997. Melanocortin receptors, red hair, and skin cancer. J. Invest. Dermatol. **2:** 94–98.
49. HUNT, G. 1995. Melanocyte stimulating hormone: A regulator of human melanocyte physiology. Pathobiol. **63:** 12–21.
50. CHLUBA-DE TAPIA, J., C. BAGUTTI, R. COTTI et al. 1996. Induction of constitutive melanogenesis in amelanotic mouse melanoma cells by transfection of the human melanocortin-1 receptor gene. J. Cell Sci. **109:** 2023–2030.
51. SUZUKI, I., R.C. CONE, S. IM et al. 1996. Binding of melanotropic hormones to the melanocortin receptor MC1-R on human melanocytes stimulates proliferation and melanogenesis. Endocrinology **137:** 1627–1633.
52. JOHNSON, G.S. & I. PASTAN. 1972. N_6,O_2-dibutyryl adenosine 3′-5′-mono-phosphate induces pigment production in melanoma cells. Nature N.B. **237:** 267–269.
53. GERST, J.E., J. SOLE, J.P. MATHER et al. 1986. Regulation of adenylate cyclase by beta-melanotropin in the M2R melanoma cell line. Mol. Cell. Endocrin. **46:** 137–147.
54. GERST, J.E., J. SOLE & Y. SOLOMON. 1987. Dual regulation of beta-melanotropin receptor function and adenylate cyclase by calcium and guanosine nucleotides in the M2R melanoma cell line. Mol. Pharm. **31:** 81–88.
55. VARGA, J.M., A. DIPASQUALE, J. PAWELEK et al. 1974. Regulation of melanocyte-stimulating hormone (MSH) action at the receptor level: discontinuous binding of MSH to synchronized mouse melanoma cells during the cell cycle. Proc. Natl. Acad. Sci. USA **71:** 1590–1593.
56. WONG, G., J. PAWELEK, M. SANSONE et al. 1974. Response of mouse melanoma cells to melanocyte-stimulating hormone. Localization in the G2 phase of the cell cycle. Nature **248:** 351–354.
57. MCLANE, J.A. & J. PAWELEK. 1988. Receptors for β-MSH in synchronized Cloudman melanoma cells exhibit positive cooperativity in the late S and G2 phase of the cell cycle. Biochem. **27:** 3743–3747.
58. MCLANE, J., M. OSBER & J. PAWELEK. 1987. Phosphorylated isomers of L-Dopa stimulates MSH binding capacity and responsiveness to MSH in cultured melanoma cells. Biochem. Biophys. Res. Comm. **145:** 719–725.
59. SLOMINSKI, A. & J. PAWELEK. 1987. MSH binding in Bomirski amelanotic hamster melanoma cells is stimulated by L-tyrosine. Biosci. Rep. **7:** 949–954.
60. SLOMINSK, A., P. JASTREBOFF & J. PAWELEK. 1989. L-Tyrosine stimulates induction of tyrosinase activity by MSH and reduces cooperative interactions between MSH receptors in hamster melanoma cells. Biosci. Rep. **9:** 579–586.
61. BIRCHALL, N., S.J. ORLOW, T. KUPPER et al. 1991. Interactions between ultraviolet light and interleukin-1 on MSH binding in both mouse melanoma and human squamous carcinoma cells. Biochem. Biophys. Res. Comm. **175:** 839–845.
62. KAMEYAMA, K., S. TANAKA, Y. ISHIDA et al. 1989. Interferons modulate the expression of hormone receptors on the surface of murine melanoma cells. J. Clin. Invest. **83:** 213–221.
63. ORLOW, S.J., S. HOTCHKISS & J. PAWELEK. 1990. Internal binding sites for MSH in wild type and variant Cloudman melanoma cells. J. Cell Physiol. **142:** 129–136.
64. CHAKRABORTY, A.K. & J. PAWELEK. 1992. Up-regulation of MSH receptor by MSH in Cloudman melanoma cells. Biochem. Biophys. Res. Comm. **188:** 1325–1331.
65. SIEGRIS, W. & A.N. EBERLE. 1993. Homologous regulation of the MSH receptors in melanoma cells. J. Recept. Res. **13:** 263–281.
66. SLOMINSKI, A. & J. PAWELEK. 1998. Animals under the sun: Effects of ultraviolet radiation on mammalian skin. Clinics in Dermatology **16:** 503–515.

67. SMITH, A.I. & J.E. FUNDER. 1988. Pro-opiomelanocortin processing in the pituitary, central nervous system, and peripheral tissues. Endocrine Rev. **9:** 159–179.

68. INOUE, A., T. KITA, M. NAKOMURA *et al.*, 1979. Nucleotide sequence of cloned cDNA for bovine corticotrophin-beta-lipotropin precursor. Nature **278:** 423–427.

69. ALLEN, B.M. 1916. The results of extirpation of the anterior lobe of the hypophysis and of the thyroid of Rana pipens larvae. Science **44:** 755–758.

70. ATWELL, W.J. 1916. On the nature of the pigmentation changes following hypophysectomy in the frog larvae. Science **49:** 48–50.

71. TSONG, S.D., D. PHILLIPS, N. HALMI *et al.* 1982. ACTH and beta-endorphin-related peptides are present in multiple sites in the reproductive tract of the male rat. Endocrinol. **110:** 2204–2206

72. THODY, A.J., K. RIDLEY, R.J. PENNY *et al.* 1983. MSH peptides are present in mammalian skin. Peptides **4:** 813–816.

73. LOLAIT, S.J., J.A. CLEMENTS, A.J. MARKWICK *et al.* 1986. Proopiomelanocortin messenger ribonucleic acid and posttranslational processing of beta endorphin in spleen macrophages. J. Clin. Invest. **77:** 1776–1779.

74. LUNEC J., C. PIERON, G.V. SHERBET *et al.* 1990. Alpha-melanocyte stimulating hormone immunoreactivity in melanoma cells. Pathobiol. **58:** 193–197.

75. SLOMINSKI, A. 1991. POMC gene expression in mouse and hamster melanoma cells. FEBS Lett. **291:** 165–168.

76. SLOMINSKI, A., R. PAUS, J. WORTSMAN *et al.* 1993. Detection of proopio-melanocortin–derived antigens in normal and pathologic human skin. J. Lab. Clin. Med. **122:** 658–666.

77. SLOMINSKI, A., R. PAUS & J. WORTSMAN. 1993. On the potential role of proopiomelanocortin in skin physiology and pathology. Mol. Cell Endocrinol. **93:** C1–C6.

78. FAROOQUI, J.Z., E.E. MEDRANO, Z. ABDEL-MALEK *et al.* 1993. The expression of proopiomelanocortin and various POMC-derived peptides in mouse and human skin. Ann. N.Y. Acad. Sci. **680:** 508–510.

79. SLOMINSKI, A., R. PAUS & J. MAZURKIEWICZ. 1992. Pro-opiomelanocortin expression in the skin during induced hair growth in mice. Experientia **48:** 50–54.

80. SLOMINSKI, A., G. ERMAK, J. HWANG *et al.* 1995. Pro-opiomelanocortin, corticotrophin releasing hormone and corticotrophin releasing hormone receptor genes are expressed in human skin. FEBS Lett. **374:** 113–116.

81. CRAMER, S.F. 1991. The origin of epidermal melanocytes. Implications for the histogenesis of nevi and melanomas. Arch. Pathol. Lab. Med. **115:** 115–119.

82. KUPPER, T.A., F. LEE, N. BIRCHALL *et al.* 1988. Interleukin-1 binds to specific receptors on human keratinocytes and induces granulocytes macrophage colony-stimulating factor mRNA and protein. A potential autocrine role for interleukin-1 in epidermis. J. Clin. Invest. **82:** 1787–1792.

83. JONES, M.T. & B. GILLHAM. 1988. Factors involved in the regulation of adreno-corticotropic hormone/ beta lipotropic hormone. Physiol. Rev. **68:** 743–818.

84. SCHUER, E., F. TRAUTINGER, A. KOCK *et al.* 1994. Pro-opiomelanocortin-derived peptides are synthesized and released by human keratinocytes. J. Clin. Invest. **93:** 2258–2262.

85. WINTZEN, M & B.A. GILCHREST. 1996. Proopiomelanocortin, its derived peptides, and the skin. J. Invest. Dermatol. **106:** 3–10.

86. KIPPENBERGER, S., A. BERNAD., S. LOITSCH *et al.* 1995. α-MSH is expressed in cultured human melanocytes and keratinocytes. Eur. J. Dermatol. **5:** 395-397.

87. Black, H.S. 1987. Potential involvement of free radical reactions in ultraviolet light-mediated cutaneous damage. Photochem. Photobiol. **46:** 213–221.

88. LAUTIER, D., P. LUSCHER & R.M. Tyrell. 1992. Endogenous glutathione levels modulate both constitutive and UVA radiation/hydrogen peroxides inducible expression of the human heme oxygenase. Carcinogenesis **13:** 227–232.
89. TOBIN, D. & A.J. THODY. 1994. The superoxide anion may mediate short- but not long-term effects of ultraviolet radiation on melanogenesis. Exp. Dermatol. **3:** 99–105.
90. MEISTER, A. 1991. Glutathione deficiency produced by inhibition of its synthesis, and its reversal: applications in research and therapy. Pharmacol. Therap. **51:** 155–194.
91. ELLER, M.S., M. YAAR & B.A. GILCHREST. 1992. DNA damage and melanogenesis. Nature **372:** 413–414.
92. ABDEL-MALEK, Z.A., V.B. SWOPE, L.S. TRINKLE et al. 1989. Stimulation of Cloudman melanoma tyrosinase activity occurs predominantly in G2 phase of the cell cycle. Exp. Cell Res. **180:** 198–208.
93. BOLOGNIA, J.L., S.A. SODI, A.K. CHAKRABORTY et al. 1994. Effects of ultraviolet light irradiation on the cell cycle. Pigment Cell Res. **7:** 73–80.
94. ROBERTSON, B., K. DOSTAL; & R.A. DAYNES. 1988. Neuropeptide regulation of inflammatory and immunologic responses. The capacity of alpha-melanocyte-stimulating hormone to inhibit tumor necrosis factor and IL-1-inducible biologic response. J. Immunol. **140:** 4300–4307.
95. KUPPER, T.S., A.O. CHUA, P. FLOOD et al. 1987. Interleukin-1 gene expression in cultured human keratinocytes is augmented by ultraviolet irradiation. J. Clin. Invest. **80:** 430–436.
96. GORDON, P.R., C.P. MANSUR & B.A. GILCHREST. 1989. Regulation of human melanocytes growth, dendricity, and melanization by keratinocyte derived factors. J. Invest. Dermatol. **92:** 565–572.
97. HALABAN, P.R., R. LANGDON, N. BIRCHALL et al. 1988. Basic fibroblast growth factor from human keratinocytes is a natural mitogen for melanocytes. J. Cell Biol. **107:** 1611–1619.
98. KOCK, A., E. SCHAUER, T. SCHWARZ et al. 1990. MSH and ACTH production by human keratinocytes: A link between the neuronal and the immune system. (Abstract). J. Invest. Dermatol. **94:** 543.
99. KIRNBAUER, R., B. CHARVAT, E. SCHAUER et al. 1992. Modulation of intracellular adhesion molecule-1 expression on human melanocytes and melanoma cells: Evidence for a regulatory role of IL-6, IL-7, TNFβ, and UVB light. J. Invest. Dermatol. **98:** 320–326.
100. URBANSKI, A., T. SCHWARZ, P. NEUNER et al. 1990. Ultraviolet light induces increased circulating interleukin-6 in humans. J. Invest. Dermatol. **94:** 808–811.
101. CHAKRABORT, A.K. & J. PAWELEK. 1992. MSH receptors in immortalized human epidermal keratinocytes: a potential mechanism for coordinated regulation of the epidermal-melanin unit. J. Cell Physiol. **157:** 344–350.
102. JIANG, J., S.D. SHARMA, V.J. HRUBY et al. 1997. Human epidermal melanocytes and keratinocytes melanotropin receptors: Visualization by melanotropic peptide conjugated macrospheres (polyamide beads). Exp. Dermatol. **6:** 6–12.
103. JIANG, J., S.D. SHARMA, V.J. HRUBY et al. 1996. Human epidermal melanocyte and keratinocyte melanocortin receptors: visualization by melanotropic peptide conjugated microspheres (latex beads). Pigment Cell Res. **9:** 240–247.
104. OREL, L., M.M. SIMON, J. KARLSEDER et al. 1997. α-Melanocyte stimulating hormone downregulates differentiation-driven heat shock protein 70 expression in keratinocytes. J. Invest. Dermatol. **108:** 410–405.
105. BHARDWAJ, R., E. BECHER, K. MAHNKE et al. 1997. Evidence for the differential expression of the functional alpha-melanocyte-stimulating hormone receptor MC1-R on human monocytes. J. Immunol. **158:** 3378–3384.
106. CHAKRABORTY, A.K., Y. FUNASAKA, J.M. PAWELEK et al. 1999. Enhanced expression of melanocortin-1 receptor (MC1-R) in normal human keratinocytes during differentiation: Evidence for increased expression of POMC peptides near suprabasal layer of epidermis. J. Invest. Dermatol. **112:** 853–860.

The Melanocortin-1 Receptor and Human Pigmentation

ZALFA ABDEL-MALEK,[a,b] ITARU SUZUKI,[c] AKIHIRO TADA,[c] SUNGBIN IM,[d] AND CAN AKCALI

[b]Department of Dermatology, University of Cincinnati, Cincinnati, Ohio 45267, USA

[c]POLA Laboratories, Yokohama, Japan

[d]Ajou University, Seoul, Korea

ABSTRACT: α-Melanocyte stimulating hormone (α-MSH) is known to be the main physiologic regulator for integumental pigmentation of various vertebrate species. However, the role of α-MSH and related melanocortins in the regulation of human cutaneous pigmentation is only beginning to be understood. Cloning of the melanocortin-1 receptor (MC1R), and the feasibility of establishing normal human epidermal melanocyte cultures have made it possible to demonstrate direct and specific biological effects of α-MSH on these cells. It is now recognized that both α-MSH and ACTH have similar mitogenic and melanogenic effects on human epidermal melanocytes. These effects are mediated by binding of these hormones to the specific MC1R that recognizes them both with similar affinity. Human MC1R is homologous to its mouse counterpart in that its activation leads to stimulation of eumelanin synthesis. MC1R is also the binding site for agouti signaling protein (ASP), the product of the agouti locus. Human epidermal melanocytes respond to purified recombinant mouse or human ASP, with a reduction in basal tyrosinase activity, and complete abrogation of the mitogenic and melanogenic effects of α-MSH. These results suggest that ASP induces pheomelanin synthesis by competing with α-MSH for binding to the MC1R. This receptor seems to be subject to regulation by a variety of paracrine and/or autocrine factors that are synthesized in response to exposure of the skin to ultraviolet radiation (UVR). Activation of MC1R seems to be pivotal for UV-induced melanogenesis, since stimulation of the cAMP pathway plays a key role in the melanogenic response of human epidermal melanocytes. The melanogenic response to UVR might be influenced by the presence of allelic variants of the MC1R gene. Allelic variants have been identified and shown to be associated with red hair, poor tanning ability, and possibly melanoma. The possible influence of these variants on the function of the MC1R needs to be investigated, in order to understand the physiological consequence of these mutations. Also, the interaction of α-MSH with other factors that are known to affect pigmentation needs to be better understood in order to define the role possible of this hormone and its receptor in acquired human cutaneous hyper- or hypopigmentation.

[a]Address for Correspondence: Zalfa Abdel-Malek, Ph.D., Department of Dermatology, University of Cincinnati, PO Box 670592, Cincinnati, OH 45267-0592, USA. 513-558-6242 (voice); 513-558-0198 (fax); abdelmza@email.uc.edu (e-mail).

PROOPIOMELANOCORTIN SYNTHESIS AND PROCESSING

Proopiomelanocortin (POMC), a 31–36-Kd protein, is the precursor for the family of melanotropic hormones, or melanocortins, that includes adrenocorticotropic hormone (ACTH), α-, β-, and γ-melanocyte–stimulating hormone (MSH), as well as the bioactive peptides, β-lipotropic hormone, and β-endorphin.[1] Proopiomelanocortin was first identified in the pituitary gland, where it was found to be cleaved by prohormone convertase (PC-1) into ACTH; and subsequently, by PC-2 into α-MSH.[1] It is recognized that POMC is also synthesized in different regions of the brain, the hypothalamus, as well as a variety of peripheral tissues that include the gastrointestinal tract, the gonads, and, of particular interest to us, the skin.[2,3] Reports from different investigative groups have demonstrated that POMC is synthesized by human epidermal keratinocytes and melanocytes.[4–6] The presence of ACTH and α-MSH has also been demonstrated by immunostaining cultured melanocytes and keratinocytes. The synthesis of these peptides has been shown to be stimulated by exposure to ultraviolet radiation (UVR), or to the epidermally derived factor interleukin-1, and by activation of the cAMP pathway.[6] Immunostaining of human skin revealed the presence of PC-1 and PC-2.[7] In human skin, immunoreactivity with α-MSH-specific antibody was observed in keratinocytes, and a stronger signal was detected in melanocytes and Langerhans cells. By comparison, the strongest immunoreactivity with ACTH-specific antibody was observed in differentiated keratinocytes. These findings, together with the ability of α-MSH and ACTH to stimulate human melanocyte proliferation and melanogenesis, suggest a paracrine/autocrine role of these hormones in the regulation of human pigmentation.[8–11]

GENETIC REGULATION OF INTEGUMENTAL PIGMENTATION BY *EXTENSION* AND *AGOUTI* LOCI

Classically, the melanotropic hormone α-MSH is known for its melanogenic effect on the integument of various vertebrate species.[12,13] α-Melanocyte stimulating hormone induces rapid color change in fish, amphibians, and reptiles; and it stimulates *de novo* melanin synthesis in mammalian melanocytes. The two major forms of pigment synthesized by mammalian melanocytes are the dark brown/black eumelanin and the yellowish reddish pheomelanin.[14] In the mouse, the most extensively used mammalian model for investigating the effects of α-MSH on pigmentation, α-MSH induces the synthesis of eumelanin in follicular melanocytes, resulting in black hairs.[15–17] Genetic studies on mouse coat color revealed that eumelanin synthesis is induced by its ligand α-MSH upon activation of the MSH receptor.[15,18] This receptor is encoded by the *extension* locus.[16] Mutations at this locus have been identified and found to affect eumelanin formation in mouse hair follicles.[17] For example, in recessive yellow (C57BL6J e/e) mice, loss of function mutation due to a frameshift results in a receptor that can bind α-MSH, but is functionally uncoupled from adenylate cyclase.[19] Since the cAMP pathway is the main signaling pathway that mediates the biological effects of α-MSH, this mutation renders the receptor nonfunctional and results in a yellow coat color, due to the absence of eumelanin synthesis.[20,21] On the other hand, in the somber (C57BL6J E^{so}/E^{so}) mouse, gain of function mutation, due to a point mutation results in the expression of a receptor that is constitutively active in the absence of ligand binding.

The synthesis of melanin is also regulated by the *agouti* locus that codes for a soluble factor, the agouti signaling protein (ASP).[22,23] This protein is synthesized in dermal papilla cells within the hair follicle, and its expression results in pheomelanin synthesis.[24] Agouti signaling protein is a physiologic antagonist for α-MSH, and its inhibitory effects on α-MSH action on melanocytes are mediated by its ability to compete with α-MSH for receptor binding. Dominant mutations of *agouti* that cause ectopic expression of ASP result in a mouse that is yellow and obese. The obese phenotype is now recognized to be due to the binding of ASP to the melanocortin-4 receptor, the α-MSH receptor that is expressed in the hypothalamus and participates in regulating feeding behavior.[25,26] Excessive amounts of ASP block the inhibitory effect of α-MSH on food intake.[26] In the wild type agouti mouse, the switch from eumelanin to pheomelanin and back to eumelanin reflects the temporal expression or repression of the *agouti* gene within the hair follicle, which accounts for the banded pattern in hairs.[27]

In conclusion, eumelanin and pheomelanin synthesis in mouse follicular melanocytes is subject to regulation by the proper expression of the *extension* locus that codes for the MSH receptor. In addition, the synthesis of eumelanin and pheomelanin is regulated by the normal expression of the *agouti* locus that codes for ASP. Inability of the MSH receptor to be activated by α-MSH, or ectopic expression and excessive availability of ASP in the hair follicle results in a yellow coat color. A third gene that might modulate eumelanin/pheomelanin synthesis is the *POMC* gene.[28] So far, little is known about the regulation of expression for this gene, the nature of the melanotropic hormones, or their concentrations in the immediate environment of the melanocyte.

BINDING OF MELANOTROPIC HORMONES
TO THE HUMAN MELANOCORTIN-1 RECEPTOR

Cloning the genes that code for the melanocortin receptors (MCR) made it feasible to understand the diverse biological effects of the various melanotropic hormones. There are five known MCRs, each of which is coded for by a separate gene.[29–34] These receptors belong to a distinct family of G-protein coupled receptors with seven transmembrane domains, and they differ from each other in their tissue distribution and in their relative affinities to the various melanotropins. The first MCR (MC1R) was cloned from mouse melanoma cells and normal human melanocytes.[29] This receptor has highest affinity for α-MSH and least affinity for γ-MSH, unlike MC2R which has highest affinity for ACTH, or MC3R that has a high affinity for γ-MSH.[11,30,33]

The physiologic role of α-MSH in regulating mouse follicular melanocytes is unequivocal. However, its role in regulating human pigmentation remained controversial for many years.[35,36] In the early 1960s, Lerner and McGuire reported that injection of human subjects with high concentrations of α- and β-MSH resulted in skin darkening.[37, 38] More recently, injection of volunteers with the potent and stable synthetic α-MSH analog, Nle[4],D-Phe[7]-α-MSH (NDP-MSH), increased skin pigmentation in the absence of sun exposure, but only in areas that were habitually sun exposed.[39] These studies, however, did not prove a direct effect of melanotropic hormones on human melanocytes, or the existence of specific melanocortin receptors on these cells. Only in the early 1990s were human epidermal melanocytes found to express MC1R.[9,29,40] Shortly thereafter, these cells were shown to respond to α-MSH with either increased proliferation or melanogenesis.[8,9] We were the first to demonstrate that human melanocytes respond equally well to α-MSH and ACTH with an increase in proliferation as well as stimulation of the activity of tyrosinase, the rate-limiting enzyme in the melanin synthetic pathway.[10,11] The minimal effective dose of either hormone on human epidermal melanocytes was 0.1 nM, as opposed to 1 nM on mouse melanoma cells.[11,41] The equal potency of α-MSH and ACTH on human melanocytes was accounted for by the similar affinity of these hormones for human MC1R, and by their similar capacity to activate adenylate cyclase and stimulate the synthesis of the second messenger cAMP.

The finding that the human MC1R has a higher binding affinity for α-MSH than the mouse MC1R, led to the proposal that human MC1R has "evolved to become supersensitive to α-MSH."[42] Moreover, human, but not mouse MC1R, binds ACTH and α-MSH with the same affinity.[11] Various investigators have found that normal human epidermal melanocytes express a very low number of MC1R—not exceeding 1000 binding sites/cell[40] (Abdel-Malek et al., unpublished data). In comparison, primary melanocyte cultures from C57 black mice express more than 100,000 sites/cell (our unpublished results). We observed that α-MSH binding to human MC1R on human epidermal melanocytes results in prolonged stimulation of cAMP formation that continues to increase for at least 24 hours.[11] In contrast, in mouse Cloudman melanoma cells, activation of cAMP formation by α-MSH was short-lived and persisted for less than ninety minutes.[21]

An interesting property of human MC1R is that, unlike other G-protein coupled receptors, it does not undergo desensitization. Treatment of human epidermal melanocytes with either α-MSH or ACTH resulted in increased MC1R mRNA.[11] Chronic treatment of these cells with either hormone resulted in sustained mitogenic and melanogenic response. Therefore, we hypothesize that the sparse expression of the human MC1R on human melanocytes is compensated for by its high affinity for α-MSH and ACTH, its ability to respond equally to both hormones, and its lack of desensitization by chronic exposure to its ligands.

Our studies on normal human epidermal melanocytes suggest that among the various melanotropic hormones, α-MSH and ACTH are the best candidates for physiologic regulators of human pigmentation.[11] Human epidermal melanocytes have a lower binding affinity for β-MSH than to either α-MSH or to ACTH, and have least affinity for γ-MSH.[11]. In addition, β-MSH is less effective than either α-MSH or ACTH in increasing cAMP synthesis, or stimulating melanocyte proliferation and melanogenesis. γ-Melanocyte stimulating hormone is least effective in these assays, suggesting that this hormone may not have significant relevance to human pigmentation.

It is known that cutaneous pigmentation results from stimulation of melanin synthesis by melanocytes and the transfer of melanin containing granules, or melanosomes, to surrounding keratinocytes.[43] Activation of the MC1R on human epidermal melanocytes by α-MSH results in stimulation of dendrite formation, a process thought to accompany increased melanogenesis and to facilitate melanosome transfer to keratinocytes.[44] We have shown that α-MSH induces the reorganization of cytoskeletal actin stress fibers, and that this is associated with increased adhesion to fibronectin.[45] These responses were most evident in human melanocytes with a high constitutive melanin content, derived from skin types V or VI, that constitutively have a higher eumelanin to pheomelanin ratio than melanocytes from skin types I, II, or III.[46] As reported for mouse follicular melanocytes, human epidermal melanocytes respond to α-MSH with stimulation of eumelanin synthesis.[47] This involves increased formation of eumelanosomes that are characterized by their elliptical shape and highly organized matrix.[48] The increase in eumelanin synthesis following α-MSH treatment is expected to confer photoprotection against the DNA damaging effects of sun exposure. Eumelanin is thought to be superior to pheomelanin in its ability to quench reactive oxygen radicals and in its resistance to degradation by exposure to UVR.[49] In addition, eumelanosomes form melanin supranuclear caps that partially shield the nuclei of melanocytes and keratinocytes from UVR.[50]

Although, human epidermal melanocytes express MC1R and respond to its activation by α-MSH or ACTH with increased proliferation and melanogenesis, proliferating human epidermal keratinocytes lack functional MCR. We were unable to detect any MC1R mRNA by Northern blotting, any specific binding to α- or γ-MSH or ACTH, as determined by receptor binding assays, or any stimulation of cAMP formation in response to the above melanotropins (unpublished results). These results indicate that human keratinocytes do not constitutively express functional MCR.

BINDING OF AGOUTI SIGNALING PROTEIN
TO THE HUMAN MELANOCORTIN-1 RECEPTOR

Human MC1R is also the receptor for ASP[25,51,52] (see FIGURE 1). We were the first to demonstrate that normal human epidermal melanocytes respond to purified recombinant mouse or human ASP with downregulation of basal tyrosinase activity—indicating that ASP acts as an inverse agonist of the MC1R, inhibiting the basal activity of the receptor in the absence of α-MSH.[53,54] Agouti signaling protein also abrogates the stimulatory effects of α-MSH on proliferation and tyrosinase activity and drastically inhibits the expression of tyrosinase related protein (TRP)-1, as determined by Western blot analysis.[53] As with mouse follicular melanocytes, ASP elicits its antagonistic effects on α-MSH induced proliferation and melanogenesis in human melanocytes by competing with α-MSH for binding to MC1R.[53] Using competitive binding assays, we showed that ASP competes with ^{125}I-NDP-MSH for MC1R binding, and has a similar affinity for the MC1R as does α-MSH. Moreover, we found that ASP inhibits the α-MSH induced stimulation of cAMP synthesis. Earlier studies showed that in mouse hair follicles, eumelanin synthesis is associated with increased expression of tyrosinase, TRP-1 and TRP-2, whereas pheomelanin synthesis is associated with a reduction in the protein level of tyrosinase, and almost complete abrogation of TRP-1 and TRP-2 expression.[55] Based on this, we suggest that treatment of human epidermal melanocytes with ASP results in abrogation of eumelanin and induction of pheomelanin synthesis. These results indicate that hu-

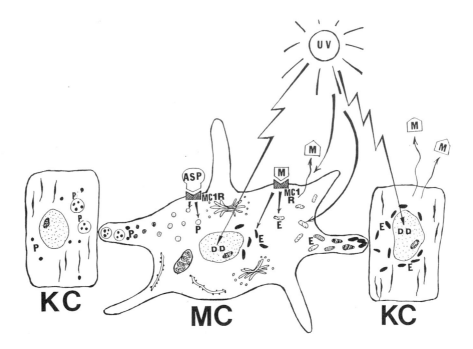

FIGURE 1. MC1R expressed on normal human epidermal melanocytes is the binding site for α-MSH, ACTH, and ASP. Activation of MC1R by α-MSH (M) or ACTH binding results in stimulation of eumelanin synthesis, increased eumelanosome (E) formation in melanocytes (MC), and enhanced transfer of eumelanosomes to keratinocytes (KC). Binding of ASP to MC1R inhibits eumelanin synthesis and induces pheomelanin synthesis in pheomelanosomes (P). Irradiation with UVR results in DNA damage (DD) and in increased synthesis of α-MSH and ACTH by melanocytes and keratinocytes. These hormones upregulate the expression of MC1R mRNA and possibly enhance the responsiveness to melanocortins.

man MC1R is a key regulator of eumelanin and pheomelanin synthesis in human epidermal melanocytes.

ACTIVATION OF THE MELANOCORTIN-1 RECEPTOR AND THE RESPONSE OF HUMAN MELANOCYTES TO UVR

Pawelek and coworkers were the first to propose that the MSH receptor on melanocytes acts as a transducer for the effects of UVR.[56] Using mouse Cloudman melanoma cells, it was demonstrated that irradiation of these cells with UVR, increased the binding of α-MSH and the cooperativity of its receptor, and upregulated MSH receptor expression.[57,58] To investigate the possible role of MC1R in the response of human melanocytes to UVR, we compared the responses of irradiated melanocytes in the presence or absence of α-MSH. We found that, in the absence of α-MSH from the growth medium, tyrosinase activity was inhibited, rather than stimulated by UVR.[59] Only in the presence of α-MSH or another cAMP inducer could we detect an increase in tyrosinase activity in UV-irradiated melanocytes. Using Western blot analysis, we found that the level of tyrosinase was drastically reduced in UV-irradiated melanocytes in the absence of α-MSH or any other cAMP inducer, and was increased following treatment of irradiated melanocytes with α-MSH. As we have previously reported, UV irradiation resulted in the arrest of human melanocytes in G1 phase of the cell cycle.[60] Treatment with α-MSH enabled melanocytes to partially overcome the UV-induced growth arrest and to enter S phase.[59] Whether or not this proliferative response is the result of enhanced repair of UV-induced DNA damage, is currently being investigated.

It has been reported that exposure to the sun increased the serum level of α-MSH in human volunteers.[61] Also, exposure of keratinocytes to UVR increased the production of the primary cytokine interleukin-1.[62] This in turn stimulated the synthesis of endothelin-1 by keratinocytes, and of α-MSH and ACTH by keratinocytes and melanocytes.[4,6,63] All four factors were found to upregulate the level of MC1R mRNA.[6,11,64] Based on these findings, we conclude that MC1R expression is subject to regulation by paracrine and autocrine factors that are induced in the epidermis in response to sun exposure. Activation of the MC1R on epidermal melanocytes leads to increased eumelanin formation, and contributes to photoprotection against repetitive sun exposure (FIG. 1).

THE MELANOCORTIN-1 RECEPTOR, HUMAN PIGMENTARY PHENOTYPES, AND SKIN CANCER

Human MC1R is homologous to its mouse counterpart in that its activation results in stimulation of eumelanin synthesis.[47] Therefore, mutations in the human MC1R gene are expected to affect the function of the receptor, as has been shown to be the case with loss- or gain-of-function mutations in the mouse *MC1R* gene.[19] In humans, total melanin, as well as the ratio of eumelanin to pheomelanin in the skin, differ among individuals with different skin phenotypes.[46] Individuals with skin types I or II have a low total melanin content and a low eumelanin to pheomelanin ratio, whereas those with skin types V or VI have a high total melanin content and a high eumelanin to pheomelanin ratio. Individuals with skin types I or II exhibit a poor tanning response to sun exposure and a high risk of skin cancer developement.[65,66] Moreover, eumelanin in the skin is thought to be photoprotective, whereas pheomelanin acts as a photosensitizer that contributes to the generation of reactive oxygen radicals when exposed to UVR.[49] Whether or not individuals with skin types I or II harbor loss of function mutations in their MC1R gene that render them more sensitive to the carcinogenic effects of UVR, is an important question that is being addressed by several investigative groups.

The first report on the presence of allelic variants in the human MC1R gene identified nine different point mutations. Eight of these variants were clustered in a region of 42 amino acids spanning the second transmembrane domain of MC1R.[67] This domain, together with the first extracellular loop, represents a critical region of the MC1R, since all of the three dominant gain-of-function mutations in the mouse involve missense mutations in this region.[19] The ninth variant, namely Asp249His, was located in the seventh transmembrane domain. In the above study, 60 unrelated British or Irish individuals were included, 30 had red hair and poor tanning response, and the remaining 30 had brown or black hair and a good tanning response. The above nine variants were found in over 80% of individuals with red hair and/or fair skin and a poor tanning response, and in fewer than 20% of individuals with brown or black hair. This gave the first clue that the *MC1R* gene-sequence variants might be associated with red hair color, fair skin and poor tanning ability, and thus possibly greater susceptibility to skin cancer.

In a subsequent study at the University Hospital in Portland, Oregon, in which a random group of 60 individuals with different skin and hair pigmentation were included, the presence of two *MC1R* gene-sequence variants was confirmed.[68] These were Val92Met and Asp84Glu. Four out of the 60 individuals had the Val 92Met allele, and three out of these four had skin type I, with blond hair and blue eyes. Two of these three were heterozygous, and one was homozygous for this allele. The fourth individual, who was heterozygous for this allele, had skin type II phenotype, with brown eyes and hair.

The significance of Val92Met allele on the function of the MC1R has been investigated. This change resulted in the generation of a *NSPI* restriction site, and unique restriction fragments of 359 and 724 base pairs.[68] Transfection of heterologous cells with the Val92Met MC1R allele did not cause a significant change in receptor function, as measured by stimulation of cAMP formation. In contrast, another study reported a reduction in the binding affinity for α-MSH in cells expressing Val92Met allele.[69] It is very likely that this variant is not a determinant of red hair, since it was expressed at a high frequency in Chinese individuals.[70]

In a study that was carried out in Australia on eight monozygotic twins with red hair and 17 dizygotic twins with one or both having red hair, a total of 12 amino acid substitutions at 11 different sites of the MC1R were identified.[70] Nine of these substitutions were novel variants that had not previously been described. Only some of the individuals with red haid expressed double variant haploids, namely Val92Met/Asp294His, Arg160Trp/Ala299Thr, Val92Met/Arg151Cys, and Val92Leu/Arg151Cys. None of the red-haired individuals had a wild-type MC1R genotype, and each was a homozygous or compound heterozygous variant. These results strongly suggest the association of MC1R variants with red hair.

More recently, a population study that included 102 Irish individuals, was carried out to identify existing MC1R gene variants and correlate these variants with hair color and skin type.[71] In the Irish population, eight variants were identified, three of which—Arg151Cys, Arg160Trp, and Asp294His—were over-represented in individuals with red hair. The presence of any variant, the Arg151Cys variant in particular, was significantly more common in individuals with a poor tanning ability and in individuals with freckles. In the same study, the Asp294His variant was examined in 95 Dutch individuals, including 33 individuals with red hair; and in 91 Swedish subjects, including 20 with red hair. This variant was found to be significantly more common in red-headed Dutch individuals, but not in red-headed Swedish individuals, compared to the respective control subjects from either country.

TABLE 1. List of the variants identified in the coding region of the MC1R gene

Ala 64 ser[67]	Val 60 Leu[70,71]
Phe 76 Tyr[67]	Arg 151 Cys[70,71]
Asp 84 Glu[67,70,71]	Ile 155 Thr[70,71]
Val 92 Met[67,70,71]	Arg 160 Trp[70,71]
Thr 95 Met[67]	Arg 163 Glu[70,71]
Val 97 Ile[67]	Hys 65 Asn[70]
Ala 103 Val[67]	Val 92 Leu[70]
Leu 106 Glu[67]	Arg 142 His[70]
Asp 294 His[67,70,71]	Ala 299 Thr[70]

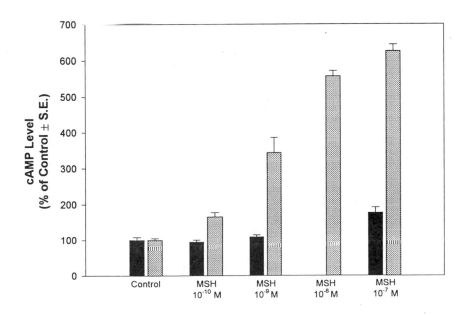

FIGURE 2. Dose-dependent effects of α-MSH on cAMP formation in responsive (*dotted bars*) and nonresponsive (*black bars*) human epidermal melanocytes. Melanocytes were treated with increasing concentrations of α-MSH ranging from 10^{-10} M to 10^{-7} M, for 40 minutes, in the presence of the phosphodiesterase inhibitor isobutyl methylxanthine. cAMP levels were determined by radioimmunoassay.

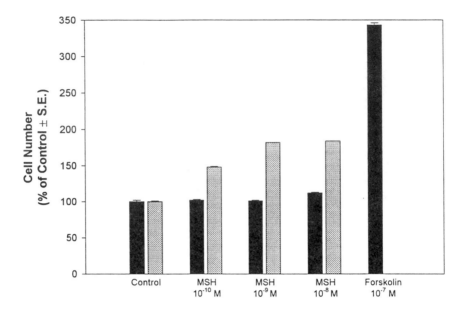

FIGURE 3. Dose-dependent effects of α-MSH on the proliferation of responsive (*dotted bars*) and nonresponsive (*black bars*) human epidermal melanocytes. Melanocytes were treated with 10^{-10}, 10^{-9}, or 10^{-8} M α-MSH; or 10^{-7} M forskolin every other day for a total of 6 days. Cell number was determined 48 hours after the final treatment with α-MSH or forskolin.

Unlike the previous studies in which the entire coding region of the MC1R gene was sequenced, in this study only the regions representing the first transmembrane domain/first intracellular loop/second transmembrane domain and intracellular loop were sequenced. This might have excluded possible mutations in other parts of the coding region that were not sequenced.

Based on the association of melanoma with skin type I phenotype, it was anticipated that *MC1R* gene variants would be over represented in melanoma patients. To determine whether or not this is the case, the frequency of MC1R variants in the second and seventh transmembrane domains was compared in 43 melanoma cases and 44 controls.[72] The results of this study showed that Asp84Glu variant was present only in melanoma cases, and was detected in 23% of the tumors tested. This and the studies described above suggest the possibility that the *MC1R* gene acts as a tumor susceptibility gene, and that allelic variants of this gene might be associated with red hair, poor tanning, and increased risk for skin cancers, including melanoma.[67,68,71,72]

So far, only the coding region of the *MC1R* gene has been analyzed, and the known variants are localized in this region (see TABLE 1). Virtually nothing is known about the regulatory region of this gene, or how any possible genetic alterations in this region might affect the expression and/or function of the MC1R. Also, little is known about the association of most of the variant *MC1R* alleles with the function

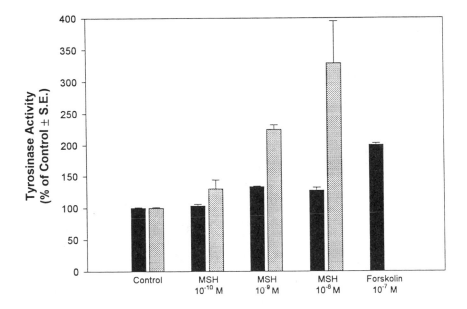

FIGURE 4. Dose-dependent effects of α-MSH on tyrosinase activity of responsive (*dotted bars*) and nonresponsive (*black bars*) human epidermal melanocytes. Melanocytes were treated with increased doses of α-MSH or 10^{-7} M forskolin for six days, as described in the legend for FIGURE 3. Tyrosinase activity was determined 48 hours after the final treatment, as described by Suzuki *et al.*[11]

of the MC1R. We speculate that some of these allelic variants represent polymorphisms that cause no significant change in the binding or signaling of the resulting MC1R. In one study, the Arg151Cys variant of MC1R was identified in a skin type I individual with red hair.[73] When expressed in heterologous cells, this variant MC1R was comparable to the wild-type MC1R in its binding affinity to α-MSH, but differed from the wild-type receptor in its inability to stimulate cAMP formation. Such studies are useful in delineating how a variant allele might perturb the function of MC1R. However, the use of heterologous cells to express the allelic variants of the *MC1R* gene might not be the same as the use of melanocytes, since these two cell types might differ in their intracellular milieu and in the regulatory genes that might affect the expression of *MC1R*.

We have been interested in comparing the responsiveness of cultured human melanocytes derived from different skin types to α-MSH. While comparing the responses in five cultures derived from very lightly pigmented skin (skin type I or type II donors), we found that one of these cultures had a significantly reduced response to α-MSH. Experiments aimed at determining the stimulation of cAMP formation, tyrosinase activity, and proliferation by α-MSH revealed that in this particular culture, there was a shift to the right in the dose-response curves (see FIGURES 2–4). Although the remaining four cultures demonstrated a significant response to α-MSH, commencing at a dose of 0.1 nM, only a minimal response was achieved upon treatment of the less responsiveness culture with 10 nM α-MSH. Genetic-sequencing of *MC1R* in this less responsive melanocyte culture, revealed the presence of a homozygous point mutation, namely Arg160Trp, which was previously reported in three independent studies.[67,70,71] Further studies are required to determine whether or not this and other allelic variants might influence the responsiveness of melanocytes to UVR, the extent of DNA damage, and/or DNA repair.

MELANOTROPINS, MC1R, AND OTHER PIGMENTARY HORMONES

There is increasing evidence for the existence of a paracrine/autocrine network in the human epidermis that regulates the survival and function of melanocytes, as well as their response to UVR.[6,62,63,74] Human melanocytes express receptors for a variety of growth factors and hormones.[11,40,64,75] Among these receptors, the MC1R seems to be a key regulator of the cAMP pathway that is pivotal for stimulating human melanocyte proliferation and melanogenesis.[11] We have reported that α-MSH interacts synergistically with other growth factors and hormones, such as endothelin-1 and basic fibroblast growth factor, to induce human melanocyte proliferation and melanogenesis.[64,76] Interestingly, endothelin-1 upregulates the expression of MC1R mRNA, and thus enhances the responsiveness of melanocytes to α-MSH and ACTH.[64] Furthermore, interleukin-1 and UVR have been shown to increase the synthesis of α-MSH and ACTH in human melanocytes and keratinocytes.[6] In turn, these two hormones increase the level of MC1R mRNA.[11] Other endocrine factors that are thought to regulate human pigmentation are the steroid hormones estrogen, progesterone, and testosterone.[77,78] The association of the cutaneous hyperpigmentation seen in melasma with pregnancy and sun exposure suggests the involvement of these steroid hormones, α-MSH and ACTH, in stimulation of melanogenesis. Further studies on the interactions of α-MSH and ACTH with steroid hormones, as well as with immune inflammatory cytokines, are needed in order to clarify the role of melanotropins and MC1R in cutaneous hyper- or hypopigmentation.

REFERENCES

1. EIPPER, B.A. & R.E. MAINS. 1980. Structure and biosynthesis of pro-adrenocorticotropin/endorphin and related peptides. Endocr. Rev. **1:** 1–27.
2. O'DONOHUE, T.L. & D.M. Dorsa. 1982. The opiomelanotropinergic neuronal and endocrine systems. Peptides **3:** 353–395.
3. THODY, A.J., K. RIDLEY, R.J. PENNY, R. CHALMERS, C. FISHER & S. SHUSTER. 1983. MSH peptides are present in mammalian skin. Peptides **4:** 813–816.
4. SCHAUER, E., F. TRAUTINGER, A. KOCK, A. SCHWARZ, R. BHARDWAJ, M. SIMON, J.C. ANSEL, T. SCHWARZ & T.A. LUGER. 1994. Proopiomelanocortin-derived peptides are synthesized and released by human keratinocytes. J. Clin. Invest. **93:** 2258–2262.
5. KIPPENBERGER, S., A. BERND, S. LOITSCH, A. RAMIREZ-BOSCA, J. BEREITER-HAHN & H. HOLZMANN. 1995. α-MSH is expressed in cultured human melanocytes and keratinocytes. Eur. J. Dermatol. **5:** 395–397.

6. CHAKRABORTY, A.K., Y. FUNASAKA, A. SLOMINSKI, G. ERMAK, J. HWANG, J.M. PAWELEK & M. ICHIHASHI. 1996. Production and release of proopiomelanocortin (POMC) derived peptides by human melanocytes and keratinocytes in culture: regulation by ultraviolet B. Biochim. Biophys. Acta **1313**: 130–138.

7. WAKAMATSU, K., A. GRAHAM, D. COOK & A.J. THODY. 1997. Characterisation of ACTH peptides in human skin and their activation of the melanocortin-1 receptor. Pigment Cell Res. **10**: 288–297.

8. HUNT, G., C. TODD, J.E. CRESSWELL & A.J. THODY. 1994. α-Melanocyte stimulating hormone and its analogue Nle^{4}DPhe$^7\alpha$-MSH affect morphology, tyrosinase activity and melanogenesis in cultured human melanocytes. J. Cell Sci. **107**: 205–211.

9. DE LUCA, M., W. SIEGRIST, S. BONDANZA, M. MATHOR, R. CANCEDDA & A.N. EBERLE. 1993. α-Melanocyte stimulating hormone (αMSH) stimulates normal human melanocyte growth by binding to high-affinity receptors. J. Cell Sci. **105**: 1079–1084.

10. ABDEL-MALEK, Z., V.B. SWOPE, I. SUZUKI, C. AKCALI, M.D. HARRIGER, S.T. BOYCE, K. URABE & V.J. HEARING. 1995. Mitogenic and melanogenic stimulation of normal human melanocytes by melanotropic peptides. Proc. Natl. Acad. Sci. USA **92**: 1789–1793.

11. SUZUKI, I., R. CONE, S. IM, J. NORDLUND & Z. ABDEL-MALEK. 1996. Binding capacity and activation of the MC1 receptors by melanotropic hormones correlate directly with their mitogenic and melanogenic effects on human melanocytes. Endocrinology **137**: 1627–1633.

12. SAWYER, T.K., V.J. HRUBY, M.E. HADLEY & M.H. ENGEL. 1983. α-Melanocyte stimulating hormone: Chemical nature and mechanism of action. Am. Zool. **23**: 529–540.

13. SHERBROOKE, W.C., M.E. HADLEY & A.M.L. CASTRUCCI. 1988. Melanotropic peptides and receptors: an evolutionary perspective in vertebrate physiologic color change. *In* Melanotropic Peptides, Vol. II. M.E. Hadley, Ed: 175–190. CRC Press. Washington.

14. PROTA, G. 1980. Recent advances in the chemistry of melanogenesis in mammals. J. Invest. Dermatol. **75**: 122–127

15. GESCHWIND, I.I. 1966. Change in hair color in mice induced by injection of alpha-MSH. Endocrinology **79**: 1165–1167

16. SILVERS, W.K., Ed. 1979. The Coat Colors of Mice. A Model for Mammalian Gene Action and Interaction. 6–44. Springer-Verlag. New York.

17. TAMATE, H.B. & T. TAKEUCHI. 1984. Action of the *e* locus of mice in the response of phaeomelanic hair follicles to α-melanocyte-stimulating hormone in vitro. Science **224**: 1241–1242.

18. TAKEUCHI, T., T. KOBUNAI & H. YAMAMOTO. 1989. Genetic control of signal transduction in mouse melanocytes. J. Invest. Dermatol. **92**: 239S–242S.

19. ROBBINS, L.S., J.H. NADEAU, K.R. JOHNSON, M.A. KELLY, L. ROSELLI-REHFUSS, E. BAACK, K.G. MOUNTJOY & R.D. CONE. 1993. Pigmentation phenotypes of variant extension locus alleles result from point mutations that alter MSH receptor function. Cell **72**: 827–834

20. WONG, G., J. PAWELEK, M. SANSONE & J. MOROWITZ. 1974. Response of mouse melanoma cells to melanocyte stimulating hormone. Nature **248**: 351–354.

21. FULLER, B.B., J.B. LUNSFORD & D.S. IMAN. 1987. Alpha-melanocyte-stimulating hormone regulation of tyrosinase in Cloudman S91 mouse melanoma cell cultures. J. Biol. Chem. **262**: 4024–4033.

22. BULTMAN, S.J., E.J. MICHAUD & R.P. WOYCHIK. 1992. Molecular characterization of the mouse agouti locus. Cell **71**: 1195–1204.

23. WILSON, B.D., M.M. OLLMANN, L. KANG, M. STOFFEL, G.I. BELL & G.S. BARSH. 1995. Structure and function of *ASP,* the human homolog of the mouse *agouti* gene. Hum. Mol. Genet. **4**: 223–230.

24. YEN, T.T., A.M. GILL, L.G. FRIGERI, G.S. BARSH & G.L. WOLFF. 1994. Obesity, diabetes, and neoplasia in yellow A^{vy}/-mice: Ectopic expression of the *agouti* gene. FASEB J. **8:** 479–488.

25. LU, D., D. WILLARD, I.R. PATEL, S. KADWELL, L. OVERTON, T. KOST, M. LUTHER, W. CHEN, R.P. WOYCHIK, W.O. WILKISON & R.D. CONE. 1994. Agouti protein is an antagonist of the melanocyte-stimulating-hormone receptor. Nature **371:** 799–802.

26. HUSZAR, D., C.A. LYNCH, V. FAIRCHILD-HUNTRESS, J.H. DUNMORE, Q. FANG, L.R. BERKEMEIER, W. GU, R.A. KESTERSON, B.A. BOSTON, R.D. CONE, F.J. SMITH, L.A. CAMPFIELD, P. BURN & F. LEE. 1997. Targeted disruption of the melanocortin-4 receptor results in obesity in mice. Cell **88:** 131–141.

27. BARSH, G.S. 1996. Genetics of pigmentation: From fancy genes to complex traits. Trends Genet. **12:** 299–305.

28. KRUDE, H. H. BIEBERMANN, W. LUCK, R. HORN, G. BRABANT & A. GRÜTERS. 1998. Severe early-onset obesity, adrenal insufficiency and red hair pigmentation caused by *POMC* mutations in humans. Nat. Genet. **19:** 155–157.

29. MOUNTJOY, K.G., L.S. ROBBINS, M.T. MORTRUD & R.D. CONE. 1992. The cloning of a family of genes that encode the melanocortin receptors. Science **257:** 1248–1251.

30. CHHAJLANI, V., R. MUCENIECE & J.E.S. WIKBERG. 1993. Molecular cloning of a novel human melanocortin receptor. Biochem. Biophys. Res. Commun. **195:** 866–873.

31. GANTZ, I., Y. KONDA, T. TASHIRO, Y. SHIMOTO, H. MIWA, G. MUNZERT, S.J. WATSON, J. DELVALLE & T. YAMADA. 1993. Molecular cloning of a novel melanocortin receptor. J. Biol. Chem. **268:** 8246–8250.

32. GANTZ, I., H. MIWA, Y. KONDA, Y. SHIMOTO, T. TASHIRO, S.J. WATSON, J. DELVALLE & T. YAMADA. 1993. Molecular cloning, expression, and gene localization of a fourth melanocortin receptor. J. Biol. Chem. **268:** 15174–15179.

33. ROSELLI-REHFUSS, L., K.G. MOUNTJOY, L.S. ROBBINS, M.T. MORTRUD, M.J. LOW, J.B. TATRO, M.L. ENTWISTLE, R.B. SIMERLY & R.D. CONE. 1993. Identification of a receptor for gamma-melanotropin and other proopiomelanocortin peptides in the hypothalamus and limbic system. Proc. Natl. Acad. Sci. USA **90:** 8856–8860.

34. LABBÉ, O., F. DESARNAUD, D. EGGERICKX, G. VASSART & M. PARMENTIER. 1994. Molecular cloning of a mouse melanocortin 5 receptor gene widely expressed in peripheral tissues. Biochem. **33:** 4543–4549.

35. FRIEDMANN, P.S., F. WREN, J. BUFFEY & S. MACNEIL. 1990. α-MSH causes a small rise in cAMP but has no effect on basal or ultraviolet-stimulated melanogenesis in human melanocytes. Br. J. Dermatol. **123:** 145–151.

36. HALABAN, R., L. TYRRELL, J. LONGLEY, Y. YARDEN & J. RUBIN. 1993. Pigmentation and proliferation of human melanocytes and the effects of melanocyte-stimulating hormone and ultraviolet B light. Ann. N.Y. Acad. Sci. **680:** 290–301.

37. LERNER, A.B. & J.S. MCGUIRE. 1961. Effect of alpha- and beta-melanocyte stimulating hormones on the skin colour of man. Nature **189:** 176–179.

38. LERNER, A.B. & J.S. MCGUIRE. 1964. Melanocyte-stimulating hormone and adrenocorticotrophic hormone. Their relation to pigmentation. N. Engl. J. Med. **270:** 539–546.

39. LEVINE, N., S.N. SHEFTEL, T. EYTAN, R.T. DORR, M.E. HADLEY, J.C. WEINRACH, G.A. ERTL, K. TOTH & V.J. HRUBY. 1991. Induction of skin tanning by the subcutaneous administration of a potent synthetic melanotropin. JAMA **266:** 2730–2736.

40. DONATIEN, P.D., G. HUNT, C. PIERON, J. LUNEC, A. TAÏEB & A.J. THODY. 1992. The expression of functional MSH receptors on cultured human melanocytes. Arch. Dermatol. Res. **284:** 424–426.

41. MARWAN, M.M., Z.A. ABDEL-MALEK, K.L. KREUTZFELD, A.M. CASTRUCCI, M.E. HADLEY, B.C. WILKES & V.J. HRUBY. 1985. Stimulation of S91 melanoma tyrosinase activity by superpotent α-melanotropins. Mol. Cell Endocrinol. **41:** 171–177.

42. MOUNTJOY, K.G. 1994. The human melanocyte stimulating hormone receptor has evolved to become "super-sensitive" to melanocortin peptides. Mol. Cell Endocrinol. **102:** R7–R11.

43. PATHAK, M.A., K. JIMBOW & T. FITZPATRICK. 1980. Photobiology of pigment cells. *In* Phenotypic Expression in Pigment Cells. M. Seiji, Ed.: 655–670. University of Tokyo Press, Tokyo.

44. JIMBOW, K., M.A. PATHAK & T.B. FITZPATRICK. 1973. Effect of ultraviolet on the distribution pattern of microfilaments and microtubules and on the nucleus in human melanocytes. Yale J. Biol. Med. **46:** 411–426.

45. SCOTT, G., L. CASSIDY & Z. ABDEL-MALEK. 1997. α-Melanocyte-stimulating hormone and endothelin-1 have opposing effects on melanocyte adhesion, migration, and pp125^{FAK} phosphorylation. Exp. Cell Res. **237:** 19–28.

46. HUNT, G., S. KYNE, S. ITO, K. WAKAMATSU, C. TODD & A.J. THODY. 1995. Eumelanin and pheomelanin contents of human epidermis and cultured melanocytes. Pigment Cell Res. **8:** 202–208.

47. HUNT, G., S. KYNE, K. WAKAMATSU, S. ITO & A.J. THODY. 1995. Nle^{4}DPhe^7 α-Melanocyte-stimulating hormone increases the eumelanin: Phaeomelanin ratio in cultured human melanocytes. J. Invest. Dermatol. **104:** 83–85.

48. PROTA, G., M.L. LAMOREUX, J. MULLER, T. KOBAYASHI, A. NAPOLITANO, M.R. VINCENSI, C. SAKAI & V.J. HEARING. 1995. Comparative analysis of melanins and melanosomes produced by various coat color mutants. Pigment Cell Res. **8:** 153–163.

49. MENON, A., A. PERSAD, N.S. RANADINE & H.F. HABERMAN. 1983. Effects of ultraviolet-visible radiation in the presence of melanin isolated from human black or red hair upon Ehrlich ascites carcinoma cells. Cancer Res. **43:** 3165–3169.

50. KOBAYASHI, N., A. NAKAGAWA, T. MURAMATSU, Y. YAMASHINA, T. SHIRAI, M.W. HASHIMOTO, Y. ISHIGAKI, T. OHNISHI & T. MORI. 1998. Supranuclear melanin caps reduce ultraviolet induced DNA photoproducts in human epidermis. J. Invest. Dermatol. **110:** 806–810.

51. BLANCHARD, S.G., C.O. HARRIS, O.R.R. ITTOOP, J.S. NICHOLS, D.J. PARKS, A.T. TRUESDALE & W.O. WILKISON. 1995. Agouti antagonism of melanocortin binding and action in the $B_{16}F_{10}$ murine melanoma cell line. Biochem. **34:** 10406–10411.

52. SIEGRIST, W., D.H. WILLARD, W.O. WILKISON & A.N. EBERLE. 1996. Agouti protein inhibits growth of B16 melanoma cells in vitro by acting through melanocortin receptors. Biochem. Biophys. Res. Commun. **218:** 171–175.

53. SUZUKI, I., A. TADA, M.M. OLLMANN, G.S. BARSH, S. IM, M.L. LAMOREUX, V.J. HEARING, J. NORDLUND & Z.A. ABDEL-MALEK. 1997. Agouti signaling protein inhibits melanogenesis and the response of human melanocytes to α-melanotropin. J. Invest. Dermatol. **108:** 838–842.

54. SIEGRIST, W., R. DROZDZ, R. COTTI, D.H. WILLARD, W.O. WILKISON & A.N. EBERLE. 1997. Interactions of α-melanotropin and agouti on B16 melanoma cells: evidence for inverse agonism of agouti. J. Recept. Signal Trans. Res. **17:** 75–98.

55. KOBAYASHI, T., W.D. VIEIRA, B. POTTERF, C. SAKAI, G. IMOKAWA & V.J. HEARING. 1995. Modulation of melanogenic protein expression during the switch from eu- to pheomelanogenesis. J. Cell Sci. **108:** 2301–2309.

56. PAWELEK, J.M., A.K. CHAKRABORTY, M.P. OSBER, S.J. ORLOW, K.K. MIN, K.E. ROSENZWEIG & J.L. BOLOGNIA. 1992. Molecular cascades in UV-induced melanogenesis: A central role for melanotropins? Pigment Cell Res. **5:** 348–356.

57. BOLOGNIA, J., M. MURRAY & J. PAWELEK. 1989. UVB-induced melanogenesis may be mediated through the MSH-receptor system. J. Invest. Dermatol. **92:** 651–656.
58. CHAKRABORTY, A., A. SLOMINSKI, G. ERINAK, J. HWANG & J. PAWELEK. 1995. Ultraviolet B and melanocyte stimulating hormone (MSH) stimulate mRNA production for α-MSH receptors and proopiomelanocortin-derived peptides in mouse melanoma cells and transformed keratinocytes. J. Invest. Dermatol. **105:** 655–659.
59. IM, S., O. MORO, F. PENG, E.E. MEDRANO, J. CORNELIUS, G. BABCOCK, J. NORDLUND & Z. ABDEL-MALEK. 1998. Activation of the cAMP pathway by α-melanotropin mediates the response of human melanocytes to UVB light. Cancer Res. **58:** 47–54.
60. BARKER, D., K. DIXON, E.E. MEDRANO, D. SMALARA, S. IM, D. MITCHELL, G. BABCOCK & Z.A. ABDEL-MALEK. 1995. Comparison of the responses of human melanocytes with different melanin contents to ultraviolet B irradiation. Cancer Res. **55:** 4041–4046.
61. ALTMEYER, P., L. STÖHR & H. HOLZMANN. 1986. Seasonal rhythm of the plasma level of alpha-melanocyte stimulating hormone. J. Invest. Dermatol. **86:** 454–456.
62. KUPPER, T.S., A.O. CHUA, P. FLOOD, J. MCGUIRE & U. GUBLER. 1987. Interleukin-1 gene expression in cultured human keratinocytes is augmented by ultraviolet irradiation. J. Clin. Invest. **80:** 430–436.
63. IMOKAWA, G., Y. YADA & M. MIYAGISHI. 1992. Endothelins secreted from human keratinocytes are intrinsic mitogens for human melanocytes. J. Biol. Chem. **267:** 24675–24680.
64. TADA, A., I. SUZUKI, S. IM, M.B. DAVIS, J. CORNELIUS, G. BABCOCK, J.J. NORDLUND & Z.A. ABDEL-MALEK. 1998. Endothelin-1 is a paracrine growth factor that modulates melanogenesis of human melanocytes and participated in their response to ultraviolet radiation. Cell Growth Differ. **9:** 575–584.
65. EPSTEIN, J.H. 1983. Photocarcinogenesis, skin cancer and aging. J. Am. Acad. Dermatol. **9:** 487–502.
66. PATHAK, M.A. 1995. Functions of melanin and protection by melanin. *In* Melanin: Its Role in Human Photoprotection. L. Zeise, M.R. Chedekel & T.B. Fitzpatrick, Eds.: 125–133. Valdenmar Publishing Company, Overland Park.
67. VALVERDE, P., E. HEALY, I. JACKSON, J.L. REES & A.J. THODY. 1995. Variants of the melanocyte-stimulating hormone receptor gene are associated with red hair and fair skin in humans. Nat. Genet. **11:** 328–330.
68. KOPPULA, S.V., L.S. ROBBINS, D. LU, E. BAACK, C.R. WHITE, JR., N.A. SWANSON & R.D. CONE. 1997. Identification of common polymorphisms in the coding sequence of the human MSH receptor (MC1R) with possible biological effects. Hum. Mutat. **9:** 30–36.
69. XU, X., M. THÖRNWALL, L.-G. LUNDIN & V. CHHAJLANI. 1996. Val92Met variant of the melanocyte stimulating hormone receptor gene. Nat. Genet. **14:** 384.
70. BOX, N.F., J.R. WYETH, L.E. O'GORMAN, N.G. MARTIN & R.A. STURM. 1997. Characterization of melanocyte stimulating hormone receptor variant alleles in twins with red hair. Hum. Mol. Genet. **6:** 1891–1897.
71. SMITH, R., E. HEALY, S. SIDDIQUI, N. FLANAGAN, P.M. STEIJLEN, I. ROSDAHL, J.P. JACQUES, S. ROGERS, R. TURNER, I.J. JACKSON, M.A. BIRCH-MACHIN & J.L. REES. 1998. Melanocortin 1 receptor variants in Irish population. J. Invest. Dermatol. **111:** 119–122.
72. VALVERDE, P., E. HEALY, S. SIKKINK, F. HALDANE, A.J. THODY, A. CAROTHERS, I.J. JACKSON & J.L. REES. 1996. The Asp84Glu variant of the melanocortin 1 receptor (*MC1R*) is associated with melanoma. Hum. Mol. Genet. **5:** 1663–1666.

73. FRÄNDBERG, P.-A., M. DOUFEXIS, S. KAPAS & V. CHHAJLANI. 1998. Human pigmentation phenotype: A point mutation generates nonfunctional MSH receptor. Biochem. Biophys. Res. Commun. **245:** 490–492.
74. HALABAN, R., R. LANGDON, N. BIRCHALL, C. CUONO, A. BAIRD, G. SCOTT, G. MOELLMANN & J. MCGUIRE. 1988. Basic fibroblast growth factor from human keratinocytes is a natural mitogen for melanocytes. J. Cell Biol. **107:** 1611–1619.
75. PITTELKOW, M.R. & G.D. SHIPLEY. 1989. Serum-free culture of normal human melanocytes: Growth kinetics and growth factor requirements. J. Cell. Physiol. **140:** 565–576.
76. SWOPE, V.B., E.E. MEDRANO, D. SMALARA & Z. ABDEL-MALEK. 1995. Long-term proliferation of human melanocytes is supported by the physiologic mitogens α-melanotropin, endothelin-1, and basic fibroblast growth factor. Exp. Cell Res. **217:** 453–459.
77. SNELL, R.S. 1964. Effect of the alpha melanocyte-stimulating hormone of the pituitary on mammalian epidermal melanocytes. J. Invest. Dermatol. **42:** 337–347.
78. WILSON, M.J. & E. SPAZIANI. 1976. The melanogenic response to testosterone in scrotal epidermis; the effects on tyrosinase activity and protein synthesis. Acta Endocrin. **81:** 435-448.

Genetic Studies of the Human Melanocortin-1 Receptor

JONATHAN L. REES,[a] MARK BIRCH-MACHIN, NIAMH FLANAGAN,
EUGENE HEALY, SIÔN PHILLIPS, AND CAROLE TODD

*Department of Dermatology, Medical School, Framlington Place,
Newcastle-upon-Tyne NE1 4LP, United Kingdom*

ABSTRACT: Genetic approaches have suggested a critical role for the melanocortin-1 receptor in the control of pigmentation. We showed that this gene is unusually polymorphic in European populations and that, of the many variants, three in particular appear to be associated with red hair or fair skin. Family studies suggest these are inherited as an autosomal recessive trait (or at least approximate to this in many families). To date all individuals with two of these three changes (homozygote or compound heterozygote) have red hair. Early functional studies are in keeping with defective signalling through MC1R. An interested and perhaps unexpected question relates to the evolutionary factors that have given rise to such variants. Two models can be proposed, that are based on multiple alleles with minor changes in function or genetic hitch-hiking.

There are at least two good reasons for being interested in the genetics of human pigmentation. First, pigmentation is perhaps the main world-wide determinant of both melanoma and nonmelanoma skin cancer. One can consider the causes of skin cancer as being primarily either genetic or environmental: both views are in reality correct, since the effects of a particular environment, or of a particular gene, are contingent on each other.[1–3] For instance, within a relatively homogeneous genetic population such as that in the UK, or among those Anglo-Saxons who migrated to Australia, differences in ambient ultraviolet exposure and associated lifestyle account for most of the differences in nonmelanoma skin cancer rates. By contrast, between the original inhabitants of Australia and the later, predominantly Anglo-Saxon, invaders, the large — perhaps up to 100-fold—difference in skin cancer rates is mainly genetic, and probably accounted for in terms of differences in pigmentation. (One should add, for completeness, that pigment is only one method of physiological adaptation to ultraviolet radiation. Very little is know about the genetics of the other method, namely that of epidermal thickening.[4])

A second reason for interest in the genetics of pigmentation is that variation in pigmentation is one of the most polymorphic human characteristics. Variation in cutaneous characteristics have been of profound social and cultural importance; arguably they have perhaps exerted more influence on human history than even infectious diseases. Why do humans from different regions vary so much in appearance? Can these differences in pigmentation be accounted for in terms of evolutionary fitness,

[a]Address for correspondence: +44 191 222 8936 (voice); +44 191 222 7094 (fax); jonathan.rees@ncl.ac.uk (e-mail).

because of the physical environment, or are there other more conscious factors at work?

Pigmentation of humans can be viewed as either facultative or constitutive. The latter is reflected by the degree and type of pigmentation in sun protected sites, whereas the former is the result of exposure to repeated ultraviolet exposure. There does seem to be a large covariance between these states: in general, those with high constitutive pigmentation develop further pigmentation in response to ultraviolet radiation and to a greater degree than those with low or particular types of constitutive pigmentation. Obviously pigmentation cannot be simply viewed as unidimensional; thus, there are different types of pigment between individuals rather than just differences in the absolute amount. For instance, and of relevance to this paper, alterations in the amount, or in the ratio, of the two major pigment types, eumelanin (black) and phaeomelanin (red or yellow), determine whether the individual has red hair or not. However, this axis of control does not explain differences between blond and dark haired individuals.

Skin pigmentation and hair color is genetically complex. In other words, most aspects of the phenotype do not follow a simple Mendelian pattern and we consider that a large number of loci influence these characteristics. This is not to deny that mutations at some loci can result in a phenotype that behaves as a Mendelian recessive—for example, many types of albinism;[5,6] but rather, that to try and explain the variation between the majority of members of a population requires more complex models of gene action.

Given the complexity of cutaneous pigmentation, one successful strategy has relied on comparative genetic approaches, using discoveries in the more experimentally tractable mouse as a basis for restricted studies in man.[5,7,8] Studies of the role of the melanocortin-1 receptor, and the role of mutations at this locus in causing red hair, provide one such example.

MURINE COAT COLOR

A large number (> 50) of loci are known to be involved in the control of coat color in the mouse.[8,9] Two particular loci have attracted considerable attention recently, *extension* and *agouti*. Loss of function mutants at the *extension* locus result in mice with yellow hair, whereas dominant gain of function mutants show black hair. Conversely, wild-type *agouti* mice show a subapical band of yellow hair against a darker background, and overexpression of the agouti product results in yellow-haired mice.[8,9] The cloning of the melanocortin-1 receptor (MC1R) by two independent groups, has allowed mechanistic insight into these changes and has provided a candidate for red hair in man (red in man can be considered analogous to yellow in the mouse).[10,11]

CLONING THE MELANOCORTIN-1 RECEPTOR

Two groups, using degenerate primers for conserved sequences in G-coupled proteins, identified a cDNA for what subsequently turned out to be the melanocortin-1 receptor (MC1R) (reviewed by Cone, see Refs. 12 and 13). The MC1R was subsequently shown to map to the *extension* locus. The human MC1R is a 317-amino-acid, seven-pass transmembrane, G-coupled receptor that signals by modulation of cAMP. In the mouse, at least, the natural ligand for this receptor is αMSH, a tridecapeptide cleavage product of POMC. ACTH is apparently also able to act through this receptor, but its chief receptor is MC2R, which shows a very different pattern of expression from MC1R, and whose major function is in the regulation of corticosteroid secretion from the adrenal cortex. The expression pattern of MC1R, which is expressed on melanocytes and other epidermal cells, is compatible with its physiological role in pigmentation.[12,13]

αMSH acts through the receptor to increase the ratio of eumelanin to phaeomelanin, thus resulting in a dark rather than red/yellow phenotype. By contrast, agouti acts as an inverse agonist with the result that it has opposite physiological effects to those of αMSH at the MC1R.[14] Agouti is produced in paracrine manner by other cells in the dermal papilla to exert effects on the MC1R of the melanocyte. One could, therefore, envisage, with varying degrees of likelihood, either POMC products, MC1R or agouti as candidates for red hair in man.

THE MC1R AS A CANDIDATE GENE FOR RED HAIR

The cloning of the human MC1R, and previous work in the mouse, together with experiments showing a pigmentary action of αMSH in man,[15,16] all suggested that the MC1R was a candidate gene for red hair. Indeed this hypothesis was implicit, if not explicit, in the paper from Cone's group.[17] In order to examine this hypothesis, we originally performed a case control study, sequencing only limited parts of MC1R.[18] The choice of a case control design may have been important. Given the complex nature of pigmentation, this approach has greater statistical power than does linkage–based approaches. We initially compared the MC1R sequence in individuals with red hair, and with a strong family history of red hair and pale skin, with those of individuals who did not possess the traits. A number of findings were of immediate interest. First, variation in MC1R was extremely common, with subsequent studies showing that over 75% of the UK population harbour coding region variants.[19] Second, some of these variants appeared to be more common in individuals with red hair (for instance the D294H).[18–20] Third, without further clarification of the functional status of particular variants, it was difficult to determine the mode of inheritance.[18,20] This is because, in many individuals with red hair, there was more than one variant on a particular allele and although many, if not most, individuals with red hair showed variants on both alleles, some did not.

SOME METHODOLOGIC PROBLEMS

Although our initial study suggested a role for this locus in determining human hair color, it had a number of limitations.[18] Assessment of phenotype was rudimentary, cloning out alleles to allow haplotype analysis was only performed in a few cases, and the entire gene was not sequenced. We therefore extended this work to

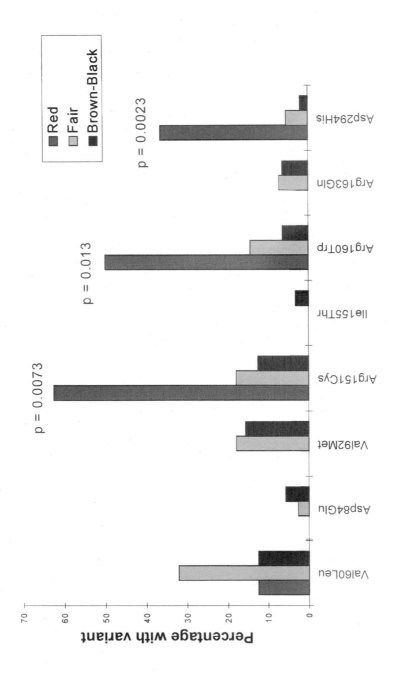

FIGURE 1. Results of population study ($n = 100$ showing a relation between possession of certain MC1R alleles and hair color (red, fair, or brown-black). Note the high relative risks for alleles ARG151Cys, Arg160Trp, and Asp294His and individuals with red hair.

include a population based study and family studies; subsequently sequencing a large number of alleles.[19]

A population based study conducted in Ireland showed that three particular variants of MC1R (R151C, R160W, and D294H) are strongly associated with red hair, each with a relative risk of 8–15 (see FIGURE 1).[19] Thus, although 75% of the population harbour at least one coding region variant, and 30% show two variants. On the basis of this study, most of the variants are not causally associated with red hair.[19] A point of caution is necessary: testing the effects of rare alleles will have little significance in a study of only 100 individuals. Of the 13 red-haired (or auburn) individuals, eight were homozygous or compound heterozygous for the R151C, R160W, and D294H changes. Conversely, in this study, every individual with this genotype had red hair (although we have subsequently identified this genotype without red hair, but very rarely). Some red-haired persons did however only show a change on one allele. A relation was also seen between the ability to tan and the possession of freckles.[19]

Ongoing family studies are in keeping with these results. We have now screened over 220 individuals from eight families with an index case of red hair. These families contain over 70 individuals with red hair. In most instances, the trait appears to follow an approximately autosomal recessive pattern, in that about 85% of the red-haired individuals are homozygotes, or compound heterozygotes, for the R151C, R160W, and D294H changes. This, at a descriptive level, is in keeping with a body of older literature suggesting that the red-hair trait, although not perfectly autosomal recessive, is close to one.[21–24] We have found two families of particular interest. In one such family we are unable to find any of the changes we observed in other individuals with red hair. Although, given the size of the family and potential penetrance

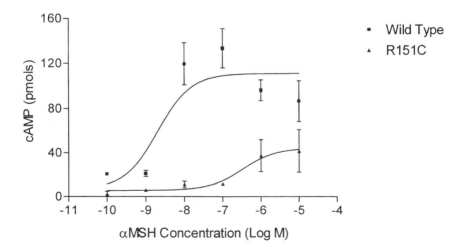

FIGURE 2. Functional expression of human Mc1R in human embryonic kidney cells. *Data points* indicate the mean of duplicate incubations and *bars* indicate SEM. Data has been normalised for cell number.

estimates for MC1R, it is not possible to exclude the locus. Sturm's group, in a twin study, also showed that siblings, identical by descent for MC1R, could possess different hair color; and more recently a family with red hair and a variety of gross endocrine abnormalities that are secondary to a mutation in the POMC gene, have been described.[20] The family we have identified is, however, phenotypically otherwise normal. In one other family, changes at codon 142 of MC1R seem to be associated with red hair, although since this allele is uncommon in the general population it has been impossible to test in a population study.

Our early and limited functional studies are in keeping with the suggested role of the R151C, R160W, and D294H changes. Frändberg has suggested that the R151C variant is functionally defective in signalling through cAMP.[25] Using transient transfection of A293 cells, we have found similar results for this change and the R160W, and for the D294H, although our results for the later two alleles are still preliminary and require confirmation (see FIGURE 2).

THE MC1R AND SKIN CANCER

Given the relation between skin type and both melanoma and nonmelanoma skin cancer, it is not surprising that overrepresentation of particular MC1R alleles occurs in the case of skin cancer. In nonmelanoma skin cancer this is indeed the case, at least with respect to the D294H allele.[19] It is easy to explain this relation on the basis of sun phototype.[19] By contrast we have reported that other alleles, including Asp84Glu, are associated with melanoma.[26] Here, interpretation is not so straightforward. First, this effect has not been seen in subsequent studies[27] (or in our own unpublished results). Therefore, the effect may represent a confounding of differences between controls and cases. Alternatively, because of the large number of alleles screened, the original result may stem from statistical artefacts due to multiple testing. Second, interpretation of any putative relation between MC1R and melanoma is hard to interpret. This is because, as with nonmelanoma skin cancer, melanoma is more common in those with fair skin, but there is also evidence that αMSH may act as a growth factor for melanocytes and, therefore, influence tumour development via this route. Our guess is that the magnitude of any effect between particular alleles and tumours will be lower for melanoma than for nonmelanoma skin cancer.

POPULATION STUDIES OF THE MC1R

The high coding diversity of MC1R may mean that the gene will be of interest, not only to pigment biologists and dermatologists, but also to population biologists and geneticists. Our unpublished studies show extensive coding region diversity in Northern European Caucasian populations. As could be expected, the changes associated with red hair (R151C, R160W, and D294H) are rarely, if ever, found in other populations, such as Africans, Japanese, Eskimos, and Melanesians. We do however find these changes in red-haired individuals from different parts of Northern Europe. Whether changes, other than those identified as being functionally significant, are more common awaits study, but this would of importance in attempting to understand evolution at this locus and human migration in the recent evolutionary past. Our early results do, however, suggest increased coding differences in MC1R in European populations for changes other than those associated with red hair, and for nonsynonymous changes. These studies may cast light on the selective pressures that have led to development of the red-hair–phenotype and pale skin. The standard explanation for the development of the pale-skin–phenotype in Northern Europe is that there is selection against dark skin in places where levels of ambient UVR are low.[28] UVR is required for vitamin D synthesis in the skin, and if the diet is poor in vitamin D, as is the case if the diet is predominantly cereal based, then rickets will result.[29] Whether red-hair can be viewed as an extension of the pale-skin–phenotype is not clear. Alternative explanations are related to sexual or social selection—explanations that have been convincingly argued for other geographical patterns of skin color distribution.[30,31]

One particular interesting question relates to heterozygote effect. The frequency of red-hair-alleles perhaps argues for a heterozygote effect. Is this compatible with our proposed recessive model of red hair based on family studies? Reanalysis of the population data carried out in Ireland, together with examination of subjects in the United Kingdom does indeed suggest that, with respect to tanning ability, there is a heterozygote effect. These questions and studies highlight the inadequacies of our phenotyping ability. Thus, although we have used hair charts, these are extremely crude, as is questioning about behavior in the sun. For instance, the original Fitzpatrick questionnaire has a low reproducibility.[32] Thus, that the red hair trait as defined may approximate to an autosomal recessive, is not incompatible with a heterozygote effect of some aspects of pigmentary status. There are other factors that now also need to be considered. Although, in general, red-haired individuals have pale skin, there is considerable heterogeneity within the red-haired group. Conversely, there are individuals with dark or black hair who have pale skin. What are the frequencies of the R151C, R160W, and D294H in this group? It is also clear that hair color can vary considerably throughout life, and with body site. In the mouse, body site variation may be accounted for in terms of differences in agouti expression.[33] Is this also the case in man?

We would argue that detailed genetic analysis is going to be hindered until quantitative measures are used for both hair color and cutaneous response to ultraviolet radiation. For instance HPLC analysis of phaeomelanin and eumelanin, or spectroscopic analysis, could be carried out.[34,35] With respect to the cutaneous response to UVR, whereas development of erythema after single exposure to UVR is inadequate, quantitative measures such as transmission of UVR, or again assessment of eumelanin and phaeomelanin after repeated experimental radiation, seem likely to increase our ability to define phenotype. Certainly these quantitative techniques offer a great opportunity to study the physiology of gene action, and the interrelation between genotype and the environment, quantitatively in man.

ACKNOWLEDGMENTS

Our work on this topic was supported by grants from the Leech Trust, MRC, CRC, and Department of Health (UK). We also acknowledge our collaborators Dr. Ian Jackson, M.R.C. H.G.U. and Dr. Rosalind Harding, M.R.C. Molecular Haematology Unit, I.M.M., Oxford.

REFERENCES

1. ARMSTRONG, B.K. & B. KRICKER. 1996. Epidemiology of non-melanoma skin cancer. *In* Skin Cancer. I.M. Leigh, J.A. Newton Bishop & M.L. Kripke, Eds.: 89–114. ICRF, Cold Spring Harbour Press.
2. GALLAGHER, R.P. & V.C. HO. 1998. Environmental and host risk factors. *In* Epidemiology, Causes and Prevention of Skin Diseases. J.J. Grob, R.S. Stern, R.M. MacKie & M.A. Weinstock, Eds.: 235–242. Blackwell.
3. MARKS, R. 1995. An overview of skin cancers: Incidence and causation. Cancer, **75:** Suppl. 607–612.
4. PATHAK, M.A. & T.B. FITZPATRICK. 1974. Sunlight and Man. 725. University of Tokyo Press, Tokyo.
5. STURM, R.A., N.F. BOX & M. RAMSAY. 1998. Human Pigmentation genetics: the difference is only skin deep. Bioessays. **20**(9): 712–721.
6. HEARING, V.J., W.S. OETTING, D.J. CREEL & R.A. KING. Albinism. 1997. *In* Metabolic and Molecular Basis of Inherited Diseases. C.R. Scriver, A.L. Beaudet, W.S. Sly & D. Valle, Eds.: CD-ROM Version. McGraw-Hill, New York.
7. JACKSON, I.J. 1991. Mouse coat colour mutations: a molecular genetic resource which spans the centuries. Bioessays **13**: 439–446.
8. JACKSON, I.J. 1994. Molecular and developmental genetics of mouse coat color. Annu. Rev. Genet. **28**: 189–217.
9. BARSH, G.S. 1996. The genetics of pigmentation: from fancy genes to complex traits. Trends. Genet. **12**(8): 299–305.
10. CHHAJLANI, V. & J.E. WIKBERG. 1992. Molecular cloning and expression of the human melanocyte stimulating hormone receptor cDNA. FEBS Lett. **309**: 417–420.
11. MOUNTJOY, K.G., L.S. ROBBINS, M.T. MORTRUD & R.D. CONE. 1992. The cloning of a family of genes that encode the melanocortin receptors. Science **257**: 1248–1251.
12. CONE, R.D., D. LU, S. KOPPULA, D.I. VAGE, H. KLUNGLAND, B. BOSTON, W. CHEN, D.N. ORTH, C. POUTON & R.A. KESTERSON. 1996. The melanocortin receptors: agonists, antagonists, and the hormonal control of pigmentation. Rec. Prog. Horm. Res. **51**: 287–317.
13. LU, D., W. CHEN & R.D. CONE. 1998. Regulation of melanogenesis by the MSH receptor. *In* The Pigmentary System: Physiology and Pathophysiology. J.J. Nordlund, R.E. Boissy, V.J. Hearing, R.A. King & J.P. Ortonne, Eds.: 183–198. Oxford, New York.
14. OLLMANN, M.M., M.L LAMOREUX, B.D. WILSON & G.S. BARSH. 1998. Interaction of agouti protein with the melanocortin 1 receptor *in vitro* and *in vivo*. Genes Dev. **12**: 316–330.
15. Lerner, A.B. 1993. The discovery of the melanotropins. Ann. N.Y. Acad. Sci. **680**: 1–12.
16. LERNER, A.B. & J.S. MCGUIRE. 1998. Effect of alpha and beta-melanocyte stimulating hormones on the skin colour of man. Nature **189**: 176–179.
17. ROBBINS, L.S., J.H. NADEAU, K.R. JOHNSON, M.A. KELLY, L. ROSELLI-REHFUSS, E. BAACK, K.G MOUNTJOY & R.D. CONE. 1993. Pigmentation phenotypes of variant extension locus alleles result from point mutations that alter MSH receptor function. Cell **72**: 827–834.
18. VALVERDE, P., E. HEALY, I. JACKSON, J.L. REES & A.J. THODY. 1995. Variants of the melanocyte-stimulating hormone receptor gene are associated with red hair and fair skin in humans. Nature Genet. **11**: 328–330.
19. SMITH, R., E. HEALY, S. SIDDIQUI, N. FLANAGAN, P.M. STEIJLEN, I. ROSDAHL, J.P. JACQUES, S. ROGERS, R. TURNER, I.J. JACKSON, M.A. BIRCH-MACHIN & J.L REES. 1998. Melanocortin 1 receptor variants in an Irish population. J. Invest. Dermatol. **111**: 119–122.

20. BOX, N.F., J.R. WYETH, L.E. O'GORMAN, N.G. MARTIN & R.A. STURM. 1997. Characterization of melanocyte stimulating hormone receptor variant alleles in twins with red hair. Hum. Mol. Genet. **6:** 1891–1897.
21. SINGLETON, W.R. & B. ELLIS. 1964. Inheritance of red hair for six generations. J. Heredity **55:** 261–261.
22. MICHELSON, N. 1934. Distribution of red hair according to age. American J. Phys. Anthropology **18:** 407–413.
23. NEEL, J.V. 1943. Concerning the inheritance of red hair. J. Heredity **34:** 93–96.
24. REED, T.E. 1952. Red hair colour as a genetical character. Ann. Eugenics **20:** 312–320.
25. FRÄNDBERG, P.A., M. DOUFEXIS, S. KAPAS & V. CHHAJLANI. 1998. Human pigmentation phenotype: A point mutation generates nonfunctional MSH receptor. Biochem. Biophys. Res. Commun. **245:** 490–492.
26. VALVERDE, P., E. HEALY, S. SIKKINK, F. HALDANE, A.J. THODY, A. CAROTHERS, I.J. JACKSON & J.L REES. 1996. The Asp84Glu variant of the melanocortin 1 receptor (MC1R) is associated with melanoma. Hum. Mol. Genet. **5:** 1663–1666.
27. ICHII-JONES, F., J.T. LEAR, A.H.M HEAGERTY, A.G. SMITH, P.E. HUTCHINSON, J. OSBORNE, B. BOWERS, P.W. JONES, E. DAVIES, W.E.R. OLLIER, W. THOMSON, L YENGI, J. BATH, A.A. FRYER & R.C. STRANGE, 1998. Susceptibility to melanoma: Influence of skin type and polymorphism in the melanocyte stimulating hormone receptor gene. J. Invest. Dermatol. **111:** 218–221.
28. BODMER, W.F. & L.L. CAVALLI-SFORZA. 1976. Genetics, Evolution and Man. W.H. Freeman, San Fransisco.
29. LOOMIS, W.F. 1967. Skin-pigment regulation of vitamin-D biosynthesis in man. Science **157:** 501–506.
30. DIAMOND, J.M. 1994. Race without color. Discovery (November) 83–89.
31. KINGDON, J. 1993. Self-Made Man. Simon and Schuster, London.
32. RAMPEN, F.H., B.A. FLEUREN, T.M. DE BOO & W.A. LEMMENS, 1988. Unreliability of self-reported burning tendency and tanning ability. Arch. Dermatol. **124:** 885–888.
33. VRIELING, H., D.M. DUHL, S.E. MILLAR, K.A. MILLER & G.S. BARSH. 1994. Differences in dorsal and ventral pigmentation result from regional expression of the mouse agouti gene. Proc. Nat. Acad. Sci. USA **91:** 5667–5671.
34. ITO, S. 1998. Advances in chemical analysis of melanins. *In* The Pigmentary System: Physiology and Pathophysiology. J.J. Nordlund, R.E. Boissy, V.J. Hearing, R.A. King & J.P. Ortonne, Eds.: 439-450. Oxford, New York.
35. OZEKI, H., S. ITO, K. WAKAMATSU & A.J. THODY. 1996. Spectrophotometric characterization of eumelanin and pheomelanin in hair. Pigment Cell Res. **9:** 265–270.

Molecular Pharmacology of Agouti Protein
in Vitro and *in Vivo*

GREGORY S. BARSH,[a] MICHAEL M. OLLMANN, BRENT D. WILSON,
KIMBERLY A. MILLER, AND TERESA M. GUNN

*Departments of Pediatrics and Genetics, and the Howard Hughes Medical Institute,
Stanford University School of Medicine, Stanford, California, USA*

ABSTRACT: Agouti protein and Agouti-related protein (Agrp) are paracrine
signaling molecules that act by antagonizing the effects of melanocortins, and
several alternatives have been proposed to explain their mechanisms of action.
Genetic crosses in a sensitized background uncover a phenotypic difference
between overexpression of Agouti and loss of Mc1r function, demonstrate that
a functional Mc1r is required for the pigmentary effects of Agouti, and suggest
that Agouti protein can act as an agonist of the Mc1r in a way that differs
from α-MSH stimulation. *In vitro*, Agouti protein inhibits melanocortin action
by two mechanisms: competitive antagonism that depends on the carboxy-
terminus of the protein, and downregulation of melanocortin receptor signaling that depends on the aminoterminus. Our findings provide evidence of a
novel signaling mechanism whereby α-MSH and Agouti protein function as independent ligands that inhibit each other's binding and transduce opposite signals through a single receptor.

INTRODUCTION

The genetics of mouse coat color offers a model system for studying gene action
and interaction. There are nearly 100 known, or so-called classical, coat color mutations; many of which have been cloned and characterized.[1,2] The relative accessibility of skin and hair to experimental manipulation allows one to determine the cell
type in which a particular gene is required. Finally, the ability to generate and analyze double mutants permits the construction of a genetic framework to build biochemical and cell-biologic pathways.

Studies carried out in our laboratory and those of others over the past decade have
demonstrated that the mouse *Agouti* gene represents the fulcrum for a new signaling
pathway in which independent ligands, the Agouti protein and melanocortin peptides, inhibit each other's binding and transduce opposite signals through a single receptor.[3–10] In what follows, we review briefly the molecular genetics of Agouti
protein and Agouti-related protein (Agrp), highlight recent studies from our laboratory that bear on their biochemical mechanism of action, and present data that implicate additional gene products in Agouti and melanocortin receptor signaling.

[a]Address for Correspondence: Greg Barsh, Beckman Center B271A, Stanford University
School of Medicine, Stanford, CA 94305-5323, USA. 650-723-5035 (voice); 650-723-1399
(fax); gbarsh@cmgm.stanford.edu (e-mail).

MOLECULAR GENETICS OF AGOUTI AND
AGOUTI-RELATED PROTEIN

The *Agouti* gene takes its name from the native language of a South American Indian tribe where these rodents, also know as the Paca, exhibit a stereotypic coat color pattern in which individual hairs display a subapical band of yellow pigment on an otherwise black background. This pattern develops dynamically during the anagen phase of hair growth, when melanocytes at the base of each follicle briefly switch from synthesizing black pigment, so-called eumelanin, to yellow pigment (pheomelanin), then back to eumelanin again as anagen hair growth is completed.[11] Most *Agouti* alleles affect only hair color, but several have dominant pleiotropic effects that include a completely yellow coat, obesity, increased linear growth, premature infertility, and immune abnormalities.[12,13] The prototype for obesity-associated *Agouti* alleles, *lethal yellow* (A^y), is one of the oldest known mouse mutations. It differs from other obesity-associated *Agouti* alleles in that homozygosity for A^y causes embryonic death around the time of implantation.[5,14]

Agouti alleles associated with yellow pigment production are generally dominant to those associated with black pigment production. The dominant-recessive relationships apply to individual hair follicles and not the entire animal. For example, *black-and-tan* (a^t/a^t) mice, which have yellow ventral hairs and black dorsal hairs, crossed with *Agouti* (*A/A*) mice, which have banded hairs on both ventrum and dorsum, produce A/a^t mice, which have yellow ventral hairs and banded dorsal hairs—the so-called light-bellied Agouti phenotype. The genetic relationships between different *Agouti* alleles suggest that production of black pigment was a "default" state in which Agouti protein activate yellow pigment synthesis.[1] In addition, elegant transplanation studies carried out by Silvers and colleagues more than thirty years ago[15,16] indicate that *Agouti* caused cells in the dermis to release a paracrine molecule that act on nearby melanocytes in the epidermal portion of hair follicles.

These predictions from early genetic and embryologic studies were confirmed when *Agouti* was cloned and found to encode a 131-amino-acid secreted protein in which two domains were predicted: a basic region of approximately 60 amino acids and a cysteine-rich carboxy-terminal region of approximately 40 amino acids[17,18] (see FIGURE 1). Expression of *Agouti* RNA is normally limited to dermal papillae cells and its timing correlates with the synthesis of yellow pigment; i.e. follicles with banded hairs express *Agouti* RNA at postnatal days 4–7, midway through anagen, whereas follicles with hairs that are completely yellow express *Agouti* RNA throughout the entire hair growth cycle.[19,20] Transgenic studies confirmed that *Agouti* had a very limited sphere of action, possibly because the highly charged amino-terminus limited diffusion through the extracellular matrix (FIG. 1). Surprisingly, A^y and other obesity-associated *Agouti* alleles were found to be caused by genomic rearrangements leading to ubiquitous expression of one or more transcripts predicted to encode the normal open reading frame.[5,6,21] The ability of Agouti protein to elicit nonpigmentary phenotypes in alleles such as A^y is likely explained by the recent discovery of Agrp, whose RNA is expressed mainly in the hypothalamus and the adrenal gland.[3,4] Although Agrp exhibits less than 20% identity with Agouti protein overall, it has the exact same size and genomic structure, and a nearly identical spacing of cysteine residues in the carboxy terminus (FIG. 1).

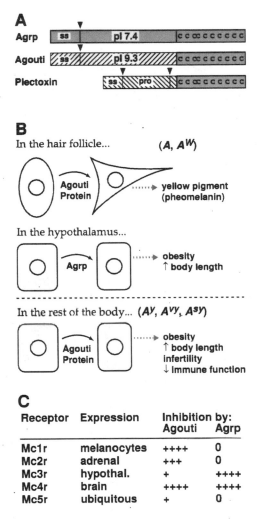

FIGURE 1. Molecular genetics and pharmacology of Agouti and Agrp. **A.** Agouti protein and Agrp are of identical size and exon structure, but primary sequence similarity between the two protein is restricted to the cysteine-rich carboxy-terminal region, where there are 10 cysteines with a characteristic pattern of spacing that is also found in plectoxins. Agouti, Agrp, and plectoxins have a cleavable signal sequence; however, plectoxins undergo additional processing at the amino- and carboxy-termini to yield the cysteine-rich segment as the active molecule *in vivo*. **B.** In most animals, expression of Agouti protein is restricted to the hair follicle where it causes melanocytes to produce yellow pigment via a paracrine mechanism. In mutant animals carrying A^y or similar mutations, ubiquitous expression of transcripts that encode a normal Agouti protein cause pleiotropic effects due to the ability of Agouti protein to mimic Agrp. **C.** Comparison of Agouti protein to Agrp in their ability to inhibit α-MSH-induced accumulation of cAMP shows that Agouti protein is a potent antagonist of the human Mc1r, Mc2r, and Mc4r, but has little effect on the Mc3r or Mc5r. By contrast, Agrp is a potent antagonist only at the Mc3r and Mc4r. Experiments supporting these findings are described in References 3, 17, and 21.

BIOCHEMICAL MECHANISM OF AGOUTI SIGNALING

The similarity in cysteine spacing between Agouti protein and Agrp is also shared by plectoxins and, to a lesser extent, omega-conotoxins, that are used by primitive hunting spiders and cone snails, respectively, to immobilize their prey.[22,23] Because these molecules are thought to act by inhibiting neuronal voltage-gated calcium channels, initial speculation regarding the mechanism of Agouti protein action focused on the possibility of a specific Agouti receptor that modulated calcium flux.[9,24] Although there is limited experimental support for a direct action of Agouti protein on calcium channels,[8,25,26] most evidence indicates that Agouti protein and Agrp require melanocortin receptors for signal transduction.[27–32] This family of G-protein-coupled receptors was first recognized by the ability of small circulating peptides, such as alpha-melanocyte stimulating hormone (α-MSH) or adrenocorticotrophic hormone (ACTH), to activate adenylate cyclase in pigment cells or the adrenal cortex, respectively. More recently, α-MSH was recognized as an important neurotransmitter in the regulation of stereotypic behavior, central pathways governing the inflammatory response, and feeding.[33–35]

A turning point in understanding the biochemical mechanism of Agouti protein action stems from the observation of Geschwind that administration of α-MSH to A^y animals causes a switch of pigment synthesis from yellow to black;[36,37] in hindsight, Agouti protein action is clearly opposite that of α-MSH. This opposite relationship was underscored by the recent observation of Cone and colleagues,[38] that the *recessive yellow* mutation, in which animals display mostly yellow pigment, is caused by a loss-of-function in the melanocyte receptor for α-MSH, the melanocortin-1 receptor (Mc1r).

These observations set the stage for pharmacologic studies demonstrating that Agouti protein (and later Agrp) would inhibit activation of adenylate cyclase by melanocortin peptides.[27–30,39,40] However, the exact mechanism of Agouti and Agrp action has been difficult to unravel, in part because direct binding assays for Agouti have been difficult to develop. We recently developed a direct binding assay for recombinant Agouti protein in which an epitope-tagged form of the molecule (HA-Agouti) was first incubated with heterologous cells engineered to express the Mc1r, then, after a brief wash and fixation, cell surface binding of the epitope was detected immunohistochemically.[32] Using this so-called "overlay" assay, we found that α-MSH or other melanocortin agonists would inhibit cell surface binding of HA-Agouti to cells that express the Mc1r (see FIGURE 2A). These observations, and their converse,[27,28,30] argue strongly that Agouti protein is a competitive antagonist of melanocortin peptides, but do not distinguish between competition for the identical site versus induction of a conformational change that prevents binding of the alternative ligand, so-called allosteric competition. The carboxy-terminal portion of Agouti or Agrp is sufficient for melanocortin receptor binding,[3,32,39] and it is likely to fold into a compact globular structure with five pairs of intrachain disulfide bonds in a 40-amino-acid segment. By contrast, the active core of melanocortin agonists is a seven-residue, relatively hydrophobic, peptide that is thought to interact with the membrane-spanning portion of the receptor. The question of whether Agouti protein and α-MSH bind to the same, different, or overlapping sites is of practical as well as

A

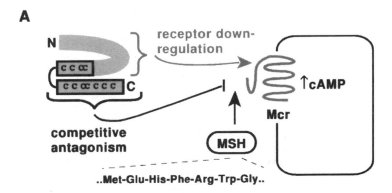

B

Interaction of Agouti and Mc1r on a sensitized (*Tyr^ch*) background

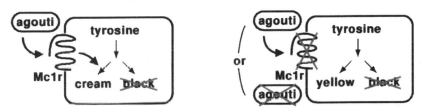

FIGURE 2. Mechanism of Agouti protein signaling *in vitro* and *in vivo*. **A.** Epitope-tagged full-length Agouti protein binds directly to the Mc1r and can be displaced either by excess melanocortin peptide or by the cysteine-rich carboxy-terminal fragment of Agouti protein. However, pharmacologic studies of full-length Agouti protein on *Xenopus* melanophores indicate a time- and temperature-dependent potentiation of melanocortin inhibition that is likely explained by receptor downregulation or desensitization. **B.** *In vivo, Agouti* inhibits expression of tyrosinase, and low levels of tyrosinase are associated with synthesis of yellow pigment. In a genetic background, where tyrosinase activity is compromised because of the *chinchilla* (*Tyr^ch*) mutation, expression of *Agouti* causes a further reduction in tyrosinase activity such that very little pigment of any type can be made, leading to a cream color. The cream-colored phenotype observed in *A^y*; *chinchilla* mice is clearly distinct from the pale yellow phenotype observed in *Mc1r^e/Mc1r^e*; *chinchilla* mice, and suggests that Agouti causes a greater inhibition of tyrosinase activity than does loss-of-function at the Mc1r. Experiments supporting these findings are described in References 32 and 42.

theoretical importance, because small molecule pharmaceutical agents targeted to a binding site specific for Agouti protein or Agrp might not have the same physiologic effects as melanocortin peptide mimetics.

Pharmaologic studies can sometimes provide insight into mechanisms of receptor antagonism, since increasing concentrations of an antagonist that competes for the same site as agonist will cause a proportionate and parallel rightward shift of the agonist dose-response curve. Most of our work on Agouti protein pharmacology has utilized the endogenous melanocortin receptor present on a *Xenopus* pigment cell line, melanophores, developed by Dr. Michael Lerner.[41] This assay system is extremely sensitive, robust, and offers an opportunity to study the effects of melanocortins or Agouti protein in real time. We find that the effects of Agouti protein cannot be explained solely by agonist displacement, since full-length Agouti protein exhibts a time- and temperature-dependent potentiation of melanocortin inhibition that suggests a direct effect of Agouti protein on receptor downregulation[32] (FIG. 2A). For example, increasing concentrations of Agouti protein cause a reduction in the maximum level of α-MSH–induced pigment dispersion, and the level of reduction depends on time, temperature, and Agouti protein concentration. Surprisingly, these noncompetitive effects are observed only with intact full-length Agouti protein.[42] The carboxy-terminal cysteine-rich domain by itself, or full-length Agouti protein treated with a protease that cleaves between the amino- and carboxy-terminal domains, have no effect on the maximum level of α-MSH–induced pigment dispersion.

We have also used pigmentation genetics to examine the relationship between Agouti protein signaling and Mc1r function *in vivo*.[32] Decreased Mc1r signaling in melanocytes, whether caused by increased Agouti expression or decreased Mc1r expression, leads to reduced activity of tyrosinase, a rate-limiting enzyme for synthesis of all pigment types.[43,44] On an appropriate genetic background provided by the *chinchilla* (Tyr^{ch}) mutation, A^y/a mutant mice exhibit a greater reduction of tyrosinase activity then $Mc1r^e/Mc1r^e$ mutant mice, leading to an obvious coat color difference, cream-colored versus yellow[32] (FIG. 2B). Animals, mutant for both mutations (A^y/a and $Mc1r^e/Mc1r^e$), exhibit a pigmentation phenotype identical to the single $Mc1r^e/Mc1r^e$ mutants; therefore, the ability of Agouti expression to depress tyrosinase activity below a level associated with Mc1r deficiency requires a functional Mc1r receptor. Taken together with the *in vitro* studies, these findings suggest that Agouti protein transduces a signal via the Mc1r independent of that caused by α-MSH displacement.

OTHER COAT COLOR GENES AND
THE AGOUTI SIGNALING PATHWAY

Many of the critical tools and key insights for understanding the pathways described above are based on previously existing mutations, recognized by their effects on pigmentation. Two additional coat color mutations that provide insight into Agouti signaling are *mahogany* and *mahoganoid*.[45] Each produces a similar phenotype; an increased amount of black/brown pigment, eumelanin, compared to red/yellow pigment, pheomelanin (see FIGURE 3). These effects are similar to those caused by loss-of-function *Agouti* mutations or constitutively activating *Mc1r* mutations and, *a priori,* might be explained by decreased production or cell surface binding of Agouti protein, increased production of α-MSH, or defects in the melanocyte enzymes or structural proteins required to produce yellow pigment granules. Plasma levels of α-MSH and ACTH are not altered by the *mahogany* or *mahoganoid* mutations;[46] we and others[47,48] have used double mutant studies to distinguish among the other alternatives. If *mahogany* were caused by defects in the melanocyte machinery required for yellow pigment synthesis, one would expect *mahogany* to suppress the

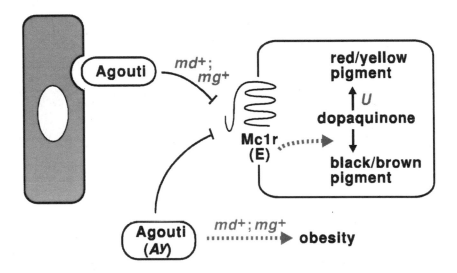

FIGURE 3. Genetic pathway for Agouti signaling. *Mahogany* (*mg*) and *mahoganoid* (*md*) are each required for Agouti signaling, since presumptive loss-of-function mutations in either gene cause a phenotype similar to that caused by a loss-of-function *Agouti* mutation. Double mutant studies, as described in the text and in the references, place *mg* and *md* downstream of Agouti transcription but upstream of the Mc1r. Experiments supporting these findings are described in Reference 46.

pigmentation phenotype of *recessive yellow*, a loss of function mutation of the Mc1r. However, animals doubly mutant for *mahogany* and *recessive yellow* are indistinguishable from single mutant *recessive yellow* animals.[46] Similarly, if *mahogany* were caused by reduced transcription of *Agouti* RNA in the hair follicle, one would expect that *mahogany* should have no effect on the yellow coat color caused by A^y, resulting from a deletion that places *Agouti* RNA under control of a ubiquitously expressed promoter. However, animals doubly mutant for A^y and *mahogany* exhibit a darkened coat color.[46] Thus, *mahogany* and *mahoganoid* lie downstream of *Agouti* transcription but upstream of the *Mc1r*, and therefore may be required for posttranslational processing, secretion, or binding of Agouti protein to the cell surface (FIG. 3).

ACKNOWLEDGMENTS

We are grateful to Chris Kaelin and Julie Kerns for their help and criticism. This work was supported in part by Grant DK28506 from the National Institutes of Health. G.S.B. is an Associate Investigator of the Howard Hughes Medical Institute.

REFERENCES

1. SILVERS, W.K. 1979. The Agouti and Extension Series of Alleles, Umbrous and Sable. 6–44. Springer-Verlag, New York.
2. JACKSON, I.J. 1994. Molecular and developmental genetics of mouse coat color. Annu. Rev. Genet. **28:** 189–217.
3. OLLMANN, M.M., B.D. WILSON, Y.K. YANG, *et al.* 1997. Antagonism of central melanocortin receptors *in vitro* and *in vivo* by agouti-related protein. Science **278:** 135–138.
4. SHUTTER, J.R., M. GRAHAM, A.C. KINSEY, S. SCULLY, R. LUTHY & K.L. STARK. 1997. Hypothalamic expression of ART, a novel gene related to agouti, is up-regulated in obese and diabetic mutant mice. Genes Dev. **11:** 593–602.
5. DUHL, D.M.J., M.E. STEVENS, H. VRIELING *et al.* 1994. Pleiotropic effects of the mouse lethal yellow (A(y)) mutation explained by deletion of a maternally expressed gene and the simultaneous production of agouti fusion RNAs. Development **120:** 1695–1708.
6. MICHAUD, E.S., S.J. BULTMAN, M.L. KLEBIG *et al.* 1994. A molecular model for the genetic and phenotypic characteristics of the mouse lethal yellow (Ay) mutation. Proc. Natl. Acad. Sci. USA **91:** 2562–2566.
7. MILTENBERGER, R.J., R.L. MYNATT, J.E. WILKINSON & R.P. WOYCHIK. 1997. The role of the agouti gene in the yellow obese syndrome. J. Nutr. **127:** 1902S–1907S.
8. Michaud, J., R.L. MYNATT, R.J. MILTENBERGER *et al.* 1997. Role of the agouti gene in obesity. J. Endocrinol. **155:** 207-209.
9. MANNE, J., A.C. ARGESON & L.D. SIRACUSA. 1995. Mechanisms for the pleiotropic effects of the agouti gene. Proc. Natl. Acad. Sci. USA **92:** 4721–4724.
10. PERRY, W.L., N.G. COPELAND & N.A. JENKINS. 1994. The molecular basis for dominant yellow agouti coat color mutations. Bioessays **16:** 705–707.
11. SEARLE, A.G. 1968. Comparative Genetics of Coat Color in Mammals. Academic Press, New York.
12. YEN, T.T., A.M. GILL, L.G. FRIGERI, G.S. BARSH & G.L. WOLFF. 1994. Obesity, diabetes, and neoplasia in yellow A(vy)/- mice: ectopic expression of the agouti gene. Faseb. J. **8:** 479–488.
13. WOLFF, G.L., D.W. ROBERTS & D.B. GALBRAITH. 1986. Prenatal determination of obesity, tumor susceptibility, and coat color pattern in viable yellow (A^{vy}/a) mice. The yellow mouse syndrome. J. Heredity **77:** 151–158.
14. CUÉNOT, L. 1905. Les races pures et leurs combinaisons chez les souris (4me note). Arch. Zool. Exp. Gen. 4e Ser **3:** cxxiii–cxxxii.
15. POOLE, T.W. 1980. Dermal-epidermal interactions and the action of alleles at the agouti locus in the mouse. II. The viable yellow (Avy) and mottled agouti (am) alleles. Dev. Biol. **80:** 495–500.
16. POOLE, T.W. 1975. Dermal-epidermal interactions and the action of alleles at the *agouti* locus in the mouse. Dev. Biol. **42:** 203–210.
17. MILLER, M.W., D.M.J. DUHL, H. VRIELING *et al.* 1993. Cloning of the mouse agouti gene predicts a secreted protein ubiquitously expressed in mice carrying the Lethal-Yellow mutation. Genes Dev. **7:** 454–467.
18. BULTMAN, S.J., E.J. MICHAUD & R.P. WOYCHIK. 1992. Molecular characterization of the mouse agouti locus. Cell **71:** 1195–1204.
19. Millar, S.E., M.W. MILLER, M.E. STEVENS & G.S. BARSH. 1995. Expression and transgenic studies of the mouse agouti gene provide insight into the mechanisms by which mammalian coat color patterns are generated. Development **121:** 3223–3232.
20. VRIELING, H., D.M. DUHL, S.E. MILLAR, K.A. MILLER & G.S. BARSH. 1994. Differences in dorsal and ventral pigmentation result from regional expression of the mouse agouti gene. Proc. Natl. Acad. Sci. USA **91:** 5667–5671.
21. DUHL, D.M.J., H. VRIELING, K.A. MILLER, G.L. WOLFF & G.S. BARSH. 1994. Neomorphic agouti mutations in obese yellow mice. Nat. Genet. **8:** 59–65.

22. QUISTAD, G.B. & W.S. SKINNER. 1994. Isolation and sequencing of insecticidal peptides from the primitive hunting spider, Plectreurys tristis (Simon). J. Biol. Chem. **269:** 11098–11101.

23. OLIVERA, B.M., J. RIVIER, J.K. SCOTT, D.R. HILLYARD & L.J. CRUZ. 1991. Conotoxins. J. Biol. Chem. **266:** 22067–22070.

24. ZEMEL, M.B., J.H. KIM, R.P. WOYCHIK et al. 1995. Agouti regulation of intracellular calcium: role in the insulin resistance of viable yellow mice. Proc. Natl. Acad. Sci. USA **92:** 4733–4737.

25. JONES, B.H., J.H. KIM, M.B. ZEMEL et al. 1996. Upregulation of adipocyte metabolism by agouti protein: possible paracrine actions in yellow mouse obesity. Amer. J. Physiol.-Endocrinol. Met. **33:** E192–E196.

26. XUE, B., N. MOUSTAID-MOUSSA, W.O. WILKISON & M.B. ZEMEL. 1998. The agouti gene product inhibits lipolysis in human adipocytes via a Ca^{2+}-dependent mechanism. Faseb. J. **12:** 1391–1396.

27. LU, D.S., D. WILLARD, I.R. PATEL et al. 1994. Agouti protein is an antagonist of the melanocyte-stimulating-hormone receptor. Nature **371:** 799–802.

28. BLANCHARD, S.G., C.O. HARRIS, O.R.R. ITTOOP et al. 1995. Agouti antagonism of melanocortin binding and action in the B16F10 murine melanoma cell line. Biochem. **34:** 10406–10411.

29. SIEGRIST, W., R. DROZDZ, R. COTTI, D.H. WILLARD, W.O. WILKISON & A.N. EBERLE. 1997. Interactions of alpha-melanotropin and agouti on B16 melanoma cells: evidence for inverse agonism of agouti. J. Receptor Signal Transd. Res. **17:** 75–98.

30. YANG, Y.K., M.M. OLLMANN, B.D. WILSON et al. 1997. Effects of recombinant agouti-signaling protein on melanocortin action. Mol. Endocrinol. **11:** 274–280.

31. SIEGRIST, W., D.H. WILLARD, W.O. WILKISON & A.N. EBERLE. 1996. Agouti protein inhibits growth of b16 melanoma cells in vitro by acting through melanocortin receptors. Biochem. Biophys. Res. Commun. **218:** 171–175.

32. OLLMANN, M.M., M.L. LAMOREUX, B.D. WILSON & G.S. BARSH. 1998. Interaction of Agouti protein with the melanocortin 1 receptor in vitro and in vivo. Genes Dev. **12:** 316–330.

33. O'DONOHUE, T.L. & D.M. DORSA. 1982. The opiomelanotropinergic neuronal and endocrine systems. Peptides **3:** 353–395.

34. DE WIED, D. 1993. Melanotropins as neuropeptides. Ann. N.Y. Acad. Sci. **680:** 20–28.

35. CONE, R.D., D. LU, S. KOPPULA et al. 1996. The melanocortin receptors: agonists, antagonists, and the hormonal control of pigmentation. Recent Prog. Horm. Res. **51:** 287–318.

36. GESCHWIND, I.I. 1966. Change in hair color in mice induced by injection of α-MSH. Endocrinol. **79:** 1165–1167.

37. GESCHWIND, I.I., R.A. HUSEBY & R. NISHIOKA. 1972. The effect of melanocyte-stimulating hormone on coat color in the mouse. Rec. Prog. Horm. Res. **28:** 91–130.

38. ROBBINS, L.S., J.H. NADEAU, K.R. JOHNSON et al. 1993. Pigmentation phenotypes of variant extension locus alleles result from point mutations that alter MSH receptor function. Cell **72:** 827–834.

39. WILLARD, D.H., W. BODNAR, C. HARRIS et al. 1995. Agouti structure and function: characterization of a potent alpha-melanocyte stimulating hormone receptor antagonist. Biochem. **34:** 12341–12346.

40. KIEFER, L.L., J.M. VEAL, K.G. MOUNTJOY & W.O. WILKISON. 1998. Melanocortin receptor binding determinants in the agouti protein. Biochem. **37:** 991–997.

41. POTENZA, M.N. & M.R. LERNER. 1992. A rapid quantitative bioassay for evaluating the effects of ligands upon receptors that modulate cAMP levels in a melanophore cell line. Pigment Cell. Res. **5:** 372–378.

42. OLLMANN, M. 1998. Mechanisms of Agouti protein signaling. Ph.D. Thesis, Stanford University School of Medicine, Stanford.
43. KOBAYASHI, T., W.D. VIEIRA, B. POTTERF, C. SAKAI, G. IMOKAWA & V.J. HEARING. 1995. Modulation of melanogenic protein expression during the switch from eu- to pheomelanogenesis. J. Cell Sci. **108:** 2301–2309.
44. PROTA, G., M.L. LAMOREUX, J. MULLER *et al.* 1995. Comparative analysis of melanins and melanosomes produced by various coat color mutants. Pigm. Cell Res. **8:** 153–163.
45. LANE, P.W. & M.C. GREEN. 1960. Mahogany, a recessive color mutatioin in linkage group V of the mouse. J. Hered. **51:** 228–230.
46. MILLER, K.A., T.M. GUNN, M.M. CARRASQUILLO, M.L. LAMOREUX, D.B. GALBRAITH & G.S. BARSH. 1997. Genetic studies of the mouse mutations mahogany and mahoganoid. Genetics **146:** 1407–1415.
47. BEECHEY, C.V. & A.G. SEARLE. 1978. Epistasy of extension alleles. Mouse News Lett. **59:** 19.
48. BEECHEY C.V. & A.G. SEARLE. 1979. Epistasy of nc over Ay. Mouse News Lett. **60:** 45–47.

Synthetic Melanocortin Receptor Agonists and Antagonists

MICHAEL R. LERNER[a]

F4. 100, Department of Dermatology, University of Texas Southwestern Medical Center,
5323 Harry Hines Boulevard, Dallas, Texas 75235, USA

ABSTRACT: Multiple melanocortin receptor subtypes with distinct cell and
tissue distribution patterns have recently been identified, thereby presenting
numerous opportunities for biological investigation. Many of these studies
could benefit from the availability of subtype selective or specific agonists and
antagonists. The purpose of this report is to summarize the state of available
melanocortin receptor agonists and antagonists.

INTRODUCTION

Identification and cloning of the genes that encode four discreet melanocortin
(MC) receptors—MC1, 3, 4, and 5—initiated by Cone, Wikberg, Gantz, and their respective collaborators, has engendered an explosion of interest in the biological effects of melanocortin–stimulating hormones.[1–5] Several types of cells in different
organs, including the central nervous system, the gastrointestinal tract, melanocytes,
adrenal cortex, and adipocytes,[6] express specific MC receptors. However, the existence of a common natural stimulatory ligand; that is, alpha melanocyte stimulating
hormone (α-MSH), presents challenges for *in vivo* studies into the biological effects
of receptor activation or blockade. The availability of both agonist and antagonist
ligands that are highly selective or even specific for each of the MC receptor subtypes could facilitate animal studies.

Over the past two decades, a handful of investigators have pioneered the development of MC receptor agonists and antagonists. This research started well prior to
the cloning of MC receptors. Initial studies were directed at the MSH receptor expressed on melanocytes, now known as the MC1 receptor. In 1979, Herbert and his
colleagues identified and cloned cDNA for proopiomelanocortin (POMC).[7] This research enabled better understanding of the relationships between the peptides, α-,
β-, and γ-MSH, and adrenal cortical trophic hormone (ACTH). By examining the sequences of these peptides, Hruby *et al.*, were able to identify a common core in all
four peptides; namely, His-Phe-Arg-Trp, which acts as a message sequence. When
acetylated at its amino terminus and amidated at its carboxyl end, this sequence exhibits biological agonist activity at the MC1 receptor in *Rana pipiens* melanocytes.[8]
Work was also begun on the development of novel synthetic melanocortin analogues
that show increased agonist activity at the amphibian MC1 receptor when compared
with the natural linear tridecapeptide molecule α-MSH.

[a]Address for corespondence: 214-648-7115 (voice); 214-648-9292 (fax); mrlerner@aol.com
(e-mail).

TABLE 1. NDP-MSH, comparison with the four natural melanocortin peptides

ACTH$_{1-39}$	SYSMEHFRWGKPVGKKRRPVKVYPNGAEDESAEAFPLEF
α-MSH	SYSMEHFRWGKPV-NH$_2$
β-MSH	DEGPYRMEHFRWGSPPKD
γ-MSH	YVMGHFRWDRF
NDP-MSH	SYSnLEHDFRWGKPV

NOTE: nL, norleucine; DF, D-phenylalanine.

NDP-MSH—A POTENT SYNTHETIC MSH

Acetylated NDP-MSH; that is, α-MSH in which norleucine has been substituted at position four and D-phenylalanine substituted at position seven, was identified almost 20 years ago.[9] The synthetic peptide (see TABLE 1) was found to exceed the potency of its counterpart at melanocortin receptors on amphibian and lizard melanocytes by a factor greater than 10. In comparison with α-MSH and the other natural melanotropins, it was also demonstrated to have prolonged activity.

The next step, in defining the structure of peptides of minimal size with agonist activity at the melanocyte MC1 receptor, was to perform truncation studies on NDP-MSH and to compare the results with the α-MSH core message sequence His-Phe-Arg-Trp.[10] Successive truncations from both the N and C termini were coupled with limited changes in the central sequence. In all cases, the peptides were acetylated and examined for agonist activity using a frog skin bioassay. The results are summarized in FIGURE 1. They reveal that the tripeptide sequence of peptide

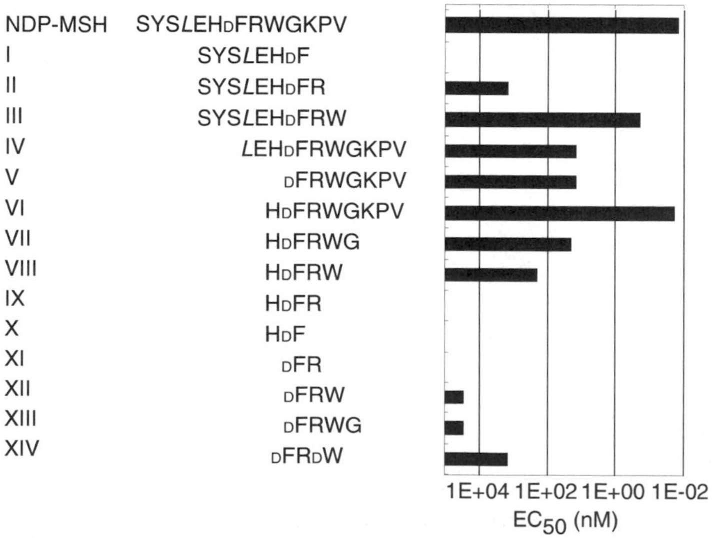

NDP-MSH	SYS*L*EHDFRWGKPV
I	SYS*L*EHDF
II	SYS*L*EHDFR
III	SYS*L*EHDFRW
IV	*L*EHDFRWGKPV
V	DFRWGKPV
VI	HDFRWGKPV
VII	HDFRWG
VIII	HDFRW
IX	HDFR
X	HDF
XI	DFR
XII	DFRW
XIII	DFRWG
XIV	DFRDW

1E+04 1E+02 1E+00 1E-02
EC$_{50}$ (nM)

FIGURE 1. Tripeptide peptidomimetics with agonist activity at the *Rana pipiens* MC1R, identified by NDP-MSH truncation studies. (Modified, with permission, from TABLE 2 in Ref. 9.)

XIV, Ac-DPhe-Arg-DTrp-NH$_2$, possess weak but detectable agonist activity, with an EC$_{50}$ on the order of 1 uM. By substituting D-amino acids at two positions in the core sequence, Hruby and his colleagues were able to eliminate the need for histidine, thereby shortening the overall sequence and forming the basis for potential melanocortin receptor peptidomimetic agonists.

PEPTIDOMIMETICS WITH SELECTIVE BINDING PROPERTIES AT MELANOCORTIN RECEPTOR SUBTYPES

With the availability of clones for the human melanocortin receptors 1, 3, 4, and 5, NDP-MSH was investigated for its binding specificity and strength, in comparison with α-MSH at each protein (see FIGURE 2).[11] In every case, its Ki was superior to that of the natural molecule. Also, in every case, the rank order for binding to the receptors was the same; MC1R > MC2R > MC3R > MC4R. Wikberg and colleagues then asked whether it was possible to develop cyclic analogues of NDH-MSH that showed increased selectivity for binding to one of the melanocortin receptors, other than MC1R. Using both cysteine disulphide based and lactam based peptides, they

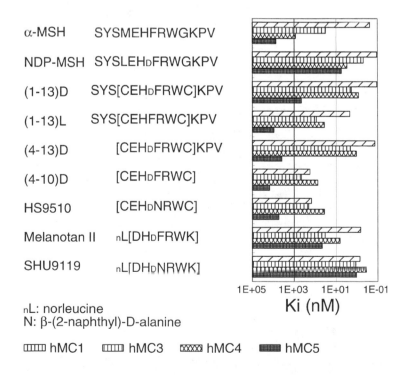

FIGURE 2. Development of cyclic melanotropins and analysis of their binding capabilities at the human melanocortin receptors 1, 3, 4, and 5. (Modified, with permission, from FIGURE 1 and TABLE 1 in Ref. 10.)

identified molecules with a small preference for MC4R. The molecule with the greatest relative MC4R selectivity was HS9510, which contains the bulky hydrophobic amino acid β-(2-naphthyl)-D-alanine at position seven in place of the original D-phenylalanine in NDP-MSH.

The development of cyclic melanocortin analogues based on cysteine disulphide bridges was then extended, to discover peptidomimetics such as HSO14 (see FIGURE 3)[12] with approximately tenfold greater selectivity for binding at human MC4R when compared with any of the human MC1, MC3, or MC5 receptors. This novel compound, which binds 300 times more effectively to MC4R than to MC1R, was determined by cAMP based bioassay to be an MC4R antagonist. The same study

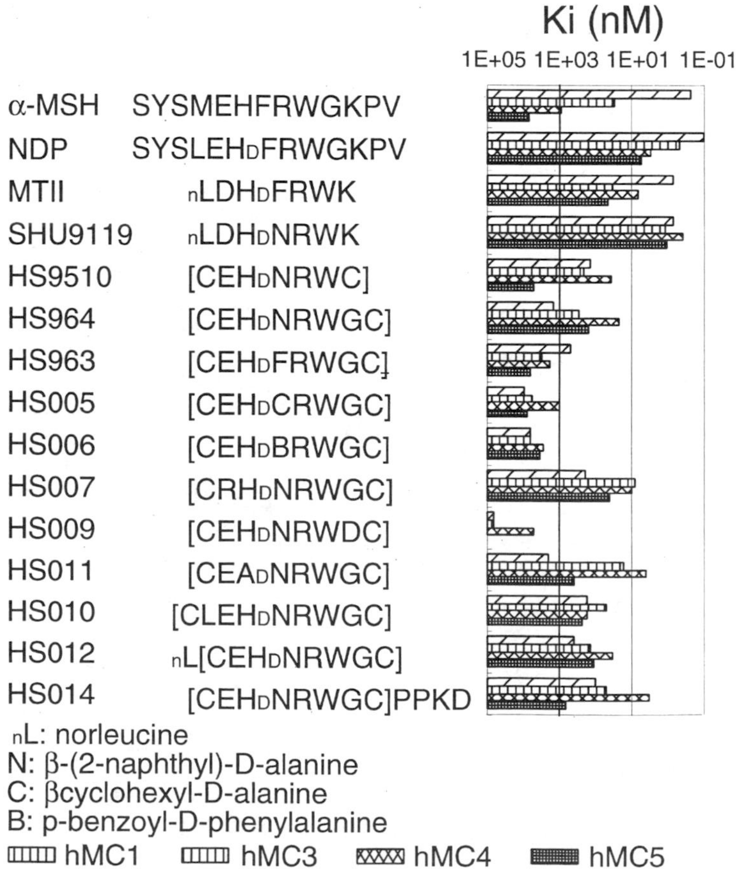

FIGURE 3. Development of cyclic melanocortin receptor subtype selective antagonists. (Modified, with permission, from TABLES 1 and 2 in Ref. 11.)

also identified a novel compound, HSO11, with binding selectivity that was greatest at MC3R, as well as several molecules with preferences for MC5R.

PEPTIDOMIMETICS WITH SELECTIVE AGONIST AND ANTAGONIST PROPERTIES AT MELANOCORTIN RECEPTOR SUBTYPES

Using bioassays based on cloned receptors, cyclic lactam melanocortin analogues were examined for their functional activities as agonists or antagonists at human melanocortin receptors (see FIGURE 4).[13] For example, cyclic peptide 3 was demonstrated to act as an antagonist at both the MC3R and MC4R, and to behave as an agonist at MC1R. Meanwhile, heptapeptide 8, with the addition of an alanine within the ring structure, was found to be a somewhat selective agonist at MC4R. The reported results showed that small changes in peptide structure could lead to differences in relative receptor binding strengths as well as changes in activity between agonism and antagonism.

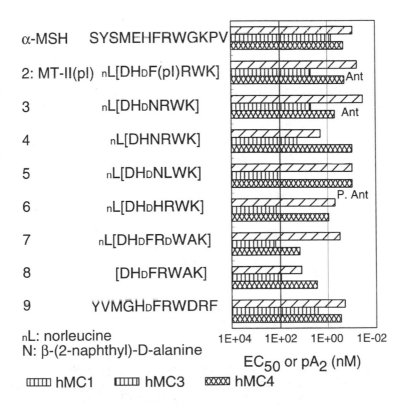

FIGURE 4. Design of cyclic lactam melanocortin receptor subtype selective agonists and antagonists. (Modified, with permission, from Table 1 in Ref. 12.)

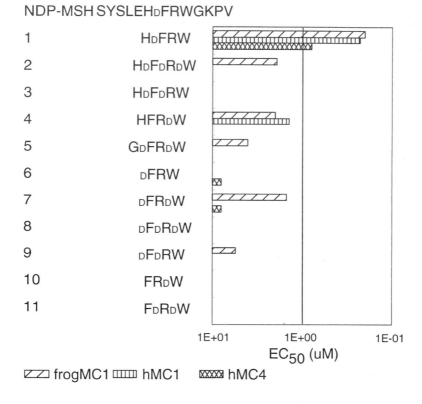

FIGURE 5. Structures of linear melanocortin receptor subtype selective peptidomimetic agonists. (Modified, with permission, from Tables 2 and 3 in Ref. 13.)

Linear molecules can also have melanocortin subtype receptor agonist selectivity (see FIGURE 5).[14] For example, Ac-DPhe-Arg-DTrp-NH$_2$, described above for its minimal size, although active at the frog MC1 receptor, it is also a weak agonist at human MC4R. Interestingly, the molecule Ac-DPhe-Arg-Trp-NH$_2$ is also an agonist at MC4R, but exhibits no activity against frog MC1R.

COMBINATORIAL LIBRARIES CAN AID IN THE IDENTIFICATION OF MELANOCORTIN RECEPTOR ANTAGONISTS

To date, all melanocortin peptidomimetics known to have receptor subtype specificities in terms of either binding, agonist, or antagonist capabilities, have ultimately been derived from an analysis of α-MSH and or NDP-MSH. In principle, it is possible to identify molecules that act as agonists or antagonists to melanocortin receptors, without requiring prior knowledge about the structure of natural ligands. The

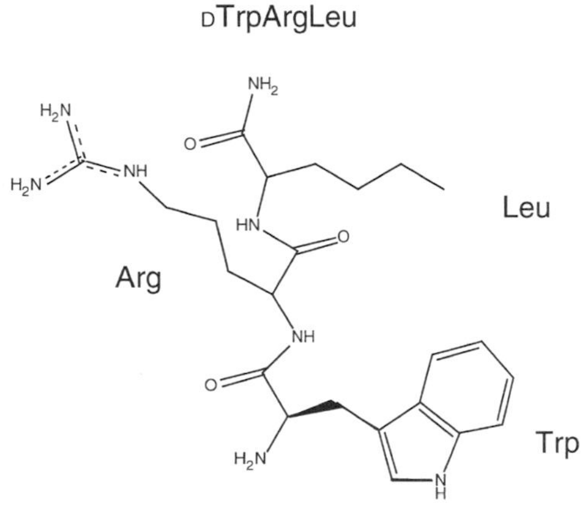

FIGURE 6. Structure of a peptidomimetic antagonist at the Xenopus laevis melano-phore melanocortin receptor.[15]

key to this approach is the ability to be able to screen a large number of molecules quickly, because the hit rate is low. An example of this method was the use of a lawn-based screen of molecules derived from a random combinatorial tripeptide library, with a complexity on the order of 400,000 components.[15,16] The lawn, composed of *Xenopus laevis* melanophores, made it possible to screen the many thousands of pep-tides that had been synthesized on polystyrene beads, so as to identify those that blocked the ability of α-MSH to mediate pigment dispersion. The most potent MC1R antagonist identified had the sequence D-Trp-Arg-Leu (see FIGURE 6). In light of the discovery that Ac-DPhe-Arg-Trp-NH$_2$ is an agonist at the *Rana pipiens* MC1R, it is interesting that an entirely random screen led to a molecule that was closely related to an agonist derived from the core melanotropin message sequence.

GOALS FOR THE FUTURE

Over the past several years, much has been learned about the structures of syn-thetic melanotropins in terms of the features that are important for imparting selec-tivity for the different melanocortin receptor subtypes, MC1, MC3, MC4, and MC5R. Most of these efforts have come from Hruby, Wikberg, Gantz, Hadley, and their colleagues. This research consists of a careful analysis of α-MSH, and the con-struction and testing of cyclically constrained peptidomimetics against recombinant melanocortin receptors. As well as the natural molecules that exhibit selectivity for the MC1 receptor, the published literature now contains examples of molecules with primary selectivity for MC4R and MC3R, and also molecules that prefer MC5R to MC1R. In the not distant future, we will probably be treated to the availability of molecules with high agonist or antagonist selectivity for each of the melanocortin receptors. These new structures will be a boon to pharmacological and physiological investigations in the proopiomelanocortin system.

REFERENCES

1. MOUNTJOY, K.G., L.S. ROBBINS, M.T. MORTRUD & R.D. CONE. 1992. The cloning of a family of genes that encode the melanocortin receptors. Science **257:** 1248–1251.
2. CHHAJLANI, V. & J.E.S. WIKBERG. 1992. Molecular cloning and expression of the human melanocyte stimulating hormone receptor cDNA. FEBS Lett. **309:** 417–420.
3. CHHAJLANI, V., R. MUCENIECE & J.E.S. WIKBERG. 1993. Molecular cloning of a novel human melanocortin receptor. Biochem. Biophys. Res. Commun. **195:** 866–873.
4. GANTZ, I., Y. KONDA, T. TASHIRO, Y. SHIMOTO, H. MIWA, G. MUNZERT, S.J. WATSON, J. DELVALLE & T. YAMADA. 1993. Molecular cloning of a novel melanocortin receptor. J. Biol. Chem. **268:** 8246–8250.
5. GANTZ, I., H. MIWA, Y. KONDA, Y. SHIMOTO, T. TASHIRO, S.J. WATSON, J. DELVALLE & T. YAMADA. 1993. Molecular cloning, expression and gene localization of a fourth melanocortin receptor. J. Biol. Chem. **268:** 15174–15179.
6. BOSTON, B.A. & R.D. CONE. 1996. Characterization of melanocortin receptor subtype expression in murine adipose tissues and in the 3T3-L1 cell line. Endocrinology **137:** 2043–2050.
7. ROBERTS, J.L., P.H. SEEBURG, J. SHINE, E. HERBERT, J.D. BAXTER & H.M. GOODMAN. 1979. Corticotropin and beta-endorphin: construction and analysis of recombinant DNA complementary to mRNA for the common precursor. Proc. Natl. Acad. Sci. USA **76:** 2153–2157.
8. CASTRUCCI, A.M.L., M.E. HADLEY, T.K. SAWYER, B.C. WILKES, F. AL-OBEIDI, D.J. STAPLES, A.E. DEVAUX, O. DYM, M.F. HINTZ, J. RIEHM, K.R. RAU, & V.J. HRUBY. 1989. α-Melanotorpin: the minimal active sequence in the lizard skin bioassay. Gen. Comp. Endocrinol. **73:** 157–163.
9. SAWYER, T.K., P.J. SANFILLIPPO, V.J. HRUBY, M.H. ENGOEL, C.B. HEWARD, J.B. BURNETT & M.E. HADLEY. 1980. 4-Norleucine, 7-D-phenylalanine-α-melanocyte–stimulating hormone: a highly potent α-melanotropin with ultra long biological activity. Proc. Natl. Acad. Sci. USA **77:** 5754–5758.
10. HASKEL-LUEVANO, C.H., T.K. SAWYER, S. HENDRATA, C. NORTH, L. PANAHINIA, M. STUM, D.J. STAPLES, A.M. CASTRUCCI, M.E. HADLEY & V.J. HRUBY. 1996. Truncation studies of α-melanotropin peptides identify tripeptide analogues exhibiting prolonged agonist bioactivity. Peptides **17:** 995–1002.
11. SCHIOTH, H.B., R. MUCENIECE, F. MUTULIS, P. PRUSIS, G. LINDEBERG, S.D. SHARMA, V.J. HRUBY & J.E.S. WIKBERG. 1997. Selectivity of cyclic [D-Nal^7] and [D -Phe^7] substituted MSH analogues for the melanocortin receptor subtypes. Peptides **18:** 1009–1013.
12. SCHIOTH, H.B., F. MUTULIS, R. MUCENIECE, P. PRUSIS & J.E.S. WIKBERG. 1998. Discovery of novel melanocortin receptor selective MSH analogues. Br. J. Pharmacology **124:** 75–82.
13. HRUBY, V.J., S.D. SHARMA, S. LIM, W. YUAN, C. HASKELL-LUEVANO, G. HAN, M.E. HADLEY, R.D. CONE & I. GANTZ. 1996. Design of potent and specific melanotropin agonists and antagonists: investigating ligands for new receptors. Peptides **17:** 485–486.
14. HASKEL-LUEVANO, C.H., S. HENDRATA, C. NORTH, T.K. SAWYER, M.E. HADLEY, V.J. HRUBY, C. DICKINSON & I. GANTZ. 1997. Discovery of prototype peptidomimetic agonists at the human melanocortin receptors MC1R and MC4R. J. Med. Chem. **40:** 2133–2139.
15. JAYAWICKREME, C.K., J.M. QUILLAN, G.F. GRAMINSKI & M.R. LERNER. 1994. Discovery and structure-function analysis of α-melanocyte–stimulating hormone antagonists. J. Biol. Chem. **269:** 29846–29854.
16. QUILLAN, J.M., C.K. JAYAWICKREME & M.R. LERNER. 1995. Combinatorial diffusion assay used to identify topically active melanocyte-stimulating hormone receptor antagonists. Proc. Natl. Acad. Sci. USA **92:** 2894–2898.

Proopiomelanocortin and the Immune–Neuroendocrine Connection

J. EDWIN BLALOCK[a]

Department of Physiology and Biophysics, University of Alabama at Birmingham, 1918 University Boulevard, MCLM896, Birmingham, Alabama 35294, USA

ABSTRACT: This presentation will cover the history, recent developments in, and implications of the ability of both the immune and neuroendocrine systems to produce POMC. The discovery of POMC in immune cells was one of the events that heralded a molecular understanding of neuroimmunomodulation. This, together with the presence of opiate and ACTH receptors on lymphocytes and macrophages, provided the first biochemical circuit for which the same signal molecules and receptors could be used for intrasystem regulation, as well as bidirectional communication between the immune and neuroendocrine systems. Today we have a quite good understanding of the regulation and processing of POMC in immune cells, as well as the interaction of its product peptides with other cytokines. For instance, IL-1 causes POMC production by immune cells, and the POMC product, α-MSH, in turn, acts functionally as an IL-1 antagonist. In the past year, the expression of full-length POMC mRNA has been reported and this solved one of the paradoxes with respect to POMC production, processing, and secretion. We provide data on these developments together with quite startling findings on the physiologic function of POMC peptides in the immune system. Among these are the local antinociceptive effects of immune cell–derived β-endorphin, altered hematopoiesis in opiate receptor-deficient animals, and the diagnosis of ACTH insensitivity by a deficiency of ACTH receptors on lymphocytes.

INTRODUCTION

The discovery of proopiomelanocortin (POMC) in immune cells[1,2] was one of the events that heralded a molecular understanding of neuroimmunomodulation. The presence of POMC–derived peptides, together with the observations of opiate and corticotropin (ACTH) receptors on lymphocytes and macrophages, provided the first biochemical circuit in which the same signal molecules and their receptors could be used for both intersystem regulation and bidirectional communication between the immune, nervous, and endocrine systems. Thus, a molecular rationale for neuroimmunomodulation became apparent. This paper explores the history, certain controversies, and recent developments relating to the role of POMC in neuroimmunomodulation.

[a]Address for correspondence: 205-934-6439 (voice); 205-934-1446 (fax); Blalock@UAB.edu (e-mail).

DISCOVERY OF POMC IN THE IMMUNE SYSTEM

ACTH production by human leukocytes was discovered in the late 1970s, somewhat serendipitously, during the course of studies related to the hormonal activities of interferon (IFN)-α. My laboratory and others had reported on the ability of IFN-α to mimic the activity of a number of hormones, including ACTH (for a review, see Ref. 3). We were particularly interested in whether ACTH bioactivity was intrinsic to the IFN-α molecule itself, or was due to another entity in IFN-α preparation. Since our initial studies preceded the routine use of molecular biologic techniques, and since IFN-α had been neither cloned nor sequenced when we began these studies, we used the routine biochemical means available at the time to address this issue. We reasoned that since IFN-α bioactivity is sensitive to the action of pepsin, whereas ACTH–mediated steroidogenesis is not, then if ACTH activity remained after pepsin digestion of IFN-α preparations, this would provide evidence that a molecule other than intact IFN-α was responsible. The results showed that pepsin destroyed IFN-α activity, but not that of ACTH.[1,2] We concluded that the IFN-α molecule either: (1) contained an ACTH sequence, (2) was tightly but noncovalently associated with an ACTH-like molecule, or (3) copurified with a lymphocyte–derived precursor for ACTH and endorphins.[2] This constituted the first controversy in the field, and it was partially resolved when human IFN-α was cloned in the very same year. Sequence analysis showed that the IFN-α molecule did not contain ACTH.[4] Thus, the first of the three possibilities was untenable. Although we favored the second, in fact the third was ultimately proved to be correct. In retrospect, we suspect that we may have been studying copurification of the 22-Kd biosynthetic intermediate of POMC with the 23-Kd form of natural IFN-α. This, of course, did not exclude the noncovalent, perhaps nonspecific, association of POMC peptides with IFN-α, for which we also had evidence.

Once it was established that immune cells made ACTH and endorphin-like substances, the second controversy revolved around whether they represented the authentic peptides.[5] Among earlier evidence that they were one in the same, were the many shared characteristics between immune system and pituitary–derived ACTH and endorphins; including, shared antigenicity as determined by using monospecific antibodies against synthetic peptides hormones; identical retention times on reverse-phase, high-pressure liquid chromatographic (HPLC) columns; identical molecular weights; shared biological activities;[6,7] and the presence of POMC-related mRNA in lymphocytes and macrophages.[8–15] The identity between pituitary and leukocyte ACTH has now been unequivocally established by demonstrating that the amino acid and nucleotide sequences of mouse splenic and pituitary ACTH are identical.[13,14] Thus, ACTH and endorphins were the first neuroendocrine peptides, synthesized *de novo,* to be identified in the immune system.

In the history of POMC production by the immune system, a final lingering dilemma was only resolved during the last year. Specifically, the inability of ourselves[15] and others (see References 16 and 17 for reviews) to demonstrate the presence of the full-length mRNA for POMC by polymerase chain reaction (PCR) techniques, had led to the commonly held notion that only truncated POMC transcripts lacking information for the signal peptide were present in immune cells. This led to the puzzle of how ACTH and endorphins, that could be found outside of immune cells, were secreted, when their precursor lacked a signal sequence. Recently, using primer extension and RNAse protection assays we were able to demonstrate full-length POMC mRNA in rat mononuclear leukocytes; and this has an identical sequence to that derived from the pituitary gland (see FIGURES 1 and 2).[18] The immune cell–derived POMC transcript is spliced in the same way as in the pituitary and, consequently, contains the sequence for the signal peptide (see FIGURES 2 and 3). As was expected from the presence of full-length POMC mRNA, its product, the 31-Kd POMC protein, was observed by Western blotting and was proteolytically processed in a way that is consistent with the pituitary gland (see FIGURES 3 and 4).[18] Thus, apparent technical differences—PCR versus primer extension/RNAse protection—led to the erroneous conclusion that only truncated POMC transcripts and

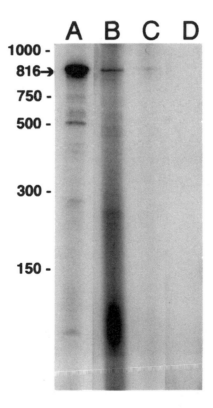

FIGURE 1. Primer extension products observed with 7 μg of the following templates; anterior pituitary total RNA (*lane A*), mRNA of ConA-treated (5 h) splenocytes (*lane B*), mRNA of untreated splenocytes (*lane C*), and tRNA (*lane D*). The observed band has size (816 nt), as expected for extension of full-length POMC mRNA with a radiolabeled primer to the 3′-end of the coding region for POMC exon 3. Lane A represents a 15 min autoradiograph and lanes B–D represent a 2 h exposure of the same acrylamide/urea gel. Radiolabelled ss DNA markers were run along with the samples. (Reprinted, with permission, from Lyons and Blalock.[18])

```
I
AAA CGG GAG GCG ACG GAG GAG AAA AGA GGT TAA GGA GCA GTG ACT AAG
▲(CAP)
AGA GGC CAC TGA ACA TCT TCG TCC TCA GAG AGC TGC CTT TCC GCG ACA
   II                              ▼(SIGNAL PEPTIDE)
G   AGC CTC AGC CAC CTG GAA G   ATG CCG AGA TTC TGC TAC AGT CGC
   ▲(alternative splice point)   MET PRO ARG PHE CYS TYR SER ARG

TCA GGG GCC CTG CTG CTG GCC CTC CTG CTT CAG ACC TCC ATA GAC GTG
SER GLY ALA LEU LEU LEU ALA LEU LEU LEU GLN THR SER ILE ASP VAL
          ▼(POMC)
TGG AGC TGG TGC CTG GAG AGC AGC CAG TGC CAG GAC CTC ACC ACG GAA
TRP SER TRP CYS LEU GLU SER SER GLN CYS GLN ASP LEU THR THR GLU
        III
AGC AAC CTG CTG GCT TGC ATC CGG GCC TGC AGA CTC GAC CTC TCG GCG
SER ASN LEU LEU ALA CYS ILE ARG ALA CYS ARG LEU ASP LEU SER ALA

GAG ACG CCC GTG TTT CCA GGC AAC GGA GAT GAA CAG CCC TTG ACT GAA
GLU THR PRO VAL PHE PRO GLY ASN GLY ASP GLU GLN PRO LEU THR GLU

AAT CCC-3'
ASN PRO
```

FIGURE 2. The nucleotide sequence of a rat splenocyte POMC cDNA is identical to that of the anterior pituitary POMC cDNA. The primer sequence (AS2) used in PCR amplification of 5′ poly dc-tailed cDNA is *underlined*. *Roman numerals* I–III mark the three exons of the POMC sequence. Both rat splenocytes and anterior pituitary corticotrophs use an alternative splice at the 5′ end of exon 2, resulting in the deletion of 30 nucleotides. (Reprinted, with permission, from Lyons and Blalock.[18])

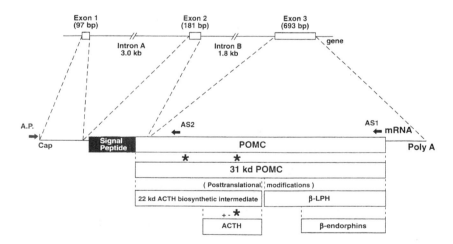

FIGURE 3. Structure of rat POMC gene, and schematic of POMC mRNA and protein processing. The POMC mRNA diagrams the regions present in each exon. The translated part of the mRNA is shown as an *open box*. Cleavage of the signal peptide generates POMC prohormone, encoded by exons 2 and 3. POMC processing is tissue-specific. The major peptide hormones in the anterior pituitary are ACTH and β-lipotropic hormone (βLPH). β-endorphins are the major cleavage products from βLPH in the intermediate pituitary, along with other proteolytic products not shown. *Asterisks* designate sites of N-linked glycosylation. (Reprinted, with permission, from Lyons and Blalock.[18])

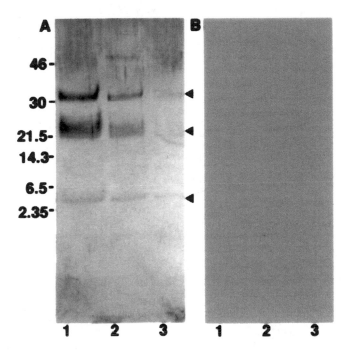

FIGURE 4. Anti-ACTH$_{1-24}$ immunoblot of cell lysates of anterior pituitary (*Lane 1,* 1×10^5 cells/lane), mitogen-stimulated splenocytes (*Lane 2,* 5×10^6 cells/lane), and untreated splenic macrophages (*Lane 3,* 5×10^6 cells/lane). (**A**) Western blot with anti-ACTH$_{1-24}$ identified POMC (31-Kd), ACTH biosynthetic intermediate (22-Kd), and nonglycosylated mature ACTH (4.5-Kd) with M$_R$ identified by *arrowheads* (◀). Immunoblots of all three samples with preimmune antibody (**B**) failed to identify any molecular species. Amersham rainbow markers were run along with samples and used to calculate M$_R$. (Reprinted, with permission, from Lyons and Blalock.[18])

their translation products are present in immune cells. They also led to questions about secretion. We now assume that ACTH and endorphin secretion from immune cells is via the signal peptide. In contrast, there continues to be no evidence for lymphocyte storage of these peptides in granules, such as occurs in corticotrophs of the pituitary gland.

ACTH AND OPIOID RECEPTORS IN THE IMMUNE SYSTEM

Opioid receptors predominantly belong to three classes; μ, δ, and κ. Early investigations indicated that both μ- and δ-class opioid receptors were expressed on T-cells, as assessed by functional assays.[19,20] These initial studies were confirmed and extended using dihydromorphine, naloxone, and [leu]-enkephalin in radioreceptor assays.[21] A saturable, high affinity binding site (Kd = 8–10 nM) was also reported on granulocytes and monocytes using [^{3}H]dihydromorphine.[22] Subsequently, a high affinity (Kd = 17 nM) enantioselective κ-like binding site was identified on the macrophage cell line, P388.[23] Activation of the macrophage opioid binding site increased Ca^{2+} mobilization in a time-dependent manner.[24] A saturable, naloxone-selective binding site was also identified on rat lymphocyte membranes (Kd = 960 nM) and this is sensitive to morphine (IC$_{50}$ = 130 nM), but not to [leu]-enkephalin, [met]-enkephalin, or β-endorphin.[25]

The binding studies were followed by structural studies that supported the presence of opioid receptors on immune cells. Specifically, using [^{3}H]cis-(+)-3-methylfentanyl-isothiocyanate (a δ-class-selective ligand), a binding site with a molecular weight of 58 kDa was specifically labeled on murine lymphocytes[26] and the P388d$_1$ macrophage cell line.[23] The μ-selective, site-directed acylating agent, [^{3}H]2-(ρ-ethoxybenzyl)-l-[N,N-diethylamino]ethyl-5-isothiocyanato-benzimidazole, labeled a lymphocyte membrane protein, exhibiting μ-class selectivity, that also had a molecular weight of 58 kDa.[27] In addition to the μ- and δ-opioid-receptors, the κ-selective, site-directed acylating agent, [^{3}H](1s,2s)-(−)-trans-2-isothiocyanato-N-methyl-N-[2-(1-pyrrolidinyl)cyclohexyl]benzeneacetamide, labeled a protein on lymphocytes that exhibited κ-class selectivity and had a molecular weight of 38–42 kDa.[28]

These early studies, that suggested the existence of opioid receptors on immune cell, have now received conclusive support as a result of cloning brain δ-,[29,30] κ-,[31] and μ-opioid[32,33] receptors. Opioid receptor transcripts in cells of the immune system were initially described in 1994 using primary and immortalized hematopoietic-derived cells.[34–39] Although these studies only determined partial sequences of the open reading frame for each of the opioid receptor types, and were found to be 98–99% homologous to the brain opioid receptor sequences, a full-length κ-opioid receptor cDNA expressed by cells of the immune system was found in the T-cell lymphocyte R1.1.[40] These results confirmed previous pharmacological studies showing the existence of a κ-opioid receptor on the R1.1 cells that was coupled to guanine nucleotide–binding protein.[41,42] A full-length δ-opioid receptor cDNA in thymocytes has also been identified and sequenced.[43] A nonopioid "orphan" receptor, having sequence homology (60%) with the "classic" opioid receptors, has also recently been cloned and sequenced in murine lymphocytes.[44] The receptor is upregulated following cell activation with mitogens. The receptor also has functional significance in mitogen–induced lymphocyte proliferation and polyclonal antibody production, but not in IL-5 production, as determined by antisense experiments.[44,45] A similar "orphan" opioid receptor, whose ligand was recently isolated,[46,47] has also been observed in activated human lymphocytes.[48]

As with opioid receptors, the earliest evidence for ACTH receptors on immune cells was functional. For example, ACTH was reported to stimulate B-cell growth[49,50] and antibody synthesis[51] at low concentrations, but at high concentrations it suppressed cytokine synthesis[52] and antibody synthesis.[21] These studies were followed by others that demonstrated ACTH binding sites on B- and T-lymphocytes but not on thymocytes, by means of a radioreceptor assay.[53] Today, although ACTH and other melanocortin receptors have been cloned, there is limited molecular biologic evidence for their presence in immune cells. Specifically, expression of α-MSH receptor mRNA was observed in monocyte/macrophage–like cells.[54] Based on the findings with opioid receptors, it will be quite surprising if there are not a plethora of future reports on this receptor mRNA in immune cells.

In hindsight, considering that we now have irrefutable data that opioid and ACTH receptors are identical in the immune and neuroendocrine systems, its not particularly surprising that they couple to the same second-messaging systems. Thus, in immune cells, opioid receptor activation leads to the stimulation of guanylate cyclase,[55] inhibition of adenylatecyclase,[55,56] reduction in potassium conductance,[57] and enhancement in Ca^{2+} uptake.[24,58] Likewise, activation of the ACTH receptor stimulated the expected Ca^{2+} uptake and cAMP synthesis in immune cells.[59,60]

A SENSORY FUNCTION FOR THE IMMUNE SYSTEM

The most important aspect of the above findings was that, for the first time, these results provide a biochemical rationale for bidirectional communication between the immune and neuroendocrine systems. Put most simply, these two systems contain and use the same set of signal molecules in the form of hormones, lymphokines, and monokines, for inter- and intrasystem communication and regulation. Furthermore, they harbor the same array of receptors for the shared ligands. Thus, in retrospect, it would seem virtually impossible for there not to be "cross talk" between the immune and neuroendocrine systems.

The realization of this biochemical circuit led, in turn, to the most interesting conceptual advance; that is, an important function of the immune system is to serve as a sensory organ. It has been proposed that the immune system may sense stimuli that are not recognized by the central and peripheral nervous systems.[61] These stimuli have been termed noncognitive, and include those things (bacteria, tumors, viruses, antigens, etc.,) that would pass unnoticed by our classic senses of touch, taste, sight, sound, and smell, were it not for their recognition by the immune system. The recognition of such noncognitive stimuli by immunocytes is then converted into information, in the form of peptide hormones, neurotransmitters, lymphokines, and monokines; this information is conveyed to the neuroendocrine system, and a physiological change occurs. Conversely, recognition of cognitive stimuli by the central and peripheral nervous system results in similar hormonal and neurotransmitter information being conveyed to, and recognized by, receptors on immunocytes, and an immunologic change results.

RECENT DEVELOPMENTS

The potential medical relevance of understanding the biochemical basis for the immune/neuroendocrine circuit is now becoming clear. For instance, the elegant studies of Stein and colleagues have defined a new analgesic pathway that is initiated in the immune system rather than the nervous system. Specifically, activation of endogenous opioids in rats by a cold-water swim results in a local antinociceptive effect on inflamed peripheral tissue. This local antinociception in the inflamed tissue is, apparently, the result of production by immune cells of endogenous opioids-that interact with opioid receptors on peripheral sensory nerves.[62] This strongly suggests that the immune system plays an essential role in pain control.[63] Locally expressed corticotroph releasing factor (CRF) was identified as the main agent inducing opioid release within the inflamed tissue. The opioid receptor-specific anti-nociception in inflamed paws of rats could be blocked by interplanar α-helical CRF (a CRF antagonist), or antiserum to CRF, or CRF-antisense oligodeoxynucleotides. The latter treatment reduced the amount of CRF extracted from inflamed paws, as well as the number of CRF-immunostained cells.[63] These observations seem to offer new potential insights into pain occurring in normal and immunosuppressed conditions. Furthermore, they provide a vivid example of the sensory function of the nervous system.

On the other hand, endogenous opiates exert profound autocrine, paracrine, and endocrine effects on immune function and development. For instance, an opiate antagonist was shown to indirectly block CRF enhancement of NK cell activity by inhibiting the action of immunocyte-derived opioid peptides.[64] Similarly, an opiate antagonist was more effective than cyclosporin in prolonging allograft survival.[65] In the most recent finding in the area, μ-opioid receptor–deficient mice displayed not only the expected behavioral abnormalities, but also showed altered hematopoiesis.[66] Specifically, these animals were observed to have increased numbers of, and proliferation rates for, granulocyte-macrophage, erythroid, and multipotential progenitor cells, in both bone marrow and spleen. Thus, in conclusion, it is not difficult to envision how a basic understanding of the role of POMC in neuroimmunomodulation may lead to profound advances in medicine, which include, but are not limited to, analgesia, transplantation, and hematopoiesis. Indeed, the ability to detect a form of glucocorticoid deficiency due to ACTH insensitivity syndrome by testing for the absence of high affinity ACTH binding sites on peripheral blood mononuclear cells of a patient may represent the first example.[67,68]

ACKNOWLEDGMENTS

The author thanks Diane Weigent for expert editorial assistance. This work was supported in part by NIH Grants A137670, MH52527, and NS2971; and a grant from the Muscular Dystrophy Association.

REFERENCES

1. BLALOCK, J.E. & E.M. SMITH. 1980. Human leukocyte interferon: structural and biological relatedness to adrenocorticotropic hormone and endorphins. Proc. Natl. Acad. Sci. USA 77: 5972–5974.
2. SMITH, E.M. & J.E. BLALOCK. 1981. Human lymphocyte production of corticotropin and enclorphin-like substances: association with leukocyte interferon. Proc. Natl. Acad. Sci. USA 78: 7530–7534.
3. BLALOCK, J.E. 1984. Relationships between neuroendocrine hormones and lymphokines. In Lymphokines. E. Pick, Ed: 1–13. Academic Press, Orlando.
4. EPSTEIN, L.B., M.E. ROSE, N.H. McMANUS & C.H. LL. 1982. Absence of functional and structural homology of natural and recombinant human leukocyte interferon (IFN-alpha) with human alpha-ACTH and beta-endorphin. Biochem. Biophys. Res. Commun. 104: 341–346.

5. BLOOM, F.E. 1987. Molecular markers of neuronal specificity. *In* Molecular Neuroscience: Expression of Neural Genes. F. Wong, D.C. Eaton, D.A. Konkel & J.R. Perez-Pola, Eds.: 1–10. Alan R. Liss. New York.

6. BLALOCK, J.E. & E.M. SMITH. 1985. A complete regulatory loop between the immune and neuroendocrine systems. Fed. Proc. **44:** 108–111.

7. SMITH, E.M., W.J. MEYER, & J.E. BLALOCK. 1982. Virus-induced corticosterone in hypophysectomized mice: a possible lymphoid adrenal axis. Science **218:** 1311–1312.

8. ENDO, Y., T. SAKATA & S. WATANABE. 1985. Identification of proopiomelanocortin-producing cells in the rat pyloric antrum and duodenum by *in situ* mRNA-cDNA hybridization. Biomed. Res. **6:** 253–256.

9. WESTLY, H.J., A.J. KLEISS, K.W. KELLEY, P.K.Y. WONG & P.H. YUEN. 1986. Newcastle disease virus-infected splenocytes express the proopiomelanocortin gene. J. Exp. Med. **163:** 1589–1594.

10. LOLAIT, S.J., J.A. CLEMENTS, A.J. MARKWICK, C. CHENG, M. MCNALLY, A.I. SMITH & J.W. FUNDER. 1986. Pro-opiomelanocortin messenger ribonucleic acid and post-translational processing of beta endorphin in spleen macrophages. J. Clin. Invest. **77:** 1776–1779.

11. OATES, E.L., G.P. ALLAWAY, G.R. ARMSTRONG, R.A. BOYAJIAN, J.H. KEHR & B.S. PROBHAKAR. 1988. Human lymphocytes produce pro-opiomelanocortin gene-related transcripts. Effects of lymphotropic viruses. J. Biol. Chem. **263:** 10041–10044.

12. BUZZETTI, R., L. MCLOUGHLIN, P.M. LAVENDER, A.J. CLARK & L.H. REES. 1989. Expression of pro-opiomelanocortin gene and quantification of adrenocorticotropic hormone-like immunoreactivity in human normal peripheral mononuclear cells and lymphoid and myeloid malignancies. J. Clin. Invest. **83:** 733–737.

13. SMITH, E.M., F.S. GALIN, R.D. LEBOEUF, D.H. COPPENHAVER, D.V. HARBOUR & J.E. BLALOCK. 1990. Nucleotide and amino acid sequence of lymphocyte-derived corticotropin: endotoxin induction of a truncated peptide. Proc. Natl. Acad. Sci. USA **87:** 1057–1060.

14. GALIN, F.S., R.D. LEBOEUF & J.E. BLALOCK. 1990. A lymphocyte mRNA encodes the adrenocorticotropin β-lipotropin region of the pro-opiomelanocortin gene. Prog. Neuro. Endocrin. Immunol. **3:** 205–208.

15. GALIN, F.S., R.D. LEBOEUF & J.E. BLALOCK. 1991. Corticotropin-releasing factor upregulates expression of two truncated pro-opiomelanocortin transcripts in murine lymphocytes. J. Neuroimmunol. **31:** 51–58.

16. PANERAI, A.E. & P. SACERDOTE. 1997. Beta-endorphin in the immune system: a role at last? Immunol. Today **18:** 317–319.

17. SHARP, B. & T. YAKSH. 1997. Pain killers of the immune system. Nature Med. **3:** 831–832.

18. LYONS, P.D. & J.E. BLALOCK. 1997. Pro-opiomelanocortin gene expression and protein processing in rat mononuclear leukocytes. J. Neuroimmunol. **70.** 47–56.

19. WYBRAN, J., T. APPELBOOM, J.-P. FAMAEY & A. GOVAERTS. 1979. Suggestive evidence for receptors for morphine and methionine-enkephalin on normal human blood T lymphocytes. J. Immunol. **123:** 1068–1070.

20. MCDONOUGH, R.J., J.J. MADDEN, A. FALEK, D.A. SHAFER, M. PLINE, D. GORDON, P. BOKOS, J.C. KUEHNLE & J. MENDELSON. 1980. Alteration of T and null lymphocyte frequencies in the peripheral blood of human opiate addicts: *In vivo* evidence for opiate receptor sites on T lymphocytes. J. Immunol. **125:** 2539–2543.

21. JOHNSON, H.M., E.M. SMITH, B.A. TORRES & J.E. BLALOCK. 1982. Neuroendocrine hormone regulation of *in vitro* antibody formation. Proc. Natl. Acad. Sci. USA **79:** 4171–4174.

22. LOPKER, A., L.G. ABOOD, W. HOSS & F.J. LIONETTI. 1980. Stereoselective muscarinic acetylcholine and opiate receptors in human phagocytic leukocytes. Biochem. Pharm. **29:** 1361–1365.
23. CARR, D.J., B.R. DECOSTA, C.H. KIM, A.E. JACOBSON, V. GUARCELLO, K.C. RICE & J.E. BLALOCK. 1989. Opioid receptors on cells of the immune system: evidence for delta- and kappa-classes. J. Endocrinol. **122:** 161–168.
24. CARR, D.J.J. & J.E. BLALOCK. 1989. Neuroendocrine characteristics of the immune system. EOS J. Immunol. Immunopharmacol. **IX:** 195–199.
25. OVADIA, H., P. NITSAN & O. ABRAMSKY. 1989. Characterization of opiate binding sites on membranes of rat lymphocytes. J. Neuroimmunol. **21:** 93–102.
26. CARR, D.J., C.H. KIM, B. DECOSTA, A.E. JACOBSON, K.C. RICE & J.E. BLALOCK. 1988. Evidence for a delta-class opioid receptor on cells of the immune system. Cell Immunol. **116:** 44–51.
27. RADULESCU, R.T., B.R. DECOSTA, A.E. JACOBSON, K.C. RICE & J.E. BLALOCK. 1991. Biochemical and functional characterization of a mu-opioid receptor binding site on cells of the immune system. Prog. Neuro. Endocrin. Immunol. **4:** 166–179.
28. CARR, D.J., B.R. DECOSTA, A.E. JACOBSON, K.C. RICE & J.E. BLALOCK. 1991. Enantioselective kappa opioid binding sites on the macrophage cell line, P388dl. Life Sci. **49:** 45–51.
29. KIEFFER, B.L., K. BEFORT, C. GAVERIAUX-RUFF & C.G. HIRTH. 1992. The delta-opioid receptor: Isolation of a cDNA by expression cloning and pharmacological characterization. Proc. Nad. Acad. Sci. USA **89:** 12048–12052.
30. EVANS, C.J., D. KEITH, K. MAGENDZO, H. MORRISON & R.H. EDWARDS. 1992. Cloning of a delta opioid receptor by functional expression. Science **258:** 1952–1955.
31. YASUDA, K., K. RAYNOR, H. KONG, C.D. BREDER, J. TAKEDA, T. REISINE & G.I. BELL. 1993. Cloning and functional comparison of κ and δ opioid receptors from mouse brain. Proc. Natl. Acad. Sci. USA **90:** 6736–6740.
32. THOMPSON, R.C., A. MANSOUR, H. AKIL & S.J. WATSON. 1993. Cloning and pharmacological characterization of a rat μ opioid receptor. Neuron **11:** 903–913.
33. WANG, J.B., Y. IMAI, C.M. EPPLER, P. GREGOR, C.E. SPIVAK & G.R. UHL. 1993. μ opiate receptor: cDNA cloning and expression. Proc. Natl. Acad. Sci. USA **90:** 10230–10234.
34. GAVERIAUX-RUFF, G., F. SIMONIN, J. PELUSO, K. DEFORT & B. KIEFFER. 1994. Expression of opioid receptors mRNAs in immune cells. Regul. Pept. **54:** 103–104.
35. CHUANG, L.F., T.K. CHUANG, K.F. KILLAM, JR., A.J. CHUANG, H. KUNG, L. YU & R.Y. CHUANG. 1994. Delta opioid receptor gene expression in lymphocytes. Biochem. Biophys. Res. Commun. **202:** 1291–1299.
36. CHUANG, L.F., T.K. CHUANG, K.F. KILLAMK, JR., Q. QIU, X.R. WANG, J. LIN, H. KUNG, W. SHENG, C. CHAO, L. YU & R.Y. CHUANG. 1995. Expression of kappa opioid receptors in human and monkey lymphocytes. Biochem. Biophys. Res. Commun. **209:** 1003–1010.
37. SEDQI, M., S. ROY, S. RAMAKRISHNAN, R. ELDE & H.H. LOH. 1995. Complementary DNA cloning of a μ opioid receptor from rat peritoneal macrophages. Biochem. Biophys. Res. Commun. **209:** 563–574.
38. GAVERIAUX, C., J. PELUSO, F. SIMONIN, J. LAFORET & B. KIEFFER. 1995. Identification of κ- and δ-opioid receptor transcripts in immune cells. FEBS Lett. **369:** 272–276.
39. CHUANG, T.K., K.F. KILLAM, JR., L.F. CHUANG, H. KUNG, W.S. SHENG, C.C. CHAO, L. YU & R.Y. CHUANG. 1995. Mu opioid receptor gene expression in immune cells. Biochem. Biophys. Res. Commun. **216:** 922–930.
40. BELKOWSKI, S.M., J. ZHU, L.-Y. LIU-CHEN, T.K. EISENSTEIN, M.W. AIDLER & T.J. ROGERS. 1995. Sequence of κ-opioid receptor cIDNA in the R1.1 thymoma cell line. J. Neuroimmunol. **62:** 113–117.

41. LAWRENCE, D.M. & J.M. BIDLACK. 1993. The kappa opioid receptor expressed on the mouse R1.1 thymoma cell line is coupled to adenyl cyclase through a pertussis toxin-sensitive guanine nucleotide-binding regulatory protein. J. Pharmacol. Exp. Ther. **266:** 1678–1683.

42. JOSEPH, D.B. & J.M. BIDLACK. 1995. The kappa opioid receptor expressed on the mouse R1.1 thymoma cell line down-regulates without desensitizing during chronic opioid exposure. J. Pharmacol. Exp. Ther. **272:** 970–976.

43. SEDQI, M., S. ROY, S. RAMAKRISHNAN & H.H. LOH. 1996. Expression cloning of a full-length cDNA encoding delta opioid receptor from mouse thymocytes. J. Neuroimmunol. **65:** 167–170.

44. HALFORD, W.P., B.M. GEBHARDT & D.J.J. CARR. 1995. Functional role and sequence analysis of a lymphocyte orphan opioid receptor. J. Neuroimmunol. **59:** 91–101.

45. CARR, D.J.J., T.J. ROGERS & R.J. WEBER. 1996. The relevance of opioids and opioid receptors on immunocompetence and immune homeostasis. Proc. Soc. Exp. Biol. Med. **113:** 248–257.

46. MEUNIER, J.C., C. MOLLEREAU, L. TOLL, C. SUAUDEAU, C. MOISAND, P. ALVINERIE, J.-L. BUTOUR, J.-C. GUILLEMOT, P. FERRARA, B. MONSARRAT, H. MAZARGULL, G. VASSART, M. PARMENTIER & J. COSTENTIN. 1995. Isolation and structure of the endogenous agonist of opioid receptor-like ORL$_1$ receptor. Nature **377:** 532–535.

47. REINSCHEID, R.K., H.-P. NOTHACKER, A. BOURSON, A. ARDATI, R.A. HENNINGSEN, J.R. BUNZOW, D.K. GRANDY, H. LANGEN, F.J. MONSMA, JR., O. CIVELLI & F.Q. ORPHANIN. 1995. A neuropeptide that activates an opioidlike G protein-coupled receptor. Science **270:** 792–794.

48. WICK, M.J., S.R. MINNERATH, S. ROY, S. RAMAKRISHNAN & H.H. LOH. 1995. Expression of alternate forms of brain opioid "orphan" receptor mRNA in activated human peripheral blood lymphocytes and lymphocytic cell lines. Mol. Brain. Res. **32:** 342–347.

49. ALVAREZ-MON, A., J.H. KEHRL & A.S. FAUCI. 1985. A potential role for adrenocorticotropin in regulating human B lymphocyte functions. J. Immunol. **135:** 3823–3826.

50. BROOKS, K.H. 1990. Adrenocorticotropin (ACTH) functions as a late-acting B cell growth factor and synergizes with interleukin 5. J. Mol. Cell Immunol. **4:** 327–335.

51. BOST, K.L., B.L. CLARKE, J. XU, H. KIYONO, J.R. MCGHEE & D. PASCUAL. 1990. Modulation of IgM secretion and H chain mRNA expression in CH12.LX.C4.5F5 B cells by adrenocorticotropic hormone. J. Immunol. **145:** 4326–4331.

52. JOHNSON, H.M., B.A. TORRES, E.M. SMITH, L.D. DION & J.E. BLALOCK. 1984. Regulation of lymphokine (gamma-interferon) production by corticotropin. J. Immunol. **132:** 246–250.

53. CLARKE, B.L. & K.L. BOST. 1989. Differential expression of functional adrenocorticotropic hormone receptors by subpopulations of lymphocytes. J. Immunol. **143:** 464–469.

54. STAR, R.A., N. RAJORA, J. HUANG, R.C. STOCK, A. CATTANIA & J.M. LIPTON. 1995. Evidence of autocrine modulation of macrophage nitric oxide synthase by alpha-melanocyte-stimulating hormone. Proc. Natl. Acad. Sci. USA **92:** 8016–8020.

55. FULOP, JR., T., D. KEKESSY & G. FORIS. 1987. Impaired coupling of naloxone sensitive opiate receptors to adenylate cyclase in PMNLs of aged male subjects. J. Immunopharmacol. **9:** 651–658.

56. CARR, D.J., K.L. BOST & J.E. BLALOCK. 1988. The production of antibodies which recognize opiate receptors on murine leukocytes. Life Sci. **42:** 2615–2624.

57. CARR, D.J., J.K. BUBIEN, W.T. WOODS & J.E. BLALOCK. 1988. Opioid receptors on murine splenocytes. Possible coupling to K$^+$ channels. Ann. N.Y. Acad. Sci. **540:** 694–697.

58. HOUGH, C.J., J.I. HALPERIN, D.L. MAZOROW, S.L. YEANDLE & D.B. MILLAR. 1990. β-Endorphin modulates T-cell intracellular calcium flux and c-myc expression via a potassium channel. J. Neuroimmunol. **27:** 163–171.
59. JOHNSON, E.W., J.E. BLALOCK & E.M. SMITH. 1988. ACTH receptor-mediated induction of leukocyte cyclic AMP. Biochem. Biophys. Res. Commun. **157:** 1205–1211.
60. CLARKE, B.L., D.R. MOORE & J.E. BLALOCK. 1994. Adrenocorticotropic hormone stimulates a transient calcium uptake in rat lymphocytes. Endocrinology **135:** 1780–1786.
61. BLALOCK, J.E. 1984. The immune system as a sensory organ. J. Immunol. **132:** 1067–1070.
62. STEIN, C., A.H.S. HASSAN, R. PRZEWLOCKI, C. GRAMSCH, K. PETER & A. HERZ. 1990. Opioids from immunocytes interact with receptors on sensory nerves to inhibit nociception in inflammation. Proc. Natl. Acad. Sci. USA **87:** 5935–5939.
63. SCHAFER, M., S.A. MOUSA, Q. ZHANG, L. CARTER & C. STEIN. 1996. Expression of corticotropin-releasing factor in inflamed tissue is required for intrinsic peripheral opioid analgesia. Proc. Natl. Acad. Sci. USA **93:** 6096–6100.
64. CARR, D.J., B.R. DECOSTA, A.E. JACOBSON, K.C. RICE & J.E. BLALOCK. 1990. Corticotropin-releasing hormone augments natural killer cell activity through a naloxone-sensitive pathway. J. Neuroimmunol. **28:** 53–61.
65. ARAKAWA, K., T. AKAMI, M. OKAMOTO, T. OKA & H. NAGASE. 1992. The immunosuppressive effect of delta-opioid receptor antagonist on rat renal allograft survival. Transplantation **53:** 951–953.
66. TIAN, M., H.E. BROXMEYER, Y. FAN, Z. LAI, S. ZHANG, S. ARONICA, S. COOPER, R.M. BIGSBY, R. STEINMETZ, S.J. ENGLE, A. MESTEK, J.D. POLLOCK, M.N. LEHMAN, H.T. JANSEN, M. YING, P.J. STAMBROOK, J.A. TISCHFIELD & L. YU. 1997. Altered hematoipoiesis, behavior, and sexual function in μ opioid receptor-deficient mice. J. Exp. Med. **185:** 1517–1522.
67. SMITH, E.M., P. BROSNAN, W.J. MEYER & J.E. BLALOCK. 1987. An ACTH receptor on human mononuclear leukocytes. Relation to adrenal ACTH-receptor activity. New Eng. J. Med. **317:** 1266–1269.
68. YAMAMOTO, Y., Y. KAWAIDA, M. NODA, M. YAMAGISHI, O. ISHIDA, T. FUJIHIRA, F. SHIRAKAWA & I. MORIMOTO. 1995. Siblings with ACTH insensitivity due to lack of ACTH binding to the receptor. Endocrine J. **42:** 171–177.

Mechanisms of Antiinflammatory Action of α-MSH Peptides

In Vivo and *in Vitro* Evidence

J.M. LIPTON,[a,b] H. ZHAO,[a] T. ICHIYAMA,[a] G.S. BARSH,[c] AND A. CATANIA[d]

[a]*Department of Physiology, University of Texas Southwestern Medical Center, 5323 Harry Hines Boulevard, Dallas, Texas 75235, USA*

[b]*Department of Anesthesiology and Pain Management, University of Texas Southwestern Medical Center, 5323 Harry Hines Boulevard, Dallas, Texas 75235, USA*

[c]*Departments of Genetics and Pediatrics, Howard Hughes Medical Institute, Stanford University School of Medicine, Stanford, California 94305, USA*

[d]*Third Division of Internal Medicine, IRCCS Ospedale Maggiore, Milan, Italy 20122*

ABSTRACT: α-Melanocyte stimulating hormone (α-MSH) modulates all forms of inflammation by acting on peripheral inflammatory cells, glial inflammatory cells, and on CNS receptors that activate descending antiinflammatory neural pathways. The multiple actions of this ancient peptide suggest that there is no singular biochemical mechanism through which it exerts its antiinflammatory activity. However, research on IL-10 deficient and Agouti protein hypersecreting mice provide new insights into the actions of the peptide in living animals. Studies of cultured human astrocytes, whole murine brain, and human monocyte/macrophages indicate that a primary effect of the peptide is modulation of activation of the nuclear transcription factor κB. The latter influence may underlie the established reduction of gene expression and production of proinflammatory peptides and inducible nitric oxide by α-MSH peptides.

A key scientific question for all effective agents concerns their mechanism of action. The question is a major one for the antiinflammatory neuroimmunomodulatory peptide, α-MSH, and related molecules. α-MSH inhibits all forms of inflammation against which it has been tested.[1] It is clear that the peptide can inhibit inflammation by acting directly upon peripheral host cells to modulate release of inflammatory substances, and by acting on receptors within the brain that drive descending antiinflammatory pathways. It is, therefore, likely that the peptide has multiple actions in inhibition of inflammation. However, it is possible that in inflammatory cells the peptide acts at a pivotal point in the inflammation cascade, a point that is common to all forms and in all sites of inflammation. The studies outlined below were designed to test hypotheses of specific actions of the peptide *in vivo* and *in vitro*.

[b]Address for correspondence: 214-648-2357 (voice); 214-648-4703 (fax); james.lipton@email.swmed.edu (e-mail).

IN VIVO SIGNIFICANCE OF ENDOGENOUS IL-10 TO THE ANTIINFLAMMATORY EFFECTS OF α-MSH

α-MSH inhibits both the induction and elicitation of contact sensitivity and can lead to hapten-specific tolerance.[2] These effects of α-MSH are presumed to involve an interleukin-10 (IL-10) antiinflammatory cytokine intermediate, because treatment with an IL-10 antibody reduced the effects of α-MSH. If α-MSH does act through release of an essential IL-10 intermediate, the peptide should be relatively ineffective in controlling inflammation in animals that are deficient in the gene for IL-10. In tests of this idea, IL-10 deficient mice had greater acute inflammatory reactions to irritant applied to the ear (see FIGURE 1). Despite the greater inflammatory reactions in IL-10–deficient mice, α-MSH given systemically effectively modulated them—much as in control mice. The relative inhibition (percent of percent change) with α-MSH was virtually the same in both IL-10–deficient and in control animals (approximately 70%). Examination of the influence of α-MSH in systemic inflammation was hampered by the markedly greater reactions of IL-10–deficient mice to challenge with LPS. In standard tests of survival in response to LPS, 67% of IL-10–deficient mice died within 6–24 h whereas all background control mice were still alive at 24 h. This result is consistent with the original observations of Berg *et al.*,[3] indicating that the lethal dose of LPS for IL-10–deficient mice is 20-fold lower than for wild-type mice. There is also recent evidence of increased susceptibility to staphylococcal enterotoxin B–induced lethal shock in IL-10–deficient mice.[4] In our experiments, blood samples taken from IL-10–deficient mice 6 h post-LPS injection

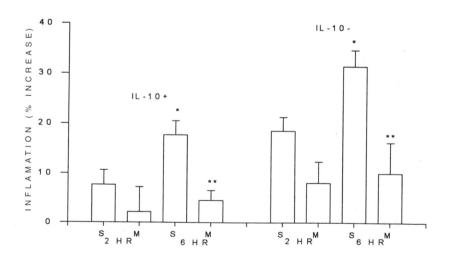

FIGURE 1. Acute inflammatory reactions to application of irritant (picryl chloride 0.5% in acetone, 10 μl applied to both surfaces of a single ear) in background control and IL-10–deficient mice. Measurements were made at 2 and 6 h after application of irritant. *S*, i.p. injection of saline (0.2 ml) at the time irritant was applied; *M*, i.p. injection of α-MSH (50 μg/0.2 ml saline). *, $p < 0.05$; **, $p < 0.01$.

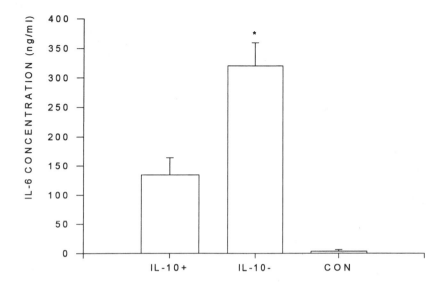

FIGURE 2. IL-6 concentrations of blood samples (tail vein) measured 6 h after i.p. ad ministration of 200 μg *E. coli* LPS in IL-10 background control (*IL-10+*) and IL-10– deficient (*IL-10–*) mice. *CON*, baseline IL-6 measures for all mice before injection of LPS. All scores are means ± SEM. *, $p < 0.05$ versus IL-10+.

contained markedly elevated concentrations of proinflammatory IL-6 (see FIGURE 2). This result is also consistent with recent findings of elevated IL-6, other cytokines, and nitric oxide in IL-10–deficient mice.[4] Thus, although IL-10–deficient mice have reduced capacity to modulate both peripheral local and systemic inflammatory reactions, they are capable of reacting to exogenous α-MSH with reduced acute inflammatory reactions. These results indicate that, at least for acute inflammation, no IL-10 intermediate is required for the antiinflammatory effect of α-MSH. It should be noted that acute inflammation is marked by local extravasation of fluid and the appearance of neutrophils with a smaller contribution from monocyte/ macrophages. It remains to be seen whether chronic inflammation associated with increased monocyte/macrophage infiltration is likewise modulated by α-MSH in IL-10–null animals.

TESTS OF INFLAMMATORY RESPONSES IN MICE
THAT OVERSECRETE AGOUTI PROTEIN
AN ENDOGENOUS MODULATOR OF α-MSH

Agouti protein is a paracrine signaling molecule that antagonizes the effects of α-MSH and other melanocortins. There is evidence that the molecule competes with α-MSH for the melanocortin receptor MC-1R although the action of Agouti protein cannot be explained solely by inhibition of α-MSH binding. It appears that there is a novel signaling mechanism whereby α-MSH and Agouti protein function as independent ligands, with each inhibiting the binding of the other and transducing opposite signals through a single receptor. It is believed likely that the interaction between Agouti protein and MC-1R represents interactions that occur between the other melanocortin receptor subtypes and Agouti-related molecules in the regulation of other biological processes.

The *Agouti* gene has been found to encode a small, secreted, highly basic protein that is approximately twice the size of insulin.[5] Agouti protein, produced and secreted by specialized cells in the skin, causes neighboring melanocytes, which normally produce black pigment, to synthesize yellow pigment instead.[6] Although originally related to coat color, agouti alleles such as aA^y and A^{vy} are associated with pleiotropic effects, indicating that ectopic expression of normal Agouti protein is responsible for obesity, increased tumor susceptibility, and premature infertility.[7] The results indicate that Agouti protein binds to receptors in nonpigmentary tissues as well; thus, there is reason to suspect that interactions between Agouti protein and melanocortin receptors occur in the regulation of other biological processes.[8,9] For example, many of the phenotypes that occur in mice carrying the dominant *Agouti* allele *lethal yellow* (A^y) are thought to be caused by inhibition of CNS-specific melanocortin receptors.[10]

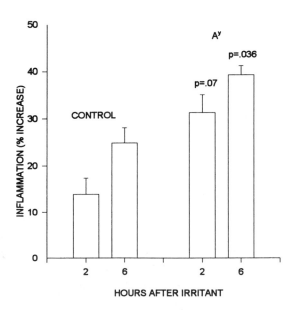

FIGURE 3. Inflammatory responses to dermal application of picryl chloride were greater in Agouti protein–secreting mice (A^y, $n = 4$) than in controls ($n = 8$). The Mann-Whitney U-test techniques are described in FIGURE 1.

That Agouti protein may be important in control of inflammation is supported by our recent data, in which A^y mice showed greater acute inflammatory responses than background animals (see FIGURE 3).

That Agouti protein secreting mice have other differences in inflammatory response was indicated by their reaction to challenge with systemic endotoxin (see FIGURE 4). Similar to the IL-10–deficient mice described above, A^y mice had greater increases in serum IL-6 after i.p. injection of LPS. From this result it appears that hypersecretion of Agouti protein promotes proinflammatory IL-6 responses to challenge. This may occur by modulation of the influence of endogenous α-MSH at the level of the melanocortin receptor.

The combined results of acute inflammation and endotoxemia studies suggest that Agouti protein must be considered in theories of the mechanism of action of α-MSH peptides. Our results indicate that this protein is important to peripheral and systemic inflammatory processes that have no *prima facie* link with pigmentation, thereby supporting a pleiotropic role for this protein. It has been established that α-MSH can overcome the influence of Agouti protein at melanocortin receptors by simply increasing α-MSH concentration.[9] To determine whether greater quantities of α-MSH are required to overcome inflammation in Agouti protein–secreting mice is the next step toward understanding the involvement of the α-MSH/Agouti protein relations in control of the inflammatory response.

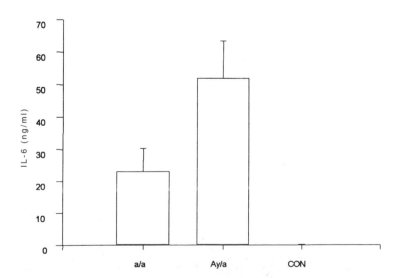

FIGURE 4. Serum IL-6 in background (*a/a*, $n = 7$) and Agouti protein secreting (A^y/a, $n = 6$) mice injected 3 h previously with *E. coli* LPS (200 μg, i.p.). Baseline, serum IL-6 (*CON*) was negligible.

INFLUENCE OF MELANOCORTIN PEPTIDES ON
INFLAMMATORY PROCESSES WITHIN THE BRAIN

Inflammation occurs in neurological disorders that are associated with infectious agents (bacteria, viruses, fungi, etc.,) but also in other disorders including CNS AIDS, multiple sclerosis, Alzheimer's disease, stroke, and neurodegenerative disorders. It is important to control such inflammation and, thereby, to preserve neurons and the functions they mediate. α-MSH is known to modulate CNS inflammation: it inhibits production of TNFα induced in murine brain both *in vivo* and *in vitro*,[11] and it modulates the functional disturbance associated with stroke in models of posterior circulation ischemia and reperfusion.[12] The mechanism (or mechanisms) underlying the anti-inflammatory influence of α-MSH has not been established, but it is clear that the influence is extremely rapid. It may be that the peptide modulates a process that is very basic to the inflammatory pathway—a process that is common to inflammation of all types and in all sites. One possibility that has recently arisen, is modulation of translocation of nuclear factor κB (NFκB). This agent is involved in the inducible regulation of a wide variety of genes involved in the inflammatory response.[13] Recent studies from this laboratory[14] indicate that α-MSH modulates LPS-induced NFκB activation in both human anaplastic astrocytoma cells in culture and in murine brain *in vivo*. These results, related to the concentration of α-MSH, we believe occur because the peptide modulates degeneration of IκBα. IκBα normally binds to NFκB within the cell, thereby preventing migration of NFκB to the nucleus and subsequent production of proinflammatory cytokines. Ichiyama *et al.*, found that LPS-induced degradation of IκBα in a human glioma cell line (A172) and in murine brains was prevented by incubation (cells) or by cerebral ventricular injection (brains) of α-MSH. Melanocortin receptors are known to occur within the brain. In addition to receptors MC-3R, -4R, and -5R previously shown to exist in brain,[15] we recently found evidence for MC-1R expression in both murine brain[11] and in human A-172 cells.[16] The combined results suggest that α-MSH modulates CNS inflammation by acting directly on melanocortin receptors in glial cells.

EVIDENCE THAT α-MSH$_{11-13}$ MODULATES NFκB
ACTIVATION IN HUMAN ASTROCYTES

The tripeptide KPV that occurs in the COOH-terminal region of α-MSH has antiinflammatory properties that parallel those of the parent molecule.[1] These parallel effects in multiple models of inflammation suggest that the tripeptide amino acid sequence is the message sequence that underlies the antiinflammatory properties of α-MSH. Our recent research indicates that the parallel effects of the tripeptide and α-MSH extend to modulation of NFκB activation. A172 cells stimulated with LPS showed marked activation of NFκB, as indicated above. Treatment with high concentrations of the tripeptide inhibited this activation (see FIGURE 5). This result suggests that the tripeptide modulates proinflammatory processes by acting, like α-MSH$_{1-13}$, on transcription of inflammatory agents, and extends the parallel effects of the two antiinflammatory peptides to yet another instance.

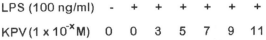

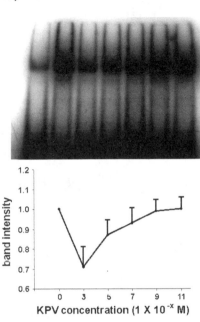

FIGURE 5, Modulation of NFκB activation by the tripeptide KPV (α-MSH$_{11-13}$) in human glioma cells (A172) stimulated with LPS. **Upper part,** representative EMSA showing Ac KPV NH$_2$–induced inhibition of NFκB activation 2 h after stimulation with LPS. **Lower part,** densitometric values derived from the EMSA illustrating effectiveness of 10^{-3} and 10^{-5} M concentrations of KPV.

MELANOCORTIN PEPTIDE INFLUENCE ON MACROPHAGES

Macrophages are prominent in the chronic inflammation that occurs in disorders such as arthritis and inflammatory bowel disease. Our previous research indicated that α-MSH peptides modulate proinflammatory mediators: nitric oxide, TNFα, and IL-1β. Recent research indicates that this inhibition extends to an influence on IL-8, a chemoattractant cytokine of great significance in inflammation. THP-1 cells, a human monocytic cell line, show marked release of IL-8 within 4 h of stimulation with LPS. This increase is modulated when the cells are incubated with LPS in the presence of α-MSH$_{1-13}$.[17] As in other instances cited above, α-MSH$_{11-13}$ had a parallel influence (see FIGURE 6), although in this case very low concentrations of the tripeptide were effective—an illustration of biphasic influences common with peptides. The results further indicated that NFκB activation was modulated in the same cells in the presence of α-MSH. Thus, just as for results with glial cells and whole brain samples described above, it may be that the primary influence of α-MSH in host in-

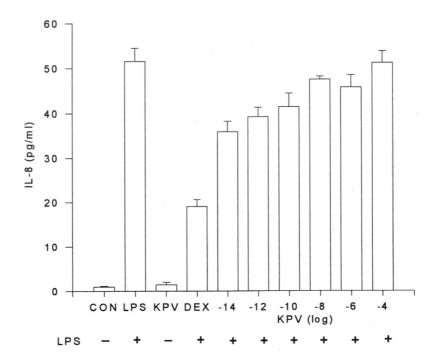

FIGURE 6. Inhibition by KPV of IL-8 production by THP-1 cells stimulated with LPS. *CON*, media alone; *KPV*, tripeptide 10^{-3} M alone; *DEX*, 10^{-6} M.

flammatory cells is inhibition of translocation of transcription factor κB to the nucleus. This modulation of transcription could account for the multiple inhibitory effects of the peptides on induction of proinflammatory agents *in vitro* and *in vivo*.

SUMMARY

The search for biochemical explanations for the antiinflammatory actions of α-MSH continues. New evidence from knockout, transgenic, and normal mice, and from *in vitro* studies of cultured CNS and peripheral inflammatory cells, suggests several leads. First, it appears that IL-10 is not an essential mediator of the antiinflammatory effects of α-MSH in acute inflammation because it occurs in mice that are IL-10–deficient. These deficient mice are highly susceptible to endotoxin and show marked increases in serum IL-6 and in death rate after LPS administration. Second, Agouti protein appears to be an important factor in endogenous control of both acute and systemic inflammatory responses; hypersecretion of this protein results in greater acute inflammatory reactions to challenge, and to greater concentrations of IL-6, in systemic inflammation. This result indicates that the influence of Agouti protein extends beyond its role in skin pigmentation. Third, in human glioma cells and in whole mouse brain, inflammatory reactions are modulated by α-MSH peptides, apparently by modulating NFκB activation through preventing IκB degradation. This result in nervous system cells could account for the antiinflammatory influence of the peptides on brain TNFα production induced by LPS in previous experiments. Finally, α-MSH$_{11-13}$ exerts an inhibitory effect on IL-8 production by macrophages, an influence that may occur via modulating NFκB activation, much as in glial cells and whole brain. These new observations clarify the influence of melanocortins in the control of inflammation.

ACKNOWLEDGMENTS

This research was supported by NIH Grant NS10046 from the National Institute of Neurological Diseases and Stroke, Grant IX Progetto AIDS (9403-30) from Progetto Sclerosi Multipla (96/J/19), Istituto Superiore di Sanita', Italy, and by NATO Collaborative Research Grant No. CGR. 950556.

REFERENCES

1. LIPTON, J.M. & A.P. CATANIA. 1997. Antiinflammatory actions of the neuroimmuno-modulator α-MSH. Immunol. Today **18:** 140–145.
2. GRABBE, S. *et al.* 1996. Alpha-melanocyte–stimulating hormone induces hapten-specific tolerance in mice. J. Immunol. **156:** 473–478.
3. BERG, D.J. *et al.* 1995. Interleukin-10 is a central regulator of the response to LPS in murine models of endotoxic shock and the Shwartzman reaction but not endotoxin tolerance. J. Clin. Invest. **96:** 2339–2347.
4. HASKO, B. *et al.* 1998. The crucial role of IL-10 in the suppression of the immunological response in mice exposed to staphylococcal enterotoxin. Eur. J. Immunol. **28:** 1417–1425.
5. MILLER, M.W. *et al.* 1993. Cloning of the mouse agouti gene predicts a secreted protein ubiquitously expressed in mice carrying the Lethal-Yellow mutation. Genes & Dev. **7:** 454–467.
6. OLLMANN, M.M. *et al.* 1997. Interaction of Agouti protein with the melanocortin 1 receptor *in vitro* and *in vivo*. Genes & Dev. **12:** 316–330.
7. SILVERS, W.K. 1979. The agouti and extension series of alleles, umbrous and sable. *In* The Coat Colors of Mice. 6–44. Springer-Verlag, New York.
8. ADAN, R.A.H. *et al.* 1996. Melanocortin receptors mediate alpha-MSH-induced stimulation outgrowth in neuro 2A cells. Mol. Brain Res. **36:** 37–44.
9. OLLMANN, M.M. *et al.* 1997. Antagonism of central melanocortin receptors *in vitro* and *in vivo* by Agouti-related protein. Science **278:** 135–138.
10. HUSZAR, C. *et al.* 1997. Targeted disruption of the melanocortin 4 receptor results in obesity in mice. Cell **88:** 131–141.
11. RAJORA, N. *et al.* 1997. α-MSH modulates local and circulating TNFα in experimental brain inflammation. J. Neuroscience **17:** 2181–2186.
12. HUH, S.-K. *et al.* 1997. The protective effects of α-melanocyte stimulating hormone on canine brainstem ischemia. Neurosurgery **40:** 132–139.
13. BAEUERLE, P. & T. HENKEL. 1994. Function and activation of NF-κβ in the immune system. Annu. Rev. Immunol. **12:** 141–179.
14. ICHIYAMA, T. *et al.* Unpublished results.
15. TATRO, J.B. 1996. Receptor biology of the melanocortins, a family of neuroimmuno-modulatory peptides. NeuroImmunoModulation **3:** 259–284.

16. WONG, K.Y. *et al.* 1997. A potential mechanism of local antiinflammatory action of α-MSH peptides within the brain: modulation of TNFα production by human astrocytic cells. NeuroImmunoModulation **4:** 37–41.
17. ZHAO, H. *et al.* Unpublished results.

α-MSH in Systemic Inflammation

Central and Peripheral Actions

ANNA CATANIA,[a,b] RENÉ DELGADO,[c] LORENA AIRAGHI,[b]
MARIAGRAZIA CUTULI,[b] LETIZIA GAROFALO,[b] ANDREA CARLIN,[b]
MARIA TERESA DEMITRI,[b] AND JAMES M. LIPTON[d]

[b]Third Division of Internal Medicine, IRCCS Ospedale Maggiore di Milano,
20122 Milan, Italy

[c]Department of Biotechnology, Center of Pharmaceutical Chemistry,
16042 Havana, Cuba

[d]Department of Physiology, University of Texas Southwestern Medical Center at Dallas,
Dallas, Texas 75235

ABSTRACT: Until recently, inflammation was believed to arise from events
taking place exclusively in the periphery. However, it is now clear that central
neurogenic influences can either enhance or modulate peripheral inflammation. Therefore, it should be possible to improve treatment of inflammation by
use of antiinflammatory agents that reduce peripheral host responses and inhibit proinflammatory signals in the central nervous system (CNS). One such
strategy could be based on α-melanocyte stimulating hormone (α-MSH). Increases in circulating TNF-α and nitric oxide (NO), induced by intraperitoneal
administration of endotoxin in mice, were modulated by central injection of a
small concentration of α-MSH. Inducible nitric oxide synthase (iNOS) activity
and iNOS mRNA in lungs and liver were likewise modulated by central
α-MSH. Increase in lung myeloperoxidase (MPO) activity was significantly
less in lungs of mice treated with central α-MSH. Proinflammatory agents induced by endotoxin were significantly greater after blockade of central
α-MSH. The results suggest that antiinflammatory influences of neural origin
that are triggered by α-MSH could be used to treat systemic inflammation. In
addition to its central influences, α-MSH has inhibitory effects on peripheral
host cells, in which it reduces release of proinflammatory mediators. α-MSH
reduces chemotaxis of human neutrophils and production of TNF-α, neopterin, and NO by monocytes. In research on septic patients, α-MSH inhibited release of TNF-α, interleukin-1β (IL-1β), and interleukin-8 (IL-8) in whole
blood samples in vitro. Combined central and peripheral influences can be beneficial in treatment of sepsis.

PERIPHERAL AND CENTRAL MECHANISMS IN
DEVELOPMENT OF SYSTEMIC INFLAMMATION

Despite different etiologies, disorders such as sepsis syndrome, septic shock, and
adult respiratory distress syndrome (ARDS) are collectively classified as *systemic*

[a]Address for correspondence: Dr. Anna Catania, Padiglione Granelli, IRCCS Ospedale Maggiore di Milano, Via F. Sforza 35, 20122 Milano, Italy. +39-02-5503-3318 (voice and fax);
Anna.Catania@unimi.it (e-mail).

inflammation.[1,2] Development of systemic inflammation is promoted by interaction between external agents, such as endotoxins, and host cells that release proinflammatory mediators. Endotoxins, fragments of bacterial cell walls, are released after bacterial invasion and provoke profound responses in the host, including fever, alterations in circulating leukocytes, disseminated intravascular coagulation, and shock.[3] The host response to endotoxin results from induction of biologically active mediators such as proinflammatory cytokines and nitric oxide (NO). One of these cytokines, tumor necrosis factor α (TNF-α), plays a central role in the host response to endotoxin. The massive amount of NO produced by inducible, calcium independent NO synthase (iNOS) is largely responsible for the hypotension and vascular leak syndrome in septic shock.[4]

Until recently, systemic inflammation was believed to arise from events taking place exclusively in the periphery. However, it is now clear that central neurogenic influences can either enhance or modulate peripheral inflammation. Central injection of endogenous pyrogen, which contains cytokines and other mediators of inflammation, enhanced acute inflammation induced by pichryl chloride in the mouse ear.[5] Small concentrations of endotoxin injected intracerebroventricularly (i.c.v.) in mice induced both circulating TNF-α and NO.[6,7] From these observations it appears that endotoxin and cytokines act, not only in the periphery, but also within the brain to enhance host responses.

INHIBITION OF SYSTEMIC INFLAMMATION BY CENTRAL ACTION OF THE NEUROPEPTIDE α-MSH

Modulation of cytokine production and/or action within the brain could have beneficial effects by interrupting transmission of inflammatory signals to the periphery. One such strategy could be based on α-melanocyte stimulating hormone (α-MSH), a proopiomelanocortin-derived peptide that modulates fever and inflammatory reactions, and has both central and peripheral antiinflammatory influences.[8,9] α-MSH modulates production of mediators of inflammation by the accessory cells in the central nervous system (CNS), astrocytes,[10] and microglia.[11] α-MSH inhibits fever caused by endotoxin, endogenous pyrogen, and individual cytokines via action within the brain.[12] Endogenous α-MSH released within the brain during host challenge contributes to physiological control of fever. That is, immunoneutralization of central α-MSH markedly prolonged interleukin-1 (IL-1)–induced fever.[13] Small concentrations of α-MSH given i.c.v. markedly reduced acute inflammation in the skin and suggested that neural antiinflammatory pathways activated by the peptide could be used as a novel way to treat inflammation.[14–17]

To ascertain whether centrally administered α-MSH can reduce systemic inflammation in endotoxemic animals, we measured markers of systemic inflammation in the circulation and in lungs and livers of mice injected with lipopolysaccharide (LPS) intraperitoneally (i.p.) and treated with central α-MSH or saline.[18] Furthermore, in experiments on immunoneutralization of central α-MSH, we tested the idea that endogenous peptide induced within the brain during systemic inflammation modulates host responses to endotoxic challenge in peripheral tissues. Increases in circulating TNF-α and NO, induced by intraperitoneal administration of endotoxin in mice, were modulated by central injection of a small concentration of α-MSH.[18] iNOS activity and iNOS mRNA in lungs and liver were likewise modulated by central α-MSH. Increase in lung myeloperoxidase (MPO) activity was significantly less in lungs of mice treated with central α-MSH. Proinflammatory agents induced by endotoxin were significantly greater after blockade of central α-MSH. The results suggest that antiinflammatory influences of neural origin that are triggered by α-MSH, could be used to treat systemic inflammation.

INHIBITORY INFLUENCES OF α-MSH ON PHAGOCYTES

Although understanding of its mechanism of action is incomplete, part of the α-MSH antiinflammatory influence is exerted through reduced production of mediators by inflammatory cells.[9] α-MSH inhibits the inflammatory cascade at many sites.[19–23] It reduces production of NO, IL-1β, TNF-α, interferon-γ (IFN-γ), monocyte chemoattractant protein-1 (MCP-1), and interleukin-8 (IL-8), and it markedly decreases the number of inflammatory cells trafficking into sites of injury.[22,24–25] α-MSH has little or no stimulatory effect on adrenal steroidogenesis and it is clear that its antiinflammatory effects are exerted directly on target cells.[8] There is evidence that α-MSH has autocrine antiinflammatory influences in monocyte/ macrophages. Upon stimulation of monocytes with endotoxin or cytokines, there is upregulation of the proopiomelanocortin gene, and production of α-MSH is increased.[20] Monocyte expression of melanocortin receptors[20,26] probably forms an afferent limb of the autocrine circuit. Most of the inhibitory effects of α-MSH, including inhibition of TNF-α production[26] and antichemotactic activity,[25] are probably caused by enhancement of intracellular cAMP as the α-MSH receptors are coupled to adenylyl cyclase and induce this cellular mediator.

INHIBITION OF SYSTEMIC INFLAMMATION BY PERIPHERAL ACTION OF THE NEUROPEPTIDE α-MSH

Treatment with α-MSH increased survival in murine septic peritonitis induced by cecal ligation and puncture, and reduced leukocyte migration into lungs in a rat model of adult respiratory distress syndrome (ARDS). Furthermore, α-MSH caused increases in heart rate, mean arterial pressure, and pulse pressure in rats subjected to ventilation interruption.[27] Research in septic patients showed that addition of small concentrations of α-MSH to LPS-stimulated whole-blood samples, inhibited TNF-α production by 30–40%. The inhibitory influences exerted by α-MSH on TNF-α production in whole-blood of septic patients, suggest that this potent peptide could be beneficial in the treatment of systemic inflammation. Similar to other conditions, inhibition patterns show that in septic patients also, α-MSH does not abolish TNF-α production but only modulates it. Thirty to forty percent inhibition of TNF-α was a very consistent activity that occurred in normal blood,[28] blood from HIV-positive patients,[28] human monocytes,[26] and other cell types.[11] This degree of modulatory effect should be sufficient to reduce severity of systemic inflammation without impairing the host defense mechanisms.

CONCLUSIONS

α-MSH inhibits fever and improves outcome in models of sepsis.[29] This potent peptide combines central and peripheral antiinflammatory influences. The inhibitory influences exerted by α-MSH on TNF-α production in whole blood of septic patients suggest that this peptide could be beneficial in the treatment of systemic inflammation in humans.

ACKNOWLEDGMENTS

This research was supported by Progetto Sclerosi Multipla Grant 96/J/T9 from Istituto Superiore di Sanità, Italy; NIH Grant NS10046 from the National Institute of Neurological Diseases and Stroke; and NATO Collaborative Research Grant CGR 950556.

REFERENCES

1. NEUGEBAUER, E.A. & J.W. HOLADAY. 1993. Handbook of Mediators of Septic Shock. CRC Press, Boca Raton.
2. BAUMANN, H. & J. GAULDIE. 1994. The acute phase response. Immunol. Today **15:** 74–78.
3. WOLF S.M. 1973. Biological effects of bacterial endotoxins in man. *In* Bacterial Lipopolysaccharide. S.W. Wolff & E.H. Kass, Eds.: 251–256. University of Chicago Press, Chicago.
4. WONG, J.M. & T.R. BILLIAR. 1995. Regulation and function of inducible nitric oxide synthase during sepsis and acute inflammation. Adv. Pharmacol. **34:** 155–170.
5. DULANEY, R., J. WOERNER, A. MACALUSO, M. HILTZ, A. CATANIA & J.M. LIPTON. 1992. Changes in peripheral inflammation induced by CNS actions of an α-MSH analog and of endogenous pyrogen. Prog. Neuroendocrinommunol. **5:** 179–186.
6. RAJORA, N., G. BOCCOLI, D. BURNS, S. SHARMA, A. CATANIA & J.M. LIPTON. 1997. α-MSH modulates local and circulating tumor necrosis factor-alpha in experimental brain inflammation. J. Neurosci. **17:** 2181–2186.
7. ZINETTI, M., F. BENIGNI, S. SACCO, M. MINTO, G. GALLI, M. SALMONA, G. ANDREONI, A. VEZZANI, P. GHEZZI & M. FRATELLI. 1996. Regional production of nitric oxide after a peripheral or central low dose of LPS in mice. Neuroimmunomodulation **3:** 364–370.
8. CATANIA, A. & J.M. LIPTON. 1993. α-Melanocyte stimulating hormone in the modulation of host reactions. Endocr. Rev. **14:** 564–576.
9. LIPTON, J.M. & A. CATANIA. 1997. Anti-inflammatory actions of the neuroimmunomodulator α-MSH. Immunol. Today **18:** 140–145.
10. WONG, K.Y., N. RAJORA, G. BOCCOLI, A. CATANIA & J.M. LIPTON. 1997. A potential mechanism of local antiinflammatory action of α-MSH peptides within the brain: modulation of TNFα production by human astrocytic cells. Neuroimmunomodulation **4:** 37–41.
11. DELGADO, R., A. CARLIN, L. AIRAGHI, M.T. DEMITRI, L. MEDA, D. GALIMBERTI, P.L. BARON, J.M. LIPTON & A. CATANIA. 1998. Melanocortin peptides inhibit production of proinflammatory cytokines and nitric oxide by activated microglia. J. Leukoc. Biol. **63:** 740–745.
12. LIPTON, J.M. & A. CATANIA. 1993. Pyrogenic and inflammatory actions of cytokines and their modulation by neuropeptides: techniques and interpretations. *In* Neurobiology of Cytokines, Part B. E.B. DeSouza, Ed.: 61–79. Academic Press, Orlando.

13. SHIH, S.T., O. KHORRAM, J.M. LIPTON & S.M. MCCANN. 1986. Central administration of α-MSH antiserum augments fever in the rabbit. Am. J. Physiol. **250:** R803–R806.

14. LIPTON, J.M., A. MACALUSO, M. HILTZ & A. CATANIA. 1991. Central administration of the peptide α-MSH inhibits inflammation in the skin. Peptides **12:** 795–798.

15. WATANABE, T., M. HILTZ, A. CATANIA & J.M. LIPTON. 1993. Inhibition of IL-1β–induced peripheral inflammation by peripheral and central administration of analogs of the neuropeptide α-MSH. Brain Res. Bull. **32:** 311–314.

16. CERIANI, G., A. MACALUSO, A. CATANIA & J.M. LIPTON. 1994. Central neurogenic antiinflammatory action of α-MSH: modulation of peripheral inflammation induced by cytokines and other mediators of inflammation. Neuroendocrinology **59:** 138–143.

17. MACALUSO, A., D. MCCOY, G. CERIANI, T. WATANABE, J. BILTZ, A. CATANIA & J.M. LIPTON. 1994. Antiinflammatory influences of α-MSH molecules: central neurogenic and peripheral actions. J. Neurosci. **14:** 2377–2382.

18. DELGADO, R., M.T. DEMITRI, A. CARLIN, C. MEAZZA, P. VILLA, P. GHEZZI, J.M. LIPTON & A. CATANIA. 1999. Inhibition of systemic inflammation by central action of the neuropeptide α-MSH. Neuroimmunomodulation **6:** 187–192.

19. TAYLOR, A.W., J.W. STREILEIN & S.W. COUSINS. 1994. Alpha-melanocyte stimulating hormone suppresses antigen-stimulated T cell production of gamma interferon. Neuroimmunomodulation **1:** 188–194.

20. STAR, R.A., N. RAJORA, J. HUANG, R.C. STOCK, A. CATANIA & J.M. LIPTON. 1995. Evidence of autocrine modulation of macrophage nitric oxide synthase by α-MSH. Proc. Natl. Acad. Sci. USA **92:** 8016–8020.

21. CHIAO, H., S. FOSTER, R. THOMAS, J. LIPTON & R.A. STAR. 1996. Alpha-melanocyte stimulating hormone reduces endotoxin-induced liver inflammation. J. Clin. Invest. **97:** 2038–2044.

22. CHIAO, H., Y. KOHDA, P. MCLEROY, L. CRAIG, I. HOUSINI & R.A. STAR. 1997. Alpha-melanocyte stimulating hormone protects against renal injury after ischemia in mice and rats. J. Clin. Invest. **99:** 1165–1172.

23. RAJORA, N., G. BOCCOLI, D. BURNS, S. SHARMA, A. CATANIA & J.M. LIPTON. 1997. α-MSH modulates local and circulating tumor necrosis factor α in experimental brain inflammation. J. Neurosci. **17:** 2181–2186.

24. MASON, M.J. & D. VAN EPPS. 1989. Modulation of IL-1, tumor necrosis factor, and C5a-mediated murine neutrophil migration by α-melanocyte stimulating hormone. J. Immunol. **142:** 1646–1651.

25. CATANIA, A., N. RAJORA, F. CAPSONI, F. MINONZIO, R.A. STAR & J.M. LIPTON. 1996. The neuropeptide α-MSH has specific receptors on neutrophils and reduces chemotaxis in vitro. Peptides **17:** 675–679.

26. RAJORA, N., G. CERIANI, A. CATANIA, R.A. STAR, M.T. MURPHY & J.M. LIPTON. 1996. α-MSH production, receptors and influence on neopterin in a human monocyte/macrophage cell line. J. Leukocyte Biol. **59:** 248–253.

27. GUARINI, S., C. BAZZANI & A. BERTOLINI. 1997. Resuscitating effect of melanocortin peptides after prolonged respiratory arrest. Br. J. Pharmacol. **121:** 1454–1460.

28. CATANIA, A., L. GAROFALO, M. CUTULI, A. GRINGERI, E. SANTAGOSTINO & J.M. LIPTON. 1998. Melanocortin peptides inhibit production of proinflammatory cytokines in blood of HIV-infected patients. Peptides. **19:** 1099–1104.

29. LIPTON, J.M., G. CERIANI, A. MACALUSO, D. MCCOY, K. CARNES, J. BILTZ & A. CATANIA. 1994. Antiinflammatory effects of the neuropeptide α-MSH in acute, chronic, and systemic inflammation. Ann. N.Y. Acad. Sci. **741:** 137–148.

Human Peripheral Blood-Derived Dendritic Cells Express Functional Melanocortin Receptor MC-1R

E. BECHER,[a] K. MAHNKE,[b] T. BRZOSKA,[a] D.-H. KALDEN,[a,b]
S. GRABBE,[b] AND T.A. LUGER[a,b,c]

[a]Ludwig Boltzmann-Institut for Cell- and Immunobiology of the Skin,
University of Münster, Germany

[b]Department of Dermatology, University of Münster, Germany.

ABSTRACT: The neuropeptide, α-melanocyte-stimulating hormone (α-MSH) is well known for its immunomodulating capabilities. α-MSH antagonizes the activity of numerous proinflammatory mediators; for example, Interleukin-1 (IL-1), IL-6, tumor necrosis factor α (TNFα), and bacterial endotoxin. In vivo α-MSH has been shown to suppress a contact hypersensitivity reaction in mice, and to induce hapten-specific tolerance. Since antigen presenting cells (APC) represent key elements for tolerance induction, the effect of α-MSH, and the expression of its receptor—melanocortin receptor-1 (MC-1R), on human peripheral blood-derived monocytes and dendritic cells (DC), was investigated. Semiquantitative RT-PCR demonstrated that monocytes and DC express MC-1R, but none of the other members of the MC-receptor family. Moreover, the extent of MC-1R expression correlated with the state of activation of these cells. Since the major ligand of MC-1R is α-MSH the question of whether α-MSH affects the function of monocyte derived DC was further investigated. We found that the expression of the costimulatory molecules CD 86 and CD 40 was downregulated on DC in the presence of α-MSH. Thus, α-MSH may exert its immunosuppressive effects by altering the function of APC.

INTRODUCTION

The proopiomelanocortin (POMC)-gene-product is the precursor for the biologically active peptide-hormones adrenocorticotropin (ACTH), melanocyte stimulating hormones (α-, β-, and γ-MSH), β-endorphin, as well as lipotropins.[1] POMC-peptides are produced in the pituitary gland and also in many other tissues and cells, including leukocytes, monocytes, and Langerhans-cells.[2–8] Five different receptors for the POMC-peptides have been reported to date. They belong to a unique receptor family, but differ markedly in their ligand specificities and tissue distribution.[9] Recent studies showed that MC-1R is expressed on immune and inflammatory cells, such as monocytes, macrophages, neutrophils, endothelial cells, and others.[3,10–13] These findings further support the multiple immunomodulatory functions of α-MSH that were previously described. Accordingly, α-MSH downregulates the production

[c]Address for correspondence: Prof. Dr. med. T. Luger Department of Dermatology, University of Münster, Von-Esmarch-Str. 56, D-41849 Münster, Germany. +49-251-8356504 (voice); +49-251-8356522 (fax); luger@uni-muenster.de (e-mail).

of proinflammatory cytokines and nitric oxide synthase by monocytes and macrophages, and it antagonizes many functions of IL-1, such as fever induction, chemokine production, and thymocyte proliferation.[10,12,13] On the other hand α-MSH was found to enhance production of the suppressor factor IL-10 in monocytes.[14] *In vivo* α-MSH inhibits induction and elicitation phase of contact hypersensitivity reactions, and induces hapten specific tolerance.[15] Therefore, we investigated the question of whether human peripheral blood-derived dendritic cells, on differentiation, express melanocortin receptors; and whether α-MSH alters their capacity to express costimulatory molecules.

MATERIALS AND METHODS

Generation of Dendritic Cells

The Ficoll-Hypaque technique, and subsequently a Percoll density gradient, were applied to isolate monocytes from human buffy coats.[16] Cells (3×10^6/ml) were cultured in RPMI with antibiotics (PAA), glutamin, 1% human serum, GM-CSF (800 U/ml, Essex, Munich), and IL-4 (500 U/ml, R&D Systems) for seven days. At day seven, the medium was changed into 50% culture medium and 50% monocyte-conditioned medium (MCM).[17]

Reverse Transcription Polymerase Chain Reaction (RT-PCR)

DCs were depleted of CD14$^+$ cells with CD14-magnetobeads (Dianova, Hamburg). For RNA-isolation, guanidinium-thiocyanate–phenol–chloroform extraction was applied.[18] For reverse transcription an RT-Kit (Promega) was used. After treatment with RNAse-free DNAse 1 U/µl (Boehringer, Mannheim) (15 minutes, 37°C) and inactivation (10 minutes, 95°C) 1 µg cDNA was mixed with 200 µM dNTPs (each), 20pM primer (each), 5 µl 10× Taq buffer (Promega), 1.5 mM MgCl$_2$ and 2.5u Taq-polymerase (Promega). Primers specific for the melanocortin-receptors MC-1R to MC-5R were used.[13] After 30 cycles (95°C, 45 sec; 55°C, 45 sec; 72°C, 1 min) PCR-products were analyzed on 1% agarose-ethidiumbromide-gels.

Southern-Blot-Analysis of PCR-Gels

Ethidiumbromide-gels were blotted on nylon membranes (Amersham) and DNA fixed by UV-crosslinking for 3 minutes (λ = 254 nm). Hybridization with a ^{32}P-labeled MC-1R–specific probe and appropriate washing procedures were followed by overnight exposure to an X-ray-film at −70°C.[19]

MC Receptor Binding Studies

Cells (2.5×10^6 cells/ml) were incubated for 1 h with biotin-labeled α-MSH (Peninsula Laboratories) in RPMI/1%BSA, washed with PBS/0.1%BSA, and resuspended in PBS/1%BSA. For staining 4 µl FITC coupled streptavidin (10 µg/ml, Dianova, Hamburg) was added for 30 minutes. The binding of biotin-labeled ligand was evaluated by FACS-analysis.[13] To determine nonspecificity, binding cells were incubated with FITC-labeled streptavidin alone. Specificity of binding was demonstrated by competition assays with unlabeled α-MSH, ACTH, or β-MSH (Bachem).

Quantification of Surface Molecule Expression by FACS-Analysis

Cells (1×10^7 cells/ml) were washed twice with PBS, preincubated in PBS/1%BSA (Sigma) for 1h at 4°C, and then incubated with unconjugated (mouse antihuman CD1a, CD14, CD11b, CD14, CD40, CD80, CD83, CD86, HLA-DR, Dianova, Hamburg), or with rabbit antihuman MC-1R antiserum for 1 h at 4°C.[20] Subsequently, cells were washed once with PBS/0.1%BSA and stained with FITC coupled goat F(ab)^2 antimouse IgG (H+L) fragment (Dianova, Hamburg) for 30 minutes. Flow cytometric analysis was performed using a Coulter-MC/XL Flow cytometer.

RESULTS

To investigate the expression of melanocortin receptors on monocyte-derived DC, RT-PCR was performed. Using MC-1R specific primers, a specific product could be amplified, and expression was confirmed by Southern Blot hybridization (see FIGURE 1). In contrast, other MC-receptors (MC-2, -3, -4, and -5) were not detected by RT-PCR indicating that monocyte-derived DCs are capable of expressing MC-1R specifically (data not shown). The expression of melanocortin-

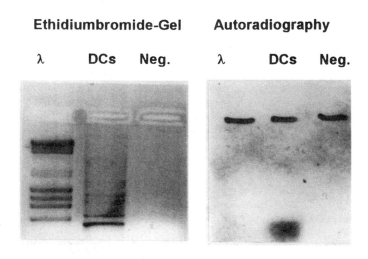

Ethidiumbromide-Gel   **Autoradiography**

λ   DCs   Neg.   λ   DCs   Neg.

416 bp—>

FIGURE 1. Expression of MC-1R–specific mRNA in human monocyte-derived dendritic cells (DCs). **Left** (Ethidiumbromide gel), PCR-products amplified from cDNA of DCs with MC-1R–specific primers were separated on an ethidiumbromid-gel (*lane 2*). Negative control, without reverse transcription (*lane 3*). **Right** (Autoradiography), hybridization with a MC-1R–specific probe revealed a positive signal in DCs (*lane 2*), but not in the negative control (*lane 3*). Marker DNA (*lane 1*), λ/HindIII/φ174/HaeIII.

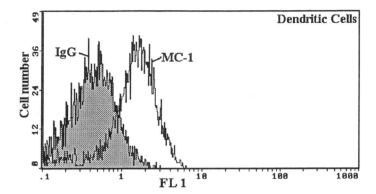

FIGURE 2. Expression of MC-1R on human monocyte-derived dendritic cells (DC). FACS analysis was performed using a polyclonal antihuman MC-1R antiserum (*MC-1*) or preimmune serum (*IgG*).

receptors on antigen presenting cells was further analyzed with a specific polyclonal antihuman–MC-1R antibody. Using this approach significant expression of MC-1R was detected on the surface of matured DC (see FIGURE 2). To study whether differentiation of monocytes into DCs affects the number of α-MSH binding sites, the α-MSH binding capacity during the maturation process of DCs was analyzed. At the beginning of DC-differentiation (day 1 of culture in GM-CSF and IL-4), no significant binding of biotinylated α-MSH to the monocytes could be detected. However, α-MSH–binding increased after five days of culture, with a maximum at day eight (see FIGURE 3). Additional incubation with monocyte-conditioned media, which has been shown to further promote maturation of DCs, had no additional effect on MC-1R-expression (data not shown).

To investigate the functional relevance of MC-1R expression on DCs, the effect of α-MSH—the major ligand for MC-1R—on the expression of T-cell-costimulatory molecules was analyzed. Incubation of DCs with α-MSH (10^{-12}M) for 48 h resulted in significant downregulation of CD86 expression and in a reproducible, but not significant manner, inhibition of CD40 expression (see FIGURE 4). Other surface molecules on DC (such as CD1a, CD80, CD83, and HLA-DR) were not affected by α-MSH (data not shown).

DISCUSSION

These results provide evidence that human DC that are generated from peripheral blood mononuclear cells (PBMC), express exclusively MC-1R. Since monocytes and macrophages have been previously shown to display MC-1R, this finding indicates that, irrespective of whether differentiation occurs into the macrophage lineage or the DC lineage, MC-1R is expressed.[12,13] However, on peripheral blood monocytes, which may be regarded as precursor for both, macrophages and DC, only a

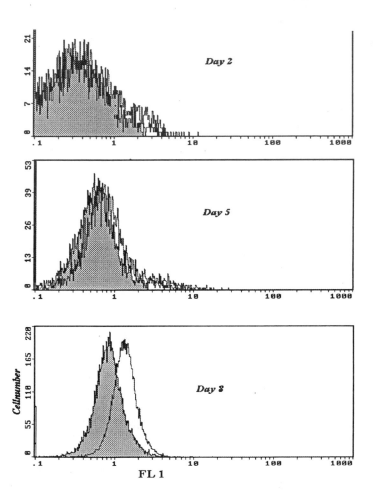

FIGURE 3. Binding of biotinylated–α-MSH to human monocyte derived dendritic cells at different days of culture in the presence of GM-CSF and IL-4. Binding increases during the maturation process, with a maximum at day eight of culture.

weak expression of MC-1R has been observed.[13] Since, among the MC-receptors, MC-1R exhibits the highest affinity for α-MSH, and since ACTH does not bind other POMC-peptides,[8] its expression on mature DC and macrophages supports the notion that α-MSH may be an important immunomodulating signal.[21] The predominant immunoregulatory function of α-MSH in comparison to the other POMC-peptides is further supported by the finding that none of the other known MC-receptors have been detected on monocytes, macrophages, or DC.[12,13]

Our investigation of the functional relevance of MC-1R expression on DC has revealed that α-MSH is able to downregulate the expression of accessory molecules,

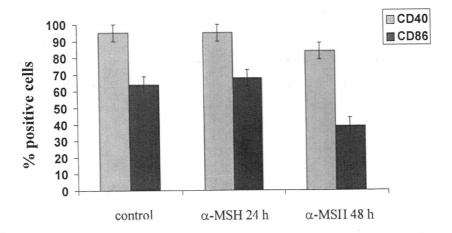

FIGURE 4. Downregulation of costimulatory molecule expression on monocyte de-rived DC. DC were stimulated with α-MSH 10^{-12}M for 24 h or 48 h; and CD40 or CD86 expression was evaluated by FACS analysis. Data are expressed as mean ± SEM of three different experiments.

such as CD86 and CD40, that are required for antigen presentation. This accords with previous data showing that α-MSH suppresses CD86 expression on monocytes.[13] Moreover, α-MSH has been shown to function as an IL-1-antagonist in keratinocytes, and to upregulate IL-10–production in monocytes and kerati-nocytes.[14,22,23] Therefore, there is circumstantial evidence that α-MSH significantly alters the function of antigen presenting cells (APC) and, via blocking accessory sig-nals, may even drive them towards tolerizing cells. This is also supported by *in vivo* studies showing that, in a mouse model of contact hypersensitivity, α-MSH is capa-ble of inducing hapten specific tolerance.[24]

The molecular mechanisms responsible for the alteration of APC-function by α-MSH are still poorly understood. However, there is recent evidence that α-MSH inhibits the activation of the nuclear factor κB (NFκB), which is responsible for the transcriptional activation of several genes, including IL-1 and adhesion molecules.[23] Accordingly, α-MSH was found to block the TNF-α, IL-1, or LPS-mediated activa-tion of NFκB in endothelial cells and keratinocytes.[22,25,26]

These results support the evidence that α-MSH, which, as a result of inflamma-tory stimuli, is released by epithelial cells, endothelial cells, fibroblasts, and inflam-matory cells; and which seems to have an important immunoregulatory function.[3] Since the antiinflammatory and tolerance-inducing capacity of α-MSH has been confirmed in an animal model,[24] further studies of the role of α-MSH in inflamma-tory or allergic diseases in humans, as well as its therapeutic potential, seem to be very promising.

ACKNOWLEDGMENTS

This work was supported by grants from the Deutsche Forschungsgemeinschaft SFB 293/B2 and from the Interdisziplinäres Klinisches Forschungszentrum IZKF/ C7.

REFERENCES

1. EBERLE, A.N. 1988. The Melanotropins. Karger, Basel.
2. BATEMAN, A., A. SINGH, T. KRAL & S. SOLOMON. 1989. The immune-hypothalamic-pituitary-adrenal axis. Endocr. Rev. **10:** 92.
3. LUGER, T.A., T. SCHOLZEN, T. BRZOSKA, E. BECHER, A. SLOMINSKI & R. PAUS. 1998. Cutaneous immunomodulation and coordination of skin stress responses by alpha-melanocyte-stimulating hormone. Ann. N.Y. Acad. Sci. **840:** 381.
4. SLOMINSKI, A., G. ERMAK, J. HWANG, A. CHAKRABORTY, J.E. MAZURKIEWICZ & M. MIHM. 1995. Proopiomelanocortin, corticotropin releasing hormone and corticotropin releasing hormone receptor genes are expressed in human skin. FEBS Lett. **374:** 113.
5. MORHENN, V.B. 1991. The physiology of scratching: involvement of proopiomelanocortin gene-coded proteins in Langerhans cells. Prog. Neuro. Endo. Immun. **4:** 265.
6. BATANERO, E., F.E. DELEEUW, G.H. JANSEN, G.F. VAN WICHEN, J. HUBER & H.J. SHUURMAN. 1992. The neuronal and neuroendocrine component of the human thymus. Brain Behav. Immun. **6:** 249.
7. GALIN, F.S., R.D. LEBOEUF & J.E. BLALOCK. 1990. Possible alternate splicing or initiation of the pro-opiomelanocortin gene in lymphocytes. Int. J. Neurosci. **51:** 171.
8. BURBACH, J.P.H. & V.M. WIEGANT. 1990. Gene expression, biosynthesis and processing of proopiomelanocortin peptides and vasopressin. *In* Neuropeptides: Basics and Perspectives. D. de Wied, Ed.: 45. Elsevier, Amsterdam.
9. CONE, R.D., D. LU, S. KOPPULA, D.I. VAGE, H. KLUNGLAND, B. BOSTON, W. CHEN, D.N. ORTH, C. POUTON & R.A. KESTERSON. 1996. The melanocortin receptors: agonists, antagonists, and the hormonal control of pigmentation. Recent. Prog. Horm. Res. **51:** 287–317.
10. LIPTON, J.M. & A. CATANIA. 1997. Antiinflammatory actions of the neuroimmuno-modulator α-MSH. Immunol. Today **18:** 140.
11. HARTMEYER, M., T. SCHOLZEN, E. BECHER, R.S. BHARDWAJ, M. FASTRICH, T. SCHWARZ & T.A. LUGER. 1997. Human microvascular endothelial cells (HMEC-1) express the melanocortin receptor type 1 and produce increased levels of IL-8 upon stimulation with αMSH. J. Immunol. **159:** 1930.
12. STAR, R.A., N. RAJORA, J. HUANG, R. CHAVEZ, A. CATANIA & J.M. LIPTON. 1995. Evidence of autocrine modulation of macrophage nitric oxide synthase by alpha-MSH. Proc. Natl. Acad. Sci. USA **92:** 8016.
13. BHARDWAJ, R.S., E. BECHER, K. MAHNKE, M. HARTMEYER, T. SCHWARZ, T. SCHOLZEN & T.A. LUGER. 1997. Evidence for the differential expression of the functional alpha melanocyte stimulating hormone receptor MC-1 on human monocytes. J. Immunol. **158:** 3378.
14. BHARDWAJ, R.S., A. SCHWARZ, E. BECHER, K. MAHNKE, H. RIEMANN, Y. ARAGANE, T. SCHWARZ & T.A. LUGER. 1996. Pro-opiomelanocortin-derived peptides induce IL-10 production in human monocytes. J. Immunol. **156:** 2517.
15. AEBISCHER, I., M. STÄMPFLI, S. MIESCHER, M. HORN, A.W. ZÜRCHER & B.M. STADLER. 1995. Neuropeptides accentuate interleukin-4 induced human immunoglobulin E synthesis *in vitro*. Exp. Derm. **4:** 418.
16. FEIGE, U., B. OVERWIEN & C. SORG. 1982. Purification of human blood monocytes by hypotonic density gradient. J. Immunol. Meth. **54:** 309.

17. BENDER, A., M. SAPP, G. SCHULER, R.M. STEINMAN & N. BHARDWAJ. 1996. Improved methods for the generation of dendritic cells from nonproliferating progenitors in human blood. J. Immunol. Meth. **196:** 121.
18. CHOMCZYNSKI, P. & N. SACCHI. 1987. Single-step method of RNA isolation by acid guanidiniumthiocyanate-phenol-chloroform extraction. Anal. Biochem. **162:** 156.
19. MANIATIS, T., E.F. FRITSCH & J. SAMBROCK. 1989. Molecular Cloning, a Laboratory Manual. Cold Spring Harbour Laboratory Press, New York.
20. BÖHM, M., T. BRZOSKA, D. METZE & T.A. LUGER. 1999. Characterization of a polyclonal antibody against the human melanocortin-1 receptor. Exp. Dermatol. In press.
21. MOUNTJOY, K.G., L.S. ROBBINS, M.T. MORTRUD & R.D. CONE. 1992. The cloning of a family of genes that encode the melanocortin receptors. Science **257:** 1248.
22. BRZOSKA, T., T. SCHOLZEN, D.H. KALDEN, E. BECHER, S. BLETZ, K. EBERT, T. SCHWARZ & T.A. LUGER. 1998. α-MSH reduces IL-1 induced chemokine expression and activation of transcription factors in human keratinocytes. FASEB J. **12:** 165.
23. SIEBENLIST, U., G. FRANZOSO & K. BROWN. 1994. Structure, regulation and function of NF-κB. Annu. Rev. Cell Biol. **10:** 405.
24. GRABBE, S., R.S. BHARDWAJ, M. STEINERT, K. MAHNKE, M.M. SIMON, T. SCHWARZ & T.A. LUGER. 1996. Alpha-melanocyte stimulating hormone induces hapten-specific tolerance in mice. J. Immunol. **156:** 473.
25. MANNA, S.K. & B.B. AGGARWAL. 1998. α-Melanocyte-stimulating hormone inhibits the nuclear transcription factor NF-κB activation induced by various inflammatory agents. J. Immunol. **161:** 2873.
26. KALDEN, D.H., M. FASTRICH, T. BRZOSKA, T. SCHOLZEN, M. HARTMEYER, T. SCHWARZ & T.A. LUGER. 1998. Alpha-melanocyte-stimulating hormone reduces endotoxin-induced activation of nuclear factor-kB in endothelial cells. J. Invest. Dermatol. **110:** 495.

Neural Influences on Induction
of Contact Hypersensitivity

J. WAYNE STREILEIN,[a] PASCALE ALARD,[b] AND HIRONORI NIIZEKI[c]

Schepens Eye Research Institute, Department of Dermatology,
Harvard Medical School, Boston, Massachusetts, USA

ABSTRACT: Contact hypersensitivity (CH)-induction begins when cutaneous antigen-presenting cells (APC) capture hapten that has been applied epicutaneously, and the process prepares hapten for presentation to T-cells. APCs are functionally plastic, are influenced by the microenvironment in which they reside, and their functional properties have a profound effect on the phenotype of the hapten-specific T-cells that they activate. Ultraviolet B radiation (UVR) distorts the cutaneous microenvironment, thereby altering local APC function, and changing the immune outcome from sensitization to unresponsiveness. Although UVR induces keratinocytes to produce TNFα and IL-10 (cytokines that have been implicated in failed CH–induction and tolerance, respectively, after UVR), dermal mast cells turn out to be the source of these immunomodulatory cytokines. Mast cell degranulation is triggered by CGRP released from UVR-exposed cutaneous nerve termini. Even in normal skin, cutaneous nerves influence the immune response to haptens. Substance P released from cutaneous nerves acts as an adjuvant, raising the immunogenicity of epicutaneously applied haptens. Thus, the nerves and the neuropeptides that these processes release contribute to the cutaneous microenvironment. By altering APC function, cutaneous nerves can dictate the quality and the quantity of immune responses to antigens of the skin.

INTRODUCTION

Because the skin forms a critical barrier between the body and the environment, an interface where potential pathogens threaten host integrity, this tissue is replete with elements of the immune system, elements designed to detect and respond to pathogenic agents that threaten to enter and cause disease. For many years experimental analysis of cutaneous immunity has been aided by the study of contact hypersensitivity, a cell-mediated immune response directed at highly reactive, small molecular weight molecules, called haptens. Epicutaneous application of a hapten, such as dinitrofluorobenzene (DNFB), results in the generation of a systemic immune response directed at this hapten, and study of this immune response is believed to be representative of immune responses directed at other types of cutaneous antigens, ranging from antigens encoded by viruses to neoantigens that accompany malignant degeneration of cutaneous parenchymal cells.

[a]Address for correspondence: Schepens Eye Research Institute, 20 Staniford Street, Boston, MA 02114, USA. 617-912-7422 (voice); 617-912-0115 (fax).
[b]Current address: Department of Pathology, University of Virginia, Charlottesville, VA, USA.
[c]Current address: Department of Dermatology, National Tokyo Medical Center, Tokyo, Japan.

Antigen (hapten) that is applied to the surface of the skin results in the derivatives of a wide array of proteins within the epidermis. These derivative molecules are captured by local antigen presenting cells, especially epidermal Langerhans cells, processed into immunogenic peptides, and loaded onto class I and class II molecules of the major histocompatibility complex.[1] Cutaneous APC are mobile, and once they have captured antigen in this manner, the cells escape from their local attachments, and migrate into lymph spaces of the dermis.[2] Eventually, lymph flow carries them to draining lymph nodes, where they come to rest in the parafollicular region of the cortex. Once the cells occupy this anatomic position, they display a diverse array of potent costimulatory properties that enable them to present the immunogenic-peptides on their surfaces to naive, antigen-specific T-cells. The latter cells proliferate, differentiate into effector cells, and then disseminate throughout the body: prepared, on subsequent encounter with the same antigen, to trigger an inflammatory response. If, subsequently, they chance to encounter the original hapten anywhere in the skin, they trigger a time-delayed, intense, inflammatory response known as contact hypersensitivity.

Cutaneous APC, which typically includes cells of the dendritic cell lineage, as well as certain macrophages, resemble APC from other regions of the body in being functionally plastic. That is to say, the capacity of cutaneous APC to capture, process, and present antigens to naive, antigen-specific T-cells is dictated by the microenvironment in which they reside. Perhaps the first indication of APC plasticity was provided by the observation of Schuler and Steinman[3] that freshly isolated epidermal Langerhans cells (LC) display less ability to activate T-cells than do LC that have been cultured for 2–3 days *in vitro* prior to their exposure to T-cells. Romani *et al.*,[4] and Streilein and Grammer[5] demonstrated that fresh epidermal LC undergo significant functional changes when cultured in the presence of GM-CSF and, to a lesser extent, IL-1β. Whereas fresh LC proved to be efficient at ingesting exogenous antigens and cleaving these molecules into immunogenic peptide fragments, the cells displayed relatively weak costimulatory properties. As a consequence, they were unable to activate naive T-cells. By contrast, LC that had been cultured with GM-CSF acquired potent costimulatory properties, such as surface expression of ICAM-1, B7-1, B7-2, and CD40, and the capacity to secrete IL-12 and IL-1β. Simultaneous with the acquisition of these costimulatory properties, GM-CSF–exposed LC lost their ability to cleave exogenous antigens efficiently into peptide fragments. In the context of induction of contact hypersensitivity, both functional phenotypes of LC are critical. On the one hand, epidermal LC are ideally prepared to capture hapten-derivative proteins, to generate therefrom immunogenic peptides, and to carry these fragments to the draining lymph node. On the other hand, once LC reach the draining lymph node, they lose their capacity to further degrade peptide fragments, thereby retaining a "snap-shot" of the cutaneous antigenic environment. At the same time, they acquire within the lymph node sufficient costimulatory properties to present the immunogenic peptide fragments to naive, hapten-specific T-cells. GM-CSF and IL-1β are key to the functional shift from "fresh" to "cultured" phenotype of LC.

When skin is bombarded by ultraviolet B radiation, many cutaneous cells change their functional properties, including cutaneous APC. In large measure, the ability of UVR to alter cutaneous APC function is directly related to the capacity of UVR to alter the cytokine milieu of the cutaneous microenvironment, and this alteration leads, necessarily, to changes in APC function.

EFFECTS OF ULTRAVIOLET B RADIATION ON
CONTACT HYPERSENSITIVITY INDUCTION

Experimental study of the effects of UVR on cutaneous immunity was initiated almost thirty years ago when Kripke[6] and Daynes[7] exposed mice to chronically large doses of UVR. This treatment not only induced cutaneous malignancies in the recipients, but it altered the immune systems of the animals, an effect that was subsequently shown to be important in the success of the skin tumors. Since those early days, a variety of UVR protocols have been studied experimentally. Two different types of protocols have been used extensively. First, mice have been exposed to acute, low-dose UVR on patches of shaved body-wall skin, and hapten has been painted immediately thereafter on the exposed site.[8] Second, mice have been exposed to a single, large dose of UVR, and hapten has been applied to unexposed skin 4–5 days later.[6,9] Not surprisingly, these two very different treatment regimens have produced similar, but distinct, alterations in the immune system of exposed mice, as well as distinct alterations in the ability of the mice to mount CH reactions to the hapten. Following acute, low-dose radiation, CH-induction to the epicutaneously applied hapten is grossly impaired in genetically defined strains of mice—termed UVB-susceptible (UVB-S).[10,11] In addition, all mice that receive hapten painted on acute, low-dose UVR–exposed skin develop hapten-specific tolerance.[12] Following treatment of mice with a single large dose of hapten, a stereotypic systemic immune deficit is produced within three to five days, a deficiency in which the ability to acquire CH is impaired, but other dimensions of immune reactivity are spared.[6] In these mice, high-dose UVR creates a systemic deficit of antigen–presenting cells, and the spleens of these animals acquire regulatory T-cells that prevent CH induction, as well as immunity to antigens expressed by UVR-induced tumors.

The pathogenesis of the immune changes that follow acute, low-dose UVR appears to turn on the local generation of immunomodulatory cytokines and other mediators that appear in the exposed skin microenvironment. Impaired CH induction in genetically susceptible mice, following acute low-dose UVR, is mediated primarily by excess local production of TNFα, and excess TNFα is somehow related to UVR-dependent isomerization of *trans*-urocanic acid (UCA) to the *cis* isoform—which is immuno suppressive.[13–17] The tolerance induced by application of hapten to skin acutely exposed to UVR is mediated primarily by IL-10.[18,19] Although TNFα appears to be the primary mediator of failed CH in this circumstance, other factors have also been implicated, including reactive oxygen intermediates,[20] and alpha-melanocyte–stimulating hormone (α-MSH).[21]

Our laboratory has confirmed the findings of Rhein *et al.*,[21] that local administration of α-MSH into a skin site robs the site of its capacity to support CH induction.[22] When DNFB was painted on skin into which α-MSH had been injected intradermally 30 minutes previously, CH induction was impaired. This was equally true whether the murine subjects were UVB-S or UVB-resistant (UVB-R). However, when the mice were subsequently tested for hapten-specific tolerance, none was found. Thus, intracutaneous administration of α-MSH impairs CH induction in a manner that resembles the effects of acute, low-dose UVR. However, there are differences in the two types of modulation. UVR only impairs CH in UVB-S mice, whereas α-MSH impairs CH in both UVB-S and UVB-R mice. Moreover, UVR promotes hapten-specific tolerance, but α-MSH does not—at least not after it has been injected intracutaneously.

We have recently demonstrated that the effect of α-MSH on CH induction is due to a direct action on epidermal LC.[23] Using epidermal cell suspensions enriched for LC, Dai and Streilein reported that LC derivatized with DNFB exposed *in vitro* to α-MSH failed to induce CH when injected intracutaneously into naive, syngeneic mice. In contrast, LC derivatized with DNFB treated with PBS and then injected intracutaneously, induced vigorous CH. As in the *in vivo* experiments, mice that received α-MSH-treated LC derivatized DNFB failed to develop tolerance. Thus, in the acute low-dose model of UVR exposure, α-MSH may contribute to the failed CH induction that is observed, but is unlikely to contribute to the hapten-specific tolerance.

Just as the immune alterations found after acute, low-dose UVR are mediated by cytokines and mediators that alter the local microenvironment, soluble factors are thought to create the immune disorder created by exposure of mice to a single, large dose of UVR. Recent evidence strongly implicates skin-derived IL-10 as the cytokine that initiates the systemic immune deficiency after high-dose UVR.[24] However, there is also good evidence to implicate α-MSH,[25] reactive oxygen intermediates,[20] and DNA photoproducts.[26] Whereas current evidence suggests that acute low-dose UVR impairs cutaneous immunity by releasing soluble factors that alter the functional properties of cutaneous APC, the cellular and molecular bases of the systemic immune deficiency, following a single, large dose of UVR, are less well defined.

LOCAL SOURCES OF UVR-DEPENDENT FACTORS THAT ALTER CUTANEOUS IMMUNITY

Because keratinocytes are unique parenchymal cells of the skin that account for many of its unique properties, and because keratinocytes bear the brunt of the energy of ultraviolet-B radiation, they have been the focus of investigators who are concerned with local sources of soluble factors following UVR. As though to reward this attention, keratinocytes exposed to UVR *in vivo* and *in vitro* have been found to produce cytokines and mediators that are implicated in the effects of UVR on cutaneous immunity.[27,28] The factors include TNFα, urocanic acid, IL-10, reactive oxygen intermediates, and α-MSH, among many others. However, other cells within the skin are also capable of producing immunomodulatory factors—although not necessarily because of exposure to UVR.

Both Langerhans cells themselves and dermal APC can produce various cytokines. In addition, fibroblasts, and endothelial cells have been found to produce similar factors, especially after exposure to UVR. Furthermore, dermal mast cells have also been considered as sources of immunomodulatory factors.[29,30] Not only do the famous granules of these cells contain histamine and other reactive bioamines, the cells also produce and store TNFα and IL-10. Thus, attention is shifting from keratinocytes to other cutaneous cells as the possible sources of the factors that modify immune reactivity following UVR, especially that delivered by acute, low-dose regimens.

Recently, one of us (Pascale Alard) found that dermal mast cells are important sources of immunomodulatory factors when skin is exposed to acute, low-dose UVR. To summarize the most critical results of these experiments, acute, low-dose UVR causes mast cells to degranulate within 30–60 minutes of exposure, and the degranulation leads to depletion of TNFα, and IL-10 from mast cell cytoplasm. As proof of this principle, mast cell secretion of TNFα and IL-10, induced by means other than UVR, has been found, respectively, to impair CH induction and to promote tolerance. Specifically, mast cell degranulation was triggered by loading the cell-surface receptors with DNP-specific IgE antibodies. The receptors were then crosslinked with DNP conjugated to human serum albumin. Crosslinking with this multivalent antigen induced the cells to release both TNFα and IL-10. When the unrelated hapten, oxazolone, was painted on skin treated in this manner, CH induction failed and the mice developed oxazolone-specific tolerance. In separate experiments, mice that were genetically deficient in dermal mast cells were exposed to acute, low-dose UVR. Epicutaneous application of hapten to the irradiated site induced intense CH and failed to promote tolerance. By infusing mast cells into the skin of mast-cell-deficient mice, susceptibility to the effects of UVR was restored. Thus, the impaired CH that follows acute low-dose UVR, and the ability of UVR-exposed skin to promote tolerance depends largely, if not exclusively, on dermal mast cells that are induced to release TNFα and IL-10 in response to UVR exposure.

EVIDENCE THAT NERVE-DERIVED PEPTIDES TRIGGER MAST CELL DEGRANULATION AFTER UVR

The epidermis absorbs the vast majority of the energy delivered to the skin during UV-B exposure. It is estimated that less than 5% of the delivered energy passes beyond the epidermis.[31] It is a paradox, therefore, that the evidence cited above reveals mast cells to be the source of factors that influence immune reactivity following acute low-dose UVR. Since only trivial amounts of UVR reach dermal mast cells *in vivo*, a direct effect of UVR on mast cells seems unlikely. Therefore, a mechanism other than direct exposure must be envisioned to account for mast-cell degranulation after UVR. One possible mechanism is related to cutaneous nerves. Granstein and his colleagues called attention to the potential for neural influence on contact hypersensitivity and cutaneous immunity, when they reported that termini of c-type nerve fibers are located directly on the surface of epidermal Langerhans cells.[32] Moreover, these nerve termini contain the neuropeptide, calcitonin gene-related peptide (CGRP). In addition to its presumed primary role as a neurotransmitter, CGRP has been found to have potent immunosuppressive and modulatory activity.[33–36] It is pertinent to this line of reasoning to mention that mast cells express surface receptors for CGRP, and that exposure of mast cells to this neuropeptide can induce degranulation.[37] Further to this point, Benrath *et al.*, recently reported that exposure of cutaneous nerve termini to UVR *in vivo* induces the release of CGRP.[38] Thus, the possibility exists that UVR triggers mast-cell release of immunomodulatory cytokines through a mechanism that involves release of CGRP from cutaneous nerves.

TABLE 1. Effects of neuropeptides on contact hypersensitivity

Manipulation	Effect on		
	Induction of CH	UVB-impaired CH induction	UVB-promoted tolerance
None	positive	not applicable	not applicable
anti-TNFα	not applicable	restores	no effect
anti-IL-10	not applicable	no effect	prevents
CGRP	suppresses	not applicable	not applicable
CGRP + anti-TNFα	positive	not applicable	not applicable
CGRP antagonist	no effect	restores	prevents
CGRP, mast-cell deficient mice	no effect	not applicable	not applicable
Subs P agon. + high dose hapten	enhances	restores	prevents

We have recently completed a series of experiments to explore the possibility that CGRP can produce similar effects to UVR on contact hypersensitivity induction.[38] The general protocol for these experiments was to inject CGRP, or its specific antagonist, into shaved abdominal skin of mice, and then paint hapten (DNFB) onto the injected site in order to determine the effect on CH induction. A summary of the results of these experiments is provided in TABLE 1. First, DNFB, painted on skin into which CGRP had been injected 30 minutes previously, failed to induce CH. Second, injection of CGRP antagonist into skin at the completion of an acute low-dose UVR regimen, restored the capacity of that skin to support CH induction. When hapten was painted on UVR-exposed skin into which CGRP antagonist had been injected, intense CH was induced. To confirm that CGRP was acting via a TNFα-dependent mechanism, neutralizing anti-TNFα antibodies were injected intraperitoneally into mice that then received an intracutaneous injection of CGRP followed by epicutaneous hapten. Intense CH developed in these mice, indicating that failed CH, after CGRP injection, was mediated by TNFα. In the final set of experiments, the ability of intracutaneously injected CGRP to impair CH induction was tested in mast-cell–deficient mice. Unlike wild-type mice, in which hapten failed to induce CH when painted on skin into which CGRP had been injected, hapten readily induced CH in mast-cell–deficient mice that had received an intracutaneous injection of CGRP. These results indicate that CGRP resembles acute low-dose UVR in its ability to impair CH induction, that the impairment is TNFα mediated, and that it depends upon dermal mast cells. The ability of CGRP antagonist to abolish the deleterious effects of UVR on CH induction proves the central role for CGRP. We have concluded from these studies that UVR impairs CH induction by first damaging cutaneous nerves. One consequence of this damage, release of CGRP, leads to mast cells being triggered in the dermis to release their granules. Since TNFα is included among the released factors, and since TNFα disarms cutaneous APC from delivering hapten-specific immunogenic signals to the draining lymph nodes,[40] CH is not induced.

EVIDENCE OF OTHER NEUROPEPTIDES THAT INFLUENCE CONTACT HYPERSENSITIVITY INDUCTION

Although c-type nerve termini in the epidermis contain CGRP, this is not the only neuropeptide/transmitter present.[41] Substance P has also been described within cutaneous nerve endings. The fact that CGRP of neural origin can influence cutaneous immunity suggests that substance P (as well as other neurotransmitters) may also be able to influence contact hypersensitivity induction. Unlike CGRP, which possesses an array of so-called immunosuppressive and antiinflammatory properties, substance P has been found to display immune enhancing properties. For example, substance P added to T-cell proliferation assays promotes T-cell mitotic activity, and it enhances IL-2 production by stimulated T-cells.[42–44] In addition, substance P acts on other cells of the lymphoreticular apparatus. Substance P promotes the production of reactive oxygen intermediates when added to macrophages that have been stimulated with LPS and interferon-gamma.[45] More importantly, substance P stimulates macrophages to produce IL-12.[46] This last property suggests that substance P might mediate its immune enhancing properties, in part by inducing APC to produce greater amounts of IL-12. IL-12 is critical to the activation of T-cells, especially Th1-type cells that are believed to be responsible for contact hypersensitivity. It is probably relevant in this context that induction of contact hypersensitivity is enhanced in neuropeptidase knockout mice.[47] Neuropeptidase is a ubiquitous enzyme that rapidly degrades substance P. One interpretation of this result is that the natural tendency of substance P is to promote CH induction and that neuropeptidases limit this function. On this point, mice treated with NK-1 receptor antagonist display reduced contact hypersensitivity.[47] Together these reports convinced us of the value of inquiring into the possibility that substance P might alter contact hypersensitivity induction.

Experiments conducted with a substance-P agonist were similar in design to the experiments described above using CGRP as a modulator of the cutaneous microenvironment. Substance P agonist was injected intracutaneously and 30 minutes later the overlying epidermis was painted with either a conventional (185 μg) or an optimal (1.5 μg) sensitizing dose of DNFB (refer to TABLE 1). Compared to controls that received intracutaneous injection of PBS alone and that displayed normal levels of CH, mice that were painted with a high dose of hapten on substance P agonist-treated skin displayed significantly exaggerated ear swelling responses. In contrast, substance P agonist-treated mice painted with a low dose of hapten displayed normal (not enhanced) CH. In separate experiments, substance P agonist was injected at one cutaneous site, and painted with hapten at a distant site. The intensity of CH induced in this experiment was no different from that of mice that received PBS alone. Therefore, the effect of substance P on CH induction is strictly local—not systemic. Since high doses of sensitizing hapten rely on dermal, rather than epidermal, APC in order to develop immunogenic hapten-bearing signals,[48,49] this evidence indicates that substance P enhances the CH-inducing properties of dermal, rather than epidermal, APC.

Acute, low-dose UVB impairs CH induction by altering, via TNFα and IL-10, the APC properties of dermal cells. Therefore, we attempted to reverse the effects of UVR in UVB-S mice by injecting substance P agonist into skin immediately after the fourth consecutive daily exposure to UVR. When DNFB was painted on the exposed and injected site 30 minutes later, CH induction was fully restored; these mice displayed an intense ear-swelling response. Moreover, when animals treated in this manner were reexposed to sensitizing doses of DNFB on previously untreated body-wall skin, they developed CH of normal intensity. This indicates that hapten-specific tolerance had not been induced.

These experimental results provide strong support for the view that substance P has the capacity to enhance CH induction. Moreover, the constitutive presence of this neuropeptide in termini of c-type cutaneous nerves implies that substance P may participate in the normal process by means of which epicutaneous application of hapten induces CH. One possibility is that the strength of a hapten may be predicated on its ability to trigger substance-P release from nerve termini; in this instance, at any given sensitizing dose of hapten, the contact hypersensitivity induced would be more intense than induction in the absence of the "adjuvant" effect of substance P. Although the result, that substance P reverses the deleterious effects of UVR on CH induction and prevents UVR-dependent tolerance, supports an adjuvant role for substance P, this presents us with a paradox. The experimental evidence presented above strongly implicates CGRP in mediating the deleterious effects of UVR on cutaneous immunity. Never does acute, low-dose UVR promote CH induction. Since both CGRP and substance P are stored in the same vesicles within c-type fiber nerve termini, we are confronted by the dilemma that only CGRP-dependent effects are observed after UVR. At this point we can only speculate. As mentioned above, neuropeptidases are ubiquitous, and have the capacity to degrade peptides such as neurotransmitters. Empirical evidence indicates that substance P is much more sensitive to neuropeptidase degradation than is CGRP.[50] Following UVB radiation of skin, both substance P and CGRP may be released simultaneously from cutaneous nerves. Given its resistance to neuropeptidase degradation, CGRP may dominate the field, since substance P is rapidly degraded. Alternatively, the cells that are relevant to induction of cutaneous immunity and tolerance may constitutively express a higher density of CGRP receptors, when compared to substance P receptors. This might also favor a CGRP-pervasive effect after UVR.

SUMMARY AND DISCUSSION

Perturbing the skin with acute, low-dose UVR has been a productive and informative approach to unmasking the factors within the cutaneous microenvironment that influence—both positively and negatively—the process by which epicutaneously applied hapten leads to CH. The results presented in this communication force us to add cutaneous nerves to the growing list of cells within the skin that can contribute immunomodulatory factors. Following acute UVR on skin, the most important cytokines identified to date that cause impaired CH induction (TNFα) and promote tolerance (IL10) are released from dermal mast cells. The factor that is responsible for triggering mast-cell degranulation in this instance is CGRP, and termini of c-type nerve fibers in the skin are the presumed source of this immunomodulatory neuropeptide. We further suspect that under physiologic circumstances, epicutaneous application of hapten fails to cause release of CGRP from nerve termini, and, in the absence of CGRP, the APC required for CH induction is able to carry out the immunogenic program.

The role of substance P is less clear. When injected into the skin, a substance-P agonist has clear, immune-enhancing effects, leading to exaggerated CH in mice that were sensitized with a conventional (high) dose of hapten. These findings do not permit us to conclude that release of substance P occurs routinely during sensitization with hapten, nor can we propose that the intensity of CH under normal circumstances is promoted by substance P. However, the report of Scholsen *et al.,* does point in that direction, since these investigators found that an NK-1 receptor-antagonist inhibited CH induction when hapten was painted on otherwise unperturbed skin.[47] Experimental study of this issue may prove to be very worthwhile, since the ability of a hapten to release substance P from cutaneous nerves may be one feature of a hapten that separates it from a simple irritant and helps to render it immunogenic.

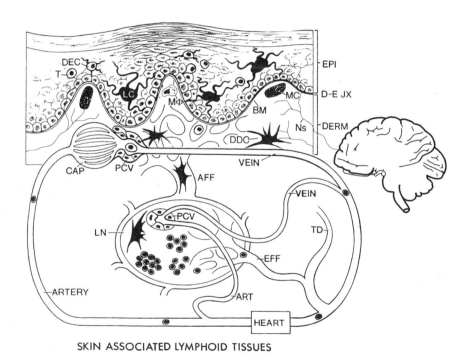

SKIN ASSOCIATED LYMPHOID TISSUES

FIGURE 1. Components of *skin associated lymphoid tissues*—1999. *EPI,* epidermis; *D-E Jx,* dermal-epidermal junction; *DERM,* dermis; *MC,* mast cells; *Ns,* cutaneous nerves; *BM,* basement membrane; *DDC,* dermal dendritic cell; *MΦ,* macrophage; *DEC,* dendritic epidermal T-cell; *T,* T lymphocyte; *PCV,* post-capillary venule; *CAP,* capillary; *LN,* lymph node; *AFF,* afferent lymphatic; *TD,* thoracic duct; *EFF,* efferent lymphatic; *ART,* artery.

In a wider sense, the data reported here indicate strongly that cutaneous nerves contribute to the local tissue microenvironment that is responsible for molding resident dendritic cells and macrophages into potent APC, capable of inducing CH. Our studies have only identified CGRP and substance P, so far, as relevant to this issue. However, there are other neuropeptides and neurotransmitters that can be released from cutaneous nerves, and these must surely be scrutinized for the capacity of modify cutaneous immunity. Specifically, α-MSH is present in certain cutaneous nerve termini. Since release of α-MSH has been implicated in some of the deleterious consequences of UVR on cutaneous immunity, the source of this potent neuropeptide may very well also be cutaneous nerve termini.

Paul Langerhans, the discoverer of the best studied antigen-presenting cells of the skin, was originally misled by the staining properties of these cells, thinking them to belong to the nervous system.[51] Although we now know that Langerhans cells are derived from the bone marrow, recent evidence has begun to link the peripheral nervous system to Langerhans cells in the function for which we believe they are designed—to act as antigen presenting cells for cutaneous antigens in the generation of cutaneous immunity. Paul Langerhans would undoubtedly have applauded these recent studies. It is perfectly possible that his belief, that these dendritic epidermal cells were part of the neurosensory system, was conceptually correct, even if the details of the relationship were beyond the grasp of science in his time.

The integrated immune system that serves the skin, sometimes referred to as *s*kin *a*ssociated *l*ymphoid *t*issues (SALT)[2] or the *s*kin *i*mmune *s*ystem,[52] has long been known to consist of a diverse set of different cells, each contributing to the capacity of this system to provide the skin with relevant immunity. The studies reported here, along with other recent reports,[53] indicate that the original formulation neglected two important cell types; mast cells and cutaneous nerves. A revised formulation of SALT, updated for 1999, is presented in FIGURE 1, and it includes both mast cells and cutaneous nerves. It is altogether likely that this revision will also fall short of the truth. However, as our understanding continues to grow, it is worthwhile periodically to take stock of current knowledge. To the best of that knowledge, the diagram in FIGURE 1 represents a reasonably current formulation of the *skin associated lymphoid tissues*.

ACKNOWLEDGMENTS

We thank Mr. Peter Mallen for preparing the artwork of FIGURE 1. The experimental work reported here was supported by USPHS Grant AR44130.

REFERENCES

1. STREILEIN, J.W., S.F. GRAMMER, T. YOSHIKAWA, A. DEMIDEM & M. VERMEER. 1990. Functional dichotomy between Langerhans cells that present antigen to naive and to memory/effector T lymphocytes. Imm. Reviews **117:** 159–184.
2. STREILEIN, J.W. 1990. Skin associated lymphoid tissues (SALT): The next generation. *In* The Skin Immune System (SIS). J. Bos, Ed.: 26–48. CRC Press, Boca Raton.
3. SCHULER, G. & R.M. STEINMAN. 1985. Murine epidermal Langerhans cells mature into potent immunostimulatory dendritic cells *in vitro*. J. Exp. Med. **161:** 526.

4. ROMANI, N., S. KOIDE, M. CROWLEY, M. WITMER-PACK, A.M. LIVINGSTON, C.G. FATHMAN, Y. INABA & R.M. STEINMAN. 1989. Presentation of exogenous protein antigens by dendritic cells to T-cell clones. Intact protein is presented best by immature, epidermal Langerhans cells. J. Exp. Med. **169:** 1169.

5. STREILEIN, J.W. & S.F. GRAMMER. 1989. In vitro evidence that Langerhans cells can adopt two functionally distinct forms capable of antigen presentation to T lymphocytes. J. Immunol. **143:** 3925–3933.

6. KRIPKE, M.L. 1984. Immunological unresponsiveness induced by ultraviolet radiation. Immunol. Rev. **80:** 87–102.

7. DAYNES, R.A., E.M. BERNHARD, M.F. GURISH & D.H. LYNCH. 1981. Experimental photoimmunology: immunologic ramifications of UV-induced carcinogenesis. J. Invest. Dermatol. **77:** 77–85.

8. BERGSTRESSER, P.R., C. FLETCHER & J.W. STREILEIN. 1980. Surface densities of Langerhans cells in relation to rodent epidermal sites with special immunologic properties. J. Invest. Derm. **74:** 77–80.

9. OKAMOTO, H. & M.L. KRIPKE. 1987. Effector and suppressor circuits of the immune response are activated in vivo by different mechanisms. Proc. Natl. Acad. Sci. USA **87:** 3841–3845.

10. STREILEIN, J.W. & P.R. BERGSTRESSER. 1988. Genetic basis of ultraviolet-B on contact hypersensitivity. Immunogenetics **27:** 252–258.

11. KURIMOTO, I. & J.W. STREILEIN. 1994. Characterization of the immunogenetic basis of ultraviolet-B light effects on contact hypersensitivity induction. Immunology **81:** 352–358.

12. TOEWS, G., P.R. BERGSTRESSER & J.W. STREILEIN. 1980. Epidermal Langerhans cell density determines whether contact sensitivity or unresponsiveness follows skin painting with DNFB. J. Immunol. **124:** 445–453.

13. YOSHIKAWA, T. & J.W. STREILEIN. 1990. Genetic basis of the effects of ultraviolet-B on cutaneous immunity. Evidence that polymorphism at the *Thfα* and *Lps* loci governs susceptibility. Immunogenetics **32:** 398–405.

14. STREILEIN, J.W. 1993. Sunlight and SALT: If UVB is the trigger, and TNFα is its mediator, what is the message? J. Invest. Dermatol. (Suppl.) **100:** 47S–52S.

15. KURIMOTO, I. & J.W. STREILEIN. 1992. *Cis*-urocanic acid suppression of contact hypersensitivity induction is mediated via tumor necrosis factor-α. J. Immunol. **148:** 3072–3078.

16. DEFABO, E.C. & F.P. NOONAN. 1983. Mechanism of immune suppression by ultraviolet irradiation *in vivo*. I. Evidence for the existence of a unique photoreceptor in skin and its role in photoimmunology. J. Exp. Med. **157:** 84–98.

17. STREILEIN, J.W., J.R. TAYLOR, V. VINCEK, I. KURIMOTO, T. SHIMIZU, C. TIE & C. GOLOMB. 1994. Review: Immune surveillance and sunlight-induced skin cancer. Immunology Today **15:** 174–179.

18. ENK, A.H., J. SALOGA, D. BECKER, M. MOHAMADZEH & J. KNOP. 1994. Induction of hapten-specific tolerance by interleukin 10 *in vivo*. J. Exp. Med. **179:** 1397–1402.

19. NIIZEKI, H. & J.W. STREILEIN. 1997. Hapten-specific tolerance induced by acute, low-dose ultraviolet B radiation of skin is mediated via Interleukin-10. J. Invest. Dermatol. **109:** 25–30.

20. NAKAMURA, T., S.R. PINNELL, D. DARR, I. KURIMOTO, S. ITAMI, K. YOSHIKAWA, J.W. STREILEIN. 1997. Vitamin C abrogates the deleterious effects of UVB radiation on cutaneous immunity by a mechanism that does not depend on TNF-α. J. Invest. Dermatol. **109:** 20–24.

21. RHEINS, L.A., A.L. COTLEUR, R.S. KLEIER, W.B. HOPPANJANS, D.N. SAUDER & J.J. NORDLUND. 1989. Alpha-melanocyte stimulating hormone modulates contact hypersensitivity responsiveness in C57BL/6 mice. J. Invest. Dermatol. **93:** 511–517.

22. SHIMIZU, T. & J.W. STREILEIN. 1994. Influence of alpha-melanocyte stimulating hormone on induction of contact hypersensitivity and tolerance. J. Dermatological Sci. **8:** 187–193.
23. DAI, R. & J.W. STREILEIN. 1997. Ultraviolet B-exposed and soluble factor-preincubated epidermal Langerhans cells fail to induce contact hypersensitivity and promote DNP-specific tolerance. J. Invest. Dermatol. **108:** 721–726.
24. RIVAS, J.M. & S.E. ULLRICH. 1992. Systemic suppression of delayed-type hypersensitivity by supernatants from UV-irradiated keratinocytes. An essential role for keratinocyte-derived IL-10. J. Immunol. **149:** 3865–3871.
25. GRABBE, S., R.S. BHARDWAJ, K. MAHNKE, M.M. SIMON, T. SCHWARZ & T.A. LUGER. 1996. α-Melanocyte-stimulating hormone induces hapten-specific tolerance in mice. J. Immunol. **156:** 473–478.
26. KRIPKE, M.L., P.A. COX, L.G. ALAS & D.B. YAROSH. 1992. Pyrimidine dimers in DNA initiate systemic immunosuppression in UV-irradiated mice. Proc. Natl. Acad. Sci. USA **89:** 7516–7520.
27. SCHWARZ, T., A. URBANSKI & T.A. LUGER. 1994. Ultraviolet light and epidermal cell-derived cytokines. *In* Epidermal Growth Factors and Cytokines. T.A. Luger & T. Schwarz, Eds.: 303–324. Marcel Dekker, New York.
28. LUGER, T.A., E. SCHAUER, F. TRAUTINGER, J. KRUTMANN, J. ANSEL & T. SCHWARZ. 1993. Production of immunosuppressive melanotropins by human keratinocytes. Ann. N.Y. Acad. Sci. **680:** 567–581.
29. WALSH, L. 1995. Ultraviolet B irradiation of skin induces mast cell degranulation and release of tumour necrosis factor-α. Immunol. Cell Biol. **73:** 226–233.
30. GORDON, J.R. & S.J. GALLI. 1990. Mast cells as a source of both preformed and immunologically inducible TNF-alpha/cachectin. Nature **346:** 274–276.
31. EVERETT, M., E. YEARGERS, R. SAYRE & R. OLSON. 1966. Penetration of epidermis by ultraviolet rays. Photochem. Photobiol. **5:** 533–538.
32. HOSOI, J., G.F. MURPHY, C.L. EGAN, E.A. LERNER, S. GRABBE, A. ASAHINA & R.D. GRANSTEIN. 1993. Regulation of Langerhans cell function by nerves containing calcitonin gene-related peptide. Nature **363:** 159–163.
33. ASAHINA, A., J. HOSOI, S. BEISSERT, A. STRATIGOS & R.D. GRANSTEIN. 1995. Inhibition of the induction of delayed-type and contact hypersensitivity by calcitonin gene-related peptide. J. Immunol. **154:** 3056–3061.
34. GOEBELER, M., U. HENSELEIT, J. ROTH & C. SORG. 1994. Substance P and calcitonin gene-related peptide modulate leukocyte infiltration to mouse skin during allergic contact dermatitis. Arch. Dermatol. Res. **286:** 341–346.
35. GUTWALD, J., M. GOEBELER & C. SORG. 1991. Neuropeptides enhance irritant and allergic contact dermatitis. J. Invest. Dermatol. **96:** 695–698.
36. LOTZ, M., J.H. VAUGHAN & D.A. CARSON. 1988. Effect of neuropeptides on production of inflammatory cytokines by human monocytes. Science **241:** 1218–1221.
37. WILLE, J., F. NJIEHS, P. AMIN & A. KYDONIEUS. 1995. Topical delivery of mast cell degranulating agents for treatment of transdermal drug-induced hypersensitivity. Proceed. Intern. Symp. Controll. Rel. Bioact. Matter. **22:** 119–120.
38. BENRATH, J., C. ESCHENFELDER, M. ZIMMERMANN & F. GILLARDON. 1995. Calcitonin gene-related peptide, substance P and nitric oxide are involved in cutaneous inflammation following ultraviolet irradiation. Eur. J. Pharmacol. **293:** 87–96.
39. NIIZEKI, H., P. ALARD & J.W. STREILEIN. 1997. Calcitonin gene-related peptide is necessary for ultraviolet B-impaired induction of contact hypersensitivity. J. Immunol. **159:** 5183–5186.
40. BACCI, S., T. NAKAMURA & J.W. STREILEIN. 1996. Failed antigen presentation after UV13 radiation correlates with modifications of Langerhans cell cytoskeleton. J. Invest. Dermatol. **107:** 838–843.

41. ANSEL, J.C., A.H. KAYNARD, C.A. ARMSTRONG, J. OLERUD, N. BUNNETT & D. PAYAN. 1996. Skin-nervous system interactions. J. Invest. Dermatol. **106:** 198–204.
42. CALVO, C.-F., G. CHAVANEL & A. SENIK. 1992. Substance P enhances IL-2 expression in activated human T cells. J. Immunol. **148:** 3498–3504.
43. PAYAN, D.G., D.R. BREWSTER, A. MISSIRIAN-BASTIAN & E.J. GOETZL. 1984. Substance P recognition by a subset of human T lymphocytes. J. Clin. Invest. **74:** 1532–1539.
44. RAMESHWAR, P., P. GASCON & D. GANEA. 1993. Stimulation of IL-2 production in murine lymphocytes by substance P and related tachykinins. J. Immunol. **151:** 2484–2496.
45. HARTUNG, H.T. & K.V. TOYKA. 1983. Activation of macrophages by substance P: Induction of oxidative burst and thromboxane release. Eur. J. Pharmacol. **89:** 301–305.
46. KINCY-CAIN, T. & K.L. BOST. 1997. Substance P-induced IL-12 production by murine macrophages. J. Immunol. **158:** 2334–2339.
47. SCHOLZEN, T., C.A. ARMSTRONG, N.W. BUNNETT, T.A. LUGER, J.E. OLERUD & J.C. ANSEL. 1998. Neuropeptides in the skin: interactions between the neuroendocrine and the skin immune systems. Exp. Dermatol. **7:** 81–96.
48. BACCI, S., P. ALARD, R. DAI, T. NAKAMURA & J.W. STREILEIN. 1997. High and low doses of haptens dictate whether dermal or epidermal antigen-presenting cells promote contact hypersensitivity. Eur. J. Immunol. **27:** 442–448.
49. KURIMOTO, I. & J.W. STREILEIN. 1993. Studies of contact hypersensitivity induction in mice with optimal sensitizing doses of hapten. J. Invest. Dermatol. **101:** 132–136.
50. MATSAS, R., J. KENNY & A.J. TURNER. 1984. The metabolism of neuropeptides. The hydrolysis of peptides, including enkephalins, tachykinins and their analogues, by endopeptidase-24.11. Biochem. J. **223:** 433–440.
51. LANGERHANS, P. 1868. Ueber die Nerven der meschlichen. Haut. Virch. Arch. Pathol. Anat. Physiol. **44:** 325–337.
52. BOS, J.D., DAS, P.K. & M.L. KAPSENBERG. 1989. The skin immune system (SIS). *In* Skin Immune System. J. Bos, Ed.: 3–8. CRC Press, Boca Raton.
53. HART, P.H., M.A. GRIMBALDESTON, G.J. SWIFT, A. JAKSIC, F.P. NOONAN & J.J. FINLAY-JONES. 1998. Dermal mast cells determine susceptibility to ultraviolet B induced systemic suppression of contact hypersensitivity responses in mice. J. Exp. Med. **187:** 2045–2054.

Role of Epidermal Cell-Derived α-Melanocyte Stimulating Hormone in Ultraviolet Light Mediated Local Immunosuppression

T.A. LUGER,[a] T. SCHWARZ, H. KALDEN, T. SCHOLZEN,
A. SCHWARZ, AND T. BRZOSKA

*Department of Dermatology and Ludwig Boltzmann Institute of
Cell Biology and Immunobiology of the Skin,
University of Münster, Münster, Germany*

ABSTRACT: Irradiation of the skin with ultraviolet light (UV) results in profound alterations of both local and systemic immune responses. These effects are largely mediated by soluble mediators released from epidermal cells in response to UV. It is well known that keratinocytes release increased amounts of cytokines upon UV-irradiation. UV-light also induces the release of the proopiomelanocortin (POMC)–derived peptide, α-melanocyte-stimulating hormone (αMSH), from keratinocytes, and upregulates the expression of POMC mRNA. αMSH exerts a variety of immunomodulating and antiinflammatory effects, mainly by virtue of its capacity to alter the function of antigen presenting cells and vascular endothelial cells. Within an *in vivo* mouse model, both intravenous and topical application of αMSH resulted in inhibiting the induction, eliciting a contact hypersensitivity reaction, and inducing hapten-specific tolerance. These findings indicate that αMSH, released in the epidermis after UV irradiation, may contribute to UV-mediated immunosuppression. The therapeutic application of αMSH or αMSH-derived peptides may prove to be a useful approach for treating inflammatory skin diseases.

INTRODUCTION

Ultraviolet (UV) irradiation of the skin is known to cause both local and systemic immunosuppression.[1] Accordingly, UV has been shown to inhibit cellular immune reactions, including contact hypersensitivity (CHS) responses, and to induce allergen specific tolerance.[2] The immunosuppressive effects of UV-light are mainly caused by the short wave lengths (UVB 290–320 nm) that are predominantly absorbed by the epidermis. Therefore, one of the mechanisms involved in these events appears to be the release of immunosuppressive cytokines by epidermal cells as a result of UV-radiation.[3] Together with release of inflammatory mediators, UV treatment of keratinocytes also leads to an increased production of immunosuppressing cytokines, such as interleukin-1 receptor antagonist (IL-1RA), transforming growth factor β (TGFβ), and IL-10.[4–8] Epidermal cells have also been shown to release

[a]Address for correspondence: Prof. Dr. med. T. Luger, Department of Dermatology, University of Münster, Von-Esmarch-Str. 56, D-48149 Münster, Germany. +49-251-8356504 (voice); +49-251-8356522 (fax); luger@uni-muenster.de (e-mail).

proopiomelanocortin (POMC)-derived peptides that exert a variety of immunomodulating activities.[9–11] The POMC precursor undergoes tissue-specific cleavage achieved by prohormone-converting enzymes (PC) that results in the release of adrenocorticotropin (ACTH), β-endorphin, and melanocyte-stimulating-hormones (α-, β-, and γMSH).[12] To exert their multiple activities, POMC-peptides need to bind to one of the melanocortin receptors (MC-R1 to MC-R5). These receptors belong to the family of G-protein coupled receptors and are expressed on many different cell types.[13]

There is strong evidence that neuropeptides function not only as neurotransmitters, but also as mediators of immunity and inflammation.[14] Among the different POMC-peptides, αMSH has been found to exert a variety of immunomodulation effects.[9] αMSH antagonizes the effects of proinflammatory cytokines such as IL-1, IL-6, and tumor necrosis factor α (TNFα) and it downregulates the production of immunostimulatory cytokines, such as interferon-γ by mitogen or antigen-stimulated T-lymphocytes.[15,16] In contrast, αMSH upregulates the production of the immunosuppressive cytokine IL-10 by monocytes and keratinocytes.[17,18] In addition to modulating the production and functions of cytokines, αMSH was also found to affect the expression of surface molecules on antigen presenting cells and endothelial cells. αMSH downregulates the expression of costimulatory molecules such as CD86 on monocytes, and it suppresses the expression of adhesion molecules such as E-selectin and VCAM, on human dermal vascular endothelial cells.[19,20] These data suggest that αMSH may contribute to the network of mediators regulating immune and inflammatory reactions in several ways. This paper summarizes the mechanism of POMC-peptide production by keratinocytes in response to UV-light, and the possible *in vivo* relevance of these findings.

EFFECT OF UV-IRRADIATION ON THE EXPRESSION OF POMC MRNA AND THE RELEASE OF αMSH IN KERATINOCYTES

Human keratinocytes including normal cells and several transformed keratinocyte cell lines (KB, A431, and HaCaT), have been shown to express POMC mRNA and to release POMC-peptides such as αMSH, ACTH, and β-endorphin.[11,21] To generate POMC-peptides the POMC precursor needs to be cleaved by specific prohormone convertases (PC), including PC1 and PC2. To give rise to β-endorphin and ACTH, PC1 is required, whereas PC2 is responsible for cleavage yielding αMSH.[12] Therefore, the regulation of convertase production in the skin is important. Thus, PC1 and the PC2-specific binding protein, 7B2, which is involved in the activation of proPC2 into PC2, have been detected in keratinocytes, and PC1 expression is upregulated as a result of UVB irradiation.[22,23] Therefore, UVB is able to induce the production of convertases in the skin, as is required for the cleavage of POMC-peptides.

In unstimulated keratinocytes, no (or very low levels of) POMC-peptides can be detected. However, on stimulation with endotoxin, tumor promoters, or the proinflammatory cytokine, IL-1, significant upregulation of POMC production is observed at both the transcriptional and translational level.[9,11,21] Similarly, UV-

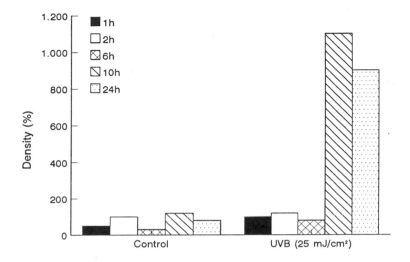

FIGURE 1. Effect of UVB on POMC-mRNA production by KB cells. KB cells were treated with UVB (25 mJ/cm²), and RT-PCR was performed after 1, 2, 6, 10, and 24 h. Amplification products of POMC and β-actin cDNA were evaluated densitometrically in order to semiquantify POMC expression.

irradiation of human normal-keratinocytes and keratinocyte cell lines in culture, significantly upregulates POMC mRNA expression and the release of αMSH. Moreover, both short-wave UVB (290–320 nm) and long-wave UVA (340–400 nm) stimulate POMC synthesis in keratinocytes. Maximum production was obtained when 25 mJ/cm² UVB or 10 J/m² UVA were applied.[24,25] Using the keratinocyte cell line KB, it can be demonstrated by semiquantitative RT-PCR that POMC mRNA upregulation, following UVB irradiation, is time-dependent with maximum induction 10 and 24 h after UV exposure (see FIGURE 1). In contrast, the production of proinflammatory mediators is generally already upregulated 1–2 h after UVB exposure, and at 12 h post-UV irradiation serum levels of circulating cytokines were detected.[4,26,27] Moreover, proinflammatory mediators such as IL-1 enhance the production of αMSH by keratinocytes.[21] In the presence of IL-1RA, UVB failed to stimulate POMC mRNA expression and αMSH release, suggesting that UVB indirectly upregulates αMSH production via IL-1 (Brzoska *et al.*, unpublished observation). On the other hand, αMSH antagonizes in particular activities of IL-1 such as fever, thymocyte proliferation, and chemokine production, possibly by inhibiting the binding of IL-1β to the IL-1 receptor of type I.[15,28] These findings suggest that αM-H, released at later times after injury by UV-irradiation, is responsible for the downregulation of inflammatory responses, preventing the host from deleterious consequences of an overshoot in the inflammatory response (see FIGURE 2). However, due to the multiple antiinflammatory and immunosuppressive effects exerted by αMSH, it may also belong to the group of mediators that are responsible for UV-mediated immunosuppression.

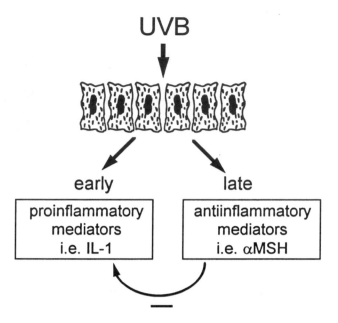

FIGURE 2. Effect of UV-irradiation on mediator production by keratinocytes. Soon after (1–2 h) UVB irradiation, the production of proinflammatory mediators is induced, whereas at later times (10–24 h) the production of suppressor factors, required for the down-regulation of inflammation, is upregulated.

IN VIVO IMMUNOMODULATORY EFFECTS OF αMSH—ROLE IN CHS

Systemic administration of αMSH in several animal models has been shown to cause antiinflammatory and immunosuppressive activities. Thus, αMSH inhibits the development of adjuvant induced arthritis, reduces endotoxin mediated fever, and reduces liver inflammation and vasculitis in the local Shwartzman reaction.[29–32] Since UV has been shown to inhibit CHS most likely via the release of suppressor factors such as IL-10 and αMSH, the effect of intravenous application of αMSH on the outcome of CHS responses was investigated.[2,5] For this purpose, mice (Balb/c) were sensitized with trinitrochlorobenzol (TNCB) at the shaved abdomen, seven days later they were challenged at one ear, and the ear swelling was evaluated after 24 h. αMSH (80 µg/kg), when injected 2 h before sensitization or challenge, significantly inhibited the ear swelling response, indicating that this peptide is able to inhibit both sensitization and elicitation phase of CHS. In contrast, αMSH has no effect on dermatitis caused by irritants such as croton oil.[33] To distinguish between a state of temporary immunosuppression and specific immunologic tolerance, mice were sensitized and challenged a second time. Only animals that had been injected with αMSH before the first sensitization were unable to develop a CHS response after additional sensitization and challenge with the same allergen. In contrast, the same mice could be sensitized with an unrelated allergen such as dinitrofluorobenzene.

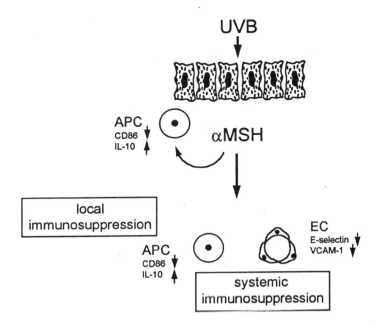

FIGURE 3. Role of αMSH in UVB mediated immunosuppression. αMSH is involved in local and systemic immunosuppression by the downregulation of accessory molecules (CD86) and upregulation of suppressor factors (IL-10) on antigen-presenting cells (APC). αMSH also suppresses the expression of adhesion molecules (P-selectin, ELAM) on vascular endothelial cells (EC).

These data indicate that αMSH, when administered i.v. 24 h before sensitization, induces hapten-specific tolerance.[33] The same animal model provides evidence that topical treatment of mice with αMSH at the site of sensitization results in the inhibition of both the sensitization and elicitation phases of CHS, and it induces allergen specific tolerance (Brzoska *et al.*, unpublished observation).

The underlying mechanisms of αMSH–mediated immunosuppression and tolerance induction are not yet clear. There is evidence that αMSH may cause these effects indirectly by affecting the function of antigen presenting cells. This includes the induction of IL-10 which was previously shown to exert the same effects on CHS as does αMSH.[17,34,35] Increased levels of IL-10 have been detected in the sera of αMSH-treated mice and administration of neutralizing antibodies against IL-10 resulted in the restoration of sensitization.[33] Moreover, αMSH was found to downregulate the expression of accessory molecules on professional APC such as CD86 which is required for a successful sensitization[19] (see FIGURE 3). Although these data provide a possible explanation for the tolerance-inducing capacity of αMSH, they are unable to interpret the inhibition of elicitation of CHS. However, αMSH has been shown to downregulate the expression of adhesion molecules, such as VCAM and E-selectin on vascular endothelial cells, that are required for the adhesion and transmigration of inflammatory cells.[20] Therefore, it may be speculated that the antiinflammatory effect of αMSH, as seen in the elicitation phase of CHS, is mediated by the downregulation of adhesion molecules on dermal microvascular endothelial cells. This notion is further supported by the finding that αMSH is able to suppress vasculitis in the local Shwartzman reaction.[32]

CONCLUSION

Our data emphasize the immunomodulatory and antiinflammatory capacity of neuropeptides, such as αMSH, that are produced in the epidermis following UV-irradiation. The effect of αMSH on APC and endothelial cells may offer one possible physiologic explanation for the well documented effects of UV on the immune system. The antiinflammatory effects of αMSH also suggest a possible role of this peptide in future treatment of inflammatory or allergic skin diseases.

ACKNOWLEDGMENTS

This work was supported by the Deutsche Forschungsgemeinschaft (So 87/11-4 E), Volkswagenstifung (I/74 582), and Centre de Recherche et d'Investigations Epidermiques et Sensorielles (C.E.R.I.E.S.), Paris.

REFERENCES

1. KRIPKE, M.L. 1990. Photoimmunology. Photochem. Photobiol. **52:** 919.
2. KIM, T.Y., M.L. KRIPKE & S.E. ULLRICH. 1990. Immunosuppression by factors released from UV-irradiated epidermal cells: selective effects on the generation of contact and delayed hypersensitivity after exposure to UVA or UVB radiation. J. Invest. Dermatol. **94:** 26.
3. LUGER, T.A., S. BEISSERT & T. SCHWARZ. 1997. The epidermal cytokine network. *In* Skin Immune System (SIS). J.D. Bos, Ed.: 271. CRC Press, Boca Raton.
4. LUGER, T.A. & T. SCHWARZ. 1995. Effects of UV-light on cytokines and neuroendocrine hormones. *In* Photoimmunology. J. Krutmann & C. Elmets, Eds.: 55. Blackwell, Oxford.
5. RIVAS, J.M. & S.E. ULLRICH. 1992. Systemic suppression of delayed-type hypersensitivity by supernatants from UV-irradiated keratinocytes. An essential role for keratinocyte-derived IL-10. J. Immunol. **149:** 3865.
6. BEISSERT, S., S.E. ULLRICH, J. HOSOI & R.D. GRANSTEIN. 1995. Supernatants from UVB radiation-exposed keratinocytes inhibit Langerhans cell presentation of tumor-associated antigens via IL-10 content. J. Leukoc. Biol. **58:** 234.
7. KONDO, S., S. PASTORE, H. FUJISAWA, G.M. SHIVJI, R.C. MCKENZIE, C.A. DINARELLO & D.N. SAUDER. 1995. Interleukin-1 receptor antagonist suppresses contact hypersensitivity. J. Invest. Dermatol. **105:** 334.
8. LEE, H.S., F. KOOSHESH, D.N. SAUDER & S. KONDO. 1997. Modulation of TGF-beta 1 production from human keratinocytes by UVB. Exp Dermatol. **6:** 105.
9. LUGER, T.A., T. SCHOLZEN & S. GRABBE. 1997. The role of α-melanocyte stimulating hormone in cutaneous biology. J. Invest. Dermatol. Derm. Symp. Proc. **2:** 87–93.
10. LUGER, T.A., T. SCHOLZEN, T. BRZOSKA, E. BECHER, A. SLOMINSKI & R. PAUS. 1998. Cutaneous immunomodulation and coordination of skin stress responses by alpha-melanocyte-stimulating hormone. Ann. N.Y. Acad. Sci. **840:** 381.

11. WINTZEN, M. & B.A. GILCHREST. 1996. Proopiomelanocortin, its derived peptides, and the skin. J. Invest. Dermatol. **106:** 3.

12. SEIDAH, N.G., R. DAY, S. BENJANNET, N. RONDEAU, A. BOUDREAULT, T. REUDELHUBER, M.K. SCHAFER, S.J. WATSON & M. CHRETIEN. 1992. The prohormone and proprotein processing enzymes PC1 and PC2: structure, selective cleavage of mouse POMC and human renin at pairs of basic residues, cellular expression, tissue distribution, and mRNA regulation. NIDA. Res. Monogr. **126:** 132.

13. CONE, R.D., D. LU, S. KOPPULA, D.I. VAGE, H. KLUNGLAND, B. BOSTON, W. CHEN, D.N. ORTH, C. POUTON & R.A. KESTERSON. 1996. The melanocortin receptors: agonists, antagonists, and the hormonal control of pigmentation. Recent. Prog. Horm. Res. **51:** 287–317.

14. SCHOLZEN, T., C.A. ARMSTRONG, N.W. BUNNETT, T.A. LUGER, J.E. OLERUD & J.C. ANSEL. 1998. Neuropeptides in the skin: interactions between the neuroendocrine and the skin immune systems. Exp. Dermatol. **7:** 81.

15. LIPTON, J.M. & A. CATANIA. 1997. Antiinflammatory actions of the neuroimmunomodulator α-MSH. Immunol. Today **18:** 140.

16. TAYLOR, A.W., J.W. STREILEIN & S.W. COUSINS. 1994. Alpha-melanocyte-stimulating hormone suppresses antigen-stimulated T cell production of gamma-interferon. Neuroimmunomodulation **1:** 188.

17. BHARDWAJ, R.S., A. SCHWARZ, E. BECHER, K. MAHNKE, H. RIEMANN, Y. ARAGANE, T. SCHWARZ & T.A. LUGER. 1996. Pro-opiomelanocortin-derived peptides induce IL-10 production in human monocytes. J. Immunol. **156:** 2517.

18. REDONDO, P., J. GARCIA FONCILLAS, I. OKROUJNOV & E. BANDRES. 1998. α-MSH regulates interleukin-10 expression by human keratinocytes. Arch. Dermatol. Res. **290:** 425.

19. BHARDWAJ, R.S., E. BECHER, K. MAHNKE, M. HARTMEYER, T. SCHWARZ, T. SCHOLZEN & T.A. LUGER. 1997. Evidence for the differential expression of the functional alpha melanocyte stimulating hormone receptor MC-1 on human monocytes. J. Immunol. **158:** 3378.

20. KALDEN, D.H., M. FASTRICH, T. BRZOSKA, T. SCHOLZEN, M. HARTMEYER, T. SCHWARZ & T.A. LUGER. 1998. Alpha-melanocyte-stimulating hormone reduces endotoxin-induced activation of nuclear factor-kB in endothelial cells. J. Invest. Dermatol. **110: 110:** 495.

21. SCHAUER, E., F. TRAUTINGER, A. KÖCK, R.S. BHARDWAJ, M. SIMON, A. SCHWARZ, J.C. ANSEL, T. SCHWARZ & T.A. LUGER. 1994. Proopiomelanocortin derived peptides are synthesized and released by human keratinocytes. J. Clin. Invest. **93:** 2258.

22. BRZOSKA, T., T. SCHOLZEN, E. BECHER, M. HARTMEYER, T. BLETZ, T. SCHWARZ & T.A. LUGER. 1997. UVB irradiation regulates the expression of proopiomelanocortin, prohormone convertase 1 and melanocortin receptor 1 by human keratinocytes. J. Invest. Dermatol. **108:** 622.

23. FIDDCCK, T., M. SCHILLER, D.H. KALDEN, T. BRZOSKA, T. SCHWARZ, M. BÖHM & T.A. LUGER 1999. Human skin cells *in vitro* express the neuroendocrine-specific prohormone convertase 2 cofactor 7B2. J. Invest. Dermatol. **110:** 600.

24. BRZOSKA, T., T. SCHOLZEN, E. BECHER & T.A. LUGER. 1997. Effect of UV light on the production of proopiomelanocortin-derived peptides and melanocortin receptors in the skin. *In* Skin Cancer and UV-Radiation. P. Altmeyer, K. Hoffmann & M. Stücker, Eds.: 227. Springer-Verlag, Berlin.

25. LUGER, T.A., A. KÖCK, E. SCHAUER, A. URBANSKI, F. TRAUTINGER & T. SCHWARZ. 1994. Cytokine neuropeptide interactions in the skin. *In* Basic Mechanism of Physiological and Aberrant Lymphoproliferation in the Skin. W.A. Van Vloten & W.C. Lambert, Eds.: 95. Plenum Press, New York.

26. SCHWARZ, T., A. URBANSKI & T.A. LUGER. 1993. Ultraviolet light and epidermal cell derived cytokines. *In* Epidermal Cytokines and Growth Factors. T.A. Luger & T. Schwarz, Eds.: 303. Marcel Decker, New York.

27. GAHRING, L., M. BALTZ, M.B. PEPYS & R. DAYNES. 1984. Effect of ultraviolet radiation on production of epidermal cell thymocyte-activating factor/interleukin 1 *in vivo* and *in vitro*. Proc. Natl. Acad. Sci. USA **81:** 1198.

28. MUGRIDGE, K.G., M. PERRETTI, P. GHIARA & L. PARENTE. 1991. Alpha-melanocyte-stimulating hormone reduces interleukin-1 beta effects on rat stomach preparations possibly through interference with a type I receptor. Eur. J. Pharmacol. **197:** 151.

29. LABBE, O., F. DESARNAUD, D. EGGERICKX, G. VASSART & M. PARMENTIER. 1994. Molecular cloning of a mouse melanocortin 5 receptor gene widely expressed in peripheral tissues. Biochemistry **33:** 4543.

30. CHIAO, H., S. FOSTER, R. THOMAS, J. LIPTON & R.A. STAR. 1996. Alpha-melanocyte-stimulating hormone reduces endotoxin-induced liver inflammation. J. Clin. Invest. **97:** 2038.

31. CERIANI, G., J. DIAZ, S. MURPHREE, A. CATANIA & J.M. LIPTON. 1994. The neuropeptide alpha-melanocyte-stimulating hormone inhibits experimental arthritis in rats. Neuroimmunomodulation **1:** 28.

32. KALDEN, D.H., S. MERFELD, T. BRZOSKA, C. SORG, T.A. LUGER & C. SUNDERKÖTTER. 1998. α-melanocyte stimulating hormone (α-MSH) reduces vasculitis in the local Shwartzman reaction. Exp. Dermatol. **7:** 225.

33. GRABBE, S., R.S. BHARDWAJ, M. STEINERT, K. MAHNKE, M.M. SIMON, T. SCHWARZ & T.A. LUGER. 1996. Alpha-melanocyte stimulating hormone induces hapten-specific tolerance in mice. J. Immunol. **156:** 473.

34. SCHWARZ, A., S. GRABBE, H. RIEMANN, Y. ARAGANE, M. SIMON, S. MANON, S. ANDRADE, T.A. LUGER, A. ZLOTNIK & T. SCHWARZ. 1994. *In vivo* effects of interleukin-10 on contact hypersensitivity and delayed-type hypersensitivity reactions. J. Invest. Dermatol. **103:** 211.

35. ENK, A.H., J. SALOGA, D. BECKER, M. MOHAMADZADEH & J. KNOP. 1994. Induction of hapten-specific tolerance by interleukin 10 *in vivo*. J. Exp. Med. **179:** 1397.

36. MURPHY, M.T., D.B. RICHARDS & J.M. LIPTON. 1983. Antipyretic potency of centrally administered alpha-melanocyte stimulating hormone. Science **221:** 192.

37. HILTZ, M.E. & J.M. LIPTON. 1990. Alpha-MSH peptides inhibit acute inflammation and contact sensitivity. Peptides **11:** 979.

38. KÖCK, A., T. SCHWARZ, R. KIRNBAUER, A. URBANSKI, P. PERRY, J.C. ANSEL & T.A. LUGER. 1990. Human keratinocytes are a source for tumor necrosis factor alpha: evidence for synthesis and release upon stimulation with endotoxin or ultraviolet light. J. Exp. Med. **172:** 1609.

39. HARTMEYER, M., T. SCHOLZEN, E. BECHER, R.S. BHARDWAJ, M. FASTRICH, T. SCHWARZ & T.A. LUGER. 1997. Human microvascular endothelial cells (HMEC-1) express the melanocortin receptor type 1 and produce increased levels of IL-8 upon stimulation with αMSH. J. Immunol. **159:** 1930.

α-MSH and the Regulation of Melanocyte Function

ANTHONY J. THODY[a]

Department of Biomedical Sciences, University of Bradford,
West Yorkshire, BD7 1DP, United Kingdom

ABSTRACT: α-MSH, has numerous actions in the skin and by activating the MC1 receptor (MC1-R) on melanocytes it stimulates melanogenesis. Rather than producing large increase in melanin production α-MSH acts specifically to stimulate eumelanin synthesis. Although this could be important in determining skin color and tanning there is debate as to the pigmentary significance of α-MSH in humans. Circulating levels of α-MSH are negligible and although it is produced in the skin by different cell types, including melanocytes, the major skin form is desacetyl α-MSH, and this is a weak agonist at MC1-R. Certain ACTH peptides, notably $ACTH_{1-17}$, are more potent agonists at the MC1-R and, since their skin concentrations exceed those of α-MSH, they could serve as natural ligands at this receptor and regulate pigmentary responses in humans. Activation of MC1-R does, however, produce other responses in human melanocytes. Thus, α-MSH stimulates melanocyte dendricity and attachment to extracellular matrix proteins. It also protects melanocytes from the damaging effects of oxidative stress, and regulates their production of NO by modulating the induction of iNOS—as it does within macrophages. α-MSH clearly affects various aspects of melanocyte behavior and its melanogenic effects could be the consequence of a more fundamental role in the melanocyte. The precise nature of this role is unclear, but it could be part of a generic role that α-MSH and other POMC peptides have in skin homeostasis.

INTRODUCTION

α-Melanocyte-stimulating hormone is produced, together with several other peptides, following the proteolytic cleavage of proopiomelanocortin (POMC). Its main site of production is the pituitary gland, but it has been known for sometime that α-MSH and related ACTH peptides are produced at other sites, including the skin.[1,2] Keratinocytes comprise a major source of these peptides, although α-MSH is present in higher concentrations in melanocytes.[2] Thus, as well as functioning as hormones in the skin, POMC peptides are produced locally and many of their cutaneous effects are presumably mediated via paracrine and/or autocrine mechanisms. Such mechanisms are important in melanocyte regulation and may have special significance in humans, where the levels of circulating α-MSH are extremely low.

Stimulation of pigment cells is a well known action of α-MSH. It is accepted that in lower vertebrates and many mammals the peptide has an important pigmentary role. However, although α-MSH increases skin darkening in human,[3,4] and is capa-

[a]Address for correspondence. 01274-236212 (voice); 01274-309742 (fax);
a.j.thody@bradford.ac.uk (e-mail).

ble of stimulating melanogenesis in human melanocytes in culture,[5,6] there is still uncertainty as to its pigmentary significance in humans. α-MSH affects melanocytes in numerous ways and, rather than simply increasing melanogenesis, it may have a more fundamental role in controlling the behavior of these cells. The purpose of this article is to discuss the various effects that α-MSH has in human melanocytes, and to consider what role it has in these cells.

EFFECTS OF α-MSH IN HUMAN MELANOCYTES

The receptor that mediates the actions of α-MSH and other POMC peptides on melanocytes is a member of a family of G-protein-coupled receptors.[7,8] At least five subtypes have been cloned and sequenced, but only one is expressed by melanocytes; this is referred to as the melanocortin-1 (MC-1) receptor.[8] The MC-1 receptor is coupled to adenylate cyclase and, after binding with α-MSH, there is an increase in intracellular cyclic AMP. Other signalling pathways might also be activated in response to α-MSH; there is, for instance, evidence that protein kinase C is involved in mediating its melanogenic actions.[9,10] These same pathways probably mediate the other effects of α-MSH in melanocytes.

Melanogenesis

The melanogenic action of α-MSH is mediated via tyrosinase (see FIGURE 1). Evidence suggests that α-MSH increases both the expression and activation of this enzyme.[11,12] The resulting increase in melanogenesis in human melanocytes is, nevertheless, quite small and this has led some investigators to conclude that α-MSH has little or no significance in regulating pigmentation.[13] The magnitude of the melanogenic response in human melanocytes certainly does not compare with that in

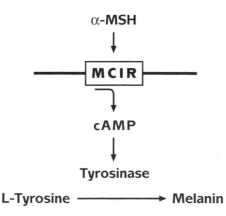

FIGURE 1. α-MSH acts via the cAMP-coupled MC1 receptor to activate tyrosinase and to stimulate melanogenesis.

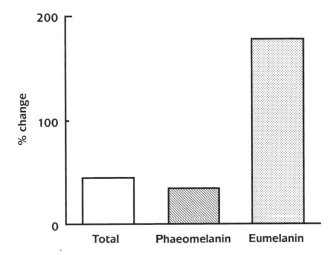

FIGURE 2. Changes in eumelanin and phaeomelanin levels in human melanocytes in response to Nle⁴DPhe⁷ α-MSH. The values are the means from six cultures and are expressed as percentages relative to untreated controls. Data taken from Hunt *et al.*[18]

murine melanoma cells, and this response is probably explained by the smaller number of binding sites in human melanocytes.[14,15] However, as in the hair follicular melanocytes of viable yellow mice,[16,17] α-MSH acts preferentially in human epidermal melanocytes to stimulate the synthesis of eumelanin[18] (see FIGURE 2).

Not all melanocytes show a melanogenic response to α-MSH. This unresponsiveness to α-MSH is particularly prevalent in melanocytes from red-haired individuals[19,20] (see TABLE 1). In animals, responsiveness to α-MSH is determined by alleles at the MC-1 receptor, and these are associated with distinct pigmentation patterns.[21] The same may be true in humans. Thus, different MC-1 receptor alleles

TABLE 1. Responsiveness of human melanocyte cultures to α-MSH[a]

Hair color	Number of cultures	Responsive			Nonresponsive
		↑ dendricity	↑ melanin	↑ dendricity ↑ melanin	
Red	10	2 (20)	0	0	8 (80)
Fair	32	10 (31)	4 (13)	11 (34)	7 (22)
Dark	36	10 (280)	3 (8)	20 (56)	3 (8)

[a]NOTE: The results are given as numbers of responsive and nonresponsive cultures, with percentages in parentheses. Responsiveness is related to pigmentation phenotype; cultures from red-haired individuals are usually nonresponsive, whereas those from dark-haired individuals are almost always responsive. (Data from Hunt *et al.*,[19] and Graham.[20])

have been identified in humans and frequently in persons with red hair and/or fair skin.[22–24] Although there is evidence that the Va192Met variant affects the binding affinity of the receptor for α-MSH[25] little is known about the effects of variants on receptor function. The high incidence of MC-1 receptor variants in red-haired individuals reported by Valverde *et al.*,[22] does, however, correlate with the high degree of unresponsiveness to α-MSH observed by Hunt *et al.*[19] Thus, although some of the variants may turn out to be simple polymorphisms, others could cause a loss of function at the receptor and be responsible for the unresponsiveness to α-MSH seen in melanocytes from red-haired individuals. However, in the studies of Hunt *et al.*,[19] it was observed that, although a melanogenic response to α-MSH was sometimes absent in melanocytes from other pigmentation phenotypes, the cells responded to the peptide by showing an increase in dendricity (see TABLE 1 and the discussion later in this paper). This suggests that melanogenic and morphological responses to α-MSH are to some extent independent of one another, and that not all melanocytes that fail to respond melanogenically lack functional MSH receptors. It appears, therefore, that melanogenic responsiveness to α-MSH is not necessarily controlled solely at the level of the MC-1 receptor.

This view is supported by other observations showing that, although cyclic AMP is effective in stimulating melanogenesis in cultures that are responsive to α-MSH, it has little or no effect in many α-MSH-unresponsive cultures.[19] Similar results were obtained with an analogue of diacylglycerol that activates protein kinase C. Although the possibility cannot be ruled out that signalling pathways downstream of the MC-1 receptor are dependent upon the normal functioning of the receptor, it appears that in human melanocytes melanogenic responsiveness to α-MSH is determined by intracellular mechanisms in addition to those acting at the receptor level. The key factor could be tyrosinase, since the expression of this enzyme is essential for melanogenesis. It is significant that melanocytes from red-haired individuals have less tyrosinase mRNA, protein and lower activity, than melanocytes from white-skinned individuals.[26] Moreover, *de novo*-synthesis of tyrosinase in human skin correlates with skin type, and is at its lowest in individuals with skin types 1 and 2 who tan poorly.[27]

Recent findings from Schallreuter and colleagues support the view that α-MSH is able to regulate melanogenesis by mechanisms that are independent of the MC-1 receptor. These workers have shown that (6R)-L-erythro-5,6,7,8-tetrahydrobiopterin (6BH$_4$) controls melanogenesis by regulating the availability of L-tyrosine, and by inhibiting tyrosinase.[28] They have further suggested that α-MSH is able to bind to 6BH$_4$ and, by removing the pterin from its complex with tyrosinase, to bring about activation of the enzyme[29] (see FIGURE 3). Even more novel is their suggestion that if the concentrations of α-MSH exceed those of 6BH$_4$ then the peptide itself could function as a substrate for tyrosinase by virtue of its tyrosine residue in position 2. The availability of 6BH$_4$ in the melanocyte could, therefore, be important for melanogenesis and in determining responsiveness to α-MSH. Epidermal concentrations of 6BH$_4$ have been shown to vary in different skin types;[29] thus it would be of interest to see whether this relationship extends to melanocytes and melanogenic responsiveness to α-MSH.

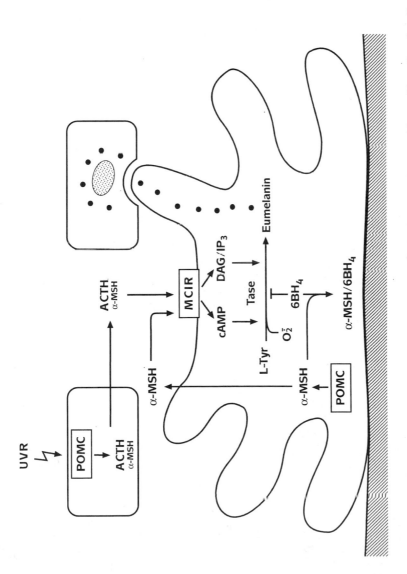

FIGURE 3. The role of POMC peptides in the regulation of skin pigmentation in humans. These peptides could mediate the effects of UVR with keratinocyte–derived ACTH peptides acting as paracrine factors and the α-MSH peptides acting predominantly via autocrine mechanisms, to activate the MC-1 receptor and regulate melanocyte morphology and eumelanin synthesis. α-MSH may also affect these processes through interactions with 6BH₄ within the melanocyte.

Dendricity

In culture, human melanocytes tend to be bipolar or tripolar in appearance. They are generally much smaller and less dendritic than those *in vivo*. In response to α-MSH the melanocytes become dendritic and more closely resemble the morphology of their counterparts *in vivo*.[2,5,11] Other factors, such as the presence of keratinocytes and growth factors, also affect melanocyte dendrite formation. Endothelin-1 (ET-1) is particularly active in this respect[30] and, in addition, enhances the effect that α-MSH has on melanocyte dendricity.[20]

It appears that different signals interact to regulate melanocyte dendricity and, in all probability, this process is dependent upon the activation of several intracellular signalling pathways. It has recently been shown that rac1 is an important signalling intermediate for dendrite formation in B16 mouse-melanoma cells. Thus, it has been suggested that this protein, which is a member of the rho subfamily of ras-related proteins, mediates the dendritic effects that α-MSH and UVR have in these cells.[31] α-MSH probably acts by stimulating the PKA and PKC pathways that serve as upstream signalling pathways for rac1-activation and, in this way, it mediates the dendritic actions of UVR.[31]

Proliferative Effects

Epidermal melanocytes proliferate slowly *in vivo*. There is no evidence at present to suggest that α-MSH regulates this process, although there are reports that the peptide stimulates the growth of human melanocytes in culture.[6,12,15] However, others have failed to observe such effects[5] and it could be that the proliferative effects of α-MSH, like the effects on melanogenesis, depend on culture conditions. If α-MSH is able to affect the proliferation of human melanocytes *in vivo*, then its action, like that on melanocyte dendricity could well be dependent upon interactions with other growth factors.[32]

Protective Actions

Of the various cell types in the skin, melanocytes are particularly vulnerable to oxidative damage. This could be related to their relatively low levels of antioxidant enzymes, in comparison with fibroblasts and keratinocytes,[33] and/or their ability to produce large amounts of superoxide anion.[34] α-MSH has been shown to protect melanocytes from the damaging effects of the superoxide anion and, thus, it has been suggested that this involves activation of tyrosinase.[35] Tyrosinase is able to utilize the superoxide anion as a substrate for melanogenesis,[36,37] hence, when activated, it could bring about a reduction in the concentrations of the potentially damaging superoxide radical. An alternative possibility is that α-MSH exerts a protective effect through its ability to complex with $6BH_4$. As discussed above, the latter controls melanogenesis, but its oxidized product, 6-biopterin, is cytotoxic to melanocytes.[38] By complexing with $6BH_4$, α-MSH could control the redox status of the pterin and in this way affect both melanogenesis and melanocyte survival.

α-MSH may also protect melanocytes from cell-mediated cytotoxicity. It has been known for sometime that α-MSH antagonizes the actions of proinflammatory cytokines on immuno competent cells,[39] and there is evidence that it has similar actions in melanocytes. Thus, α-MSH inhibits the action of tumor necrosis factor α

(TNF-α) in inducing ICAM-1 expression in melanocytes. It has been suggested that this prevents the cells from being targeted by the immune system.[40] How α-MSH antagonizes the actions of proinflammatory cytokines is not known, but it may involve nitric oxide (NO). This reactive molecule, which is produced by melanocytes,[34] has many physiological functions and has recently been shown to stimulate melanogenesis.[41] It is also capable of cell-damaging effects through its ability to react with the superoxide anion to produce peroxynitrite and the highly cytotoxic hydroxyl radical. There is evidence that α-MSH is able to modulate the production of NO in melanocytes in response to UVR and lipopolysaccharide,[42,43] but whether it acts by affecting the induction of the inducible form of nitric oxide synthase (NOS)—as it does in macrophages[44]—is not yet known. Whatever its mechanism of action, the fact that α-MSH is able to affect NO production could be of relevance with respect to both its melanogenic and protective actions in these cells.

WHAT IS THE ROLE OF POMC PEPTIDES IN MELANOCYTE?

There is a good case for accepting that α-MSH has a pigmentary function in humans. As discussed above, there is much evidence that α-MSH and related analogues are capable of stimulating melanogenesis in human melanocytes. Rather than producing large increases in melanin, α-MSH specifically stimulates the synthesis of eumelanin, resulting in an increase in the eumelanin/phaeomelanin ratio. This could have important consequences because eumelanin, not only makes the greater contribution to the tanning response, but also has the greater photoprotective capacity. Phaeomelanin, on the other hand, has a greater potential for generating free-radicals in response to UVR, and since these are capable of damaging DNA, this particular melanin may actually contribute to the phototoxic effects of UVR. By regulating the pattern of melanogenesis, α-MSH could, therefore, play a key role in the tanning response and in protecting the skin from the damaging effects of UVR. An inability of the melanocytes to respond to α-MSH might explain why certain individuals—e.g., those with red hair—are unable to tan, and also explain their increased susceptibility to UVR induced skin damage.

α-MSH may, in addition, regulate other processes associated with the pigmentary response (FIG. 3). *In vivo,* melanocytes are situated on the basement membrane but are in contact with other epidermal cells through dendrites that ramify throughout the epidermis. Such an arrangement is important for melanocyte-keratinocyte communication, and it ensures that melanin is transferred into keratinocytes, especially those that actively divide in the lower layers of the epidermis. Whether α-MSH stimulates the transfer of melanin into the keratinocyte is not yet known, but since it stimulates melanocyte dendricity, it is likely to play an important role in helping to maintain the integrity of the epidermal-melanin unit and in coordinating the events that are essential for normal pigmentation.

UVR is an important stimulator of skin pigmentation in humans. As discussed above, α-MSH may mediate the effects that UVR has on melanocyte dendricity, and it may also serve as a paracrine mediator of UVR-induced melanogenesis[45,46] (FIG. 3). Keratinocytes secrete α-MSH and related POMC peptides in response to UVR.[47–49] Similar responses have been seen in human melanocytes,[46] and this implies that autocrine mechanisms are involved in the tanning response. UVR has been shown to upregulate the function and expression of the MC-1 receptor on Cloudman melanoma cells,[46,50] and to increase the binding of α-MSH to human melanocytes in culture.[51] It is possible, therefore, that in stimulating skin pigmentation, UVR acts not only by increasing the production of α-MSH in the epidermis, but also by enhancing the responsiveness of the melanocytes to this peptide.

Even if we accept that activation of the MC-1 receptor is an important event in the pigmentary response, questions still arise as to the identity of the natural ligands at this receptor in the skin. Acetylated α-MSH is considered to be the most potent melanogenic peptide[52] and, for this reason, it is often assumed that it is this particular peptide that acts at the MC-1 receptor to regulate skin pigmentation. This may be true in some mammals, but the situation could be different in humans. In the first place, the major form of α-MSH in human epidermis is desacetyl α-MSH[2] and this peptide is considerably less potent than acetylated α-MSH in activating the human MC-1 receptor and in stimulating melanogenesis. Second, other POMC peptides, such as ACTH, are capable of stimulating melanogenesis in cultured human melanocytes[11] and their concentrations in human epidermis exceed those of α-MSH.[2] One of the most active of the ACTH peptides is $ACTH_{1-17}$. This peptide binds to the human MC-1 receptor with an affinity comparable to that of acetylated α-MSH, and is more potent than α-MSH in activating this receptor and stimulating melanogenesis.[2,53] The dose response curves to the ACTH peptides differ from those of α-MSH in that they are biphasic.[11,53] It could be that the ACTH peptides bind to two distinct receptors or, alternatively, on binding to the MC-1 receptor, activate other signalling systems that are not activated by α-MSH. Whatever the explanation, the possibility should be considered that ACTH peptides are involved in regulating melanocyte function and, since they are produced by keratinocytes in greater amounts than the α-MSH peptides, they could turn out to be more important than the latter as paracrine regulators of skin pigmentation. (FIG. 3). The α-MSH peptides, on the other hand, are present at higher concentrations in melanocytes and are, therefore, more likely to affect melanocytes via autocrine mechanisms.[2] Although the α-MSH peptides may be released from the melanocyte in order to activate the MC1 receptor, their presence within the melanocyte is consistent with an intracellular action and, as discussed above, this could involve interactions with $6BH_4$ (FIG. 3).

It is, however, clear that α-MSH is not just a pigmentary peptide and that there is a growing awareness of a number of different actions that it has in the melanocyte (see FIGURE 4). It could be that its primary role in the melanocyte is one of protection. It is recognized, for instance, that dendritic melanocytes are more resistant to apoptosis and thus α-MSH, by inducing dendritic formation, could enhance melanocyte survival. The stimulation of eumelanogensis could also have survival value in protecting melanocytes from oxidative damage and, furthermore, cause the melanocytes to be less susceptible to attack by the immune system (see FIGURE 5). It is intriguing that melanocytes not only respond to the α-MSH peptides, but are also major producers of these peptides. It is not yet clear whether these melanocyte-derived peptides are secreted and target other cells, or whether their actions are confined to melanocytes. Whatever the explanation, it is interesting that there is a reduction in the expression of α-MSH in melanocytes in vitiligo, a condition in which melanocytes become nonfunctional and may be lost from the epidermis.[54]

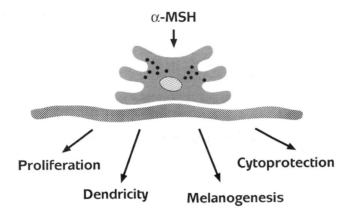

FIGURE 4. α-MSH has several effects in human melanocytes.

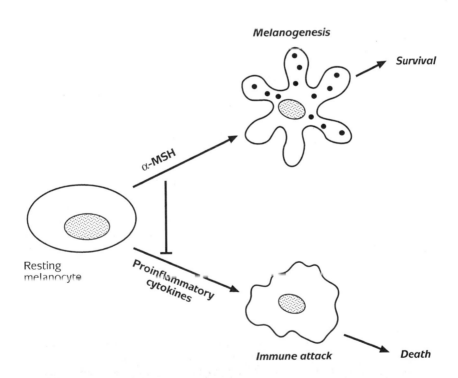

FIGURE 5. α-MSH increases melanocyte survival. By stimulating dendricity and melanogenesis, and by opposing the actions of proinflammatory cytokines α-MSH protects the melanocyte from oxidative damage and attack by the immune system.

It could be sometime before we understand the true role of α-MSH in the melanocyte. A major problem is that, although melanocytes produce melanin, they have other functions and these appear to be far more complex than hitherto imagined. A more complete understanding of melanocyte physiology is clearly required if we are to appreciate the significance of α-MSH and its different actions in this particular cell.

ACKNOWLEDGMENTS

I would like to thank the Medical Research Council and Stiefel Laboratories for their support. I am also pleased to acknowledge my many research students, colleagues, and collaborators with whom it has been a pleasure to work.

REFERENCES

1. THODY, A.J., K. RIDLEY, R.J. PENNY et al. 1983. MSH peptides are present in mammalian skin. Peptides **4:** 813–816.
2. WAKAMATSU, K., A. GRAHAM, D. COOK & A.J. THODY. 1997. Characterization of ACTH peptides in human skin and their activation of the melanocortin-1 receptor. Pigment Cell Res. **10:** 288–297.
3. LERNER, A.B. & J.S. MCGUIRE. 1961. Effect of alpha- and beta-melanocyte stimulating hormone on the skin colour of man. Nature **189:** 176–179.
4. LEVINE, N., S.N. SHEFTEL, T. EYTAN et al. 1991. Induction of skin tanning by subcutaneous administration of a potent synthetic melanotropin. JAMA. **266:** 2730–2736.
5. HUNT, G., C. TODD, J.E. CRESSWELL & A.J. THODY. 1994. α-Melanocyte stimulating hormone and its analogue Nle^{4}DPhe^7 α-MSH affect morphology, tyrosinase activity and melanogenesis in cultured human melanocytes. J. Cell Sci. **107:** 205–211.
6. ABDEL-MALEK, Z., V.B. SWOPE, I. SUZUKI et al. 1995. Mitogenic and melanogenic stimulation of normal human melanocytes by melanotropic peptides. Proc. Natl. Acad. Sci. USA **92:** 1789–1793.
7. CHHAJLANI, V. & J.E.S. WIKBERG. 1992. Molecular cloning and expression of the human melanocyte stimulating hormone receptor cDNA. FEBS Lett. **309:** 417–420.
8. MOUNTJOY, K.G., L.S. ROBBINS, M. MORTRUD & R.D. CONE. 1992. The cloning of a family of genes that encode the melanocortin receptors. Science **257:** 1248–1251.
9. BUFFEY, J.A., A.J. THODY, S.S. BLEEHEN & S. MACNEIL. 1992. α-Melanocyte-stimulating hormone stimulates protein kinase C activity in B16 melanoma. J. Endocrinol. **133:** 333–340.
10. PARK, H.-Y., V. RUSSAKOVSKY, Y. AO et al. 1996. α-Melanocyte-stimulating hormone-induced pigmentation is blocked by depletion of protein kinase C. Exp. Cell Res. **227:** 70–79.
11. HUNT, G., P.D. DONATIEN, J. LUNEC, et al. 1994. Cultured human melanocytes respond to MSH peptides and ACTH. Pigment Cell Res. **7:** 217–221.
12. SUZUKI, I., R.D. CONE, S. IM et al. 1996. Binding of melanotropic hormones to the melanocortin receptor MC1 R on human melanocytes stimulates proliferation and melanogenesis. Endocrinology **137:** 1627–1633.
13. HEDLEY, S.J., D.J. GAWKRODGER, A.P. WEETMAN & S. MACNEIL. 1998. α-MSH and melanogenesis in normal human adult melanocytes. Pigment Cell Res. **11:** 45–56.
14. DONATIEN, P.D., G. HUNT, C. PIERON et al. 1992. The expression of functional MSH receptors on cultured human melanocytes. Arch. Dermatol. Res. **284:** 424–426.

15. DE LUCA, M., W. SIEGRIST, S. BONDARIZA et al. 1993. α-Melanocyte stimulating hormone stimulates normal human melanocyte growth by binding to high affinity receptors. J. Cell Sci. **105:** 1079–1084.

16. BURCHILL, S.A., A.J. THODY & S. ITO. 1986. Melanocyte-stimulating hormone, tyrosinase activity and the regulation of eumelanogenesis and phaeomelanogenesis in the hair follicular melanocytes of the mouse. J. Endocr. **109:** 15–21.

17. BURCHILL, S.A., S. ITO & A.J. THODY. 1993. Effects of melanocyte-stimulating hormone on tyrosinase expression and melanin synthesis in hair follicular melanocytes of the mouse. J. Endocrinol. **137:** 189–195.

18. HUNT, G., S. KYNE, K. WAKAMATSU et al. 1995. Nle^{4}DPhe^7 α-melanocyte-stimulating hormone increases the eumelanin:phaeomelanin ratio in cultured human melanocytes. J. Invest. Dermatol. **104:** 83–85.

19. HUNT, G., C. TODD & A.J. THODY. 1996. Unresponsiveness of human epidermal melanocytes to melanocyte-stimulating hormone and its association with red hair. Mol. Cell. Endocrinol. **116:** 131–136.

20. GRAHAM, A.J. 1997. Skin peptides and their role in the regulation of human melanocytes. Ph.D. Thesis, University of Newcastle-upon-Tyne, U.K.

21. ROBBINS, L.S., J.H. NADEAU, K.R. JOHNSON et al. 1993. Pigmentation phenotypes of variant extension locus alleles result from point mutations that alter MSH receptor function. Cell **72:** 827–834.

22. VALVERDE, P., E. HEALY, I. JACKSON et al. 1995. Variants of the melanocyte-stimulating hormone receptor gene are associated with red hair and fair skin in humans. Nature Genet. **11:** 328–330.

23. KOPPULA, S.V., L.S. ROBBINS, D. LU, E. BAACK et al. 1995. Identification of common polymorphisms in the coding sequence of the human MSH receptor (MCIR) with possible biological effects. Human Mutation **9:** 30–36.

24. BOX, N.F., J.R. WYETH, L.E. O'GORMAN et al. 1997. Characterization of melanocyte stimulating hormone receptor variant alleles in twins with red hair. Human Mol. Genet. **6:** 1891–1897.

25. XU, X., M. THORNWALL, L.G. LUNDIN & V. CHHAJLANI. 1996. Val192Met variant of the melanocyte stimulating hormone receptor gene. Nature Genet. **14:** 384.

26. IOZUMI, K., G.E. HOGANSON, R. PENNELLA et al. 1993. Role of tyrosinase as the determinant of pigmentation in cultured human melanocytes. J. Invest. Dermatol. **100:** 806–811.

27. BURCHILL, S.A., J.M. MARKS & A.J. THODY. 1990. Tyrosinase synthesis in different skin types and the effects of α-melanocyte-stimulating hormone and cyclic AMP. J. Invest. Dermatol. **95:** 558–561.

28. WOOD, J.M., K.U. SCHALLREUTER-WOOD, N.J. LINDSEY et al. 1995. A specific tetrahydrobiopterin binding domain on tyrosinase controls melanogenesis. Biochem. Biophys. Res. Commun. **206:** 480–485.

29. SCHALLREUTER, K.U., J. MOORE, T. JENNER et al. 1997. Pterins and α-MSH in the control of pigmentation in the human epidermis. In Chemistry and Biology of Pteridines and Folates. W. Pfleiderer & H. Rokos, Eds.: 791–795. Blackwell Science, Berlin.

30. HARA, M., M. YAAR & B.A. GILCHREST. 1995. Endothelin-1 of keratinocyte origin is a mediator of melanocyte dendricity. J. Invest. Dermatol. **105:** 744–748.

31. SCOTT, G.A. & L. CASSIDY. 1998. Racl mediates dendrite formation in response to melanocyte stimulating hormone and ultraviolet light in a murine melanoma model. J. Invest. Dermatol. **111:** 243–250.

32. SWOPE, V.B., E.E. MEDRANO, D. SMALARA et al. 1995. Long-term proliferation of human melanocytes is supported by the physiologic mitogens α-melanotropin, endothelin-1 and basic fibroblast growth factor. Exp. Cell Res. **217:** 453-459.

33. YOHN, J.J., D.A. NORRIS, D.G. YRASTORZA *et al.* 1991. Disparate antioxidant enzyme activities in cultured human cutaneous fibroblasts, keratinocytes and melanocytes. J. Invest. Dermatol. **97:** 405–409.

34. VALVERDE, P., P. MANNING, A. GRAHAM *et al.* 1996. Melanocytes produce superoxide anion and nitric oxide in response to low doses of ultraviolet radiation. (Abstract). J. Invest. Dermatol. **107:** 509.

35. VALVERDE, P., P. MANNING, C.J. MCNEIL & A.J. THODY. 1996. Activation of tyrosinase reduces the cytotoxic effects of the superoxide anion in B16 mouse melanoma cells. Pigment Cell Res. **9:** 77–84.

36. WOOD, J.M. & K.U. SCHALLREUTER. 1991. Studies on the reactions between human tyrosinase, superoxide anion, hydrogen peroxide and thiols. Biochim. Biophys. Acta. **1074:** 378–385.

37. TOBIN, D. & A.J. THODY. 1994. The superoxide anion may mediate short- but not long-term effects of ultraviolet radiation on melanogenesis. Exp. Dermatol. **3:** 99–105.

38. SCHALLREUTER, K.U., G. BUTTNER, M.R. PITTELKOW *et al.* 1994. The cytotoxicity of 6-biopterin to human melanocytes. Biochem. Biophys. Res. Commun. **204:** 43–48.

39. CATANIA, A. & J.M. LIPTON. 1993. Alpha-melanocyte stimulating hormone in the modulation of host reactions. Endocrine Rev. **14:** 564–576.

40. HEDLEY, S.J., D.J. GAWKRODGER, A.P. WEETMAN *et al.* 1998. α-Melanocyte stimulating hormone inhibits tumour necrosis factor-α stimulated intercellular adhesion molecule-1 expression in normal cutaneous human melanocytes and in melanoma cell lines. Brit. J. Dermatol. **138:** 536–543.

41. ROMÉRO-GRAILLET, C., E. ABERDAM, M. CLÉMENT *et al.* 1997. Nitric oxide produced by ultraviolet-irradiated keratinocytes stimulates melanogenesis. J. Clin. Invest. **99:** 635–642.

42. GRAHAM, A., P. MANNING, U. ATIF *et al.* 1997. α-MSH induces nitric oxide production in melanocytes. (Abstract). Pigment Cell Res. **10:** 327.

43. TSATMALI, M., P. MANNING, C.J. MCNEIL *et al.* 1999. α-MSH inhibits lipopolysaccharide induced nitric oxide production in B16 mouse melanoma cells. Ann. N.Y. Acad. Sci. USA. **885:** this volume.

44. STAR, R.A., N. RAJORA, J. HUANG *et al.* 1995. Evidence of autocrine modulation of macrophage nitric oxide synthase by α-melanocyte-stimulating hormone. Proc. Natl. Acad. Sci. USA **92:** 8016–8020.

45. BOLOGNIA, J., M. MURRAY & J. PAWELEK. 1989. UVB-induced melanogenesis may be mediated through the MSH-receptor system. J. Invest. Dermatol. **92:** 651–656.

46. CHAKRABORTY, A., A. SLOMINSKI, G. ERMAK *et al.* 1995. Ultraviolet B and melanocyte-stimulating hormone (MSH) stimulate mRNA production for alpha MSH receptors and prooopiomelanocortin-derived peptides in mouse melanoma cells and transformed keratinocytes. J. Invest. Dermatol. **105:** 655–659.

47. SCHAUER, E., F. TRAUTINGER, A. KOCK *et al.* 1994. Proopiomelanocortinderived peptides are synthesized and released by human keratinocytes. J. Clin. Invest. **93:** 2258–2262.

48. CHAKRABORTY, A.K., Y. FUNASAKA, A. SLOMINSKI *et al.* 1996. Production and release of proopiomelanocortin (POMC) derived peptides by human melanocytes and keratinocytes in culture: Regulation by ultraviolet B. Biochim. Biophys. Acta. **1313:** 130–138.

49. WINTZEN, M. & B.A. GILCHREST. 1996. Proopiomelanocortin gene product regulation in keratinocytes. J. Invest. Dermatol. **106:** 673–678.

50. CHAKRABORTY, A.K., S.J. ORLOW, J.L. BOLOGNIA & J.M. PAWELEK. 1991. Structural/functional relationships between internal and external MSH receptors: Modulation of expression in Cloudman melanoma cells by UVB radiation. J. Cell. Physiol. **147:** 1–6.
51. THODY, A.J., G. HUNT, P.D. DONATIEN & C. TODD. 1993. Human melanocytes express functional melanocyte-stimulating hormone receptors. Ann. N.Y. Acad. Sci. **680:** 381–390.
52. EBERLE, A.N. 1988. The Melanotropins. Karger, Basel.
53. TSATMALI, M., K. WAKAMATSU, A. GRAHAM & A.J. THODY. 1999. Skin POMC peptides: their binding affinities and activation of the human MC1 receptor. Ann. N.Y. Acad. Sci. **885:** this volume.
54. GRAHAM, A., W. WESTERHOF & A.J. THODY. 1998. The expression of α-MSH by melanocytes is reduced in vitiligo. (Abstract). Pigment Cell Res. **11:** 252.

Molecular Basis of the
α-MSH/IL-1 Antagonism

T. BRZOSKA, D.-H. KALDEN, T. SCHOLZEN, AND T.A. LUGER[a]

*Ludwig Boltzmann Institute of Cellbiology and Immunobiology of the Skin,
Department. of Dermatology, University Muenster, Germany*

ABSTRACT: The neuropeptide α-melanocyte stimulating hormone (α-MSH) is recognized as a potent mediator of immune and inflammatory reactions. Accordingly, α-MSH *in vitro*, as well as *in vivo*, antagonizes the proinflammatory activities of cytokines such as interleukin-1 (IL-1), IL-6, and tumor necrosis factor α (TNFα). Since the molecular basis of these antiinflammatory effects is not well known, the influence of α-MSH on IL-1β–induced chemokine production and transcription factor activation was investigated in human keratinocytes. α-MSH, in a dose-dependent manner, after 48 h, significantly reduced the IL-1β mediated secretion of the C-X-C chemokines IL-8 and Groα. This was confirmed by semiquantitative RT-PCR, which revealed a marked downregulation in IL-8 and Groα mRNA expression. Furthermore, we determined the effect of α-MSH on the IL-1β–induced activation of the nuclear factor κB (NFκB)—a major transcription factor for chemokine genes. Electrophoretic mobility-shift-assays showed that α-MSH, in a dose range from 10^{-6} to 10^{-12} M, significantly downregulated the IL-1β–induced activation of NFκB 10 minutes after stimulation. Therefore, NFκB inactivation by α-MSH appears to be a crucial event, one that is responsible for the downregulation of cytokine gene transcription.

INTRODUCTION

Interleukin-1 (IL-1) is well appreciated as one of the major mediators of inflammation.[1] When IL-1 binds to the interleukin-1 receptor type-I (IL-1RI) a cascade signal is initiated via the GTPase-activity located in the intracellular portion of the receptor. The GTPase activity leads to activation of the MAP-kinase pathway and results in phosphorylation of many intracellular proteins, among them the inhibitory κB (IκB), which is rapidly degraded upon phosphorylation. Phosphorylation and degradation of IκB, in turn, lead to activation of the transcription factor nuclear factor κB (NFκB) and its subsequent translocalization into the nucleus.[2] The transcription factors NFκB and AP-1 are the main mediators of IL-1 induced biological effects. Both are present in the cytosols of unstimulated cells and, on stimulation with IL-1, they rapidly translocate into the nucleus, where they activate a wide range of target genes.[1]

To exert maximum effect it is sufficient for IL-1 to occupy only a small part of the IL-1RI. Therefore, and because the spectrum of IL-1 induced genes is very

[a]Address for correspondence: Prof. Dr. med. T. Luger, Department of Dermatology, University of Muenster, Von-Esmarch Str. 56, 48149 Münster, Germany. +49-251-8356504 (voice); +49-251-8356522 (fax); luger@uni-muenster.de (e-mail).

broad, specific inhibitors are required to hold the effects of this molecule within well defined limits. These include the IL-1 receptor type-II which, like IL-1RI, is able to bind IL-1 but, in contrast to IL-1RI, lacks a signal transduction domain. The shedded form of the type-II receptor may capture IL-1 molecules before they bind to IL-1RI. The second inhibitory protein is the IL-1 receptor antagonist (IL-1RA), which competes with IL-1 in binding to IL-1RI. In contrast to IL-1, the binding of IL-1RA to IL-1RI does not trigger the signal transduction cascade.

The proopiomelanocortin (POMC)–derived peptide α-MSH is well known for its role in pigmentation,[3–5] as well as for its immunomodulatory capacities.[6–11] Moreover α-MSH has turned out to be a very potent antagonist for IL-1. It effectively inhibits the activities of IL-1 *in vitro* and *in vivo*. Thus, α-MSH suppresses IL-1–induced fever, thymocyte proliferation, prostaglandin production, inflammation, and edema formation.[10–13] POMC–derived peptides such as α-MSH are not only expressed in the pituitary, but also in many tissues, including the skin.[14–18] In addition, epidermal cells, including melanocytes and keratinocytes, were found to express the melanocortin-1 receptor (MC-1R) that is specific for α-MSH.[5,18–21] On treatment with α-MSH, keratinocyte proliferation is induced and production of the suppressor factor IL-10 is increased.[22,23] Because of the potent antiinflammatory capacities of α-MSH, the purpose of this study was to investigate the underlying molecular mechanisms. Hence, the effect of α-MSH on IL-1β–induced transcription factor activation, and the subsequent production of chemokines by human keratinocytes, was investigated.

METHODS

Cell Culture and Chemokine Assays

HaCaT cells were cultured in DMEM with 10% FCS (PAA Laboratories GmbH, Linz, Austria). Twelve hours prior to each experiment, the growth medium was replaced by depletion medium (DMEM with 2% FCS). After 48 h of culture, supernatants were tested for IL-8 or Groα using a specific ELISA (Laboserv GmbH, Staufenberg, Germany).

Electrophoretic Mobility Shift Assays (EMSA)

Nuclear extracts of HaCaT cells were harvested 10 min after stimulation with 5 ng/ml IL-1β as described elsewhere.[24] α-MSH (10^{-8} to 10^{-12} M) was added to the cultures immediately prior to addition of IL-1β. EMSAs were performed using a ^{32}P-labeled oligonucleotide containing the NFκB binding consensus site (Santa Cruz Biotechnology, Santa Cruz, Ca.). 10 μg of each extract were used for the experiments. To determine the specificity, some samples were additionally treated with an excess of nonlabeled oligonucleotide, resulting in the loss of specific bands.

RT-PCR

mRNA was isolated using phenol–chloroform extraction, reverse transcribed (Reverse Transcription System; Promega GmbH, Mannheim, Germany) and equal amounts of each cDNA were subjected to PCR with primers specific for β-actin.

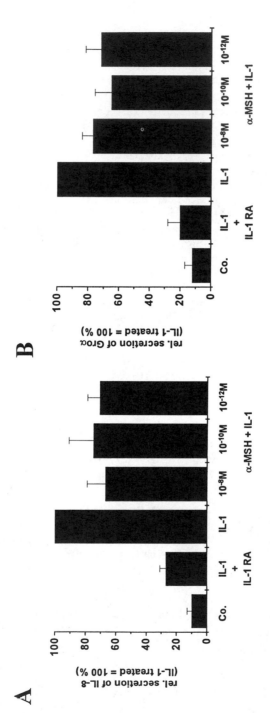

FIGURE 1. IL-8 and Groα release by HaCaT cells. Cells were left untreated (Co.) or stimulated with IL-1β (5 ng/ml); IL-1β and IL-1RA (25 U/ml); or IL-1β and α-MSH (10^{-8} to 10^{-12} M). Supernatants were analyzed for IL-8 (**A**) or Groα (**B**) after 48 h, using specific ELISAs. Results are expressed as mean ± SEM of three different experiments.

Subsequently, the amounts of cDNA were adjusted according to the results of the β-actin PCR, and corresponding volumes of the cDNA solutions were used for IL-8- or Groα-PCR.[25] Relative expression of IL-8 and Groα was determined after standardization by densitometric analysis (Bio-Profil Bio-1D; ltf Labortechnik GmbH, Wasserburg, Germany).

RESULTS

Effect of α-MSH on Keratinocyte Chemokine Release and mRNA Expression

To investigate whether α-MSH affects the IL-1β–mediated increase of IL-8 or Groα production, HaCaT-cells were treated with IL-1β (5 ng/ml) and different concentrations of α-MSH (10^{-8} to 10^{-12} M). After 48 h of culture α-MSH, at any of the concentrations used, inhibited the release of IL-8 and Groα. Although the inhibitory effect was significant, it was less pronounced than the effect of a 10-fold excess of IL-1RA (25 u/ml) (see FIGURE 1). In contrast α-MSH (10^{-8} to 10^{-12} M) was not able to alter HaCaT cell IL-8, or Groα production between 2 and 72 h of incubation (data not shown). These data were also confirmed at the transcriptional level. Hence, treatment of HaCaT cells for 48 h with IL-1β alone resulted in a significant upregulation of IL-8 mRNA, whereas α-MSH downregulated IL-8 mRNA expression in a dose-dependent manner. The IL 8 mRNA suppressing capacity of α-MSH (10^{-10} M) was comparable with that of IL-1RA (see FIGURE 2).

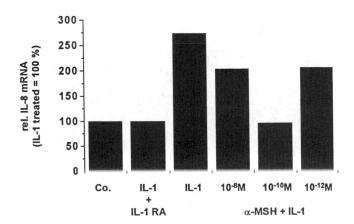

FIGURE 2. Kinetics of IL-8 mRNA expression. IL-8 mRNA was compared to β-actin expression after stimulation. HaCaT cells were left untreated (Co.) or stimulated with IL-1β (5 ng/ml) alone, or with either IL-1RA (25 U/ml) or α-MSH (10^{-8} to 10^{-12} M). After 24 h, total RNA was subjected to RT-PCR and the amplification products of IL-8 and β-actin cDNA were separated on agarose gels, followed by densitometric evaluation to semiquantify IL-8 expression.

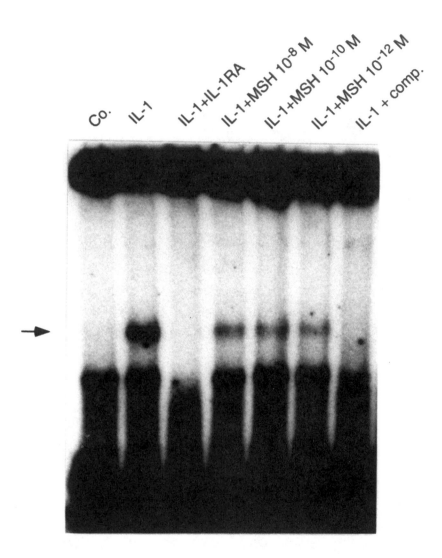

FIGURE 3. Dose response of α-MSH for the inhibition of IL-1β dependent NFκB activation. HaCaT cells were left untreated (Co.) or stimulated with IL-1β (5 ng/ml), IL-1β and IL-1RA (25 U/ml), or IL-1β and α-MSH (10^{-8} to 10^{-12} M). Nuclear extracts were prepared 10 minutes after treatment and then assayed for NFκB by EMSA. The NFκB heterodimer (p50/p65) is indicated by an *arrow*. The specificity of NFκB binding was determined by the binding reaction in the presence of an excess of unlabeled NFκB oligonucleotide (IL-1 + comp.).

Effect of α-MSH on NFκB Activation in Keratinocytes

To gain more insight into the molecular mechanisms of α-MSH–mediated effects on keratinocytes, activation of the transcription factor NFκB by IL-1β in the presence or absence of α-MSH was investigated. When HaCaT cells were treated with 5 ng/ml IL-1β, activation of NFκB was observed after 10 minutes. In keratinocytes treated with α-MSH (10^{-8} to 10^{-12} M) alone, no activation of NFκB was detected between 10 minutes and 5 hours (data not shown). Treatment of HaCaT cells with α-MSH and IL-1β, after 10 min resulted in significantly reduced nuclear translocation and activation of the NFκB heterodimer p65/p50 (see FIGURE 3). Similarly, treatment of HaCaT cells with IL-1β and a tenfold excess of IL-1RA resulted in a complete inhibition of NFκB activation. To prove the identity of NFκB heterodimer, nuclear extracts of IL-1β–treated cells were preincubated with an excess of unlabeled NFκB consensus oligonucleotide, resulting in the loss of the band specific for the p65/p50 heterodimer (FIG. 3).

DISCUSSION

This study provides first evidence that α-MSH inhibits the proinflammatory effects of IL-1β in keratinocytes. α-MSH is able to block the IL-1β–mediated synthesis and release of the chemokines IL-8 and Groα. This accords with previous findings showing that α-MSH antagonizes many of the proinflammatory effects of IL-1β, such as thymocyte proliferation, acute phase protein production, and fever.[8,10–13] Moreover, some of the antiinflammatory and immunomodulating effects of α-MSH may be explained by the result that α-MSH upregulates the production of the cytokine synthesis inhibitor IL-10 in monocytes and keratinocytes.[23,26] The concept that α-MSH is able to affect the function of monocytes, macrophages and keratinocytes was confirmed recently by the detection of binding sites specific for α-MSH on these cells.[27–29] Monocytes and keratinocytes both express MC-1R, which among the melanocortin receptors has the highest affinity for α-MSH. Other known MC-Rs (MC-R 2–5) exhibit a lower affinity for α-MSH and have not been detected on keratinocytes or monocytes.

The production of α-MSH, as well as the expression of its receptor in keratinocytes, is induced on stimulation with IL-1, ultraviolet light, or PMA.[6,30] Thus, in the absence of proinflammatory or injurious stimuli, α-MSH is not able to alter the production of cytokines by keratinocytes.[21] Therefore, α-MSH, by virtue of its potent anti IL-1 activities, may function as an important antiinflammatory mediator required for the downregulation of ongoing immune or inflammatory responses. This is supported by *in vivo* studies demonstrating that α-MSH inhibits the induction as well as the elicitation phase of contact hypersensitivity reactions, reduces vasculitis in the local Shwartzman reaction,[31] and suppresses IL-1 induced fever.[9,10,11,31]

The molecular mechanisms involved in α-MSH–mediated regulation of cytokine and chemokine production in keratinocytes, however, are not clear. One important transcription factor involved in the regulation of many cytokines, including IL-8 and Groα, is NFκB. Activation of the heterodimer NFκB in the cytoplasm occurs via dissociation of an inactive complex consisting of NFκB and its inhibitor—the protein inhibitory κB (IκB). This transcriptional activator was also shown to be the target of endotoxin, UV, and cytokines such as IL-1. However, nuclear extracts from IL-1β–treated HaCaT cells, harvested after exposure to α-MSH showed a significant decrease in NFκB activation. Therefore, NFκB inactivation by α-MSH may be a crucial event, responsible for the downregulation of cytokine gene transcription in keratinocytes. Since downregulation of NFκB activation has been also observed in LPS–stimulated endothelial cells[32] and in IL-1–treated monocytes,[33] inhibition of this transcriptional activator appears to be a common mechanism for the antiinflammatory activities of α-MSH.

ACKNOWLEDGEMENTS

This work was supported by grants from the Deutsche Forschungsgemeinschaft (SFB 293, B2) and from the Interdisziplinäres Klinisches Forschungszentrum (IKF, C7).

REFERENCES

1. DINARELLO, C.A. 1996. Biologic basis for interleukin-1 in disease. Blood **87:** 2095–2147.
2. BAEUERLE, P.A. & D. BALTIMORE. 1996. NF-κB: ten years after. Cell **87:** 13–20.
3. GILCHREST, B.A., H.Y. PARK, M.S. ELLER et al. 1996. Mechanisms of ultraviolet light-induced pigmentation. Photochem. Photobiol. **63:** 1–10.
4. ROBBINS, L.S., J.H. NADEAU, K.R. JOHNSON et al. 1993. Pigmentation phenotypes of variant extension locus alleles result from point mutations that alter MSH receptor function. Cell **72:** 827–834.
5. CONE, R.D., D. LU, S. KOPPULA et al. 1996. The melanocortin receptors: agonists, antagonists, and the hormonal control of pigmentation. Recent. Prog. Horm. Res. **51:** 287–317.
6. LUGER, T.A., T. SCHOLZEN, T. BRZOSKA et al. 1998. Cutaneous immunomodulation and coordination of skin stress responses by α-melanocyte-stimulating hormone. Ann. N.Y. Acad. Sci. **840:** 381–394.
7. HILTZ, M.E., A. CATANIA & J.M. LIPTON. 1992. Alpha-MSH peptides inhibit acute inflammation induced in mice by rIL-1 beta, rIL-6, rTNF-alpha and endogenous pyrogen but not that caused by LTB4, PAF and rIL-8. Cytokine. **4:** 320–328.
8. CATANIA, A. & J.M. LIPTON. 1991. Anti-inflammatory actions of the neuroimmunomodulator alpha-MSH. Immunol. Today **18:** 140–145.
9. GRABBE, S., R.S. BHARDWAJ, M. STEINERT et al. 1995. Alpha melanocyte-stimulating hormone induces hapten-specific tolerance in vivo. Arch. Dermatol. Res. **287:** 351.
10. CANNON, J.G., J.B. TATRO, S. REICHLIN et al. 1986. Alpha melanocyte stimulating hormone inhibits immunostimulatory and inflammatory actions of interleukin 1. J. Immunol. **137:** 2232–2236.
11. ROBERTSON, B., K. DOSTAL & R.A. DAYNES. 1988. Neuropeptide regulation of inflammatory and immunologic responses. The capacity of alpha-melanocyte-stimulating hormone to inhibit tumor necrosis factor and IL-1-inducible biologic responses. J. Immunol. **140:** 4300–4307.
12. DAYNES, R.A., B.A. ROBERTSON, B.H. CHO et al. 1987. Alpha-melanocyte-stimulating hormone exhibits target cell selectivity in its capacity to affect interleukin 1-inducible responses in vivo and in vitro. J. Immunol. **139:** 103–109.
13. WATANABE, T., M.E. HILTZ, A. CATANIA et al. 1993. Inhibition of IL-1 beta-induced peripheral inflammation by peripheral and central administration of analogs of the neuropeptide alpha-MSH. Brain Res. Bull. **32:** 311–314.

14. BLALOCK, J.E. 1994. The syntax of immune-neuroendocrine communication. Immunol. Today **15:** 504–511.

15. SLOMINSKI, A., G. ERMAK, J. HWANG *et al.* 1996. The expression of proopiomelanocortin (POMC) and of corticotropic releasing hormone receptor (CRH-R) genes in mouse skin. Biochim. Biophys. Acta **1289:** 247–251.

16. WILDER, R.L. 1996. Neuroendocrine-immune system interactions and autoimmunity. Ann. Rev. Immunol. **13:** 307–338.

17. CATANIA, A. & J.M. LIPTON. 1993. Alpha-melanocyte stimulating hormone in the modulation of host reactions. Endocr. Rev. **14:** 564–576.

18. LUGER, T.A., T. SCHOLZEN & S. GRABBE. 1997. The role of α-melanocyte stimulating hormone in cutaneous biology. J. Invest. Dermatol. Derm. Symp. Proc. **2:** 87–93.

19. ERMAK, G. & A. SLOMINSKI. 1997. Production of POMC, CRH-R1, MC1- and MC2-receptor mRNA and expression of tyrosinase gene in relation to hair cycle and dexamethasone treatment in C57BL/6 mouse skin. J. Invest. Dermatol. **108:** 160–165.

20. DE LUCA, M., W. SIEGRIST, S. BONDANZA *et al.* 1993. Alpha melanocyte stimulating hormone (alpha MSH) stimulates normal human melanocyte growth by binding to high-affinity receptors. J. Cell Sci. **105:** 1079–1084.

21. BRZOSKA, T., T. SCHOLZEN, E. BECHER *et al.* 1997. Effect of UV light on the production of proopiomelanocortin-derived peptides and melanocortin receptors in the skin. *In* Skin Cancer and UV-Radiation. P. Altmeyer, K. Hoffmann & M. Stücker, Eds.: 227–237. Springer-Verlag, Berlin.

22. OREL, L., M.M. SIMON, J. KARLSEDER *et al.* 1997. α-Melanocyte stimulating hormone downregulates differentiation-driven heat shock protein 70 expression in keratinocytes. J. Invest. Dermatol. **108:** 401–405.

23. REDONDO, P., J. GARCIA-FONCILLAS, I. OKROUNJNOV *et al.* 1998. α-MSH regulates interleukin-10 expression by human keratinocytes. Arch. Dermatol. Res. **290:** 425–428.

24. ARAGANE, Y., D. KULMS, T.A. LUGER *et al.* 1997. Down-regulation of interferon gamma-activated STAT1 by UV light. Proc. Natl. Acad. Sci. USA **94:** 11490–11495.

25. HARTMEYER, M., T. SCHOLZEN, E. BECHER *et al.* 1997. Human microvascular endothelial cells (HMEC-1) express the melanocortin receptor type 1 and produce increased levels of IL-8 upon stimulation with αMSH. J. Immunol. **159:** 1930–1937.

26. BHARDWAJ, R.S., A. SCHWARZ, E. BECHER *et al.* 1996. Pro-opiomelanocortin-derived peptides induce IL-10 production in human monocytes. J. Immunol. **156:** 2517–2521.

27. BHARDWAJ, R., E. BECHER, K. MAHNKE *et al.* 1997. Evidence for the differential expression of the functional α-melanocyte-stimulating hormone receptor MC-1 on human monocytes. J. Immunol. **158:** 3378–3384.

28. STAR, R.A., N. RAJORA, J. HUANG *et al.* 1995. Evidence of autocrine modulation of macrophage nitric oxide synthase by alpha-melanocyte-stimulating hormone. Proc. Natl. Acad. Sci. USA **92:** 8016–8020.

29. BHARDWAJ, R.S., E. BECHER, K. MAHNKE *et al.* 1996. Evidence of the expression of a functional melanocortin receptor 1 by human keratinocytes. J. Invest. Dermatol. **106:** 817.

30. SCHAUER, E., F. TRAUTINGER, A. KÖCK *et al.* 1994. Proopiomelanocortin-derived peptides are synthesized and released by human keratinocytes. J. Clin. Invest. **93:** 2258–2262.

31. KALDEN, D.-H., S. MERFELD, T. BRZOSKA *et al.* 1998. α-Melanocyte stimulating hormone (α-MSH) reduces vasculitis in the local Shwartzman reaction. (Abstract). Exp. Dermatol. **7:** 225.

32. KALDEN, D.-H., M. FASTRICH, T. SCHOLZEN *et al.* 1998. α-MSH modulates the expression of LPS-induced adhesion molecules. Abstract. Exp. Dermatol. **7:** 225.

33. LIPTON J. M., A. CATANIA & H. ZHAO. 1998. α-MSH-induced modulation of inflammation: local CNS and peripheral host cell responses. Abstract. Exp. Dermatol. **7:** 226.

Expression of Functional Melanocortin Receptors and Proopiomelanocortin Peptides by Human Dermal Microvascular Endothelial Cells

THOMAS E. SCHOLZEN,[a] THOMAS BRZOSKA,[b] DIRK-HENNER KALDEN,[b] MECHTHILD HARTMEYER,[b] MICHAELA FASTRICH,[b] THOMAS A. LUGER,[b] CHERYL A. ARMSTRONG,[a] AND JOHN C. ANSEL[a,c]

[a]Department of Dermatology, Emory University School of Medicine, Atlanta, Georgia 30322, USA

[b]Ludwig Boltzmann Institute for Cellbiology and Immunobiology of the Skin, Department of Dermatology, University of Münster, Germany

ABSTRACT: Human dermal microvascular endothelial cells (HDMEC) are capable of mediating leukocyte–endothelial interactions by the expression of cellular adhesion molecules and the release of proinflammatory cytokines and chemokines during cutaneous inflammation. Recent studies support the important role for proopiomelanocortin (POMC) peptides, such as α-melanocyte stimulating hormone (α-MSH), as immunomodulators in the cutaneous immune system. The purpose of the studies described here was to determine whether HDMEC serves as both target and source for POMC peptides. RT-PCR and Northern blot studies demonstrated the constitutive expression of mRNA for the adrenocorticotropin (ACTH) and α-MSH-specific melanocortin receptor 1 (MC-1R) in HDMEC, and the microvascular endothelial cell line HMEC-1 that could be upregulated by stimulation with IL-1β and α-MSH. HDMEC responded to stimulation by α-MSH with a dose- and time-dependent synthesis and release of the CXC chemokines, IL-8 and GROα. Likewise, α-MSH augmented HDMEC chemokine release induced by TNF or IL-1. HDMEC were found to constitutively express POMC and prohormone convertase 1 (PC-1); the latter being required to generate ACTH from the POMC prohormone. POMC and PC-1 mRNA expression are increased as a result of stimulation with UVB and UVA1 radiation, IL-1, and α-MSH. In addition, UV-radiation is capable of inducing the release of HDMEC, ACTH, and α-MSH in a time- and dose-dependent fashion. Thus, these data provide evidence that HDMEC are capable of expressing functional MC-1R, POMC, and PC-1 mRNA; and of releasing POMC peptides with UV light, IL-1, and α-MSH as regulatory factors. The expression and regulation of these peptides may be of importance, not only for the autocrine or paracrine regulation of physiologic functions of dermal endothelial cells, but also for the regulation of certain microvascular-mediated cutaneous or systemic inflammatory responses.

[c]Address for correspondence: John C. Ansel, Emory University School of Medicine, Department of Dermatology, 5313 Woodruff Memorial Building, Atlanta GA 30322, USA. 404-727-5107 (voice); 404-727-5217 (fax); jansel@emory.edu (e-mail).

INTRODUCTION

Human dermal microvascular endothelial cells (HDMEC) play a central role in mediating various types of cutaneous inflammatory responses. In addition to producing hematopoietic growth factors, HDMEC and established microvascular cell lines such as HMEC-1 are capable of producing a variety of proinflammatory cytokines or chemokines, such as IL-1, IL-6, IL-8, growth-related oncogene α (GROα), RANTES (regulated upon activation, normally T-cell expressed and secreted), or macrophage-chemoattractant protein-1 (MCP-1). These molecules are capable of triggering both local and systemic inflammatory events. In addition, microvascular endothelial cells also express cellular adhesion molecules of the integrin, immunoglobulin, and selectin families that allow the precise, regulated trafficking of leukocytes into the extravascular tissue and to the actual site of inflammation or injury. Previous studies had indicated that HDMEC cytokine and chemokine production, as well as the expression of adhesion molecules such as intercellular adhesion molecule 1 (ICAM-1) or vascular adhesion molecule 1 (VCAM-1), can be modulated by noxious external stimuli, including endotoxins or ultraviolet (UV) light; either directly or indirectly via induced proinflammatory cytokines such as IL-1 and TNFα, or by the release of neuropeptides from cutaneous sensory nerves.[1–8]

Recently, it has also been proposed that, in addition to these mediators, certain neurohormones may also be potent modulators of cutaneous inflammatory responses, including endothelial cell functions. It is now widely accepted that the skin is a source, as well as a target, for the POMC peptides ACTH, β-lipotropin (β-LPH), α-, β-, γ-melanocyte–stimulating hormones (MSH), and β-endorphin (β-END), as well as their corresponding melanocortin receptors (MC-R). The expression of these POMC peptides and receptors has been demonstrated in human and mouse skin *in vivo* and in cultured normal melanocytes, keratinocytes, fibroblasts, and adipocytes, as well as in numerous human and murine epidermoid cell lines *in vitro*.[9–12] Circulating immunocompetent cells are also capable of expressing POMC peptides and/ or MC-R.[13–16] Although only very low amounts of POMC peptides are detected in normal skin of healthy volunteers, the expression of POMC peptides in the epidermal compartment of the skin is increased as a result of external noxious stimuli, such as ultraviolet exposure *in vivo*.[9,17] Likewise, UV light is one of the few known stimuli for POMC mRNA and peptide expression in keratinocytes, epidermoid carcinoma cell lines, melanocytes, or melanoma cell lines *in vitro*.[12,18–20] It has been reported that POMC peptides such as ACTH or β-END are accumulated in lesional skin in cutaneous diseases such as psoriasis and basal cell carcinoma.[21] In this regard it is noteworthy that elevated plasma levels of α-MSH are also detected under a variety of pathological conditions. For example, one can find increased α-MSH levels in the serum of patients with metastatic melanoma, UV-induced skin inflammation,[9] and chronic inflammatory arthritis,[22] as well as parasitic and viral infections such as HIV.[23]

Previous studies demonstrated the presence of functional MC-1R on HDMEC and HMEC-1.[24] In extension of these studies we further examined the regulation and function of melanocortin receptors on endothelial cells, and addressed the possibility that HDMEC might not only serve as target but also as an important source for POMC peptides.

RESULTS

Melanocortin Receptor Expression in Human Dermal Endothelial Cells

To address the possibility that dermal endothelial cells might be a target for POMC peptides, we have analyzed the expression of MC-R by semiquantitative RT-PCR in HDMEC and HMEC-1. As indicated in FIGURE 1, HDMEC constitutively express MC-1R mRNA. In contrast, our previous studies had demonstrated that MC-2R, MC-3R MC-4R, and MC-5R mRNA are not expressed in HDMEC or HMEC-1.[24,25] We next determined whether MC-1R mRNA expression could be regulated by proinflammatory cytokines, such as IL-1β or even α-MSH itself. Densitometric evaluation of the ethidium bromide-stained agarose gels from RT-PCR studies, normalized for β-actin expression, revealed that stimulation of HDMEC with IL-1β significantly increased MC-1R mRNA expression (FIG. 1B). Likewise, α-MSH upregulated the MC-1R expression in a concentration-dependent fashion. A concentration of 10^{-8} M α-MSH was the most effective dose in increasing MC-1R mRNA (FIG. 1B). A maximum induction of the MC-1 mRNA was observed between 1 and 3 h after stimulation, both in HDMEC and in HMEC-1 (data not shown).

We next examined the interaction between α-MSH and dermal endothelial cells by competition and equilibrium saturation-binding assay studies (see TABLE 1). Our results indicate that $[^{125}I]$α-MSH binds to a single, saturable site on HDMEC and HMEC-1 with a K_D of 1.9 nM and 1.1 nM, respectively, which is comparable to the binding affinity for α-MSH observed for various human and mouse melanoma cell lines. In general, the number of α-MSH-specific binding sites detected on HDMEC and HMEC-1 was about two- to tenfold higher than the number of MC-1Rs reported for human melanoma cells.[26] In a competition binding assay study, unlabeled α-MSH, but not β-MSH, competitively inhibited binding of $[^{125}I]$α-MSH to HMEC-1. This is consistent with observations that β-MSH has an approximately 50-fold lower affinity for MC-1R when compared with α-MSH.[24,27] The functional coupling of melanocortin receptors to cellular adenylyl cyclase has been used as a tool to characterize the functional activity of MC-R expressed on a certain cell type.[28] As indicated in FIGURE 2, stimulation of HDMEC with different concentrations of α-MSH upregulated intracellular cAMP accumulation in the presence of phosphodiesterase inhibitors, such as 3-methyl-isobutyl xanthine (IBMX), indicating that the MC-1R expressed by endothelial cells are functional.

Physiologic Function of MC-1R on Dermal Endothelial Cells

MC-R expression has been localized in various parts of the CNS and in peripheral tissues including skin.[11] In addition to HDMEC, high affinity binding sites for α-MSH have also been detected on brain microvascular endothelial cells, suggesting that MC-R and their ligands may be of general importance for endothelial cell biology in a number of tissues.[29] To address the physiologic relevance of MC-1R expression on HDMEC, a series of studies were conducted to examine the cytokine and chemokine production repertoire of these cells after α-MSH stimulation. From these studies it became evident that α-MSH stimulation of HDMEC and HMEC-1 selectively upregulated the release of the CXC chemokines IL-8 and GROα.[24,30] The regulation of these endothelial derived-mediators was dependent on the α-MSH

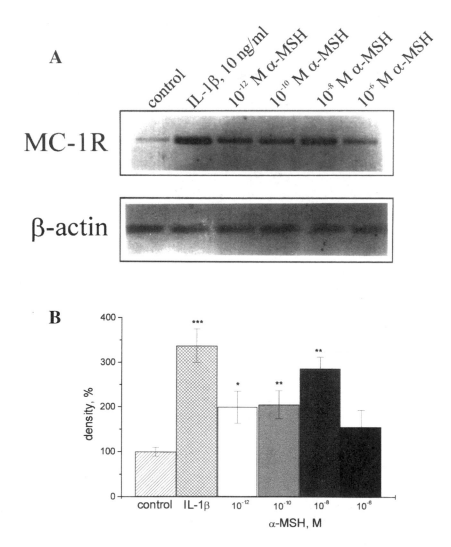

FIGURE 1. MC-1R mRNA expression and regulation in HDMEC. Cells were incubated for 2 h with α-MSH (10^{-6}, 10^{-8}, 10^{-10}, and 10^{-12} M) or IL-1β (10 ng/mL). Total RNA was subjected to RT-PCR amplification using primers specific for the MC-1R and β-actin. PCR-conditions that would allow reliable comparison of MC-1 expression with β-actin mRNA expression in different samples, were established by making serial dilutions of template cDNA at constant cycle numbers for each primer pair so as to verify the linearity of PCR amplification. Subsequently, cDNA mixtures were diluted to obtain equal amounts of PCR product specific for amplified β-actin, and subjected to amplification of MC-1-specific PCR products. Amplification products were separated on agarose gels (**A**) and the gels were evaluated densitometrically to semiquantify MC-1R-specific products in comparison with β-actin (**B**). Values are expressed in percent + SEM. *, $p < 0.05$; **, $p < 0.01$; ***, $p < 0.001$ versus control

TABLE 1. Binding of [^{125}I]α-MSH to human dermal endothelial cells in comparison with various mouse and human melanoma cell lines[a]

	K_D, nM	Binding sites/cell
HDMEC	1.90	2687
HMEC-1	1.10	13300
B16 F1 (mouse)	1.02	10300
D10 (human)	0.20	1590
LSD22 (human)	1.04	1518
ME 8 (human)	2.87	1281
A375 (human)	0.41	608
205 (human)	0.22	1053

[a]From References 24–26.

concentration and on the duration of HDMEC exposure to α-MSH. Levels of IL-8 and GROα were significantly elevated in HDMEC and HMEC-1 cell supernatants 8 h after the addition of 0.1 and 10 nM α-MSH (see TABLE 2). IL-8 induction by α-MSH could be almost completely blocked by incubating the cells with the MC-1R peptide antagonist, 153N-6 (Met-Pro-D-Phe-Arg-D-Trp-Phe-Lys Pro Val-NH$_2$), that has been demonstrated to effectively inhibit α-MSH functions *in vitro*.[31] These ob-

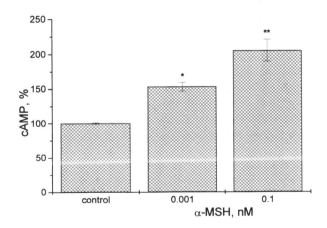

FIGURE 2. Cyclic AMP production by HDMEC after α-MSH stimulation. HDMEC were plated in six-well plates and preincubated with 1 mM IBMX for 30 min. Subsequently, cells were stimulated in the presence of IBMX for 5 min with α-MSH (10^{-12} M, 10^{-10} M) or left untreated (*control*). cAMP was extracted and analyzed using a commercially available EIA. Values are expressed in percent ± SEM. *, $p < 0.05$; **, $p < 0.01$.

TABLE 2. Expression and release of IL-8 and GROα by HMEC-1 and HDMEC after α-MSH stimulation

| | IL-8 (ng/mL) | | | | GROα (ng/mL) | | |
| | | α-MSH[a] | | | | | α-MSH[a] |
	control	10^{-8} M	10^{-8} M + antagonist	10^{-10} M	10^{-10} M + antagonist	control	10^{-8} M	10^{-10} M
HMEC-1	1.63 ± 0.15	2.58 ± 0.34	1.56 ± 0.05	3.15 ± 0.62	1.56 ± 0.07	0.81 ± 0.05	1.28 ± 0.045	1.01 ± 0.01
HDMEC	1.44 ± 0.09	2.42 ± 0.1	n.d.	2.56 ± 0.09	n.d.	1.92 ± 0.07	3.39 ± 0.10	2.79 ± 0.20

[a]Cells were stimulated for 24 h with α-MSH, in concentrations as indicated, or preincubated with the peptide antagonist, 153N-6 (10^{-5} M) for 15 min followed by α-MSH stimulation in the presence of the antagonist. Cell supernatants were harvested and analyzed by ELISA. All values are given as mean ± SEM.

servations were further confirmed by semiquantitative RT-PCR studies. Accordingly, constitutively expressed GROα and IL-8 mRNA were upregulated by stimulation with 10 nM α-MSH (see FIGURE 3A and C). To semiquantify the amounts of IL-8 or GROα mRNA expression, the signal intensity of the specific PCR was normalized to the β-actin PCR product amplified from the same cDNA in separate reactions. α-MSH treatment significantly induced HDMEC GROα mRNA expression at 1 and 3 h, whereas IL-8 mRNA was induced at 3 and 5 h (FIG. 3B and D).

HDMEC and HMEC-1 are also capable of secreting CC chemokines, such as RANTES or monocyte chemoattractant protein-1 (MCP-1), as well as proinflammatory cytokines, such as IL-1 or IL-6.[3,4] Our studies indicate that stimulation of HDMEC (data not shown) and HMEC-1[24] with α-MSH had no significant impact on the production of these mediators.

In another series of experiments we examined the effect of α-MSH on the expression of HDMEC IL-8 and GROα induced by the proinflammatory cytokines TNFα and IL-1. Our results demonstrate that α-MSH synergized with TNFα and IL-1β to augment the HDMEC production of IL-8 and GROα.[30] However, this α-MSH modulatory capacity appears to be dependent on both the concentration of the added cytokine (TNFα or IL-1β) and the duration of α-MSH stimulation. For example, α-MSH augmented the IL-1-induced HDMEC IL-8 production only when applied concomitantly with IL-1 for 8 or 24 h, whereas no effect of α-MSH was observed when cells were only incubated for 15 min with α-MSH prior to IL-1 stimulation.[30] The results of this study are not in agreement with the hypothesis that α-MSH antagonizes the effects of IL-1 by acting as an antagonist for the IL-1 type I receptor, as previously reported.[32]

The α-MSH modulatory capacity on the TNFα-induced HDMEC IL-8 expression appears to be dependent on cAMP and protein kinase A (PKA)-signaling-pathways following the activation of HDMEC MC-1R.[30] Accordingly, the α-MSH–mediated increase in TNF-induced IL-8 could be completely blocked by a combined application of the PKA inhibitors RpcAMPS (adenosine-3′, 5′-cyclic monophosphothioate) and H-89, supporting the role of PKA in mediating α-MSH induced MC-1R signaling. Likewise, indirect activation of PKA by forskolin and IBMX, both of which are potent stimuli for intracellular cAMP accumulation, mimicked not only the α-MSH induction of HDMEC IL-8 production, but also augmented the effect of α-MSH on TNF-induced HDMEC IL-8 release. Similarly, the PKA inhibitors partly inhibited HDMEC IL-8 induction by TNF and forskolin/IBMX, but did not inhibit cells stimulated with TNF alone (see TABLE 3).

POMC Expression and Regulation in Dermal Endothelial Cells

Recent studies also examined the possibility that HDMEC are not only the target, but also a source of POMC peptides.[33] In these studies HDMEC expression of POMC and specific prohormone convertases (PC), such as are required to generate POMC peptides, was examined. Semiquantitative RT-PCR studies demonstrated the constitutive expression of POMC mRNA by HDMEC *in vitro,* upregulated by IL-1β. In addition, irradiation of HDMEC with UVA1 or UVB was capable of enhancing POMC mRNA expression as well as the secretion of the POMC–derived peptides, ACTH and α-MSH. In addition to POMC, PC-1 mRNA expression was detected in HDMEC and was augmented after exposure to α-MSH, IL-1β, or irradiation with

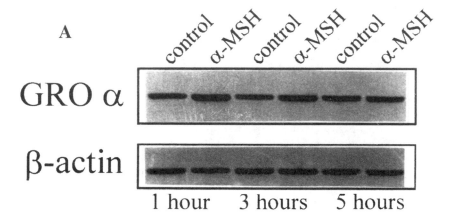

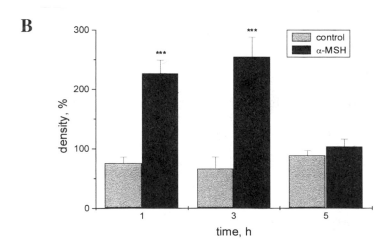

FIGURE 3. Kinetics of HDMEC GROα (**A** and **B**) and IL-8 (**C** and **D**) mRNA upregulation by α-MSH. Cells were stimulated with α-MSH (10^{-8} M). Total RNA was harvested at the indicated times and subjected to semiquantitative RT-PCR using GROα, IL-8, and β-actin–specific primer pairs.

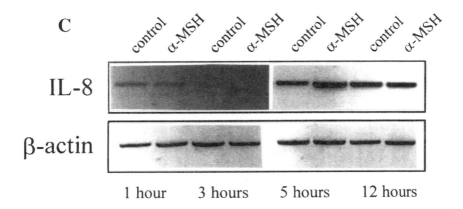

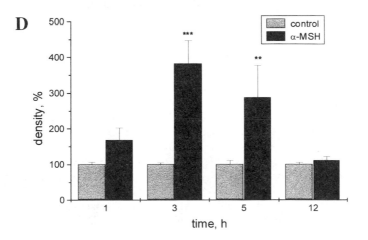

FIGURE 3/continued. Amplification products of chemokine and β-actin cDNA were separated on agarose gels (**A** and **C**) and subjected to densitometric evaluation to semiquantify IL-8 or GROα mRNA expression (**B** and **D**). The results are expressed as mean ± SEM of three individual experiments. *, $p < 0.05$; **, $p < 0.01$; ***, $p < 0.001$ versus control

TABLE 3. Inhibition of α-MSH dependent augmentation of TNFα–induced IL-8 release from HDMEC by PKA inhibitors

	IL-8 (%)
TNF	100
TNF + PKA inhibitors[a]	86.4 ± 13.9
TNF + α-MSH (10^{-8} M)	223.2 ± 4.2
TNF + α-MSH + PKA inhibitors[a]	104.4 ± 15.3
TNF + forskolin/IBMX[b]	244.8 ± 11.0
TNF + forskolin/IBMX + PKA inhibitors[b]	170.9 ± 5.6

[a]Cell were preincubated with RpcAMPS/H89 (50/10 µM) for 2 h and subsequently stimulated with TNFα and α-MSH in the presence of the PKA inhibitors.
[b]Cell were preincubated with RpcAMPS/H89 (50/10 µM) for 2 h and subsequently stimulated with TNFα and forskolin/IBMX (10/50 µM) in the presence of the PKA inhibitors.

UV. Thus, these findings demonstrate that HDMEC express POMC as well as PC-1, as is required for the generation of ACTH. However, PC-2, a necessity for POMC prohormone processing to α-MSH, could not to be detected in HDMEC, suggesting an alternative pathway for the generation of α-MSH in endothelial cells.[33]

SUMMARY AND DISCUSSION

Our observations indicate that normal human dermal microvascular endothelial cells (HDMEC) and the endothelial cell line HMEC-1 express functional MC-1R that can be regulated by IL-1 and α-MSH. HDMEC MC-1R are coupled to cellular adenylyl cyclase, and activation results in intracellular cAMP accumulation, induction of chemokine expression, and augmentation of the chemokine production induced by proinflammatory cytokines. We observed that α-MSH selectively upregulates the CXC chemokines IL-8 and GROα but not other chemokines such as RANTES or MCP-1. These results may have important implications for cutaneous inflammation. The recruitment of leukocytes to the site of inflammation, and the subsequent emigration of these cells into the extravascular tissue, are important steps during inflammatory responses of the skin. It requires the highly organized activation and attraction of leukocytes, their first weak adhesion to the vascular wall (rolling), the subsequent tight binding (adhesion), and eventually the transmigration through the vascular wall. IL-8 and other chemokines are capable of binding to cell surface proteoglycans, and heparin—which is required to establish functional chemokine gradients under blood flow conditions so as to recruit leukocytes to the site of inflammation—helps to immobilize cells and to enhance their effects on high-affinity receptors.[34–38] Both IL-8 and GROα are important chemoattractants for neutrophils and T-lymphocytes. IL-8 stimulation of neutrophils and monocytes enhances the expression of certain integrin complexes on these cells (CD11a/CD18 and CD11b/CD18), which are required for the adhesion to endothelial cells. This activation contributes to the transition from leukocyte rolling to firm adhesion.[39] Our experimental results imply that α-MSH may have an impact on the attraction and migration of selected subsets of immunocompetent cells *in vivo* by the induction of specific chemokines.

It is noteworthy that soluble chemokines, including IL-8, have been demonstrated to inhibit leukocyte adhesion to endothelial cells *in vitro*; and that intravenously injected IL-8 was capable of inhibiting neutrophil emigration *in vivo*.[40,41] These observations have lead to a refined model of leukocyte activation and adhesion in which only "rolling" leukocytes can be activated in a coordinated manner by contact with chemokines immobilized on the vessel wall. In contrast, activation of circulating leukocytes by soluble chemokines, such as IL-8, prevents rather than promotes firm leukocyte-endothelium adhesion.[36] There is evidence that α-MSH may have antiinflammatory properties, as demonstrated in studies in which intravenously injected α-MSH, like soluble IL-8, also inhibited neutrophil chemotaxis *in vitro* and neutrophil accumulation *in vivo*.[15,42] Thus, the ability of α-MSH to induce HDMEC production of the soluble chemokines IL-8 and GROα may be important in blocking leukocyte emigration in certain phases of cutaneous inflammation.

The simultaneous expression of both MC-1R and POMC–derived peptides by HDMEC has a number of implications regarding biological functions of endothelial cells in the skin. Our data suggest that UV-light is capable of upregulating POMC and PC-1 expression in HDMEC, either directly, or indirectly via the induction of IL-1 that may be derived from endothelial cells or other cutaneous cells after UV ex-

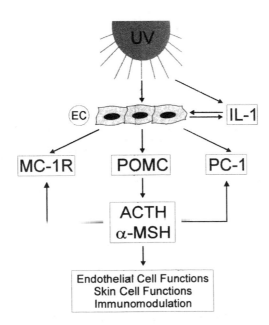

FIGURE 4. Model for the regulation of POMC, PC-1, and MC-1R expression in dermal endothelial cells by UV-light. EC, endothelial cells. For all other abbreviations see text.

posure of the skin.[4,43] However, PC-2, which is required to generate α-MSH in neuroendocrine cells, could not be detected in HDMEC. The POMC prohormone induced by UV can be posttranslationally cleaved by PC-1 to generate ACTH, and to a peptide with α-MSH immunoreactivity by a novel, or not yet identified, endothelial–derived peptidase (see FIGURE 4). One possible enzyme candidate for the production of a such a peptide could be the zinc metallo-protease, neutral-endopeptidase (NEP; EC 3.4.24.11; also known as CD10 or enkephalinase), which is capable of processing ACTH to α-MSH, and is expressed by human dermal endothelial cells.[44,45] In parallel, the HDMEC MC-1R expression is also increased by IL-1 and by α-MSH, the latter being also capable of enhancing PC-1 expression. Thus, UV-light directly or indirectly promotes the production of ACTH and α-MSH; and it may also indirectly upregulate the expression of their corresponding receptor MC-1R via induced IL-1 and α-MSH. This may in turn be important for the autocrine response of MC-1R bearing target cells to their ligands. This model may also apply to other skin cells, such as keratinocytes, since UV-light exhibits similar regulatory properties on MC-1R, POMC, and PC-1 expression in these cells.[46] In addition to the local effects POMC peptides may exert on HDMEC and surrounding skin cell functions *in vivo,* one is tempted to speculate that ACTH and α-MSH may be released into the vascular lumen resulting in increased levels of α-MSH in human plasma following UV-exposure. It is also conceivable that UV-induced POMC peptides released into the circulation directly modulate functions of circulating immunocompetent cells, and this may explain systemic immunomodulatory effects of α-MSH. Thus, expression of functional MC-1R and POMC peptides by human dermal endothelial cells offers the potential to alter cutaneous as well as systemic inflammatory events.

REFERENCES

1. SWERLICK, R.A. & T.J. LAWLEY. 1993. Role of microvascular endothelial cells in inflammation. J. Invest. Dermatol. **100:** 111S–115S.

2. ADES, E.W., F.J. CANDAL, R.A. SWERLICK, V.G. GEORGE, S. SUMMERS, D.C. BOSSE & T.J. LAWLEY. 1992. HMEC-1—establishment of an immortalized human microvascular endothelial cell line. J. Invest. Dermatol. **99:** 683–690.

3. GOEBELER, M., T. YOSHIMURA, A. TOKSOY, U. RITTER, E.B. BROCKER & R. GILLITZER. 1997. The chemokine repertoire of human dermal microvascular endothelial cells and its regulation by inflammatory cytokines. J. Invest. Dermatol. **108:** 445–451.

4. SCHOLZEN, T., M. HARTMEYER, M. FASTRICH, T. BRZOSKA, E. BECHER, T. SCHWARZ & T.A. LUGER. 1998. Ultraviolet light and interleukin-10 modulate expression of cytokines by transformed human dermal microvascular endothelial cells (HMEC-1). J. Invest. Dermatol. **111:** 50–56.

5. XU, Y., R.A. SWERLICK, N. SEPP, D. BOSSE, E.W. ADES & T.J. LAWLEY. 1994. Characterization of expression and modulation of cell adhesion molecules on an immortalized human dermal microvascular endothelial cell line (HMEC-1). J. Invest. Dermatol. **102:** 833–837.

6. CORNELIUS, L.A., N. SEPP, L.J. LI, K. DEGITZ, R.A. SWERLICK, T.J. LAWLEY & S.W. CAUGHMAN. 1994. Selective upregulation of intercellular adhesion molecule (ICAM-1) by ultraviolet B in human dermal microvascular endothelial cells. J. Invest. Dermatol. **103:** 23–28.

7. QUINLAN, K.L., I.-S. SONG, N.W. BUNNETT, E. LECTRAN, B. HARTEN, J. OLERUD, C.A. ARMSTRONG, S.W. CAUGHMAN & J.C. ANSEL. 1998. Neuropeptide regulation of human dermal microvascular endothelial cells ICAM-1 expression and function. Am. J. Physiol. **275:** C1580–C1590.

8. SCHOLZEN, T., C.A. ARMSTRONG, N.W. BUNNETT, T.A. LUGER, J.E. OLERUD & J.C. ANSEL. 1998. Neuropeptides in the skin: interactions between the neuroendocrine and the skin immune systems. Exp. Dermatol. **7:** 81–96.

9. LUGER, T.A., T. SCHOLZEN & S. GRABBE. 1997. The role of alpha-melanocyte-stimulating hormone in cutaneous biology. J. Invest. Dermatol. Symp. Proc. **2:** 87–93.

10. BRZOSKA, T., T. SCHOLZEN, E. BECHER & T.A. LUGER. 1997. Effect of UV light on the production of proopiomelanocortin- derived peptides and melanocortin receptors in the skin. *In* Skin Cancer and UV Irradiation. P. Altmeyer, K. Hoffmann & M. Stuecker, Eds.: 227–237. Springer Verlag, Berlin.

11. CONE, R.D., D. LU, S. KOPPULA, D.I. VAGE, H. KLUNGLAND, B. BOSTON, W. CHEN, D.N. ORTH, C. POUTON & R.A. KESTERSON. 1996. The melanocortin receptors: agonists, antagonists, and the hormonal control of pigmentation. Rec. Prog. Hormone Res. **51:** 287–317.

12. WINTZEN, M., M. YAAR, J.P. BURBACH & B.A. GILCHREST. 1996. Proopiomelanocortin gene product regulation in keratinocytes. J. Invest. Dermatol. **106:** 673–678.

13. CABOT, P.J., L. CARTER, C. GAIDDON, Q. ZHANG, M. SCHAFER, J.P. LOEFFLER & C. STEIN. 1997. Immune cell-derived beta-endorphin. Production, release, and control of inflammatory pain in rats. J. Clin. Invest. **100:** 142–148.

14. GAILLARD, R.C., T. DANEVA, R. HADID, K. MULLER & E. SPINEDI. 1998. The hypothalamo-pituitary-adrenal axis of athymic Swiss nude mice. The implications of T lymphocytes in the ACTH release from immune cells. Ann. N.Y. Acad. Sci. **840:** 480–490.

15. CATANIA, A., N. RAJORA, F. CAPSONI, F. MINONZIO, R.A. STAR & J.M. LIPTON. 1996. The neuropeptide alpha-MSH has specific receptors on neutrophils and reduces chemotaxis *in vitro*. Peptides **17:** 675–679.

16. BHARDWAJ, R., E. BECHER, K. MAHNKE, M. HARTMEYER, T. SCHWARZ, T. SCHOLZEN & T.A. LUGER. 1997. Evidence for the differential expression of the functional alpha-melanocyte–stimulating hormone receptor MC-1 on human monocytes. J. Immunol. **158:** 3378–3384.

17. FAROOQUI, J.Z., E.E. MEDRANO, Z. ABDEL-MALEK & J. NORDLUND. 1993. The expression of proopiomelanocortin and various POMC-derived peptides in mouse and human skin. Ann. N.Y. Acad. Sci. **680:** 508–510.

18. CHAKRABORTY, A.K., Y. FUNASAKA, A. SLOMINSKI, G. ERMAK, J. HWANG, J.M. PAWELEK & M. ICHIHASHI. 1996. Production and release of proopiomelanocortin (POMC) derived peptides by human melanocytes and keratinocytes in culture: regulation by ultraviolet B. Biochim. Biophys. Acta **1313:** 130–138.

19. CHAKRABORTY, A., A. SLOMINSKI, G. ERMAK, J. HWANG & J. PAWELEK. 1995. Ultraviolet B and melanocyte-stimulating hormone (MSH) stimulate mRNA production for alpha MSH receptors and proopiomelanocortin-derived peptides in mouse melanoma cells and transformed keratinocytes. J. Invest. Dermatol. **105:** 655–659.

20. SCHAUER, E., F. TRAUTINGER, A. KOCK, A. SCHWARZ, R. BHARDWAJ, M. SIMON, J.C. ANSEL, T. SCHWARZ & T.A. LUGER. 1994. Proopiomelanocortin-derived peptides are synthesized and released by human keratinocytes. J. Clin. Invest. **93:** 2258–2262.

21. SLOMINSKI, A., J. WORTSMAN, J.E. MAZURKIEWICZ, L. MATSUOKA, J. DIETRICH, K. LAWRENCE, A. GORBANI & R. PAUS. 1993. Detection of proopiomelanocortin-derived antigens in normal and pathologic human skin. J. Lab. Clin. Med. **122:** 658–666.

22. CATANIA, A., V. GERLONI, S. PROCACCIA, L. AIRAGHI, M.G. MANFREDI, C. LOMATER, L. GROSSI & J.M. LIPTON. 1994. The anticytokine neuropeptide alpha-melanocyte-stimulating hormone in synovial fluid of patients with rheumatic diseases: comparisons with other anticytokine molecules. Neuroimmunomodulation 1: 321–328.

23. CATANIA, A., M.G. MANFREDI, L. AIRAGHI, M.C. VIVIRITO, A. CAPETTI, F. MILAZZO, J.M. LIPTON & C. ZANUSSI. 1994. Plasma concentration of cytokine antagonists in patients with HIV infection. Neuroimmunomodulation 1: 42–49.

24. HARTMEYER, M., T. SCHOLZEN, E. BECHER, R.S. BHARDWAJ, T. SCHWARZ & T.A. LUGER. 1997. Human dermal microvascular endothelial cells express the melanocortin receptor type 1 and produce increased levels of IL-8 upon stimulation with alpha-melanocyte-stimulating hormone. J. Immunol. 159: 1930–1937.

25. HARTMEYER, M., E. BECHER, D.-H. KALDEN, T. BRZOSKA, M. FASTRICH, T. SCHOLZEN & T.A. LUGER. 1997. Expression and function of the melanocortin receptor type 1 (MC-1) on human dermal microvascular endothelial cells (HDMEC). Abstract. Exp. Dermatol. 6: 279.

26. EBERLE, A.N., W. SIEGRIST, C. BAGUTTI, J. CHLUBA-DE TAPIA, F. SOLCA, J.E. WIKBERG & V. CHHAJLANI. 1993. Receptors for melanocyte-stimulating hormone on melanoma cells. Ann. N.Y. Acad. Sci. 680: 320–341.

27. SCHIOTH, H.B., R. MUCENIECE, J.E. WIKBERG & V. CHHAJLANI. 1995. Characterisation of melanocortin receptor subtypes by radioligand binding analysis. Eur. J. Pharmacol. 288: 311–317.

28. MOUNTJOY, K.G. 1994. The human melanocyte stimulating hormone receptor has evolved to become "super-sensitive" to melanocortin peptides. Mol. Cell. Endocrinol. 102: R7–11.

29. DE ANGELIS, E., U.G. SAHM, A.R. AHMED, G.W. OLIVIER, L.J. NOTARIANNI, S.K. BRANCH, S.H. MOSS & C.W. POUTON. 1995. Identification of a melanocortin receptor expressed by murine brain microvascular endothelial cells in culture. Microvasc. Res. 50: 25–34.

30. SCHOLZEN, T., D.-H. KALDEN, T.A. LUGER, C.A. ARMSTRONG & J.C. ANSEL. 1998. α-melanocyte-stimulating hormone (α-MSH) modulates TNFα or IL-1β–induced production of interleukin-8 and GROα by human dermal microvascular endothelial cells. Abstract. Arch. Dermatol. Res. 290: 104.

31. JAYAWICKREME, C.K., J.M. QUILLAN, G.F. GRAMINSKI & M.R. LERNER. 1994. Discovery and structure-function analysis of alpha-melanocyte–stimulating hormone antagonists. J. Biol. Chem. 269: 29846–29854.

32. MUGRIDGE, K.G., M. PERRETTI, P. GHIARA & L. PARENTE. 1991. Alpha-melanocyte-stimulating hormone reduces interleukin-1 beta effects on rat stomach preparations possibly through interference with a type I receptor. Eur. J. Pharmacol. 197: 151–155.

33. SCHOLZEN, T., T. BRZOSKA, D.-H. KALDEN, M. HARTMEYER, M. FASTRICH, E. BECHER, T.A. LUGER, C.A. ARMSTRONG & J.C. ANSEL. 1998. Expression of pro-opiomelanocortin (POMC) peptides by human dermal microvascular endothelial cells (HDMEC) is transcriptionally and posttranslationally regulated by UV-light and IL-1. Abstract. Exp. Dermatol. 7: 229.

34. HOOGEWERF, A.J., G.S. KUSCHERT, A.E. PROUDFOOT, F. BORLAT, I. CLARK-LEWIS, C.A. POWER & T.N. WELLS 1997. Glycosaminoglycans mediate cell surface oligomerization of chemokines. Biochemistry 36: 13570–13578.

35. KOOPMANN, W. & M.S. KRANGEL. 1997. Identification of a glycosaminoglycan-binding site in chemokine macrophage inflammatory protein-1alpha. J. Biol. Chem. 272: 10103–10109.

36. ROT, A., E. HUB, J. MIDDLETON, F. PONS, C. RABECK, K. THIERER, J. WINTLE, B. WOLFF, M. ZSAK & P. DUKOR. 1996. Some aspects of IL-8 pathophysiology. III: Chemokine interaction with endothelial cells. J. Leukoc. Biol. **59:** 39–44.

37. TANAKA, Y., D.H. ADAMS & S. SHAW. 1993. Proteoglycans on endothelial cells present adhesion-inducing cytokines to leukocytes. Immunol. Today **14:** 111–115.

38. SPILLMANN, D., D. WITT & U. LINDAHL. 1998. Defining the interleukin-8-binding domain of heparan sulfate. J. Biol. Chem. **273:** 15487–15493.

39. ISSEKUTZ, T.B. 1993. The contributions of integrins to leukocyte infiltration in inflamed tissues. Curr. Top. Microbiol. Immunol. **184:** 177–185.

40. LEY, K., J.B. BAKER, M.I. CYBULSKY, M.A. GIMBRONE, JR. & F.W. LUSCINSKAS. 1993. Intravenous interleukin-8 inhibits granulocyte emigration from rabbit mesenteric venules without altering L-selectin expression or leukocyte rolling. J. Immunol. **151:** 6347–6357.

41. HECHTMAN, D.H., M.I. CYBULSKY, H.J. FUCHS, J.B. BAKER & M.A. GIMBRONE, JR. 1991. Intravascular IL-8. Inhibitor of polymorphonuclear leukocyte accumulation at sites of acute inflammation. J. Immunol. **147:** 883–892.

42. PERRETTI, M., I. APPLETON, L. PARENTE & R.J. FLOWER. 1993. Pharmacology of interleukin-1-induced neutrophil migration. Agents & Actions **38:** C64–65.

43. LUGER, T.A. & T. SCHWARZ. 1995. Effects of UV-light on cytokines and neuroendocrine hormones. *In* Photoimmunology. J. Krutmann & C. Elmers, Eds.: 55–76. Blackwell, Oxford.

44. SMITH, E.M., T.K. HUGHES, JR., F. HASHEMI & G.B. STEFANO. 1992. Immunosuppressive effects of corticotropin and melanotropin and their possible significance in human immunodeficiency virus infection. Proc. Natl. Acad. Sci. USA **89:** 782–786.

45. OLERUD, J.E., C.L. HAYCOX, M.L. USUI, J.C. ANSEL & N.W. BUNNETT. 1998. Neutral endopeptidase (NEP) expression in normal human skin and in selected skin disease states. Abstract. J. Invest. Dermatol. **110:** 655.

46. BRZOSKA, T., T. SCHOLZEN, E. BECHER, M. HARTMEYER, S. BLETZ, T. SCHWARZ & T.A. LUGER. 1997. UVB regulates the expression of proopiomelanocortin, prohormone convertase 1 and melanocortin 1 receptor by human keratinocytes. Abstract. J. Invest. Dermatol. **108:** 622.

Mechanisms of the Antiinflammatory Effects of α-MSH

Role of Transcription Factor NF-κB and Adhesion Molecule Expression

D.-H. KALDEN, T. SCHOLZEN, T. BRZOSKA, AND T.A. LUGER[a]

Ludwig Boltzmann Institute of Cellbiology and Immunobiology of the Skin, Department of Dermatology, University of Münster, Münster, Germany

ABSTRACT: The recruitment of leukocytes from the circulation to inflamed tissue is regulated by the expression of adhesion molecules on both leukocytes and endothelial cells. The proopiomelanocortin–derived peptide α-melanocyte stimulating hormone (α-MSH) is known to modulate inflammation. Thus, we investigated the influence of α-MSH on the LPS-induced expression of the adhesion molecules E-selectin and VCAM-1 on endothelial cells. Human microvascular endothelial cells (HMEC-1) were treated with LPS (100 ng/ml) alone or in the presence of α-MSH (10^{-8} to 10^{-16} M). RT-PCR analysis showed that α-MSH significantly reduced LPS-induced expression of VCAM-1 and E-selectin. Since many adhesion molecules contain regulatory NF-κB sites in their promoter region, the role of α-MSH in the activation of the transcription factor NF-αB was also investigated. α-MSH significantly downregulated the LPS–mediated activation of NF-κB, in a dose-dependent manner. These findings indicate that modulation of the transcription factor NF-κB is a crucial molecular event, one that seems to be responsible for the antiinflammatory effects of α-MSH.

INTRODUCTION

Positioned at the interface between blood and tissue, the endothelium is equipped to respond quickly to local changes in biological needs caused by trauma or inflammation. Endothelial cells (EC) express cell surface molecules that orchestrate the trafficking of circulating blood cells. These cell-associating molecules mediate the migration of leukocytes into specific organs under physiologic conditions, and accelerate migration toward sites of inflammation—in response to lipopolysaccharide (LPS), for example. During inflammation, leukocytes tether to and roll on the EC surface, then they stop, spread, and finally migrate between ECs to eventually reach the underlying tissues.[1] In most circumstances they interact with selectins; these are transmembrane glycoproteins that recognize cell-surface carbohydrate ligands found on leukocytes, and that initiate and mediate tethering and rolling of leukocytes on the EC surface.[2] However, selectin-mediated adhesion of leukocytes does not

[a]Address for correspondence: Prof. Dr. med. T. Luger, M.D., Department of Dermatology, University of Münster, Von-Esmarch-Str. 56, D-48149 Münster, Germany. +49-251-8356504 (voice); +49-251-8356522 (fax); luger@uni-muenster.de (e-mail).

lead to firm adhesion and transmigration unless members of the immunoglobulin superfamily, such as vascular cell adhesion molecule-1 (VCAM-1), are involved.[3] Therefore, the expression of various adhesion molecules on the endothelial surface changes over time, initially favoring neutrophil recruitment (e.g., dependence on E-selectin expression) and, later, recruitment of other leukocytes (e.g., dependence on VCAM-1 expression).[4,5]

Nuclear factor κB (NF-κB) is an inducible transcription factor that regulates the expression of genes; such as cytokines and their receptors, adhesion molecules, and inflammatory enzymes; that are involved in immune and inflammatory responses.[6,7] NF-κB is a heterodimeric complex consisting of a 50-kDa (p50, NF-κB1) and a 65-kDa (p65, RelA) subunit that is localized in the cytoplasm in an inactive form, in association with members of the IκB family. A number of agents, including inflammatory cytokines and endotoxin, cause translocation of NF-κB to the nucleus through phosphorylation and subsequent degradation of IκB.[8] In the nucleus NF-κB is able to activate transcription of various target genes; for example, VCAM and E-selectin.[9] NF-κB itself induces the mRNA synthesis of its inhibitor IκB to prevent an excessive activation of NF-κB inducible genes. The neuropeptide α-melanocyte-stimulating-hormone (α-MSH), a 13-amino-acid proopiomelanocortin derivative, is well known as a potent antipyretic and antiinflammatory agent in all major forms of inflammation.[10–12] α-MSH reduces acute inflammation induced by peripheral administration of inflammatory stimuli or by injection of presumed mediators of inflammation, such as cytokines.[13,14] α-MSH has been shown to inhibit nitric oxide synthesis[15] and the production of TNF-α.[16] It protects against renal injury after ischemia in mice and rats[17] and inhibits the increase in vascular permeability induced in rabbit skin by injections of histamine or endogenous pyrogen.[18] Furthermore, α-MSH prevents LPS-induced liver damage, even when it is administered 30 minutes after LPS, and it decreases LPS-induced hepatic leukocyte infiltration in mice.[19] The potent antiinflammatory capacity of α-MSH suggests that this peptide may affect the function of endothelial cells, particularly the adhesion molecule-mediated-transmigration of neutrophils. Therefore, we investigated the effect of α-MSH on the expression of adhesion molecules by endothelial cells following activation by proinflammatory stimuli.

METHODS

Cell Culture

The transformed human dermal microvascular endothelial cell line HMEC-1[20] was cultured in endothelium basal media (SFM; Life Technologies, Eggenstein, Germany) supplemented with 10% FCS (PAA Laboratories GmbH, Linz, Austria). Usually, prior to stimulation, the cells were depleted for 15 h at 2% FCS.

RT-PCR

Cells were harvested and total RNA was isolated using the acidic guanidinium thiocyanate-phenol-chloroform method.[21] After reverse transcription (Reverse Transcription System; Promega GmbH, Mannheim, Germany), equal amounts of cDNA were subjected to PCR using primer sets specific for β-actin, VCAM-1, and E-selectin. PCR products were analyzed by agarose gel electrophoresis and visualized in UV-light after ethidium bromide staining. Relative expression of VCAM-1 and E-selectin were determined by densitometric analysis (Bio-Profil Bio-1D; ltf Labortechnik GmbH, Wasserburg, Germany) after standardizing the amount of amplification product according to the expression of a constant gene, β-actin.

Electrophoretic Mobility Shift Assays (EMSA)

HMEC-1 cells were treated with 100 ng/ml LPS (Sigma, Deisenhofen, Germany) alone or in the presence of α-MSH (10^{-8} to 10^{-16} M) (Bachem Biochemica GmbH, Heidelberg, Germany). Nuclear proteins were extracted 30 minutes after stimulation, as described previously.[22] Binding reactions were carried out by addition of 3 μg of poly(dI-dC) (Boehringer Mannheim, Germany) and 10^4 cpm of ^{32}P-labeled, double-stranded oligonucleotide containing the NF-κB binding motif (Santa Cruz Biotechnology, Santa Cruz, CA) to the nuclear protein extracts. Reaction samples were separated electrophoretically on native highly ionic gels at 130 V for 3.5 h, and evaluated by autoradiography. Competition analysis was performed by adding an excess of unlabeled oligonucleotides.

RESULTS

α-MSH Modulates the Expression of Adhesion Molecules

To investigate the effect of α-MSH on the mRNA expression of VCAM-1 and E-selectin, RT-PCR was performed. Monolayer cell cultures of HMEC-1 were treated with LPS (100 ng/ml) alone or with different concentrations of α-MSH (10^{-8} to 10^{-12} M) and the mRNA was isolated after four hours. Stimulation with LPS resulted in a 12-fold and 7.5-fold induction of E-selectin and VCAM-1 mRNA expression, respectively. The expression of the tested adhesion molecules was not affected by α-MSH alone. However, α-MSH significantly downregulated the LPS-induced E-selectin mRNA expression in HMEC-1. The LPS-mediated E-selectin expression was suppressed by more that 50%, irrespective of the dose of α-MSH used. VCAM-1 expression was downregulated by α-MSH in a concentration-dependent manner with a maximum at 10^{-8} M (see FIGURE 1). Furthermore, VCAM-1 suppression by α-MSH was most pronounced after 3 h, and still detectable after 8 and 16 h (see FIGURE 2).

Effect of α-MSH on NF-κB Activation in Endothelial Cells

Regulation of the expression of adhesion molecules, such as VCAM-1 and E-selectin, depends on the activation of transcription factors—that is, NF-κB. Therefore, we set out to determine whether α-MSH affects the LPS mediated activation of NF-κB. Nuclear extracts were prepared 30 minutes after treatment of HMEC-1 with LPS and α-MSH; electrophoretic mobility shift assays were performed on these extracts. NF-κB was strongly activated 30 minutes after stimulation with LPS. However, α-MSH significantly reduced the LPS-mediated activation of NF-κB in a dose-dependent manner, whereby 10^{-8} M α-MSH nearly abolished the NF-κB transloca-

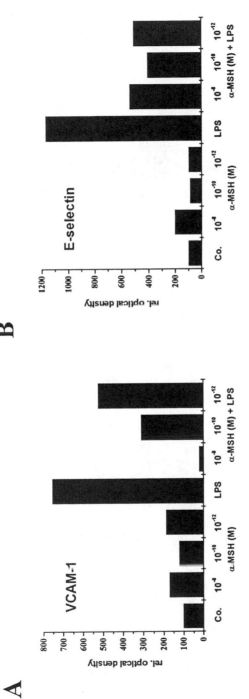

FIGURE 1. Kinetics of VCAM-1 (**A**) and E-selectin (**B**) mRNA expression in relation to β-actin expression after stimulation. HMEC-1 (2×10^6 cells) were left untreated (Co.) or treated with either α-MSH ($10^{-8} - 10^{-12}$ M) or LPS (100 ng/ml) alone or with LPS and α-MSH. Cells were harvested after 4 h, and total RNA was subjected to RT-PCR. Amplification products of VCAM-1, E-selectin, and β-actin cDNA were separated on agarose gels, followed by densitometric evaluation to semiquantify VCAM-1 and E-selectin expression. The data shown are representative of three separate experiments.

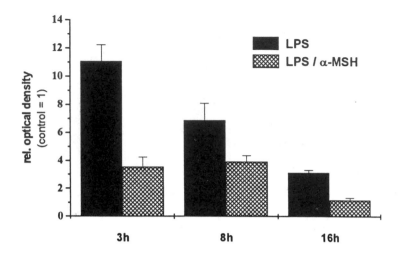

FIGURE 2. Kinetics of the inhibitory effect of α-MSH on LPS-induced expression of VCAM-1 mRNA in HMEC-1. Cells were left untreated (control) or incubated with either LPS (100 ng/ml) alone, or with LPS and 10^{-8} M α-MSH for the indicated periods of time. Amplification products of VCAM-1 and β-actin cDNA were separated on agarose gels, followed by densitometric evaluation to semiquantify VCAM-1 expression.

tion (see FIGURE 3). In contrast, other transcription factors, such as YY-1 and AP-1, were not affected after 30 minutes (data not shown). To test whether the band detected by the EMSA corresponds to the NF-κB heterodimer, nuclear extracts of LPS–treated cells were preincubated with an excess of unlabeled NF-κB consensus-oligonucleotide. This treatment resulted in the loss of the band specific for the p65/p50 heterodimer (data not shown).

DISCUSSION

Endothelial cells play a key role in the initiation of the inflammatory response by managing the crosstalk between peripheral blood mononuclear cells and the surrounding tissue. Recently, it was shown that the receptor that is specific for α-MSH (melanocortin-1 receptor, MC-1R) is expressed on endothelial cells, indicating that they may serve as a target for this peptide.[23] Accordingly, in the present study it has been shown that α-MSH strongly downregulates LPS-induced expression of adhesion molecules, such as VCAM-1 and E-selectin, on human dermal microvascular endothelial cells. This finding has been further supported by recent data showing that α-MSH *in vitro* significantly suppresses the LPS-induced adhesion of T- and B-lymphocytes to HDMEC.[24] Moreover, *in vivo* expression of E-selectin in the local Shwartzman reaction in mice is significantly reduced by application of α-MSH.[25] These data suggest that the antiinflammatory effect of

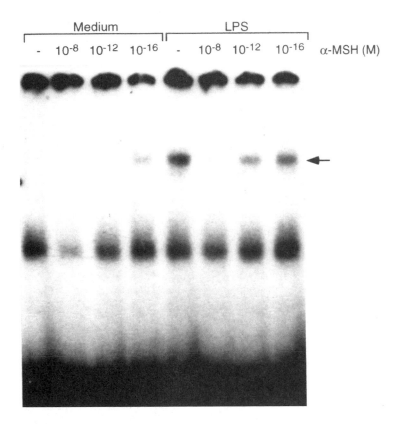

FIGURE 3. Dose response of α-MSH for the inhibition of LPS-dependent NF-κB activation. HMEC-1 cells were left untreated, or incubated with either α-MSH ($10^{-8} - 10^{-16}$ M) or LPS (100 ng/ml) alone, or with LPS and different amounts of α-MSH. Nuclear extracts were prepared 30 minutes after treatment and then assayed for NF-κB on 7% acrylamide gels as described in the Methods section of the text. The NF-κB heterodimer (p50/p65) is indicated by an *arrow*.

α-MSH may be mediated by its capacity to downregulate the expression of adhesion molecules on endothelial cells. However, α-MSH does not have any effect on cells that have not been activated by such proinflammatory stimuli as LPS or IL-1. Apparently, these signals are required to upregulate MC-1R expression on endothelial cells, as well as on inflammatory cells. Subsequently, they become responsive to α-MSH, which acts as one of the signals required for the downregulation of inflammation. Therefore, α-MSH appears to function as one of the mediators required for the neutralization of proinflammatory signals.

The regulation of adhesion-molecule expression is under the control of transcription factors, including NF-κB. α-MSH previously has been shown to inhibit the NF-κB–dependent events involved in inflammation, such as TNFα production,[16] migration of neutrophils,[26] and nitric oxide synthesis.[15] Moreover, there is evidence for a relationship between the p65 subunit of the NF-κB heterodimer and α-MSH, because both were found to be colocalized in rat brain.[27] The data of this study support the role of α-MSH as a modulator of NF-κB activity, since the LPS-induced activation of NF-κB was completely abolished by α-MSH in a dose-dependent manner. Apart from adhesion molecules, several other mediators involved in the inflammatory response, including IL-1, IL-6, TNF-α, chemokines, and nitric oxide synthase require the activation of transcription factor NF-κB. Moreover, α-MSH has recently been shown to suppress NF-κB activation induced by TNF-α in a dose- and a time-dependent manner; and to prevent IκB degradation induced by TNF-α.[28] In keratinocytes, α-MSH inhibits the NF-κB–mediated proinflammatory effects of IL-1β, such as chemokine induction.[29] In animal studies, α-MSH was found to protect against hepatic leukocyte infiltration, liver damage, and mortality of systemic endotoxemia in mice even when administered after LPS.[17] These findings suggest that α-MSH may provide an useful approach for the treatment of inflammatory diseases.

ACKNOWLEDGMENTS

This work was supported by the Deutsche Forschungsgemeinschaft (So 87/11-4 E) and the Volkswagenstiftung (I/74 582).

REFERENCES

1. AUGUSTIN, H.G., D.H. KOZIAN & R.C. JOHNSON. 1994. Differentiation of endothelial cells: analysis of the constitutive and activated endothelial cell phenotypes. Bioessays **16:** 901–906.
2. MCEVER, R.P., K.L. MOORE & A.D. CUMMINGS. 1995. Leukocyte trafficking mediated by selectin-carbohydrate interactions. J. Biol. Chem. **270:** 11025–11028.
3. ZIMMERMANN, G.A., S.M. PRESCOTT & T.M. MCINTYRE. 1992. Endothelial cell interactions with granulocytes: tethering and signaling molecules. Immunol. Today **13:** 93–100.
4. BUTCHER, E.C. & L.J. PICKER. 1996. Lymphocyte homing and homeostasis. Science **272:** 60–66.
5. SPRINGER, T.A. 1995. Traffic signals on endothelium for lymphocyte recirculation and leukocyte emigration. Annu. Rev. Physiol. **57:** 827–872.
6. MÜLLER J.M., H.W. ZIEGLER-HEITBROCK & P.A. BAEUERLE. 1993. Nuclear factor kappa B, a mediator of lipopolysaccharide effects. Immunobiology **187:** 233–256.
7. BAEUERLE, P.A. & V.R. BAICHWAL. 1997. NF-kappa B as a frequent target for immunosuppressive and anti-inflammatory molecules. Adv. Immunol. **65:** 111–137.
8. MALEK S., T. HUXFORD & G. GHOSH. 1998. Ikappa B alpha functions through direct contacts with the nuclear localization signals and the DNA binding sequences of NF-kappaB. J. Biol. Chem. **273:** 25427–25435.
9. MAY M.J. & S. GHOSH. 1998. Signal transduction through NF-kappa B. Immunol. Today **19:** 80–88.
10. LIPTON, J. M. & A. P. CATANIA. 1997. Antiinflammatory influence of the neuroimmunomodulator α-MSH. Immunol. Today **18:** 140–145.
11. LUGER, T.A., T. SCHOLZEN & S. GRABBE. 1997. The role of α-melanocyte stimulating hormone in cutaneous biology. J. Invest. Dermatol. **2:** 87–93.
12. CATANIA, A. & J.M. LIPTON. 1993. Alpha-melanocyte stimulating hormone in the modulation of host reactions. Endocr. Rev. **14:** 564–576.

13. ROBERTSON, B., K. DOSTAL & R. DAYNES. 1988. Neuropeptide regulation of inflammatory and immunologic responses. J. Immunol. **140:** 4300–4307.

14. LUGER, T.A., T. SCHOLZEN, T. BRZOSKA, E. BECHER, A. SLOMINSKI & R. PAUS. 1998. Cutaneous immunomodulation and coordination of skin stress responses by α-melanocyte-stimulating hormone. Ann. N.Y. Acad. Sci. **840:** 381–394.

15. STAR, R.A., N. RAJORA, J. HUANG, R.C. STOCK, A. CATANIA & J.M. LIPTON. 1995. Evidence of autocrine modulation of macrophage nitric oxide synthase by α-melanocyte-stimulating hormone. Proc. Natl. Acad. Sci. USA **92:** 8016–8020.

16. RAJORA N., G. CERIANI, A. CATANIA, R.A. STAR, M.T. MURPHY & J.M. LIPTON. 1996. α-MSH production, receptors, and influence on neopterin in a human monocyte/macrophage cell line. J. Leukoc. Biol. **59:** 248–253.

17. CHIAO, H., Y. KOHDA, P. MCLEROY, L. CRAIG, I. HOUSINI & R.A. STAR. 1997. α-Melanocyte-stimulating hormone protects against renal injury after ischemia in mice and rats. J. Clin. Invest. **99:** 1165–1172.

18. LIPTON, J.M. 1989. Neuropeptide alpha-melanocyte stimulating hormone in control of fever, the acute phase response and inflammation. *In* Neuroimmune Networks: Physiology and Diseases. E.J. Goetzl & N.H. Spector, Eds.: 243–250. Alan R. Liss, New York.

19. CHIAO, H., S. FOSTER, R. THOMAS, J. LIPTON & R.A. STAR. 1996. α-Melanocyte-stimulating hormone reduces endotoxin-induced liver inflammation. J. Clin. Invest. **97:** 2038–2044.

20. ADES, E.W., F.J. CANDAL, R.A. SWERLICK, V.G. GEORGE, S. SUMMERS, D.C. BOSSE & T.J. LAWLEY. 1992. IIMEC-1: establishment of an immortalized human microvascular endothelial cell line. J. Invest. Dermatol. **99:** 683–690.

21. CHOMCZYNSKI, P. & N. SACCHI. 1987. Single-step method of RNA isolation by acid guanidinium thiocyanate-phenol-chloroform extraction. Anal. Biochem. **162:** 156–159.

22. ARAGANE, Y., D. KULMS, T. A. LUGER & T. SCHWARZ. 1997. Down-regulation of interferon gamma-activated STAT1 by UV light. Proc. Natl. Acad. Sci. USA **94:** 11490–11495.

23. HARTMEYER, M., T. SCHOLZEN, E. BECHER, R.S. BHARDWAJ, T. SCHWARZ & T.A. LUGER. 1997. Human microvascular endothelial cells (HMEC-1) express the melanocortin receptor type 1 and produce increased levels of IL-8 upon stimulation with αMSH. J. Immunol. **159:** 1930–1937.

24. KALDEN, D.-H., M. FASTRICH, T. SCHOLZEN, T. BRZOSKA & T.A. LUGER. 1998. α-MSH modulates the expression of LPS-induced adhesion molecules. Abstract. Exp. Dermatol. **7:** 225.

25. KALDEN, D.-H., S. MERFELD, T. BRZOSKA, C. SORG, T.A. LUGER & C. SUNDERKÖTTER. 1998. α-Melanocyte stimulating hormone (α-MSH) reduces vasculitis in the local Shwartzman reaction. Abstract. Exp. Dermatol. **7:** 225.

26. CATANIA, A., N. RAJORA, F. CAPSONI, F. MINONZIO, R.A. STAR & J.M. LIPTON. 1996. The neuropeptide α-MSH has specific receptors on neutrophils and reduces chemotaxis *in vitro.* Peptides **17:** 675–679.

27. JOSEPH, S.A., C. TASSORELLI, A.V. PRASAD & E. LYND-BALTA. 1996. NF-κB transcription factor subunits in rat brain: colocalization of p65 and α-MSH. Peptides **17:** 655–664.

28. MANNA, S.K. & B.B. AGGARWAL. 1998. α-Melanocyte-stimulating hormone inhibits nuclear transcription factor NF-κB activation induced by various inflammatory agents. J. Immunol. **161:** 2873–2880.

29. BRZOSKA T., D.-H. KALDEN, T. SCHOLZEN, T.A. LUGER. 1998. Molecular basis of the α-MSH/IL-1 antagonism. Abstract. Exp. Dermatol. **7:** 221.

POMC and Fibroblast Biology

TORELLO LOTTI,[a] PATRIZIA TEOFOLI,[b,c] BEATRICE BIANCHI,[a] AND
ALAIN MAUVIEL[c]

[a]*Department of Dermatology, University of Florence, Italy*

[b]*Istituto Dermopatico dell'Immacolata, IDI, IRCCS, Rome, Italy*

[c]*Department of Dermatology and Cutaneous Biology, Thomas Jefferson University,
Philadelphia, Pennsylvania, USA*

ABSTRACT: We evidenced *in vitro* proopiomelanocortin (POMC) mRNA–
transcription in human dermal fibroblasts using Northern blot hybridization.
Modulation of POMC gene expression by cytokines (transforming growth
factor-β, TGF-β, and tumor necrosis factor-α, TNF-α) was investigated by incubating human normal fibroblasts with 1 and 10 ng/ml cytokines, either alone
or in combination, for 24 hours. Our results show that dermal fibroblasts express POMC at significant levels under unstimulated conditions. POMC
steady-state levels were significantly reduced by addition of TGF-β. On the
other hand, TNF-α exerted a stimulatory effect on POMC mRNA transcription, partially counteracting the effect of TGF-β. These data provide the first
demonstration of POMC gene expression in cultured skin fibroblasts. The opposite regulatory effect of TGF-β and TNF-α, two cytokines primarily involved in extracellular matrix regulation, suggests a possible role for POMC-
derived peptides in fibroblast activity. We also investigated POMC mRNA expression in keloid-derived fibroblasts in culture, and its regulation by TGF-β
added at the highest concentration documented for inhibition. Keloid-derived
fibroblasts showed clearly detectable levels of POMC mRNA in basal conditions, and no alteration of POMC gene expression was observed when TGF-β
was added in culture. The altered TGF-β regulation of POMC mRNA levels
suggest that POMC-derived peptides may play a role in the pathogenesis of keloid formation through an autocrine/paracrine network, resulting in modulation of extracellular matrix synthesis.

INTRODUCTION

POMC, initially isolated in the pituitary gland, is a precursor polypeptide whose
cleavage gives rise to the peptides corticotropin (ACTH), melanotropins (MSH), and
endorphins (EP). POMC gene expression and synthesis has been demonstrated in the
skin, where it has been suggested that POMC-derived peptides play a major role in
neuroimmune interactions (for a review see Refs. 1 and 2). We investigated POMC
gene expression in skin fibroblasts from healthy donors and from keloid-derived fibroblasts in order to evaluate POMC gene expression and its response to TNF-α and
TGF-β. The effect of TGF-β was also evaluated on human normal keratinocytes.

[c]Address for correspondence: Patrizia Teofoli, M.D., Istituto Dermopatico dell'Immacolata,
IDI, IRCCS, Via dei Monti di Creta 104, 00167, Rome, Italy. +39-6-66462981 (voice); +39-6-
66464435 (fax).

MATERIALS AND METHODS

Cell Cultures

Human normal keratinocytes, normal and keloid-derived human fibroblasts, were grown as previously described.[3]

Cytokines

Human recombinant TGF-β_2 was a generous gift from Dr. D.R. Olsen, Celtrix Laboratories, Santa Clara, CA. Human recombinant TNF-α was purchased from Boeringher Manneheim, Indianapolis, IN, USA.

Northern Analyses and cDNA Probes

See the Methods Section in Reference 3.

RESULTS AND DISCUSSION

Confluent normal skin fibroblasts were incubated, with or without TGF-β or TNF-α, either alone or in combination, for 24 hours. The total RNA was extracted and analyzed by Northern hybridization using a ^{32}P-labeled cDNA probe specific for POMC transcripts. As shown in FIGURES 1–5, the autoradiogram clearly indicates presence of significant amounts of POMC mRNA, with expected 1.3-Kb size, in unstimulated fibroblasts (FIG. 1). Total RNA from 3T3 cell line cultures was also analyzed by Northern blot analysis. We were able to detect POMC mRNA transcripts in basal conditions (data not shown). Visual analysis of the effects of the cytokines on POMC expression indicates a dose-dependent downregulation by TGF-β, whereas TNF-α exerts a stimulatory effect that partially reverses the effect of TGF-β (FIG. 1). Quantitative analysis, by scanning densitometry, of the results from three independent experiments, corrected against values for GAPDH transcripts in each RNA preparation, indicated that the inhibitory effect of TGF-β reached 80% with the highest concentration used (10 ng/ml), whereas TNF-α induction of POMC expression exceeds control levels by a factor of about 2.5 (FIG. 2). This suggests that fibroblasts may provide a significant source of POMC-derived peptides, especially on stimulation by proinflammatory cytokines, such as TNF-α, as may occur during inflammatory and repair processes.

Examination of the effect of TGF-β on keratinocytes indicates rapid, time-dependent downregulation of POMC mRNA levels in cultured keratinocytes (FIG. 3). In fact, significant (about 60%) reduction in POMC levels was observed as early as one hour after growth factor stimulation and this further increased over time, leading to almost undetectable POMC transcript levels at 24 and 48 hours (FIG. 3). The same result was also shown by scanning densitometry (FIG. 4). We conclude that TGF-β is able to inhibit POMC expression of both fibroblasts and keratinocytes, contrasting with its cell-type specific effect on the expression of both interstitial collagenase and *c-jun* genes.[4]

Significant POMC transcript levels were also detected in unstimulated keloid-derived fibroblasts from a 44-year-old donor. TGF-β did not alter POMC expression, since we observed in fibroblast cultures from healthy donors (FIG. 5A). To verify the lack of responsiveness of the keloid-derived fibroblasts, we measured the expression

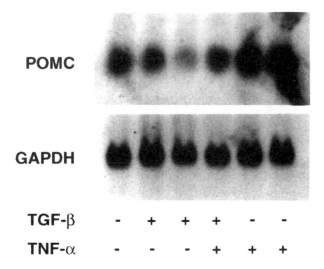

FIGURE 1. As previously described,[3] untreated normal dermal fibroblasts in cultures show a signal for POMC gene expression in detectable amounts. Modulation of POMC mRNA levels by TGF-β and TNF-α after 24 hours at different concentrations (1–10 ng/ml) document a stimulatory effect of TNF-α and inhibitory effect of TGF-β on POMC gene expression. GAPDH cDNA was used as control.

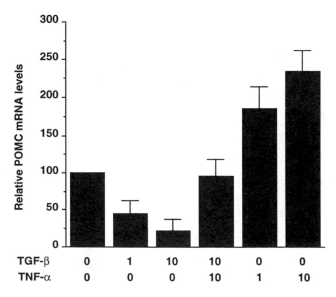

FIGURE 2. Quantitative analysis, by scanning densitometry, of results from three independent experiments (after correction against values for GAPDH transcripts in each RNA preparation) was used to evaluate relative POMC mRNA levels. We observed that the inhibitory effect of TGF-β reaches 80% at the highest concentration used (10 ng/ml), whereas TNF-α (10 ng/ml) induction of POMC expression exceeds control levels by about 2.5.

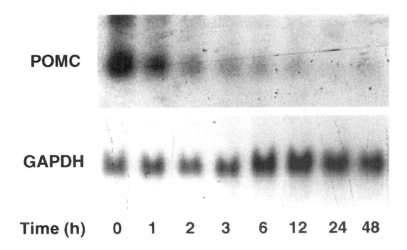

FIGURE 3. Time course effect of TGF-β (10 ng/ml) on POMC gene expression by keratinocytes after 1, 2, 3, 6, 12, 24, and 48 hours.

of several other genes known to be upregulated by TGF-β. Expression of the immediate early gene, jun-B, was induced after one hour of stimulation by the growth factor, confirming previous observations[4] (FIG. 5B). The expression of COL1A2 and fibronectin was enhanced by TGF-β, with a maximum stimulation observed 24 hours after the addition of the growth factor (FIG. 5B), in agreement with previous studies.[5,6] Collectively, these results suggest that POMC expression in keloid-derived fibroblasts is not altered by TGF-β, and this contrasts with the downregulation observed in fibroblast cultures derived from normal skin.

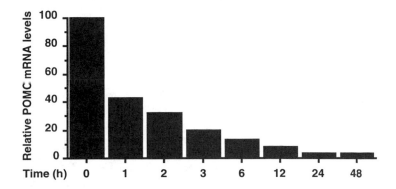

FIGURE 4. Time-dependent TGF-β inhibition-effect has been documented, as shown by quantitative analysis using scanning densitometry.

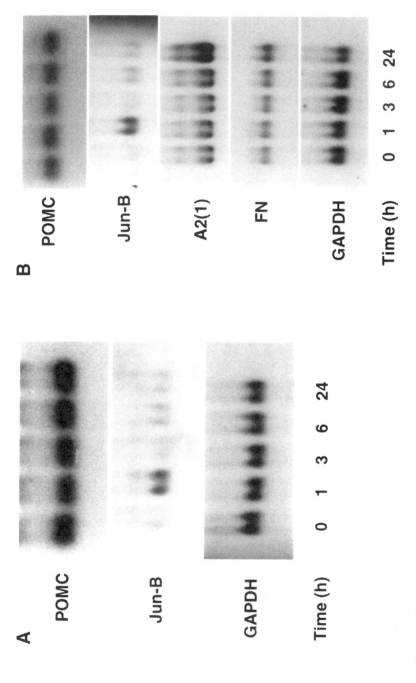

FIGURE 5. Time-course of the expression of POMC mRNA in cultured keloid fibroblasts. (**A**). Lack of effect of TGF-β (10 ng/ml). (**B**). Jun-B, COLA2(1) and fibronectin (FN) gene expression analyzed by Northern hybridization at each time in the same RNA preparations.

In this work, we have provided the first evidence for POMC expression in dermal fibroblasts, either normal fibroblasts or those derived from keloid lesions. We have shown, that POMC mRNA levels are regulated in opposite ways by TGF-β and TNF-α in normal fibroblasts. The inhibitory effect of TGF-β was also observed in epidermal keratinocytes. In contrast, TGF-β did not alter POMC transcript levels in keloid fibroblasts. Keloids are acquired cutaneous lesions, and cultured keloid-fibroblasts display increased collagen production and other extracellular matrix components.[7] It has been suggested that keloid overproduction of extracellular matrix components may be due to an inherent modification of the TGF-β regulatory program.[8] In our work, TGF-β appeared to inhibit POMC mRNA expression in both normal fibroblasts and keratinocytes, whereas in keloid fibroblast cultures, TGF-β did not alter POMC expression, although other genes known to be regulated by TGF-β were responsive to this cytokine. This attests to the specificity of our observation on POMC expression. Clinical data indicate that, at puberty and during pregnancy, the incidence of keloid increases, in parallel with the activity of the pituitary gland. This suggests that pituitary hormones, MSH in particular, could play a role in fibroblast activity.[9,10] Our data suggest the possibility that POMC-derived peptides, released from dermal fibroblasts, may play a paracrine or autocrine role on fibroblast activity and in keloid formation.

REFERENCES

1. BLALOCK, J.E. 1994. The syntax of immune-neuroendocrine communication. Immunol. Today **15:** 504–507.

2. LUGER, T.A., T. SHOLZEN & S. GRABBE. 1997. The role of α-melanocyte-stimulating hormone in cutaneous biology. J. Invest. Dermatol. Suppl. **2:** 87–93.

3. TEOFOLI, P., K. MOTOKI, T.M. LOTTI, J. UITTO & A. MAUVIEL. 1997. Proopiomelanocortin (POMC) gene expression by normal skin and keloid fibroblasts in culture: modulation by cytokines. Exp. Dermatol. **6:** 111–115.

4. MAUVIEL, A., K.Y. CHUNG, A. AGARWAL, K. TAMAI & J. UITTO. 1996. Cell-specific induction of distinct oncogenes of the jun family is responsible for differential regulation of collagenase gene expression by transforming growth factor-β in fibroblasts and keratinocytes. J. Biol. Chem. **271:** 10917–10923.

5. IGNOTZ, R., T. ENDO & J. MASSAGUÉ. 1987. Regulation on fibronectin and Type I collagen mRNA levels by transforming growth factor-β. J. Biol. Chem. **262:** 6443–6446.

6. VARGA, J., J. ROSENBLOOM & S.A. JIMENEZ. 1987. Transforming growth factor-β (TGF–β) causes a persistent increase in steady-state amounts of type I and type III collagen and fibronectin mRNA in human dermal fibroblasts. Biochem. J. **247:** 597–604.

7. UITTO, J., A.J. PEREJDA, R.P. ABERGEL, M-L. CHU & F. RAMIREZ. 1985. Altered steady-state ratio of type I/III procollagen mRNAs with selectively increased type I procollagen biosynthesis in coltered keloid fibroblasts. Proc. Natl. Acad. Sci. USA **82:** 5935–5939.

8. BABU, M., R. DIEGELMANN & N. OLIVER. 1992. Keloid fibroblasts exhibit an altered response to TGF-β. J. Invest. Dermatol. **99:** 650–655.

9. MOUSTAFA, M.F., M.A. ABDEL-FATTAH & D.C. ABDEL-FATTAH. 1975. Presumptive evidence of the effects of pregnancy estrogens on keloid growth. Plast. Reconstr. Surg. **56:** 450–453.

10. ANCES, G., & S.H. POMERANTZ. 1974. Serum concentrations of β-melanocyte-stimulating hormone in human pregnancy. Am. J. Obstet. Gynecol. **119:** 1062–1068.

The Role of Proopiomelanocortin-Derived Peptides in Skin Fibroblast and Mast Cell Functions

PATRIZIA TEOFOLI,[a] ALESSANDRA FREZZOLINI,[a] PIETRO PUDDU,[a]
ORNELLA DE PITÀ,[a] ALAIN MAUVIEL,[b] AND TORELLO LOTTI[c]

[a]Department of Immunodermatology,
Istituto Dermopatico dell'Immacolata (IDI), Rome, Italy

[b]Department of Dermatology and Cutaneous Biology, Thomas Jefferson University,
Philadelphia, Pennsylvania, USA

[c]Department of Dermatology, University of Florence, Italy

ABSTRACT: We have previously described proopiomelanocortin (POMC)
gene-expression in human normal cultured dermal fibroblasts, and its dose-
and time-dependent modulation by transforming growth factor-β (TGF-β)
and tumor necrosis factor-α (TNF-α). The aim of the work described here was
to investigate POMC-derived peptide release in vitro by cultured fibroblasts
following incubation with different concentrations of both TNF-α and TGF-β
for 24 hours (1, 5, and 10 ng/ml). The effect of simultaneous addition of both
TNF-α and TGF-β (10 ng/ml) was also evaluated. Culture supernatants of human skin fibroblasts were collected to detect adrenocorticotropin hormone
(ACTH), α-melanotropin (α-MSH), and β-endorphin (β-EP) levels by specific
immunoenzymatic assay. We investigated the in vitro histamine-releasing activity of the POMC-derived peptides, α-MSH and β-EP, on human foreskin
mast cells. Detection of cleavage products in supernatants from cultured normal human dermal fibroblasts indicated intracellular processing by POMC
protein. We were able to measure detectable levels of all peptides in basal
conditions. TNF-α addition resulted in an increase in β-EP and ACTH levels.
TGF-β–stimulated fibroblasts showed no alteration in β-EP and α-MSH
levels, whereas ACTH release was significantly enhanced. Both α-MSH and
β-EP induced histamine release from human foreskin mast cells in vitro
with β-EP-induced histamine levels as high as those observed with the calcium
ionophore, ionomycin. Our data document fibroblast POMC-derived peptide
release and modulation by cytokines, suggesting that they have a possible role
in extracellular matrix deposit regulation and skin inflammation.

INTRODUCTION

Proopiomelanocortin (POMC) is a 29-Kd polypeptide processed posttranslationally in the pituitary gland to yield the biologically active peptides adrenocorticotropin (ACTH), endorphins (α-, β-, γ-EP), and melanotropins (α-, β-, γ-MSH).[1,2]

[a]Address for correspondence: Patrizia Teofoli, M.D., Department of Immunodermatology,
Istituto Dermopatico dell'Immacolata, 104, Via dei Monti di Creta, 100167, Rome, Italy. +39-6-
66462981 (voice); +39-6-66464435 (fax).

POMC gene expression has been detected in several extrapituitary tissues, such as brain, gonads, gastrointestinal tract, placenta, and immune cells; as well as in non-pituitary tumors.[3,4] α-MSH shows a potent antiinflammatory and antipyretic activity, and it inhibits cutaneous and delayed-type hypersensitivity,[5,6] thereby preventing both sensitization and elicitation phase of cutaneous hypersensitivity. It also upregulates human monocyte interleukin 10 (IL10) synthesis.[7,8] β-EP, generated by the activation of the pituitary-adrenal axis is a 31-amino-acid peptide belonging to the endogenous opiate family; it exhibits antinociceptive and immunomodulating activity.[9–11] The skin has been suggested as a target for POMC-peptides. POMC mRNA transcriptional and translational activity has been detected in the A431 squamous carcinoma cell line, human normal keratinocytes, melanocytes, Langerhans cells, skin infiltrating mononuclear cells, endothelial cells, and anagen hair follicles (see Ref. 12 for a review).

It has been demonstrated that human normal keratinocytes produce ACTH and α-MSH after stimulation with ultraviolet light (UV), phorbol esters, interleukin-1 and interleukin-4.[13] Our group was the first to demonstrate POMC gene expression in cultured normal human skin fibroblasts, and its modulation by tumor necrosis factor-α (TNF-α) and transforming growth factor-β (TGF-β); exhibiting a dose- and time-dependent, stimulatory and inhibitory effect, respectively.[14] The expression of melanocortin receptor-1 (MC-1) by dermal fibroblasts has recently been reported.[15] The aim of this work was to investigate, by immunoenzimatic assay, the release of POMC-derived peptides adrenocorticotropin hormone (ACTH), α-melanotropin (α-MSH), and β-endorphin (β-EP) from cultured skin fibroblasts after incubation with TNF-α and/or TGF-β at different concentrations. The effect of the TNF-α and TGF-β combination on POMC-peptide production was also evaluated, as well as that of POMC-derived peptide histamine-releasing activity on human foreskin mast cells.

MATERIALS AND METHODS

Cell Cultures

Human dermal fibroblast cultures, established by explanting tissue specimens obtained from neonatal foreskin, were utilized between passages 3 to 8. Fibroblasts were maintained in the modified-Eagle's medium of Dulbecco (DMEM) supplemented with 10% fetal calf serum (FCS), 2 mM glutamine, and antibiotics (50 μg/ml streptomycin, 200 U/ml penicillin-G, 0.25 μg/ml amphotericin-B). One hour prior to the addition of growth factors, the confluent fibroblast cultures were rinsed with DMEM and placed in DMEM containing 1% FCS.

Cytokines/Growth Factors

Human recombinant TGF-β$_2$ was a generous gift from Dr. David R. Olsen, Celtrix Laboratories, Santa Clara, CA, USA. Throughout the text, it will be referred to as TGF-β. Human recombinant TNF-α was purchased from Boeringer Manneheim, Indianapolis, IN, USA.

Immunoenzymatic Evaluation of α-MSH, ACTH, and β-EP

α-MSH, ACTH, and β-EP levels in fibroblast supernatants were measured by using commercially available ELISA kits according to instructions from the manufacturer (ACTH-α-MSH-β-EP-EIA Kit, Phoenix Pharmaceutical, Mountain View, CA, USA). Each kit for peptide detection had 0.5 ng/ml sensitivity with precision specifications for intra-assay variation < 5% and inter-assay variation < 14%. The α-MSH EIA kit showed no cross-reactivity with α-MSH II, β-MSH, γ_3-MSH, ACTH, β-EP, or met-enkephalin. The ACTH assay showed 100% cross-reactivity with rat ACTH or 1–24 Human ACTH; 30% reactivity with 7–38 human ACTH; and no cross-reactivity with CRF, β-EP, α-MSH, α-ANP, or BNP-32. The β-EP EIA kit showed 100% cross-reactivity with human, porcine, and with rat β-EP; 45% cross-reactivity with camel, ovine, and bovine β-EP; and no cross-reactivity with α- or γ-endorphin or with met- and leu-enkephalin. For each assay a standard curve was constructed.

Histamine Release from Human Skin Mast Cells

Human foreskin, obtained at circumcision, was dissected free from subcutaneous tissue, and cut in slices, as described by Niimi et al.[16] Five skin slices were each washed twice in calcium/magnesium-free buffer, suspended in assay buffer with 2 mM calcium and 1 mM magnesium, and then incubated at 37°C for 30 minutes with α-MSH (10 μM/ml) or β-EP (10 μM/ml) (Sigma Chemicals, St. Louis). Samples with assay buffer alone, or with the Ca^{2+}-ionophore, ionomycin (10 μM/ml), were used as controls.

Determination of Histamine Release

Histamine release was measured with an enzyme immunoassay kit (Bouty, Milan, Italy) according to instructions provided by the manufacturer. All histamine experiments were performed in duplicate.

RESULTS

POMC-Cleavage Products Release

To investigate POMC-derived peptide production and its regulation by TNF-α and TGF-β, cultures of normal skin fibroblast were incubated with or without TNF-α and TGF-β, either alone (at three different concentrations, 1, 5, and 10 ng/ml) or in combination at the highest concentration (10 ng/ml). Conditioned media were harvested after 24 hours and tested, in duplicate, for the presence of β-EP, α-MSH, and ACTH peptides by using a specific ELISA. Human skin fibroblasts have been shown to release significant amounts of α-MSH (25 ng/ml), β-EP (18 ng/ml), and ACTH (2.8 ng/ml) in unstimulated conditions growing in plain culture medium (see FIGURE 1). As shown in FIGURE 2, β-EP concentration increased by a factor 1.7 when TNF-α was added to the culture. The β-EP increase was not dose-dependent since maximal β-EP levels were detected at the lowest concentration used (1 ng/ml), with no further increase at higher TNF-α concentrations. In contrast, TGF-β did not seem to influence β-EP production at the concentrations examined (FIG. 2). The combina-

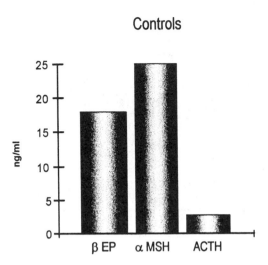

FIGURE 1. POMC-derived peptide production and its regulation by TNF-α and TGF-β in normal human dermal fibroblasts. Fibroblasts in the culture were incubated with or without TNF-α and TGF-β, either alone (at three different concentrations; 1, 5, and 10 ng/ml) or in combination at the highest concentration (10 ng/ml) for 24 hours. The conditioned media were then harvested after 24 hours and tested in duplicate for the presence of β-EP, α-MSH, and ACTH peptides using the appropriate immunoenzymatic assay. As shown, measurable levels of all peptides were detected in basal conditions.

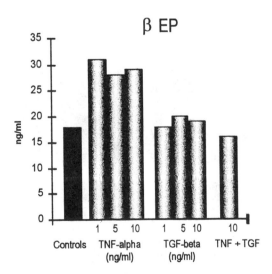

FIGURE 2. Shows the levels of β-EP after stimulation with TNF-α and TGF-β, and the effect of a combination of both cytokines. No dose-dependent pathway can be observed in POMC-derived peptide cytokine modulation.

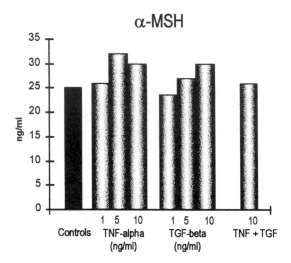

FIGURE 3. Shows the levels of α-MSH after stimulation with TNF-α and TGF-β, and the effect of a combination of both cytokines. No dose-dependent pathway can be observed in POMC-derived peptide cytokine modulation.

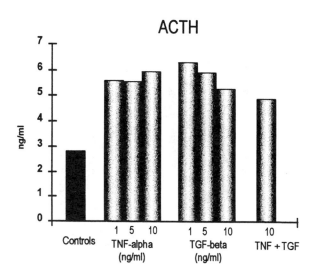

FIGURE 4. Shows the levels of ACTH after stimulation with TNF-α and TGF-β, and the effect of a combination of both cytokines. No dose-dependent pathway can be observed in POMC-derived peptide cytokine modulation.

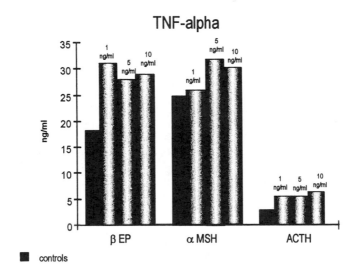

FIGURE 5. Effect of TNF-α on normal human fibroblasts. TNF-α addition resulted in an increase in β-EP and ACTH levels.

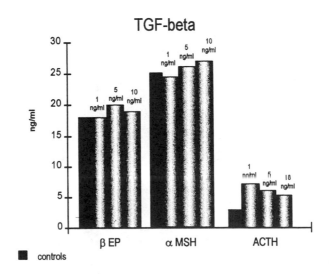

FIGURE 6. Effect of TNF-β on normal human fibroblasts. TGF-β stimulated fibroblasts showed no alteration of β-EP or α-MSH levels, whereas ACTH release was significantly enhanced.

tion of TNF-α and TGF-β resulted in β-EP values that were similar to those in the controls. Supernatants that were tested for α-MSH showed high amounts of the peptide in normal human fibroblast media, suggesting a high level of α-MSH secretion in basal conditions (FIG.1). A small increase was obtained with 5 ng/ml and 10 ng/ml TNF-α, whereas addition of TGF-β displayed no effect (see FIGURE 3). Similarly, when both cytokines were added they did not induce any variation in α-MSH levels (FIG. 3). Immunoenzymatic assay was also performed in order to investigate skin fibroblast ACTH production by skin fibroblasts. We found that untreated fibroblasts released a detectable amount of ACTH (FIG. 1). Compared to the controls, both cytokines significantly enhanced ACTH production—approximately double in each case (see FIGURE 4). We were not able to detect a significant difference when different concentrations were used. Addition of both cytokines to the cultures did not demonstrate a synergistic effect on ACTH release (FIG. 4). FIGURES 5 and 6 show the effect of TNF-α and TGF-β on the cleavage of POMC in comparison with that on the controls.

β-EP and α-MSH Induced Skin Mast Cell-Histamine Release

In our study, using two separate experiments, we detected both α-MSH and β-EP induced histamine release from human skin mast cells, in amounts different from those in control samples. Spontaneous histamine release in control samples was 14 ng/ml, whereas addition of α-MSH resulted in more than a fivefold increase (82 ng/ml). With β-EP incubation, histamine release reached the maximum (192 ng/ml) as detected by the histamine immunoenzymatic assay. β-EP histamine release levels were higher than ionomycin–induced histamine levels (162 ng/ml) (see FIGURE 7).

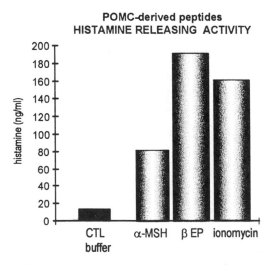

FIGURE 7. α-MSH and β-EP (both at 10 μM/ml) histamine-releasing activity. Assay buffer and ionomycin (10 μM/) were used as controls.

DISCUSSION

Our results show, for the first time, that normal human dermal fibroblasts can release the POMC-derived peptides β-EP, α-MSH, and ACTH, as measured by specific immunoenzymatic assay. Constitutive release of β-EP, α-MSH, and ACTH was detectable in the harvested media from confluent untreated fibroblasts in culture, as shown by two separate experiments. α-MSH levels indicated that the peptide is mainly expressed in untreated fibroblasts, with a minor influence when TNF-α or TGF-β were added alone or in combination. This suggests that it is near maximal production at basal conditions. β-EP immunoreactivity was found to be significant in unstimulated conditions and it was significantly upregulated by TNF-α, whereas TGF-β did not alter its release. Similarly, the combination of TNF-α and TGF-β did not modify the β-EP levels. Thus, TGF-β might counteract the TNF-α effect on β-EP release. By comparing the effect of these two cytokines on POMC cleavage-product release, our data displayed a significant induction of β-EP and ACTH by TNF-α, with no dose-dependent pathway. TGF-β induced an increase in ACTH levels, but it failed to induce any effects on β-EP and α-MSH release. As we previously described, untreated normal skin fibroblasts that express POMC mRNA transcripts are modulated in an opposite manner by TNF-α and TGF-β.[14] Cleavage product detection in supernatants of human dermal fibroblasts from healthy donors, indicate the presence of POMC protein intracellular processing in these cells, as described in the A431 cell-line, and in human normal keratinocytes.[13] Fibroblasts represent a source of POMC-cleavage products with various stimuli, including proinflammatory cytokines such as TNF-α, and these result in an increase of β-EP and ACTH as confirmed by TNF-α POMC mRNA transcript level upregulation. TGF-β did not alter β-EP or α-MSH, whereas ACTH release is enhanced. However, this observation does not apparently correlate with the documented 50% downregulation of POMC gene-expression by 1 ng/ml TGF-β observed after 24 hours incubation. The role of POMC peptides on fibroblast biology is not completely understood, but a paracrine/autocrine pathway regulation could be important by acting to bind the specific melanocortin receptor-1 (MC-1) expressed by skin fibroblasts.[15] These data show that POMC cleavage is regulated differentially by TNF-α and TGF-β, both of which are primarily involved in tissue remodelling. α-MSH is active in fibroblast synthetic activity, inducing collagenase/matrix metalloproteinase-1 release from human dermal fibroblasts. This suggests a role in UV-induced collagenolysis and cutaneous photo-ageing.[17]

Other than their role in extracellular matrix deposition, these two cytokines play an important role in modulation of inflammation. They could act *in situ*, regulating POMC-derived peptide synthesis and release. Itching may be related to β-EP levels in human skin since specific μ-receptors[18] and specific mast cell degranulation[19] have been demonstrated in this situation. The exact mechanism, however, remains to be elucidated.

REFERENCES

1. MAINS, R.A., B.A. EIPPER & N. LING. 1977. Common precursor to corticotropins and endorphins. Proc. Natl. Acad. Sci. USA **74:** 3014–3018.

2. KRIEGER, T., & A.S. LIOTTA. 1979. Pituitary hormones in brain: where, how, and why? Science **205:** 366–372.
3. LOLAIT, S.J., J.A. CLEMENTS, A.J. MARKWICK *et al.* 1986. Proopiomelanocortin messenger ribonucleic acid and posttranslational processing of beta-endorphin in spleen macrophages. J. Clin. Invest. **77:** 1776–1779.
4. HOPPENER, J.M.W., P.H. STEENBERGH, P.J.J. MOONEN *et al.* 1986, Detection of mRNA encoding calcitonin, calcitonin gene related peptide and proopiomelanocortin in human tumors. Mol. Cell. Endocrinol. **47:** 125–130.
5. LIPTON, J,M. & A. CATANIA. 1992. α-MSH peptides modulate fever and inflammation. *In* Neuroimmunology of Fever. T. Bartfai, Ed.: 123–136. Pergamon Press, Oxford.
6. CERIANI, G., A. MACALUSO, A. CATANIA & J.M. LIPTON. 1994. Central neurogenic antiinflammatory action of α-MSH: modulation of peripheral inflammation induced by cytokines and other mediators of inflammation. Neuroendocrinol. **59:** 138–143.
7. LUGER, T.A., T. SHOLZEN & S. GRABBE. 1997. The role of α-melanocyte-stimulating hormone in cutaneous biology. J. Invest. Dermatol. Suppl. **2:** 87–93.
8. BHARDWAJ, R.S., A. SCHWARZ, E. BECHER, K. MAHNKE, Y. ARAGANE, T. SCHWARZ & T.A. LUGER. 1996. Pro-opiomelanocortin-derived peptides induce IL-10 production in human monocytes. J. Immunol. **156:** 2517–2521.
9. VAN DEN BERG, P., J. ROZING & L. NAGELKERKEN. 1991. Two opposing modes of action of beta-endorphin on lymphocytes function. J. Immunol. **72:** 537–543.
10. MCCAIN, H.W., I.B. LAMSTER, J.M. BOZZONE *et al.* 1982. Beta-endorphin modulates human immune activity via non-opiate receptors mechanism. Life. Sci. **81:** 1619–1624.
11. SHAVIT, Y., J.W. LEWIS, G.W. TERMAN, R.P. GALE & J.C. LIEBESKIND. 1984. Opioid peptides mediate the suppressive effect of stress on natural killer cell cytotoxicity. Science. **223:** 188–190.
12. WITZEN, M. & B.A. GILCHREST. 1996. Proopiomelanocortin, its derived peptides, and the skin. J. Invest. Dermatol. **106:** 3–10.
13. SCHAUER, E., F. TRAUTINGER, A. KOCK, A. SCHWARZ, R. BHARDWAJ, M. SIMON, J.C. ANSEL, T. SCHWARZ & T.A. LUGER. 1994. Proopiomelanocortin-derived peptides are synthesized and released by human keratinocytes. J. Clin. Invest. **93:** 2258–2262.
14. TEOFOLI, P., K. MOTOKI, T.M. LOTTI, J. UITTO & A. MAUVIEL. 1997. Proopiomelanocortin (POMC) gene expression by normal skin and keloid fibroblasts in culture: modulation by cytokines. Exp. Dermatol. **6:** 111–115.
15. BOSTON, B.A. & R.D. CONE. 1996. Characterization of melanocortin receptor subtype expression in murine adipose tissue and 3T3-L1 cell line. Endocrinology **137:** 2043–2050.
16. NIIMI, N., D.M. FRANCIS, F. KERMANI, B.F. O'DONNELL, M. HIDE, A. KOBZA-BLACK, R.K. WILNKELMANN, M.W. GREAVES & R.M. BARR. 1996. Dermal mast cell activation by autoantibodies against the high affinity IgE receptor in chronic urticaria. J. Invest. Dermatol. **106:** 1001–1006.
17. KISS, M., M. WLASCHEK, P. BRENNEISEN, G. MICHEL, C. HOMMEL, T.S. LANGE, D. PEUS, L. KEMENY, A. DOBOZY *et al.* 1995. Alpha-melanocyte stimulating hormone induces collagenase/matrix metalloproteinase-1 in human dermal fibroblasts. Biol. Chem. Hoppe Seyler **376:** 425–430.
18. BIGLIARDI, P., M. BIGLIARDI-QI, S. BUECHNER & T. RUFIL. 1998. Expression of mu-opiate receptor in human epidermis and keratinocytes. J. Invest. Dermatol. **111:** 297–301.
19. CASALE, T.B., S. BOWMAN & M. KALINER. 1984. Induction of human cutaneous mast cell degranulation by opiates and endogenous opioid peptides: evidence for opiate and nonopiate receptor participation. J. Allergy Clin. Immunol. **73:** 775–781.

Alpha-Melanocyte-Stimulating Hormone Modulates Activation of NF-κB and AP-1 and Secretion of Interleukin-8 in Human Dermal Fibroblasts

MARKUS BÖHM,[a] URSULA SCHULTE, HENNER KALDEN, AND T.A. LUGER

Department of Dermatology and Ludwig Boltzmann Institute for Cell Biology and Immunobiology of the Skin, University of Münster, Germany

ABSTRACT: Alpha-melanocyte-stimulating hormone (α-MSH) has evolved as a mediator of diverse biological activities in an ever-growing number of non-melanocytic cell types. One mechanism by which α-MSH exerts its effects is modulation of AP-1 and NF-κB. These two transcription factors also play an important role in fibroblasts, in extracellular matrix composition, and in cytokine expression. By use of electric mobility shift assays, we demonstrate that α-MSH (10^{-6} to 10^{-14} M) activates AP-1 in human dermal fibroblasts, whereas coincubation with interleukin-1β (IL-1β) results in suppression of its activation. α-MSH also induces activation of NF-κB but does not modulate DNA binding on costimulation with IL-1β. Since AP-1 and NF-κB are key elements in controlling interleukin-8 (IL-8) transcription, human fibroblasts were treated with α-MSH and IL-1β for 24 hours, and cytokine levels in the supernatants were measured by ELISA. α-MSH alone had little effect, whereas coincubation with IL-1β led to marked downregulation of IL-8 secretion (at most 288 ± 152 ng/mL) when compared to treatment with IL-1β alone (919 ± 157 ng/mL). Our results indicate that α-MSH exerts modulatory effects on the activation of NF-κB and AP-1, and that it can regulate chemokine secretion in human dermal fibroblasts. These effects of α-MSH may have important regulatory functions in extracellular matrix composition, wound healing, or angiogenesis.

INTRODUCTION

Alpha-melanocyte-stimulating hormone (α-MSH) was originally identified as a neuropeptide derived from the pituitary gland. Its main biological function was considered to be one of regulating skin pigmentation in a number of vertebrate species. The biological effects of α-MSH and its receptor, the melanocortin-1 receptor (MC-1R), in melanogenesis, melanocyte proliferation, and coat-color regulation have been well elucidated in numerous studies *in vitro* and *in vivo*.[1–3] There is clear evidence that α-MSH, and other proopiomelanocortin (POMC)-derived peptides such as β-endorphin or adrenocotiocotropin (ACTH), are also generated at extraneu-

---

[a]Address for correspondence: M. Böhm, M.D., Department of Dermatology, Westfälische Wilhelms Universität Von Esmarch-Str. 56, D-48149 Münster, Germany. 49-251-835 8635 (voice); 49-251-835 6522 (fax); bohmm@uni-muenster.de (e-mail).

ral sites where they can exert a plethora of non-pigmentary effects in an ever-growing number of tissues and cell types.[4–6]

It has now been established that human skin, itself, is a source for POMC–derived peptides.[7–11] In undiseased human skin, α-MSH has been detected immunohistochemically, mainly in differentiated keratinocytes; whereas specific immunostaining in melanocytes, Langerhans cells, and some dermal cells was not reported by all investigators.[10] In culture, normal human fibroblasts, melanocytes, and keratinocytes express POMC at the mRNA level[12–14] and the latter two cell types can also secrete α-MSH into the culture media—especially after UVB irradiation.[13,14]. Since melanocytes and keratinocytes express MC-Rs,[15–17] it appears that α-MSH exerts its biological activities in the skin, at least in part, by autocrine and/or paracrine regulatory loops.

With regard to fibroblasts, little is known about the biological significance of POMC–derived peptides and possible expression of melanocortin receptors in these mesenchymal cells. Human dermal fibroblasts, however, are key elements in photoaged skin in which wrinkling is associated with altered extracellular matrix (EM) proteins; namely, collagen and elastin.[18,19] One mechanism through which these actinic changes are thought to accumulate is repetitive induction of interstitial collagenase, gelatinase, and stromelysin—all members of the so-called metallomatrixproteinase (MMP) family.[20,21] α-MSH itself upregulates mRNA expression and activity of interstitial collagenase in human dermal fibroblasts *in vitro*.[22] Thus, UV-induced upregulation of POMC-derived peptides in the epidermis or dermis may represent an effector mechanism by which MMP expression and subsequent EM decomposition by MMP is brought about.

We recently detected specific transcripts for MC-1R in human dermal fibroblasts as shown by RT-PCR.[23] In order to gain more insight into the biological activities of POMC-peptides in human fibroblasts, we examined a number of α-MSH-induced effects, previously reported in other cell types. We show here that α-MSH modulates interleukin-8 (IL-8) secretion and DNA-protein complex formation of two transcription factors, AP-1 and NF-κB, in human dermal fibroblasts in culture.

MATERIAL AND METHODS

Cell Culture

Normal human dermal fibroblasts derived from neonate foreskin were purchased from BioWhittaker (Walkersville, MD), established in culture according to instructions provided by the manufacturer. They were maintained in RPMI 1640 (Boehringer, Ingelheim, Germany) supplemented with 10% fetal calf serum (FCS), 1% glutamine, and 1% penicillin/streptomycin (all from Boehringer) in a humidified atmosphere of 5% CO_2. Cells were used at passages 3 to 8.

Nuclear Extract Generation

Fibroblasts were seeded into petridishes until they became subconfluent. Cells were deprived from FCS by incubating them in Ultraculture medium (Boehringer, Ingelheim) for 24 hours. They were stimulated for 30 minutes with α-MSH

(Bachem, Heidelberg, Germany) at 10^{-6} to 10^{-14} M, rhIL-1β (1 ng/mL; Biozol, Eching, Germany), or both substances, or were left untreated. After rinsing with ice-cold phosphate-buffered saline (PBS), cells were scraped into PBS and centrifuged at 1200 rpm. Cell pellets were subsequently swollen in hypotonic buffer (10 mM HEPES buffer, pH 7.9; 10 mM NaCl; 0.1 mM EDTA; 1 mM DTT; 5% glycerol; 0.5 mM PMSF; 50 mM NaF; 0.1mM sodium vanadate; 10 mM sodium molybdate; 100 μg/mL leupeptin; 4 μg/mL aprotinin, 2 μg/mL chymostatin; 1.5 μg/mL pepstatin; and 1 μg/mL antipain) for 15 minutes on ice. Cell suspensions were briefly vortexed after addition of Nonidet P-40 (Sigma Chemical Co, St. Luis, MO) to a final concentration of 0.5%, and centrifuged at 2000 rpm at 4° for 5 minutes. Supernatants were discarded and the nuclear proteins were extracted from the pellets by incubation in hypertonic buffer (hypotonic buffer with 0.04 M NaCl) for 15 minutes on ice. After centrifugation at 14,000 rpm at 4° for 10 minutes, nuclear proteins in the supernatants were measured by means of the Bio-Rad protein assay. Aliquots were prepared and the samples were stored at −80° until use.

Electric Mobility Shift Assay (EMSA)

The double-stranded oligonucleotides for AP-1 (5′-CGCTTGATGACTCAGC-CGGAA-3′) and NF-κB (5′-AGTTGAGGGGACTTTCCCAGGC-3′) were purchased from Santa Cruz Biotechnology (Santa Cruz, CA). Reactions were performed with 10 μg of nuclear protein, 20 mM HEPES, pH 7.9; 50 mM NaCl; 1 mM EDTA; 1 mM DTT; 5% glycerol and 240 μg/mL bovine serum albumin, 2 μg poly(dI-dC) (Boehringer, Mannheim, Germany) in the presence of 5–10×10^4 cpm of ^{32}P-labeled double-stranded oligonucleotides at 25° for 20 minutes. In some experiments, unlabeled double-stranded oligonucleotides were coincubated in a 50-fold molar excess for competition studies. Electrophoresis was conducted in 5% acrylamide/bisacrylamide (19/1) gels with 25 mM Tris-borate, pH 8.2 and 0.5 mM EDTA at 120 V for 2 h. Gels were dried and autoradiographied at −70° until signals became apparent.

Determination of IL-8

Cells were seeded into six-well tissue culture plates (1.5×10^6 cells per well). Subconfluent monolayer cultures were deprived from FCS, as described above and treated with α-MSH at doses ranging from 10^{-6} to 10^{-18} M, rhIL-1β (1 ng/mL), both agents, or were left untreated. After 24 hours, the supernatants were harvested. They were stored in aliquots at −80° until use. IL-8 was determined by a commercially available ELISA (Biozol). The detection limit for IL-8, according to the manufacturer, was below 2 pg/mL. Duplicate wells were used for all determinations. Mean values and standard errors (SEM) from three independent experiments were calculated. The significance of the data, as compared to the controls from untreated cells, or those treated with IL-1β alone, was assessed by the Student's *t*-test.

RESULTS AND DISCUSSION

It had been previously shown that treatment of B-16 mouse melanoma cells with the synthetic α-MSH analogue [Nle^4, D-Phe^7]α-MSH plus the cAMP-elevating agent isobutylmethylxanthine (IBMX), activated the activating protein-1 (AP-1).[24] AP-1 is a family of transcription factors that specifically bind to the TPA-response element (TRE; TGAG/CTCA) and regulate transcription of TRE containing genes by acting on their promoter.[25] Most MMPs are among the genes that contain such TRE consensus sequences, and the AP-1 site is known to play a dominant role in the transcriptional activation of MMP promoters.[26] Therefore, we attempted to establish whether α-MSH induces activation of AP-1 in human dermal fibroblasts. Cells were deprived from FCS and stimulated with α-MSH at different concentrations ranging from 10^{-6} to 10^{-14} M for 30 minutes. Nuclear extracts were prepared and gel retardation assays (EMSAs) were performed with a labeled oligonucleotide containing the TRE consensus sequence (see FIGURE 1). A single inducible band was detected

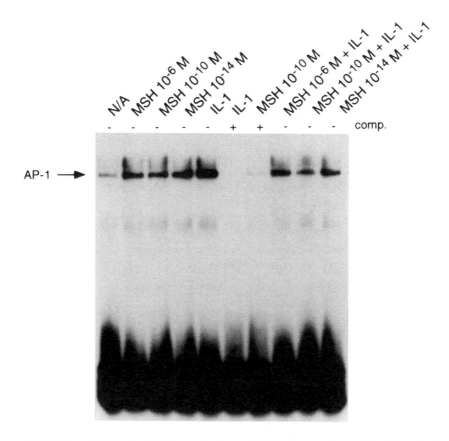

FIGURE 1. Effect of α-MSH on activation of AP-1 in human dermal fibroblasts. Cells were deprived from FCS and stimulated with 10^{-6} to 10^{-14} M α-MSH, as indicated. Unstimulated cells (N/A) served as negative controls, those stimulated with IL-1β (1 ng/mL) were used as positive control. Nuclear extracts were prepared and AP-1 activation was tested as described in the text. Specificity of the AP-1 binding was determined by EMSA in the presence of a 50-fold molar excess of unlabeled AP-1 oligonucleotide (+).

at all α-MSH concentrations tested when compared with unstimulated cells. The latter displayed a weak constitutive DNA-protein complex formation at the same location. Treatment with IL-1β (1 ng/mL) also resulted in one single band whose intensity, however, was stronger than that induced by α-MSH. In order to determine the specificity of the detected DNA protein complexes induced by α-MSH and IL-1β, competition assays with cold oligonucleotides containing TRE in a 50-fold molar excess were performed. These experiments resulted in complete disappearance of the α-MSH– and IL-1β–inducible bands indicating that these DNA-protein complexes contain AP-1 components (FIG. 1). On the other hand, when fibroblasts, were simultaneously treated with α-MSH plus IL-1, activation of AP-1 was markedly suppressed (FIG. 1). This suppressive effect of α-MSH on IL-1–induced activation of AP-1 was most apparent at a concentration of 10^{-10} M. Taken together, these findings strongly suggest that AP-1 in human dermal fibroblasts can be regulated by α-MSH, and that the particular effect of α-MSH appears to be dependent on the presence or absence of a costimulus.

We next analyzed the effect of α-MSH on the activation of NF-κB in human dermal fibroblasts. NF-κB is a ubiquitous transcription factor, that plays a central role in the immune system, by regulating many inflammatory responses through transcriptional activation of certain proinflammatory cytokines, the inducible nitric oxide synthase gene and other genes involved in inflammation.[27] Since EM synthesis in fibroblasts and enzymatic degradation by MMPs are regulated by cytokines, including IL-1, IL-6, transforming growth factor-β (TGF β), or tumor-necrosis factor-α (TGF-α),[28,29] NF-κB necessarily plays an important role in controlling the functional state of dermal fibroblasts. Recently, α-MSH was shown to inhibit NF-κB activation induced by several inflammatory agents including TNF-α, lipopolysaccharide, okadeic acid, and ceramide.[30] Thus, we wondered whether α-MSH also affects activation of NF-κB in human dermal fibroblasts. As tested by EMSA, stimulation of FCS-deprived human dermal fibroblasts with α-MSH for 30 minutes resulted in one strong band, which was abrogated by preincubation with cold oligonucleotide containing the NF-κB consensus site (see FIGURE 2). NF-κB induced by α-MSH was maximal at 10^{-10} M. A similar strong band at the same location was detected after stimulation with IL-1β for 30 minutes and was also abrogated by preincubation with a 50-fold excess of cold oligonucleotide (FIG. 2). In order to check, whether IL-1β–induced NF-κB activation is suppressed by concomitant treatment with α-MSH, nuclear extracts were prepared and analyzed by EMSA. Under the experimental conditions applied, however, we were unable to detect any effect of α-MSH on IL-1β–induced NF-κB activation in fibroblasts (FIG. 2). These findings disagree somewhat with the results of Manna *et al.*,[30] who were unable to detect any inducible effect of α-MSH on NF-κB, but rather observed significant suppression on costimulation with known NF-κB inducers. It is possible that these discrepancies are due to cell-specific differences, or reflect differences in the experimental conditions. We simultaneously treated human fibroblasts with α-MSH and IL-1β for only 30 minutes, whereas Manna and coworkers preincubated α-MSH for up to 24 hours prior to stimulation with inflammatory agents other than IL-1β. It is also possible that deprivation from FCS for 24 hours sensitized human fibroblasts to an inducible effect of α-MSH on

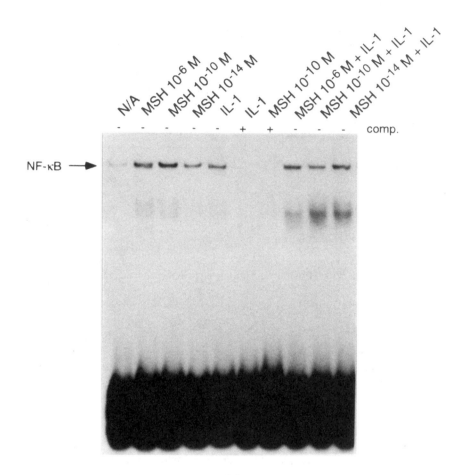

FIGURE 2. Effect of α-MSH on NF-κB activation in human dermal fibroblasts. Cells were deprived from FCS and stimulated with 10^{-6} to 10^{-14} M α-MSH, as indicated. Unstimulated cells (N/A) served as negative control, cells stimulated with IL-1β (1 ng/mL) were used as positive control. Nuclear extracts were prepared and NF-κB activation was tested as described in the text. Specificity of the NF-κB binding was determined by EMSA in the presence of a 50-fold molar excess of unlabeled NF-κB oligonucleotide (+).

NF-κB. Further studies are necessary in order to examine the possible interactions between α-MSH and inflammatory agents in more detail.

Based on the observed effects of α-MSH on AP-1 and NF-κB activation in human dermal fibroblasts, we finally examined the ability of α-MSH to modulate interleukin-8 secretion. Transcription of the IL-8 gene requires activation of the combination of NF-κB and AP-1, or that of NF-κB, and another transcription factor, NF-IL-6.[31] In addition to being a well-characterized chemoattractant for neutrophils and a regulator of angiogenesis, this chemokine has been shown to

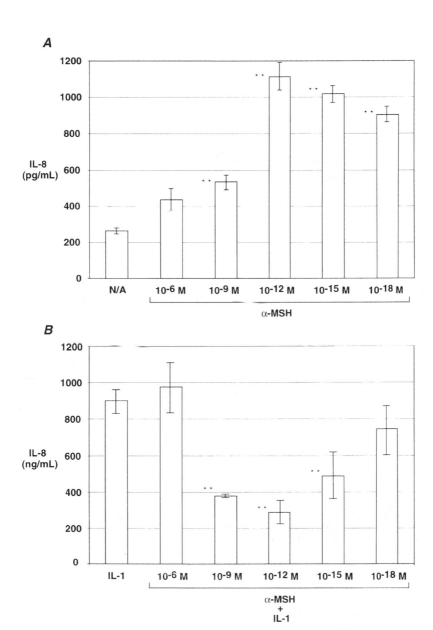

FIGURE 3. IL-8 release by human dermal fibroblasts after stimulation with α-MSH alone and in combination with IL-1β. Cells (1.5×10^6 cells) were deprived from FCS and treated with α-MSH and/or IL-1β, as indicated, for 24 hours. IL-8 in the supernatants was determined by ELISA. (**A**) Effect of α-MSH alone at 10^{-6} to 10^{-18} M on IL-8 secretion as compared to unstimulated cells. (**B**) Effect of α-MSH and IL-1β costimulation as compared to IL-1β alone. Results are expressed as mean ± SEM of three independent experiments. Significance in comparison to the control, **, $p < 0.001$.

increase the percentage of cells lacking focal adhesions consequently promoting primary fibroblasts to acquire a migratory phenotype.[32] We have recently shown that α-MSH upregulated IL-8 release and mRNA expression in transformed human microvascular endothelial cells (HMEC-1).[33] In order to check whether α-MSH has similar effects on human dermal fibroblasts, and to examine whether cytokine-induced IL-8 secretion can be modulated by α-MSH, we analyzed secretion of IL-8 after treating fibroblasts in culture with various doses of α-MSH, alone and in combination with IL-1β for 24 hours. IL-8 in the culture supernatants was determined by ELISA. α-MSH, alone induced a weak, but reproducible and statistically significant, dose-dependent increase of IL-8 release from 0.28 ± 0.03 ng/mL to 1.1 ± 0.2 ng/mL at an α-MSH concentration of 10^{-12} M (see FIGURE 3A). The α-MSH–induced IL-8 release, however, was small in comparison to the prominent effect induced by IL-1β (1 ng/mL), resulting in 919 ± 157 ng/mL (FIG. 3B). Coincubation of IL-1β and α-MSH led to a significant and dose-dependent suppression of the IL-1β–mediated IL-8 release. At an α-MSH dose of 10^{-12} M IL-1β–induced IL-8 release was suppressed to 288 ± 152 ng/mL (FIG. 3B). Taken together, our findings on the modulatory role of α-MSH on IL-8 release by human fibroblasts extend the range of observations on antagonism of α-MSH to the secretion of other proinflammatory cytokines, such as IL-1, IL-6, and TNF-α.[5] Although the bidirectional effects of α-MSH on IL-8 release and AP-1 activation are puzzling at first, it appears that the antiinflammatory effects of this neuropeptide, observed under costimulatory conditions, exceeds the weak inductive effect of α-MSH alone. We suggest, therefore, that α-MSH in the complex regulation of cutaneous inflammatory processes, such as dermal photoaging, wound healing, or angiogenesis, may act as a fine-tuning mediator whose actual contribution to individual cellular responses depends on the presence or absence of other proinflammatory cytokines.

REFERENCES

1. HUNT, G. et al. 1994. Cultured human melanocytes respond to MSH peptides and ACTH. Pigm. Res. **7:** 217–221.
2. ROBBINS, L.S. et al. 1993. Pigmentation phenotypes of variant extension locus alleles result from point mutations that alter MSH receptor function. Cell. **72:** 827–834.
3. ABDEL-MALEK, Z. et al. 1995. Mitogenic and melanogenic stimulation of normal human melanocytes by melanotropic peptides. Proc. Natl. Acad. Sci. USA **92:** 1789–1793.
4. THODY, A.J. et al. 1975. Control of sebaceous gland function in the rat by α-melanocyte-stimulating hormone. J. Endocrinol. **64:** 503–510.
5. LIPTON, J.M. et al. 1997. Antiinflammatory actions of the neuroimmunomodulator α-MSH. Immunol. Today. **18:** 140–145.
6. VAN DER REUT, R. et al. 1992. Stimulation by melanocortins of neurite outgrowth from spinal and sensory neurons in vitro. Peptides **13:** 1109–1115.
7. THODY, A.J. et al. 1983. MSH peptides are present in mammalian skin. Peptides **4:** 813–816.
8. SLOMINSKI, A. et al. 1993. Detection of proopiomelanocortin-derived antigens in normal and pathological human skin. J. Lab. Clin. Med. **122:** 658–666.
9. SLOMINSKI, A. et al. 1995. Proopomelanocortin, corticotropin releasing hormone and corticotropin releasing hormone receptor genes are expressed in human skin. FEBS Lett. **374:** 113–116.

10. WAKAMATSU, K. *et al.* 1997. Characterization of ACTH peptides in human skin and their activation of the melanocortin-1 receptor. Pigm. Cell Res. **10:** 288–297.

11. NAGAHAMA, M. *et al.* 1998. Immunoreactivity of α-melanocyte-stimulating hormone, adrenocorticotrophic hormone and β-endorphin in cutaneous malignant melanoma and benign melanocytic naevi. Brit. J. Dermatol. **138:** 981–985.

12. TEOFOLI, P. *et al.* 1997. Proopiomelanocortin (POMC) gene expression by normal skin and keloid fibroblasts in culture: modulation by cytokines. Exp. Dermatol. **6:** 111–115.

13. SCHAUER, E. *et al.* 1994. Proopiomelanocortin-derived peptides are synthesized and released by human keratinocytes. J. Clin. Invest. **93:** 2258–2262.

14. CHAKRABORTY, A.K. *et al.* 1996. Production and release of proopiomelanocortin (POMC) derived peptides by human melanocytes and keratinocytes in culture: regulation by UVB Biochim. Biophys. Acta **1313:** 130–138.

15. CHAKRABORTY, A. *et al.* 1993. MSH receptors in immortalized human epidermal keratinocytes: a potential mechanism for coordinate regulation of the epidermal-melanin unit. Cell Physiol. **157:** 344–350.

16. HUNT, G. *et al.* 1995. Nle^{4}DPhe^7-α-melanocyte-stimulating hormone increased the eumelanin:phaeomelanin ratio in cultured human melanocytes. J. Invest. Dermatol. **104:** 83–85.

17. CHHAJLANI, V. *et al.* 1992. Molecular cloning and expression of the human melanocyte stimulating hormone receptors cDNA. FEBS Lett. **309:** 417–420.

18. TALWAR, H.S. *et al.* 1995. Reduced type I and type III procollagens in photodamaged adult human skin. J. Invest. Dermatol. **105:** 285–290.

19. LAVKER, R.M. *et al.* 1979. Structural alterations in exposed and unexposed aged skin. J. Invest. Dermatol. **73:** 559–566.

20. FISHER, G.J. *et al.* 1996. Molecular basis of sun-induced premature skin aging and retinoid antagonism. Nature **379:** 335–339.

21. FISHER, G.J. *et al.* 1997. Pathophysiology of premature skin aging induced by ultraviolet light. New Engl. J. Med. **337:** 1419–1428.

22. KISS, M. *et al.* 1995. α-Melanocyte stimulating hormone induces collagenase/metallomatrix proteinase-1 in human dermal fibroblasts. Biol. Chem. Hoppe-Seyler. **376:** 425–430.

23. SCHULTE, U. *et al.* 1998. Evidence for a functional melanocortin receptor on human fibroblasts. Abstract. J. Invest. Dermatol. **110:** 479.

24. ENGLARO, W. *et al.* 1995. Mitogen-activated protein kinase pathway and AP-1 are activated during cAMP-induced melanogenesis in B-16 melanoma cells. J. Biol. Chem. **270:** 24315–24320.

25. MITCHELL, P.J. *et al.* 1989. Transcriptional regulation in mammalian cells by sequence-specific DNA binding proteins. Science **245:** 371–378.

26. BENBOW, U. *et al.* 1997. The AP-1 site and MMP gene regulation: what is all the fuss about? Matrix Biol. **15:** 519–526.

27. SIEBENLIST, U. *et al.* 1994. Structure, regulation and function of NF-κB. Ann. Rev. Cell Biol. **10:** 405–455.

28. CRAWFORD, H.C. *et al.* 1996. Mechanisms controlling the transcription of matrix metalloproteinase genes in normal and neoplastic cells. Enzyme Prot. **49:** 20–37.

29. CHUNG, K.-Y. *et al.* 1996. An AP-1 binding sequence is essential for regulation of the human α2(I) collagen (COL1A2) promoter activity by transforming growth factor-β. J. Biol. Chem. **271:** 3272–3278.

30. MANNA, S.K. *et al.* 1998. α-Melanocyte stimulating hormone inhibits the nuclear factor transcription factor NF-κB activation induced by various inflammatory agents. J. Immunol. **161:** 2873–2880.

31. MUKAIDA, N. *et al.* 1994. Molecular mechanisms of interleukin-8 gene expression. J. Leukocyte Biol. **56:** 554–558.
32. DUNLEVY, J.R. *et al.* 1995. Interleukin-8 induces motile behavior and loss of focal adhesions in primary fibroblasts. J. Cell. Sci. **108:** 311–321.
33. HARTMEYER, M. *et al.* 1997. Human microvascular endothelial cells (HMEC-1) express the melanocortin receptor type 1 and produce increased levels of IL-8 upon stimulation with α-MSH. J. Immunol. **159:** 1930–1937.

Cutaneous Expression of CRH and CRH-R

Is There a "Skin Stress Response System?"

ANDRZEJ T. SLOMINSKI,[a,b] VLADIMIR BOTCHKAREV,[c]
MASHKOOR CHOUDHRY,[d] NADEEM FAZAL,[d] KLAUS FECHNER,[e]
JENS FURKERT,[e] EBERHART KRAUSE,[e] BIRGIT ROLOFF,[e]
MOHAMMAD SAYEED,[d] EDWARD WEI,[f] BLAZEJ ZBYTEK,[g] JOSEF ZIPPER,[e]
JACOBO WORTSMAN,[h] AND RALF PAUS[c]

[b]Department of Pathology, Medical Center, Loyola University, Maywood, Illinois, USA

[c]Department of Dermatology, Charite, Humboldt University, Berlin, Germany

[d]Department of Physiology, Medical Center, Loyola University, Maywood, Illinois, USA

[e]Institute of Molecular Pharmacology, Berlin, Germany

[f]Department of Pharmacology, School of Public Health,
University of California, Berkeley, California, USA

[g]Department of Histology, Medical School of Gdansk, Gdansk, Poland

[h]Department of Medicine, Southern Illinois University, Springfield, Illinois, USA

ABSTRACT: The classical neuroendocrine pathway for response to systemic stress is by hypothalamic release of corticotropin releasing hormone (CRH), subsequent activation of pituitary CRH receptors (CRH-R), and production and release of proopiomelanocortin (POMC) derived peptides. It has been proposed that an equivalent to the hypothalamic–pituitary–adrenal axis functions in mammalian skin, in response to local stress (see Reference 1). To further define such system we used immunocytochemistry, RP-HPLC separation, and RIA techniques, in rodent and human skin, and in cultured normal and malignant melanocytes and keratinocytes. Production of mRNA for CRH-R1 was documented in mouse and human skin using RT-PCR and Northern blot techniques; CRH binding sites and CRH-R1 protein were also identified. Addition of CRH to immortalized human keratinocytes, and to rodent and human melanoma cells induced rapid, specific, and dose-dependent increases in intracellular Ca^{2+}. The latter were inhibited by the CRH antagonist α-helical-CRH(9–41) and by the depletion of extracellular calcium with EGTA. CRH production was enhanced by ultraviolet light radiation and forskolin (a stimulator for intracellular cAMP production), and inhibited by dexamethasone. Thus, evidence that skin cells, both produce CRH and express functional CRH-R1, supports the existence of a local CRH/CRH-R neuroendocrine pathway that may be activated within the context of a *skin stress response system*.

[a]Address for correspondence: Andrzej Slominski M.D., Ph.D., Department of Pathology, Loyola University Medical Center, 2160 First South Avenue, Maywood, IL 60153, USA. 708-327-2613 (voice); 708-327-2620 (fax); aslomin@wpo.it.luc.edu (e-mail)

INTRODUCTION

The most common stressors are environmental in nature. They are represented by solar radiation, biological, and chemical insults. These stressors primarily affect the skin, a strategically located protective barrier. To maintain the integrity of its diverse structures and functional domains, the skin should be able to deal with these external stresses by employing a defense mechanism that is rapid and widely distributed, but is also efficiently self-regulated in intensity and field of activation.[1–3] These local requirements are not met by the systemic stress response system.

The main adaptive response to systemic stresses is activation of the hypothalamic-pituitary-adrenal (HPA) axis.[4–6] This involves production and release of corticotropin–releasing hormone (CRH) followed by production and secretion of POMC peptides, of which the most important is ACTH. ACTH induces production and secretion of the powerful antiinflammatory factor, cortisol. This factor terminates the stress response and attenuates CRH and POMC peptide production. The HPA axis

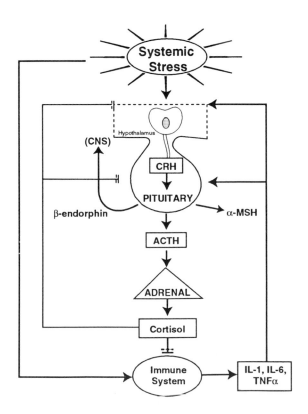

FIGURE 1. Systemic response to stress.

can also be activated by proinflammatory cytokines.[6,7] A representative model is presented illustrated in FIGURE 1.

The POMC–derived ACTH and MSH peptides have long been recognized as exerting marked effects on the skin, stimulating its pigmentary characteristics and probably suppressing the skin immune system (SIS).[2,8–13] Moreover, recent investigations from several laboratories (see References 14–17 and elsewhere in this volume for further details), including our own[18–30] have demonstrated that skin has the capacity to produce CRH and POMC peptides and to express the corresponding receptors. Similar to what is found in the production of these peptides at the central level, cutaneous CRH and POMC production is also modulated by proinflammatory cytokines. Among the proinflammatory cytokines produced by skin cells are interleukin-1 (IL-1), interleukin-6 (IL-6), tumor necrosis factor alpha (TNFα), and interferons (INF). Based on these observations, we have postulated that an equivalent to the hypothalamic–pituitary–adrenal axis might operate locally in the skin, as coordinator and executor of peripheral responses to stress.[1,3] In contrast with the central stress response system, its cutaneous equivalent—which we have called the *skin stress response system* (SSRS)—would involve only locally produced CRH, and POMC messages generated in response to external stressors or proinflammatory cytokines.

GENERAL INFORMATION ON CRH AND CRH-R

The most proximal elements of the HPA axis are CRH and its receptors (CRH-R). The gene for CRH is expressed, not only in the brain, but also in extracranial tissues,[31,32] including normal mammalian skin.[22,23,25,26,28,29] The CRH gene has two exons separated by an intron.[33,34] The first exon encodes most of the 5′-untranslated region in the mRNA, whereas the second exon contains the prohormone sequence and the 3′-untranslated region. CRH transcripts in rodent and human brains are approximately 1.4 and 1.5 Kb, respectively, and those in the testes and adrenals are longer, by about 0.2 and 0.5 Kb, respectively.[33,34] CRH is synthesized as a large 191-amino-acid precursor, from which a final 41-amino-acid CRH-peptide is subsequently cleaved.[31,32]

Receptors for CRH (CRH-R) have been identified in testes, splenic macrophages, lymphocytes, and placenta.[31,32] Two distinct genes, encoding CHR-R, have been cloned; both sharing high sequence homology and belonging to the family of seven-transmembrane-receptors coupled to the Gs signaling pathway.[35–38] Two spliced variants of CHR-R2 have been identified that differ in their amino-terminal domains and anatomical distribution.[37,38] The two main CRH-Rs differ in pharmacological profile and tissue distribution; for example, CHR-R1 is found in the pituitary and brain;[35,36] whereas CHR-R2 is present in the brain, heart, and skeletal muscle.[37,39] Following interaction with CHR-R, the CRH signal is transmitted by transduction into cAMP and calcium-sensitive metabolic pathways.[31,32]

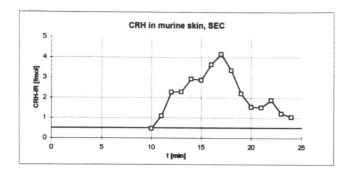

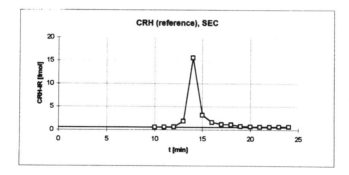

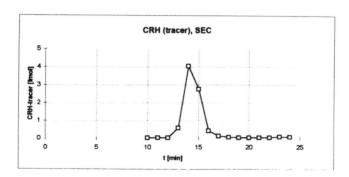

FIGURE 2A. Identification of CRH from mouse skin using acetonitrile/TFA extraction.[28] Size exclusion chromatography was carried out on a Jasco HPLC system with a Spherogel TSK-2000SW column (300 × 7.5 mm) at ambient temperature using isocratic elution. The mobile phase consisted of 0.1% TFA in 30% acetonitrile/70% water (v/v). Eluted fractions of skin extract (*upper panel*) or peptide standard (*middle panel*) were monitored for CRH using a specific RIA assay. CRH in the elution peak coeluted with ^{125}I-Tyr-oCRH tracer (*lower panel*).

EXPRESSION OF CRH AND CRH-R IN SKIN

Mouse Skin

CRH was originally detected in the skin by immunocytochemistry in the C57BL6 mouse; it was found to be localized to the pilosebaceous unit of the hair follicle and the epidermis.[23] These findings were confirmed and further extended by reversed-phase high-performance liquid chromatography (HPLC), in combination with CRH radioimmunoassays (RIA) that employ antibodies to recognize different epitopes.[28] Mouse skin was extracted using acetonitrile/TFA,[28] and CRH was purified by size exclusion chromatography (see FIGURE 2A). The fractions containing CRH were concentrated and further separated by RP-HPLC; the collected fractions were monitored for CRH-IR using antibodies that recognized CRH but not CRH-related peptides.[28] Immunoreactive peaks of CRH and CRH-S-oxide (CRH-SO) eluted

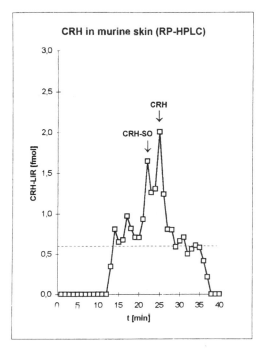

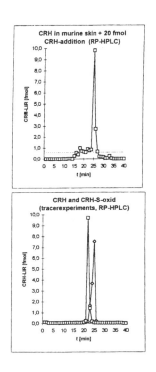

--- RIA detection limit

FIGURE 2B. The combined fractions containing CRH immunoreactivity (IR) (*upper panel* from FIGURE 2A) were further separated by RP-HPLC and the peptide identified as CRH, with a highly specific anti-CRH RIA (see Ref. 28). The CRH- and CRH-S-oxide (CRH-S-oxid)-peaks were identified by tracer experiments (^{125}I-CRH and ^{125}I-CRH-SO tracers) and by addition of 20 fmol CRH to murine skin extracts before RP-HPLC. The CRH and CRH-S-oxide (CRH-SO) immunoreactive peaks (*left panel*) eluted at the same time as corresponding ^{125}I-CRH (25 min) and ^{125}I-CRH-SO (22 min) tracers (*right panel*). Left panel is reprinted, with permission, from Reference 28).

at the same time as ^{125}I-CRH (25 min) and ^{125}I-CRH-SO (22 min) tracers (see
FIGURE 2B). Using an alternate procedure, skin was extracted with detergent and the
solute separated through a SEPCOL-1 column. The fractions obtained were further
separated by RP-HPLC with subsequent RIA for CRH-IR.[25,28] A representative
chromatogram showing the separation of CRH-peptide–related standards is presented in FIGURE 3A. Identification of CRH in anagen VI skin is illustrated in
FIGURE 3B. The highest CRH levels were found in anagen III/IV skin (67 fmols/g of
wet tissue [wt]), and the smallest values were detected in catagen and telogen skin
(36 fmols/g wt).[28] For comparison, serum CRH concentrations in telogen and
anagen III serum were 5.6 and 8.6 fmols/ml, respectively.

CRH distribution in the skin, determined by indirect immunofluorescence,[28]
showed maximal immunoreactivity (CRH-IR) in the basal epidermis, nerve bundles,
and hair follicles (the outer root sheath (ORS) and matrix region of anagen IV/VI
follicles, and their perifollicular neural network). In contrast, catagen and telogen
skin displayed minimal CRH-IR.[28] The specimens with abundant CRH immunoreactivity in the skin were simultaneously associated with comparatively low peptide
concentration in serum. This discrepancy was not due to local synthesis as the source
of CRH, because CRH mRNA was below the limit of detectability (by RT-PCR) at
all stages of the hair cycle (telogen, anagen, and catagen).[23,26] Therefore, it appears
that, by analogy with hypothalamic–pituitary axis, in mice, cutaneous CRH may
reach the skin through descending (afferent) nerves that target well-defined compartments, and thus provide a mechanism to precisely regulate local POMC production.[23] It is also possible that skin cells could express hitherto undetected CRH
variants or a related CRH gene. All of these possibilities can be subjected to experimental testing, such as examination *in situ* of the effect of sectioning descending
nerves fibers, and the molecular cloning of putative variant(s) of CRH related genes.

The gene for the CRH-R1 is expressed in the skin (RT-PCR method) throughout
the entire hair cycle in the C57BL6 mouse,[23] whereas in hairless mice expression of
the CRH-R1 gene was detected in the epidermis (see Figure 4A). In the C57BL6
mice the size of CRH-R1 mRNA transcript, detected by Northern hybridization in
anagen but not telogen skin, was 2.7 Kb.[23] The same transcript was approximately
0.2 Kb shorter in hamster melanoma cells (FIG. 4B). The translational product of
CRH-R1 mRNA, CRH-R1 protein was detected by immunofluorescence in the ORS,
hair matrix, and dermal papilla of anagen VI follicles, as well as in the inner and outer root sheaths of early catagen;[28] the protein was absent or in very low concentration in telogen skin. Taken together, these data suggest that, in mice, both
transcription and translation of CRH-R1 gene are hair-cycle dependent.

Autoradiography of telogen skin sections (see FIGURE 5) showed binding sites
specific for ^{125}I-[Tyr^0]-oCRH in hair follicles, epidermis, and panniculus carnosus
(mostly on dermal muscles).[28] The local density difference in binding sites was
suggestive of receptor heterogeneity; that is, that CRH-R2 in addition to CRH-R1
could also be present.[28] Using RT-PCR, we in fact identified CRH-R2 mRNA (see
FIGURE 6), and tentatively concluded that CRH-R2 predominates in extrafollicular
compartments such as panniculus carnosus.

A potential role for CRH in the regulation of hair growth has been tested in a well
characterized skin organ culture system in which DNA synthesis in epidermal and
dermal compartments correspond predominantly to proliferation of epidermal and

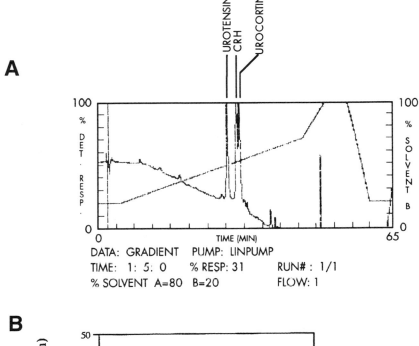

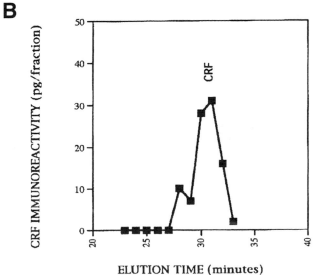

FIGURE 3. RP-HPLC identification of CRH immunoreactivity from anagen VI skin using detergent extraction.[25,28,29]). **A.** Representative separation of urotensin, CRH and urocortin peptide standards. **B.** The skin extracts were purified through SEPCOL-1 columns and elutants combined and separated by RP-HPLC.[25] CRH-1R that was detected by specific anti-CRH RIA, eluted at the same time as the CRH (CRF) standard. Column and conditions were slightly different from those in FIGURE 2B.[28,29]

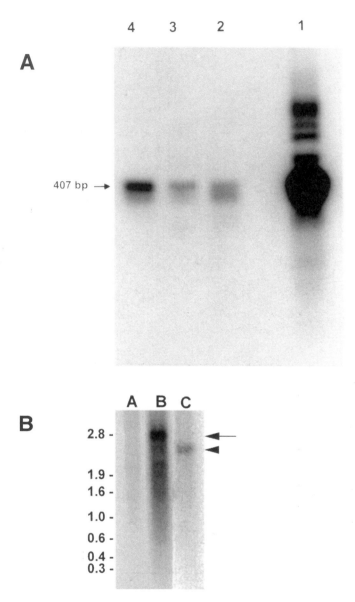

FIGURE 4. Identification of CRH-R1 mRNA in mouse skin. **A.** Detection of CRH-R1 mRNA in the epidermis of hairless mice. RT-PCR amplification and Southern hybridization were performed as previously described.[26] Poly (A⁺) mRNA (0.2 μg per samples) isolated from the epidermis of hairless mice was a gift of Dr. LaDonna Wood (VA Hospital, San Francisco). Murine pituitary control, 1; murine epidermis, 2–4. **B.** Detection of CRH-R1 mRNA using and CRH-R1 cDNA (gift from Dr. DeVita) in anagen VI mouse skin and hamster melanoma cells. Northern hybridization technique and mRNA (2 μg of poly(A⁺)), were used for assay.[26] Size markers (Kb) are on the left; *telogen, A;* anagen VI, *B;* AbC-1 hamster melanoma, *C. Arrow* and *arrowhead* represent 2.7 and 2.5 Kb CRH-R1 transcripts, respectively.

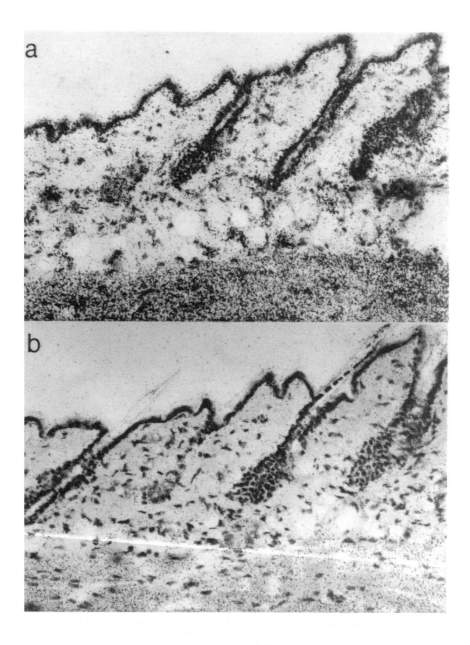

FIGURE 5. Autoradiographic distribution of CRH-binding sites (*dark grains*) in telogen mouse skin.[28] Total binding with 0.1 nM [125]I-[Tyr[0]]-*o*CRH is presented in **panel a,** and nonspecific binding determined in the presence of 1 μM of unlabeled *o*CRH is shown in **panel b.**

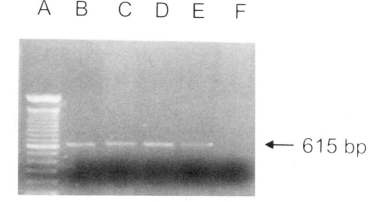

FIGURE 6. Identification of CRH-R2 mRNA in mouse skin. The sequence of primers and conditions for RT-PCR amplification (30 cycles) of a 615-bp-fragment, representative of the CRH-R2 segment common to human and mouse, followed those described by Rodriguez-Linares *et al.*[42] Note that the primers do not differentiate alpha from beta variants of the CRH-R2 gene. DNA ladder: *A*, mouse brain; *B*, anagen III; *C*, anagen IV; *D*,, anagen VI; *E*, control; *F*, no DNA template.

follicular keratinocytes.[40,41] Addition of CRH was found to stimulate DNA synthesis in epidermal keratinocytes of telogen skin and anagen IV skin, without measurable effect in the dermal compartment (see TABLE 1). In anagen II, CRH showed an opposite effect, inhibiting DNA synthesis in epidermis and stimulating it in the dermal compartment (TABLE 1). These results suggest a strong hair-cycle restriction for the expression of such CRH phenotypic effects as epidermal and follicular keratinocyte proliferation. Thus, expression of CRH related receptors determines that exogenously applied CRH may have variable effects depending on the cellular population targeted, and on the hair-cycle phase. Factors contributing to the effect of exogenous CRH include the prevailing endogenous levels of CRH-related molecules, and of POMC peptides.

Human Skin

CRH has been detected by immunocytochemistry in the epidermis, hair follicles, dermal blood vessels, skeletal muscle, and nerve bundles (see FIGURE 7). That CRH peptide was indeed present in human skin was conclusively demonstrated by using RP-HPLC separation, followed by monitoring of the eluted fractions with specific anti-CRH RIA.[25,29] From our studies we concluded that CRH peptide is present in facial skin, human melanocytes, HaCaT keratinocytes, squamous cell carcinoma, and melanoma cells. Moreover, expression of CRH protein was accompanied by the expression of CRH mRNA, since RT-PCR demonstrated the predicted 413-bp product representative of the CRH exon-2 transcript that hybridized to human CRH cDNA, whereas it was absent in control RNA amplified without RT.[22,25,29] Northern blot hybridization with human CRH cDNA showed a CRH mRNA transcript 1.5-Kb

TABLE 1. Effect of CRH on ^{3}H-thymidine incorporation in murine skin organ culture[a]

Skin compartment	Epidermis				Dermis			
CRH concentration (mol/l)	0	1×10^{-11}	1×10^{-9}	1×10^{-7}	0	1×10^{-11}	1×10^{-9}	1×10^{-7}
Telogen ($n = 16$)	100 ± 4.2	110.3 ± 8.4	120.2 ± 8.8*	103.6 ± 4.6	100 ± 25	118.2 ± 27.6	124.2 ± 30	89 ± 22.2
Anagen II ($n = 5$)	100 ± 3.1	120.4 ± 18.5	92.4 ± 7.2	68.1 ± 5.6*	100 ± 16.3	151.7 ± 8.4*	131.9 ± 25.7	109.2 ± 11.2
Anagen IV ($n = 15$)	100 ± 6.8	134.6 ± 10.5**	105.5 ± 7.5	130.9 ± 7.8*	100 ± 9.4	77.2 ± 6.8	83.7 ± 7.1	86.8 ± 9.3

[a]NOTES: Organ culture methodology and measurement of incorporation of ^{3}H-thymidine into epidermal/dermal compartment were performed as previously described.[40,41] Skin punches were cultured in William's E media in the presence of different concentrations of CRH and ^{3}H-thymidine (1 μCi/ml) for 20 h. Epidermal and dermal segments were separated, and incorporation of ^{3}H-thymidine was measured by liquid scintillation spectrometry. Data are presented as percent of control (no CRH added) from the representative experiment. CPM in epidermis control were: telogen, 584; anagen II, 20450; and anagen IV, 2151. In dermis CPM were: telogen, 1219; anagen II, 6685; and anagen IV, 3914. Each data point represents the mean ± SEM. Statistical analysis was performed with one-way ANOVA, fixed effects (Statistica, Statsoft, Tulsa, OK). The significance of differences between mean values of control and CRH treatment were tested by the *post hoc* LSD test. *$p < 0.05$; **$p < 0.01$

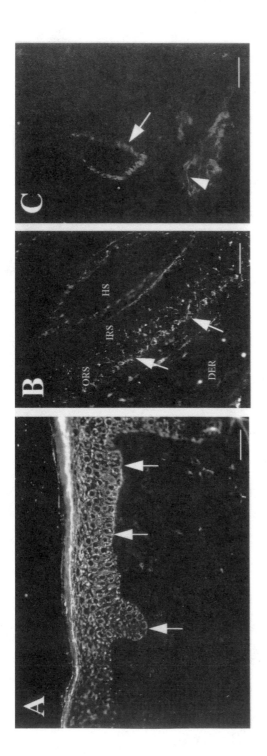

FIGURE 7. CRH-like immunoreactivity (CRH-LIR) in human scalp skin. Cryostat sections of normal human scalp skin were stained with antiserum against CRH. **A.** CRH-IR expression in basal, spinosum, and granular layers of epidermis (*arrows*). **B.** CRH-IR expression in the hair follicle outer root sheath (*arrows*). **C.** CRH-IR expression in blood vessel (*arrow*) and dermal nerve fibers (*arrowhead*). Abbreviations: DER, dermis, HS, hair shaft; IRS and ORS, inner and outer root sheath. *Scale bars:* 50 μm. CRH-IR was determined in acetone-fixed cryostat sections using rabbit antiserum against CRH (Euro-Diagnostica, Malmö, Sweden; 1:50). Specimens were incubated overnight at room temperature, and TRITC-conjugated goat-anti-rabbit IgG was used as secondary antibodies.[28]

long.[29] Studies of regulation control of CRH peptide production showed that it was stimulated by ultraviolet radiation (UV-B, wavelength 280–320 nm) and by agents that raise intracellular cAMP such as forskolin. However, it was inhibited by dexamethasone.[25,29] Interestingly, despite significant changes in CRH peptide production, the level of the corresponding CRH mRNA was similar under each of the conditions tested.

As well as CRH peptide and its mRNA, we also identified CRH-R1 mRNA *in situ* using RT-PCR followed by Southern blot hybridization in biopsy specimens from normal human scalp, compound nevus, basal cell carcinoma, and perilesional facial skin.[22,29] This was associated with expression of the CRH-R1 gene, detected in cultured normal and malignant keratinocytes and melanocytes.[22,29]

CRH Receptors in Cultured Skin Cells

Receptors for CRH were detected and characterized in established cell lines of human and hamster melanoma, and in HaCaT human keratinocytes. Specific binding sites for CRH were expressed in melanoma and HaCaT cells (see FIGURE 8), in which CRH and its related peptides sauvagine and urocortin induced rapid and significant increases in intracellular Ca^{2+} (see FIGURE 9). The effect was considered to be specific, since other neuropeptides that also interact with G protein-linked receptors showed either no effect (β-endorphin) or minimal (α-MSH and ACTH), albeit detectable, effect on melanoma cells (see FIGURE 10). ACTH and α-MSH showed no Ca^{2+} effect on HaCaT cells. Moreover, L-DOPA, a putative cutaneous neurohormone,[44–46] showed no effect on intracellular Ca^{2+} even at high concentrations (10^{-7}–10^{-4} M, not shown). On the other hand CRH produced a potent and dose dependent Ca^{2+} stimulation, already detectable at concentrations as low as 10^{-12} M and 10^{-10} M in human and hamster melanomas, respectively.[30] The induction of intracellular Ca^{2+} accumulation by CRH was inhibited by the CRH antagonist α-helical-CRH(9–41) and by depletion of extracellular calcium using EGTA.[30] Addition of CRH was associated with important phenotypic-effects; namely, the stimulation of cellular proliferation in human, but not in hamster, melanoma cells (see FIGURE 11).

The significance of CRH in cutaneous biology is underscored by our data since they show that melanoma cells and HaCaT keratinocytes express CRH binding sites, that interaction of CRH with those binding sites results in rapid increase in the intracellular calcium concentration, and that this sequence is associated with a measurable phenotypic effect on cell proliferation. Although neither the nature of those receptors, nor their mechanism of signal transduction, have yet been determined; the detection of CRH-R1 mRNA by RT-PCR in human melanoma cells[29] and by Northern hybridization in hamster melanoma (FIG. 4B) suggests that both cell lines express CRH-R1 or CRH-R1 variants. Moreover, the development of rapid, dose-dependent, and specific increases in intracellular Ca^{2+}, and the inhibition of this process by the antagonist α-helical-CRH(9–41), and by the EGTA induced extracellular calcium depletion, all suggest that transduction of CRH signal is coupled, at least in part, to activation of Ca-channels. The current research challenges in this area are: (1) To determine whether other signal transduction pathways, such as those involving adenylate cyclase, phospholipase C, or phospholipase A, are also activated by cutaneous CRH receptors. (2) To assign specific phenotypic effects that are linked to

Binding of CRH in cultured cells

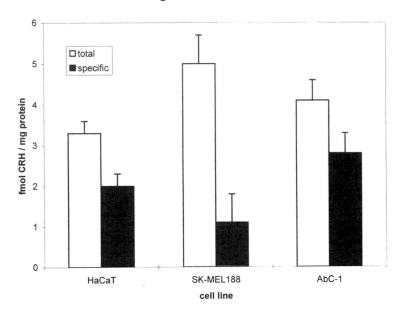

FIGURE 8. Identification of CRH binding sites in melanoma and HaCaT cells. The binding of 1 nM (2-[^{125}I-His32)-CRH (Amersham) was performed at 2–4°C (hamster melanoma and HaCaT cells) or at 12°C (human melanoma cells), in 24-well plates containing 300,000 cells in serum free Ham's F-10, in the absence (total binding) or presence of 1 μM CRH (nonspecific binding) for 90 min. The plates were washed thee times with serum free media. Cells were dissolved in 1 N NaOH and bound radioactivity was counted in a gamma counter. The specific binding is defined as the difference between total and nonspecific binding. The data represent mean ± SD (n = 2 or 3) of fmols of ^{125}I-His-CRH bound per mg protein. The specific binding (fmols) of CRH per 300,000 cells was 0.24 ± 0.03, 0.04 ± 0.01, and 0.05 ± 0.01, for HaCaT, human (SK-MEL188), and hamster (AbC-1) melanoma cells, respectively. The conditions of cell culture were as described previously.[28, 43]

stimulation of the receptors and activation of signal transduction systems. (3) To determine whether the same cells are able to coexpress variants of CRH-R1 and CRH-R2 receptors, thus implying that CRH receptor forms that are highly specific for cutaneous cells and are yet to be cloned, may exist.

CRH may also have a role in skin pathophysiology, since it has shown clear anti-inflammatory effects in models of tissue injury.[47–49] For example, in a rat with thermally-injured skin, injection of CRH (10–50 μg/kg), subcutaneously or intravenously, suppresses over 50% of the local fluid accumulation, independently of HPA axis function. The mechanism for this antiedemic action is apparently the suppression of the attracting force (negative interstitial fluid pressure) that develops in traumatized tissue. Even when administered locally, CRH still demonstrates striking

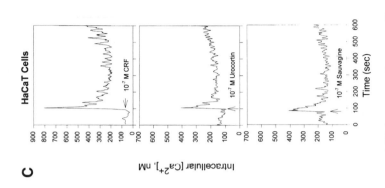

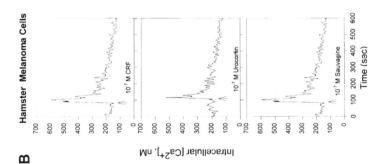

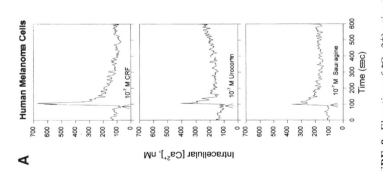

FIGURE 9. Elevation of [Ca 2+]_i stimulated by CRH (CRF), urocortin and sauvagine in (**A**) human and (**B**) hamster melanoma cells, and in (**C**) HaCaT keratinocytes. All measured by fura-labeling at the time indicated by the *arrow*. The measurements of [Ca^{2+}]_i were performed by using methods described previously.[30] Briefly, cells were loaded with Fura-2 and the fluorescence signals after stimulation of the peptide with 10^{-7} M, were recorded using Hitachi Spectrofluorometer at excitation wavelengths of 340 and 380 nm. The emission was measured at 540 nm. An elevation in [Ca^{2+}]_i occurring within seconds after the addition of peptide was used for calcium analysis.

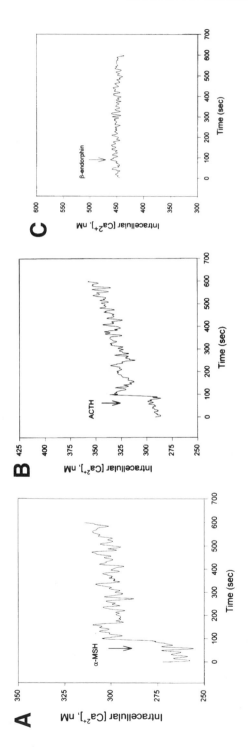

FIGURE 10. Minimal elevation of $[Ca^{2+}]_i$ in human melanoma cells after stimulation with POMC peptides. Cells were stimulated with **A**, 10^{-7} M of α-MSH; **B**, 10^{-7} M of ACTH; or **C**, 10^{-7} M of β-endorphin. Changes in $[Ca^{2+}]_i$ were measured by fura-labeling at times indicated by the *arrows*.

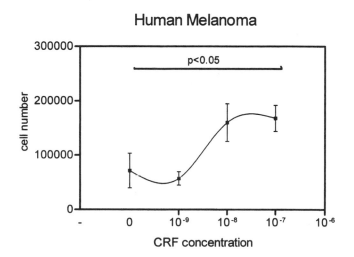

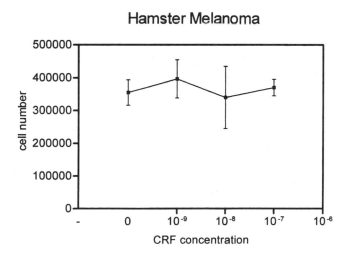

FIGURE 11. Effect of CRH on cell proliferation. 100,000 cells were seeded in six well-plates in 1 ml media composed of Ham's F-10 plus 2.5% fetal bovine serum (FBS) (human SKMEL-188 and hamster ABC-1 melanoma cells). The media were changed every day and the listed concentrations (mols/l) were added every 12 hours. After three days cells were detached by treatment with 0.25% trypsin and counted in hematocytometer. The data represent mean ± SD ($n = 3$).

antiinflammatory effects. McLoon and Wirtschafter[48] found in rabbits and monkeys, that pretreatment of the eyelid with CRH (0.075 or 0.15 mg) reduced the severity of doxorubicin-induced inflammation and accelerated wound-healing. In addition to the antiinflammatory effects, CRH displays antinociceptive actions.[49]

HYPOTHESIS

By analogy with the response to systemic stress, mediated by the neuroendocrine system and modulated by the immune system (FIG. 1), we propose that an equivalent structural organization (possible evolutionary continuum) operates in the skin as a peripheral defense against local stress (see FIGURE 12). We suggest that the response

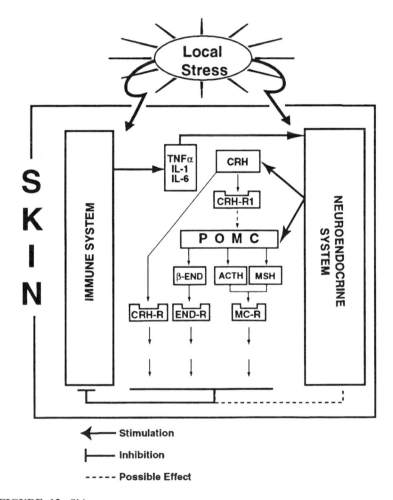

FIGURE 12. Skin stress response system.

to stressor agents by this skin neuroendocrine system (SNS) are mediated via production of CRH and POMC peptides, and modulated by the local skin immune system (SIS). Signals originating in the latter and represented by proinflammatory cytokines perhaps stimulate production of CRH and POMC peptides. In turn, the signals generated by the interaction of CRH, ACTH, MSH, and β-endorphin, with their corresponding receptors, counteract the effect of local stress. As well as modifying skin phenotype, the neuroendocrine peptides and/or, possibly, locally produced steroids, might have regulatory function to inhibit SIS and SNS activity through a feedback mechanism.

In support of the above model, we have the enhancement of CRH production by SNS-stimulation with physical energy (electromagnetic and thermal), chemical or biological insults, or signal molecules dispatched by SIS (FIG. 12). Therefore, CRH-activating CRH-R1, CRH-R2, and other putative members of the CRH-R family, could determine the local production of POMC peptides, and ultimately regulate skin functions necessary for neutralizing the triggering stress. Thus, the flow of information contained in the cutaneous response to stress could be arranged hierarchically, from CRH through CRH-R1, resulting in activation of POMC peptide production and corresponding activation of the respective receptors for these peptides (FIG. 12). Such an organization of signal transduction would provide a high degree of precision in the promotion of desirable phenotypic effects. An alternative, and perhaps less sensitive pathway could involve a direct (distal) activation of POMC production without participation of CRH and CRH-R1 (FIG. 12).

DISCUSSION

The data presented and reviewed in this paper show that mammalian skin does produce CRH peptide locally and that it expresses functional CRH receptors. Since molecular analyses demonstrate expression of CRH-R1 and CRH-R2 mRNA, it is possible that both types of receptor operate in the skin. In this respect, Theoharides *et al.*,[50] observed that skin mast cells express CRH-R1, that CRH induces their degranulation, and that the effect is specific, dose-dependent and accompanied by increased vascular permeability. Further support for the functional activity of CRH-R is the reported antiinflammatory effects of topical or systemic application of CRH to cutaneous or mucosal tissue[47–49] and direct hypotensive effect on vascular smooth muscle.[51]

Following the detection of MSH peptides in mammalian skin[52] several laboratories observed expression of the POMC gene and production of multiple POMC derived peptides such as ACTH, MSH, β-endorphin, and their variants (see References 1–3, 14–23, 26, 27, 53, 54, and elsewhere in this volume). Evidence for the trascription and translation of the POMC gene in normal mammalian skin was first obtained in C57BL6 mice.[19,20] In subsequent experiments it was shown that POMC-like immunoreactivity was frequently present in lesional and nonlesional human skin;[21] and that POMC mRNA was detectable in human skin biopsy specimens.[22] Furthermore, the production of POMC peptides in keratinocytes and melanocytes was found to be under regulatory control,[54] being stimulated by UVB, selected cytokines, and by disease processes.[1–3,14–16,21,23,53] Cutaneous receptors for POMC peptides were found to be present in melanocytes, keratinocytes, cells of SIS, and endothelial cells.[3,8–12,55–57] A functional activity for POMC peptides was also established. For example, MSH peptides in addition to regulating skin pigmentation[3,8–12] can also modify other cutaneous functions, such immune activity and keratinocyte differentiation.[11,56,57]

The evidence available from studies in mammalian skin documents the presence of elements of the postulated upper or regulatory arm of the SSRS (e.g., CRH and its functional receptors), of the lower or regulatory/executive arm (e.g., POMC derived ACTH, MSH, and endorphins), of their corresponding receptors, and of their capability to stimulate specific signal transduction pathways (FIG. 12).

We previously proposed a model whereby cutaneous stress would be managed primarily at the local level through a complex highly structured organization.[1,3] According to this scheme, stress would trigger multiple pathways, including local production of proinflammatory cytokines, stimulation of the CRH signal, and production of POMC-derived messages. This response would be susceptible to modulation (attenuation) through feedback-inhibition by a cortisol/corticosterone-like factor after restoring and/or stabilizing peripheral homeostasis.[1,24] The local effects of exogenous dexamethasone most definitively support this concept, since it inhibits POMC gene expression in murine skin[26] and CRH peptide production in cultured malignant keratinocytes and melanocytes.[29] Within the same context, our laboratory has detected the ACTH receptor in human skin and also the expression of genes that code for enzymes involved in steroid biosynthesis.[24] Currently we are testing for the actual local production of the postulated negative signal molecules—glucocorticoids.

To reiterate, the skin is exposed to multiple physical, chemical, and biological stressors that raise the need for an efficient mode of recruiting local defense mechanisms to allow for rapid reestablishment of tissue homeostasis. Therefore, our postulation of restricted, differential, and highly-regulated cutaneous expression of the CRH and POMC genes, with production of multifunctional CRH and POMC-derived peptides represents a particularly appropriate response.[1–3,13] Certainly, availability of such an optional stress-response mechanism would be a far more economical, and, would provide an effective alternative for containing localized disturbances of homeostasis, than reliance on the systemic structures (HPA axis).[1,3] Thus, in contrast to the systemic HPA axis which set, a stress response mode that abruptly affects functions in the entire organism, its cutaneous equivalent would be mobilized solely in the periphery and compartmentally restricted to a single organism—the skin. That the SSRS may be also involved in cutaneous pathology is further implied by the observed overexpression of POMC products in selected skin diseases and that could reflect a compensatory cutaneous response to unidentified stressors.[1,3] In this context the potential action of SSRS could be related to the known immunosuppressive effects of CRH, ACTH, MSH, and β-endorphin; and the analgesic properties of endorphins. Local release of CRH and POMC products could, therefore, represent an attempt to counterbalance the proinflammatory effects of cytokine and other chemical messengers generated in hyperproliferative and inflammatory skin diseases.[1,3] During oncogenesis, expression of the same markers could simply represent random derepression of the CRH and POMC genes.[1,3,18,21,22,53] Locally generated "hypothalamic-pituitary" hormones, as integral components of tissue homeostasis-maintaining mechanisms may, therefore, play an important role in skin physiology and pathology.[1-3,13]

The skin, with its extensive vascular and afferent and efferent neural networks, is in a unique position to communicate the surrounding environment to the rest of the body, complementing the function of the sensory organs. Therefore, the potential for a systemic effect of SSRS signals originating in stimulated or diseased skin raises some intriguing possibilities. For example, locally produced chemical messengers could be utilized *in situ,* targeted for delivery to distant organs through the vascular network, or transmitted centrally via the afferent neural network; all in order to preserve homeostasis.[1] This could help explain the well-documented observation of increased levels of circulating MSH and ACTH in horses and humans exposed to sunlight or whole-body UVB irradiation.[58,59] The same stimulus (high-intensity UV) stimulates production and secretion of ACTH, α-MSH,[14,54] and CRH[23] in cultured melanocytes and keratinocytes. Therefore, activation of the local cutaneous CRH–POMC axis could contribute to the systemic response to stress by the entire organism, depending on the surface area, location, and magnitude of intensity of tissue damage.[1,3]

Since the skin will not rescue the organism after the destruction of the pituitary or adrenals, cutaneous coverage of systemic requirements is unlikely. However, although the cutaneous SSRS does not replace the HPA axis, it can still react to peripheral stresses in the total absence of central stress responses, or with only minor central activation. Therefore, any potential systemic effects in response to primary peripheral, rather than central, stress will become especially manifest when cutaneous SSRS is unable to neutralize local damage because of its magnitude or complexicity. In such cases, following release by destruction of, or direct secretion from, skin cells the systemic circulation may contain cutaneously-derived CRH, endorphins, MSH, ACTH, and related local peptides. These could potentially affect the function of other organs, including endocrine glands such as the adrenals. This putative interaction between local and global stress response is a new frontier for research into the complexities of interorgan communication.[1-3]

PERSPECTIVE

The proposed model has strong physiologic implications by virtue of introducing a new element in the "fine-tuning" of a response to noxious agents. It also has pathologic and therapeutic relevance for inflammatory skin diseases with their attendant reactive responses; that is, the different forms of alopecia, and pigmentary disorders. In this respect our investigations are proceeding actively in a search for effectors that are able to regulate the local equivalent of the HPA-axis in order to suppress cutaneous inflammation, stimulate the skin pigmentary system,[1-3,13] and promote hair growth/regrowth.[13,60] This could be achieved by the development of small easily deliverable molecules for topical application and absorption, so as to regulate CRH or POMC peptide production or the activity of the corresponding receptors and achieve the desirable phenotypic effects. Furthermore, gene cloning of additional members of the CRH-R and CRH related peptides family that are specific for skin may become an exciting area. Our own data[22,23,28,29] already suggest their existence.

Finally, transfection or delivery of CRH or POMC genes into the epidermis or hair follicle, in the chosen constructs, should allow precisely regulated production (overproduction) of CRH or POMC peptides. This could represent a whole new paradigm for the treatment of skin diseases that would combine genetic and pharmacological modalities such as cotransfection with specific convertases—PC1 and PC2— to shift the processing of POMC into specific forms of MSH, ACTH, or endorphin. Thus, transfection into the epidermal genome of the main genes coding for the HPA axis, cloned under promoters responding to small molecules that can cross skin-barrier layers, may revolutionize the therapy of skin diseases; and potentially, of systemic disorders that have a significant cutaneous component.

CONCLUSION

A local CRH-CRH-R signaling system may operate as an important neuroendocrine pathway that regulates skin functions. In the context of defense against cutaneous stressors, activation of local POMC peptide production would elicit anatomical and functional tissue reaction, a process that would be terminated by glucorticoids of systemic (adrenals) or skin origin.

ACKNOWLEDGMENTS

We thank Drs. J. Curry and M. Dahiya for RT-PCR amplification of CRH-R2 fragments shown in FIGURE 6. The work was supported by Grants IBN-9405242 and IBN-9604364 from National Science Foundation, LU#9178 from Bane Charitable Trust (AS), Pa345/6-1 from Deutsche Forschunsgemeinschaft, NMBF 011ZZ9508, and Wella AG, Dermstadt (RP).

REFERENCES

1. SLOMINSKI, A. & M. MIHM. 1996. Potential mechanism of skin response to stress. Int. J. Dermatol. **35:** 849–851.
2. SLOMINSKI, A. & J. PAWELEK. 1998. Animals under the sun: effects of ultraviolet radiation on mammalian skin. Clin. Dermatol. **16:** 503–515.
3. SLOMINSKI, A. et al. 1993. On the potential role of proopiomelanocortin in skin physiology and pathology. Mol. Cell. Endocrinol. **93:** C1–C6.
4. McCUBBIN, J.A. et al. 1991. Stress, Neuropeptides, and Systemic Disease. Academic Press, San Diego.
5. AUTELITANO, D.J. et al. 1989. Hormonal regulation of POMC gene expression. Annu. Rev. Physiol. **51:** 715–726.
6. FUKATA, J. et al. 1993. Cytokines as mediators in the regulation of the hypothalamic-pituitary-adrenocortical function. J. Endocrinol. Invest. **16:** 141–145.
7. BLALOCK, J.E. 1989. Molecular basis for bidirectional communication between the immune and the neuroendocrine system. Physiological Rev. **69:** 1–69.
8. LERNER, A.B. & J. McGUIRE. 1961. Effect of alpha- and beta-melanocyte stimulating hormones on the skin color of man. Nature **189:** 176–179.
9. EBERLE, A.N. 1988. The Melanotropins: Chemistry, Physiology and Mechanism of Action. S. Karger Publ., New York.

10. PAWELEK, J. *et al.* 1992. Molecular cascades in UV-induced melanogenesis: a central role for melanotropins? Pigment Cell Res. **5:** 34–356.
11. LUGER, T.A. *et al.* 1998. Cutaneous immunomodulation and coordination of skin stress responses by alpha-melanocyte-stimulating hormone. Ann. N.Y. Acad. Sci. **830:** 381–394.
12. SLOMINSKI, A. *et al.* 1992. Melanotropic activity of gamma MSH peptides in melanoma cells. Life Sci. **50:** 1103–1108.
13. SLOMINSKI, A. & R. Paus. 1993. Melanogenesis is coupled to murine anagen: Toward new concepts for the role of melanocytes and the regulation of melanogenesis in hair growth. J. Invest. Dermatol. **101:** 90S–97S.
14. CHAKRABORTY, A. *et al.* 1996. Production an release of proopiomelanocortin (POMC)-derived peptides by human melanocytes and keratinocytes in culture: Regulation by UVB. Biochim. Biophys. Acta **1313:** 130–138.
15. WINZEN, M. *et al.* 1996. Proopiomelanocortin gene product regulation in keratinocytes. J. Invest. Dermatol. **106:** 673–678.
16. WAKAMATSU, K. *et al.* 1997. Characterization of ACTH peptides in human skin and their activation of the melanocortin-1 receptor. Pigment Cell Res. **10:** 288–297.
17. CAN, G. 1998. Identification and sequencing of a putative variant of proopiomelanocortin in human epidermis and epidermal cells in culture. J. Invest. Dermatol. **111:** 485–491.
18. SLOMINSKI, A. 1991. POMC gene expression in hamster and mouse melanoma cells. FEBS Lett. **291:** 165–168.
19. SLOMINSKI, A. *et al.* 1991. Proopiomelanocortin expression and potential function during induced hair growth in C57BL6 mouse. Ann. N.Y. Acad. Sci. **642:** 459–462.
20. SLOMINSKI, A. *et al.* 1992. Proopiomelanocortin expression in the skin during induced hair growth in mice. Experientia **48:** 50–54.
21. SLOMINSKI, A. *et al.* 1993. Detection of the proopiomelanocortin-derived antigens in normal and pathologic human skin. J. Lab. Clin. Med. **122:** 658–666.
22. SLOMINSKI, A. *et al.* 1995. Proopiomelanocortin, corticotropin releasing hormone and corticotropin releasing hormone receptor genes are expressed in human skin. FEBS Lett. **374:** 113–116.
23. SLOMINSKI, A. *et al.* 1996. The expression of proopiomelanocortin (POMC) and of corticotropin releasing hormone receptor (CRH-R) genes in mouse skin. Biochim. Biophys. Acta **1289:** 247–251.
24. SLOMINSKI, A. *et al.* 1996. ACTH receptor, CYP11A1, CYP17 and CYP21A2 genes are expressed in skin. J. Clin. Endocrinol. Metab. **81:** 2746–2749.
25. SLOMINSKI, A. *et al.* 1996. UVB stimulates production of corticotropin releasing factor (CRF) by human melanocytes. FEBS Lett. **399:** 175–176.
26. ERMAK, G. & A. SLOMINSKI 1997. Production of POMC-, CRH-, ACTH-, and α-MSH-receptor mRNA and expression of tyrosinase gene in relation to hair cycle and dexamethasone treatment in the C57BL6 mouse skin. J. Invest. Dermatol. **108:** 160–167.
27. FURKERT, J. *et al.* 1997. Identification and measurement of β-endorphin levels in the skin during induced hair growth in mice. Biochim. Biophys. Acta **1336:** 315–322.
28. ROLOFF, B. *et al.* 1998. Hair cycle-dependent expression of corticotropin releasing factor (CRF) and CRF receptors (CRF-R) in murine skin. FASEB J. **12:** 287–297.
29. SLOMINSKI, A. *et al.* 1998. Characterization of corticotropin releasing hormone (CRH) in human skin. J. Clin. Endocrinol. Metab. **83:** 1020–1024.
30. FAZAL, N. *et al.* 1998. Effect of CRF and related peptides on calcium signaling in human and rodent melanoma cells. FEBS Lett. **435:** 187–190.
31. ORTH, D.N. 1992. Corticotropin-releasing hormone in humans. Endocrine Rev. **13:** 164–191.

32. OWENS, M.J. & C.B. NEMEROFF 1991. Physiology and pharmacology of corticotropin releasing factor. Pharmacol. Rev. **43:** 425–473.
33. SHIBAHARA, S. *et al.* 1983. Isolation and sequence analysis of the human corticotropin-releasing factor precursor gene. EMBO J. **2:** 775–779.
34. THOMPSON, R.L. 1987. Rat corticotropin-releasing hormone gene: sequence and tissue-specific expression. Mol. Endocrinol. **1:** 363–390.
35. VITA, N. 1993. Primary structure and functional expression of mouse pituitary and human corticotropin releasing factors receptors. FEBS Lett. **335:** 1–5.
36. CHEN, R. *et al.* 1993. Expression cloning of human corticotropin-releasing factor receptor. Proc. Natl. Acad. Sci. USA **90:** 8967–8971.
37. KISHIMOTO, T. *et al.* 1995. A sauvagine/corticotropin-releasing factor receptor expressed in heart and skeletal muscle. Proc. Natl. Acad. Sci. USA **92:** 1108–1112.
38. LOVENBERG, T.W. *et al.* 1995. Cloning and characterization of a functionally distinct corticotropin-releasing factor receptor subtype from rat brain. Proc. Natl. Acad. Sci. USA **92:** 836–840.
39. LIAW, C.W. *et al.* 1996. Cloning and characterization of the human corticotropin-releasing factor-2 receptor complementary deoxyrubonucleic acid. Endocrinol. **137:** 72–77.
40. LI, N. *et al.* 1992. Skin histoculture assay for studying the hair cycle. In Vitro Cell Dev. Biol. **28A:** 695–698.
41. PAUS, R. *et al.* 1991. The epidermal pentapeptide pyroGlu-Glu-Asp-Ser-GlyOH inhibits murine hair growth in vivo and in vitro. Dermatologica **183:** 173–178.
42. RODRIGUEZ-LINARES, B. *et al.* 1998. Expression of corticotrophin-releasing hormone receptor mRNA and protein in human myometrium. J. Endocrinol. **156:** 15–21.
43. SLOMINSKI, A. *et al.* 1989. MSH inhibits growth in a line of amelanotic hamster melanoma cells and induces increases in cAMP levels and tyrosinase activity without inducing melanogenesis. J. Cell Sci. **92:** 551–559.
44. SLOMINSKI, A. & R. Paus. 1990. Are L-tyrosine and L-DOPA hormone-like bioregulators. J. Theor. Biol. **143:** 123–138
45. SLOMINSKI, A. & R. PAUS. 1994. Towards defining receptors for L-tyrosine and LnDOPA. Mol. Cell. Endocrinol. **99:** C7–C11.
46. SLOMINSKI, A. *et al.* 1993. Melanocytes are sensory and regulatory cells of epidermis. J. Theor. Biol. **164:** 103–120.
47. GJERDE, E.A. *et al.* 1998. Corticotropin-releasing hormone inhibit lowering of interstitial fluid pressure in rat trachea induced by neurogenic inflammation. Europ. J. Pharmacol. **352:** 99–102.
48. MCLOON, L.K. & J. WIRTSCHAFTER 1997. Local injections of corticotropin releasing factor reduce doxorubicin-induced acute inflammation in the eyelid. Invest. Ophthalmol. Vis. Sci. **38:** 834–841.
49. WEI, E.T. 1993. Peripheral anti-inflammatory actions of corticotropin-releasing factor. Ciba. Found. Symp. **172:** 258–267.
50. THEOHARIDES, T.C. *et al.* 1998. Corticotropin-releasing hormone induces skin mast cell degranulation and increased vascular permeability, a possible explanation for its proinflammatory effects. Endocrinol. **139:** 403–413.
51. ROHDE, E. *et al.* 1996 Corticotropin releasing hormone (CRH) receptors in the mesenteric small arteries of rats resemble the (2)-subtype. Biochem. Pharmacol. **52:** 829–833.
52. THODY, T. *et al.* 1983. MSH peptides are present in mammalian skin. Peptides **4:** 813–816.
53. LOIR, B. *et al.* 1997. Immunoreactive α-melanotropin as an autocrine effector in human melanoma cells. Eur. J. Biochem. **244:** 923–930.

54. SCHAUER, E. *et al.* 1994. Proopiomelanocortin-derived peptides are synthesized and released by human keratinocytes. J. Clin. Invest. **93:** 2258–2262.
55. MOUNTJOY, K.G. *et al.* 1992. The cloning of a family genes that encode melnocortin receptors. Science **257:** 1248–1251.
56. OREL, L. *et al.* 1997. α-Melanocyte-stimulating hormone down-regulates differentiation-driven heat shock protein 70 expression in keratinocytes. J. Invest. Dertmatol. **108:** 401–405.
57. CHAKRABORTY, A. & J. PAWELEK. 1993. MSH receptors in immortalized human epidermal keratinocytes: a potential mechanism for coordinated regulation of the epidermal-melanin unit. J. Cell Physiol. **157:** 344–350.
58. HOLTZMANN, H. *et al.* 1982. Der einfluss ultravioletter strtahlen auf die hypothalamus-hypophysenachse des menschen. Acta Dermatol. **8:** 119–123.
59. HOLTZMANN, H. *et al.* 1983 Die beemfussung des alpha-MSH durch UVA-bestrahlunger der hautein funktionstest. Hautarzt. **34:** 294–297.
60. PAUS, R. 1996. Control of the hair cycle and hair diseases as cycling disorders. Curr. Opinion Dermatol. **3:** 248–258.

Corticotropin Releasing Factor Receptors and Their Ligand Family

MARILYN H. PERRIN AND WYLIE W. VALE

The Clayton Foundation Laboratories for Peptide Biology,
The Salk Institute for Biological Studies, 10010 North Torrey Pines Road,
La Jolla, California 92037, USA

ABSTRACT: The CRF receptors belong to the VIP/GRF/PTH family of G-protein coupled receptors whose actions are mediated through activation of adenylate cyclase. Two CRF receptors, encoded by distinct genes, CRF-R1 and CRF-R2, and that can exist in two alternatively spliced forms, have been cloned. The type-1 receptor is expressed in many areas of the rodent brain, as well as in the pituitary, gonads, and skin. In the rodent, one splice variant of the type-2 receptor, CRF-R2α, is expressed mainly in the brain, whereas the other variant, CRF-R2β, is found not only in the CNS, but also in cardiac and skeletal muscle, epididymis, and the gastrointestinal tract. The poor correlation between the sites of expression of CRF-R2 and CRF, as well as the relatively low affinity of CRF for CRF-R2, suggested the presence of another ligand, whose existence was confirmed in our cloning of urocortin. This CRF-like peptide is found not only in brain, but also in peripheral sites, such as lymphocytes. The broad tissue distribution of CRF receptors and their ligands underscores the important role of this system in maintenance of homeostasis. Functional studies of the two receptor types reveal differences in the specificity for CRF and related ligands. On the basis of its greater affinity for urocortin, in comparison with CRF, as well as its brain distribution, CRF-R2 may be the cognate receptor for urocortin. Mutagenesis studies of CRF receptors directed toward understanding the basis for their specificity, provide insight into the structural determinants for hormone-receptor recognition and signal transduction.

INTRODUCTION

It is a matter of life or death for an organism that is exposed to environmental perturbations (stressors) to be able to respond in a manner that maintains physiological homeostasis. A major regulator of homeostasis is the corticotropin-releasing-factor (CRF), which mediates the autonomic, behavioral, and neuroendocrine responses to stress. In addition, there are many data suggesting that CRF and its family members are involved in the function of the immune, reproductive, and cardiovascular systems,[1-3] as well as in pathophysiologic states, such as depression and Alzheimer's disease.[4-8] Recently, the observation that CRF affects the growth of mammary and lung cancer cells, and that it protects neuronal cells from hypoxia-induced cell death,[9-11] suggests that CRF may play a role in cell growth and survival.

The family of CRF agonists includes (fish) urotensin, (frog) sauvagine, and the new mammalian CRF agonist, urocortin. The actions of these CRF agonists are initiated by binding and activating receptors that belong to the family of seven-transmembrane domain, G-protein–coupled receptors that activate adenylate cyclase. In order to understand the mechanism of CRF action, a detailed description of the ligand-receptor interaction at a molecular level is required. This paper describes the cloned CRF receptors and the structural determinants for ligand recognition. Data on the tissue distribution and receptor binding of urocortin are included.

CRF RECEPTOR TYPES AND VARIANTS

To date, two types of CRF receptors, each encoded by a different gene, have been cloned. Using an expression cloning approach, the cDNA for CRF-R1 was obtained from a human Cushing's tumor[12] and from the mouse AtT-20 cell line.[13] The homologous receptors in rat and human were also cloned and were found to have only minor amino acid differences.[13–15] Type-1 CRF receptors have subsequently been cloned in sheep (Meyers, Trinh, Myers, Gene Bank #AF054582), chicken,[16] and *Xenopus*.[17] A splice variant of CRF-R1, in which 29 amino acids are inserted into the first intracellular loop, was cloned from the Cushing's tumor.[12] To date, the latter variant has not been found in any other tissue. Another variant, from which the third exon—encoding amino acids 40–80—is deleted, was cloned from human hypothalamus.[18] This variant has been detected in human fetal and placental tissue,[19] as well as in rat testis.[20]

After CRF-R1 had been cloned, its expression sites in the rat brain were found to be widespread, but not completely overlapping with previously detected binding sites. For example, there are CRF binding sites in the hypothalamus,[21] but there is very little binding to CRF-R1,[22] or expression of its message.[23,24] The existence of another CRF receptor was confirmed when rodent CRF-R2 was cloned.[25–28] In the rodent, there are two splice variants, CRF-R2α and CRF-R2β, that differ in their N-terminal domains. Subsequently, the human homologs of CRF-R2α and CRF-R2β were cloned,[29,30] as well as a third N-terminal splice variant, CRF-R2γ.[31] The sequences of cloned CRF receptors are compared in FIGURE 1.

The CRF receptors belong to the family that includes the growth hormone releasing factor, parathyroid hormone, glucagon, vasoactive intestinal peptide, calcitonin, and secretin receptors. The rodent CRF-R1 and CRF-R2β are overall 68% similar, at the amino acid level, but they are 79% similar in the transmembrane domains, and 84% similar in the intracellular domains. The major sequence differences between the two types of receptors occur in the extracellular domains (FIG. 1).

All receptors have putative signal peptides, N-glycosylation sites in their N-termini, and eight conserved cysteine residues in their extracellular domains. Consistent with the signal transduction pathway of the native receptors, the cloned receptors transduce a CRF-stimulated accumulation of intracellular cAMP in transfected cells.[26] It is relevant, in this respect, that all receptors have the same sequence in the third intracellular loop, which is presumed to play an important role in coupling to the G-proteins (FIG.1).

The genomic structures of the rat and human receptors show that they contain 13 exons and 12 introns, and a general structure similar to that of the genes for parathyroid hormone and glucagon receptors.[20,32] The splice variant encoding the insertion

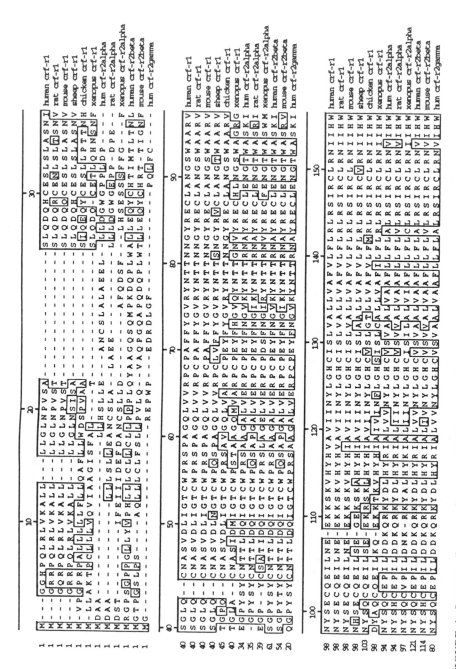

FIGURE 1. Sequence alignment of the cloned CRF receptors./Continued on next two pages.

FIGURE 1/continued.

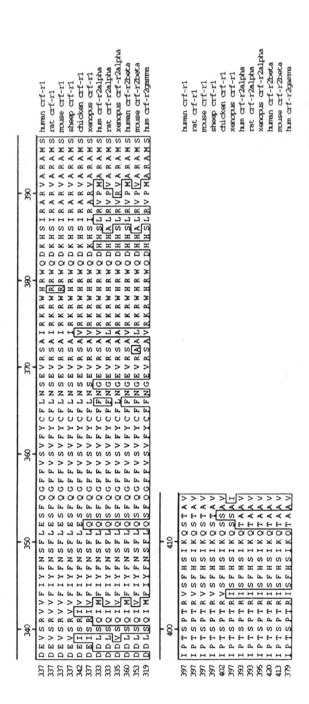

FIGURE 1/continued. Sequence alignment of the cloned CRF receptors.

in the first intracellular loop, isolated from the human Cushing's tumor, was not detected in the rat gene, but was found in the human gene.[32]

CRF RECEPTOR EXPRESSION

After the receptors had been cloned, their expression sites were determined by means of *in situ* hybridization, RNAse protection, and RT-PCR. These results show that there is a wide distribution of CRF-R1 in the rat brain, with high levels in the forebrain, subcortical limbic structures in the septal region, amygdala, cerebellar cortex, and deep nuclei; and low or no expression in the hypothalamus. In keeping with the effects of CRF on the pituitary, CRF-R1 is also expressed in the anterior and intermediate lobes of the rat pituitary.[23] Additionally, CRF-R1 expression is found in mouse testis,[33] human ovary,[34] skin,[35,36] human endometrial stromal cells,[37] human leukemic mast cells,[38] rat mammary carcinoma,[10] and melanoma cells.[39]

In the rodent, CRF-R2α is found mainly in the brain, where it is confined to subcortical structures; with high expression in the lateral septal nucleus, the ventromedial hypothalamus, and in the choroid plexus; with very low expression in the pituitary.[24] A distinct site of expression for CRF-R2β is in cerebral arterioles throughout the rat brain.[24] Interestingly, in the rodent, CRF-R2β is expressed both in the brain and in the periphery—namely, the epididymis, skeletal muscle, gastrointestinal tract, and heart.[26–28,40] Additionally, CRF-R2β is expressed in mouse AT-1 myocyte tumor cells.[41] In contrast to the rodent, the human CRF-R2α is found in the brain and periphery, whereas CRF-R2β and CRF-R2γ are found mainly in the brain.[30,31]

Using pharmacological differences in affinities for ovine CRF, the binding sites that correspond to CRF-R1 and CRF-R2 in the rat brain were shown to be in distinct, nonoverlapping regions each associated with a specific message expression.[22] Pharmacological characterization of CRF-like effects on relaxation of mesenteric small arteries of the rat suggests that the receptors that mediate these effects are CRF-R2;[42] as are the mediators for rat neonatal cardiomyocytes and a murine cardiomyocyte tumor cell line.[41]

A SECOND MAMMALIAN CRF AGONIST, UROCORTIN

The impetus behind the search for another mammalian, CRF-like ligand was based on four different observations. First, the peptides, urotensin and sauvagine, in fish and frogs, respectively, were thought to be the corresponding orthologs of CRF until peptides more closely related to CRF were cloned in these species.[43,44] Second, urotensin and sauvagine are nearly equipotent with CRF on CRF-R1, but are more potent than CRF on CRF-R2.[25–27] Third, there was specific urotensin-like immunoreactivity in rat brain and other tissues. Finally, the sites of expression of CRF-R1 and CRF-R2 in the rat brain are largely nonoverlapping,[24] showing a lack of correspondence, in some areas, with the expression of CRF. Using an antibody to urotensin, a peptide named urocortin was cloned from rat brain.[45] Subsequently, the human homolog was cloned.[46] Urocortin is 63% homologous to urotensin and 43%

CRF RAT   S E E P P I S L D L T F H L L R E V L E M A R A E Q L – A Q Q A H S N R K L M E I I
CRF HUMAN   S E E P P I S L D L T F H L L R E V L E M A R A E Q L – A Q Q A H S N R K L M E I I
CRF PIG   S E E P P I S L D L T F H L L R E V L E M A R A E Q L – A Q Q A H S N R K L M E I F
CRF SUCKER   S E E P P I S L D L T F H L L R E V L E M A R A E Q L – A Q Q A H S N R K M M E I F
CRF XENOPUS   A E E P P I S L D L T F H L L R E V L E M A R A E Q I – A Q Q A H S N R K L M D I I

CRF SHEEP   S Q E P P I S L D L T F H L L R E V L E M T K A D Q L – A Q Q A H S N R K L L D I A
CRF GOAT   S Q E P P I S L D L T F H L L R E V L E M T K A D Q L – A Q Q A H S N R K L L D I A
CRF COW   S Q E P P I S L D L T F H L L R E V L E M T K A D Q L – A Q Q A H N N R K L L D I A

UT CARP   N D D P P I S L D L T F H L L R N M I E M A R N E N Q – R E Q A G L N R K K Y L D E V
UT SUCKER   N D D P P I S I D L T F H L L R N M I E M A R I E N E – R E Q A G L N R K K Y L D E V
UT GFHin#2   N D D P P I S I D L T F H L L R N M I E M A R N E N Q – R E Q A G L N R K K Y L D E V

UT SOLE   S E E P P M S I D L T F H M L R N M I H R A K M E G E – R E Q A L I N R N L L D E V
UT FLOUNDER   S E D P P M S I D L T F H M L R N M I H M A K M E G E – R E Q A Q I N R N L L D E V

UCN RAT   – D D P P L S L E L L R T L L E L A R T Q S Q – R E R A E Q N R I H F D S V
UCN HUMAN   – D N P S L S I D L T F H L L R T L L E L A R T Q S Q – R E R A E Q N R I H F D S V

SAUVAGINE   – E G P P I S I D L S L E L L R K M I E I E K Q E K E – K Q Q A E Q N R L L D T I

MAS DH   – R M P S L S I D L P M S V L R Q K L S L E K E R K V H A L R A A N R L N D I

FIGURE 2. Sequences of CRF family members.

TABLE 1. Relative potencies of CRF ligands[a]

Compound	Inhibitory binding constant, K_i (nM)[b]						cAMP, EC$_{50}$ (nM)[c]	
	hCRF-R1[d]	hCRF-R1[e]	rCRF-R2α[d]	rCRF-R2α[e]	mCRF-R2β[d]	mCRF-R2β[e]	rCRF-R1	mCRF-R2β
Astressin	2.0 (1.8–2.3)	1.6 (0.95–2.7)	1.5 (0.81–2.8)	2.8 (1.7–4.7)	1.0 (0.39–2.8)	0.87 (0.56–1.4)	n/a	n/a
α-helical CRF(9–41)	17 (13–21)	49 (29–82)	5.0 (2.6–10)	4.1 (2.5–6.7)	0.97 (0.43–2.2)	0.81 (0.52–1.3)	n/a	n/a
[dPhe^{12},Nle^{21,38}]r/ hCRF(12–41)	56 (41–75)	75 (64–88)	5.2 (2.6–10)	31 (19–51)	8.4 (4.4–16)	6.9 (5.0–9.5)	n/a	n/a
r/hCRF	11 (8.2–15)	5.2 (2.9–9.3)	44 (26–75)	13 (7.2–22)	38 (21–67)	17 (10–29)	1.9 ± 0.8	1.7 ± 0.4
rUcn	1.3 (0.71–2.6)	0.79 (0.43–1.4)	1.5 (0.74–3.2)	0.58 (0.42–0.82)	0.97 (0.46–2.0)	0.41 (0.26–0.66)	0.8 ± 0.1	0.18 ± 0.04
sfUrotensin I	3.1 (2.4–4.0)	2.8 (2.4–3.3)	9.8 (5.5–17)	3.4 (2.6–4.4)	6.4 (3.8–11)	3.0 (1.8–4.8)	3.1 ± 1.7	0.74 ± 0.1
Sauvagine	9.4 (7–13)	11 (8.8–13)	9.9 (4.4–22)	1.4 (1.1–1.8)	3.8 (2.3–6.2)	2.0 (1.1–3.6)	2.5 ± 1.4	0.5 ± 0.2

[a] The values for this table are taken from Refs. 45 and 60.
[b] 95% confidence limits in parentheses.
[c] ± SEM.
[d] ^{125}I-[dTyr^1]Astressin as radioligand.
[e] ^{125}I-[Tyr^0]rUcn as radioligand.

homologous to CRF. The sequences for urocortin and the other CRF family members are shown in FIGURE 2, from which it can be seen that urocortin is more closely related to urotensin than to CRF.

Urocortin is detected in many regions of the rat brain, including the Edinger-Westphal nucleus, lateral superior olive,[45] substantia nigra, ventral tegmental area, linear and dorsal raphe nuclei,[47,48] and the hypothalamus.[49] In the human brain, urocortin-like immunoreactivity and message are observed in every region, with the highest concentrations found in the frontal cortex, temporal cortex, and hypothalamus.[50]

Urocortin is also found in peripheral sites. For example, immunoreactive urocortin is detected in the rat digestive system and the pituitary.[49,51] Human anterior pituitary was also found to express both the message and immunoreactivity for urocortin.[52] Other sites of expression of urocortin mRNA and of the peptide are mucosal inflammatory cells in the human gastrointestinal tract,[53] human placenta, and fetal membranes.[54] Using RT-PCR, urocortin mRNA is detected in primary cultures of rat cardiomyocytes as well as in cardiac myocyte cell lines.[55]

By combining RT-PCR and radioimmunoassay, it was found that normal human lymphocytes produce urocortin but not CRF.[56] The involvement of CRF-like ligands in immune function is further highlighted by the observation that both CRF and urocortin suppress experimental autoimmune encephalomyelitis in rats.[57] These neuropeptides may act directly on the components of the immune system, rather than indirectly through the activation of the HPA.

The regions of urocortin immunoreactivity overlap with the regions of expression of CRF-R2 in many areas of the brain[47] and some effects of urocortin appear to be mediated by CRF-R2. For example, urocortin was found to be approximately six times more potent than CRF as an inhibitor of heat-induced edema.[58] Furthermore, blockade of CRF-R1 does not affect the CRF- and urocortin-induced decrease in food intake in rats.[59] Also, urocortin protects myocytes, cells that express CRF-R2, from hypoxia-induced cell death.[55]

Pharmacologic studies have shown that urocortin is more potent than CRF on both types of CRF receptors, but in general, the difference in potencies is greater for CRF-R2.[45,60] The affinities of selected CRF ligands and the potencies in stimulating cAMP in cells expressing the two types of CRF receptors are given in TABLE 1. Astressin is a CRF peptide antagonist that has high affinity for both types of CRF receptors.[61] From TABLE 1 it can be seen that the antagonist α-helical CRF(9–41) has a greater affinity for CRF-R2 than for CRF-R1. This observation may explain the fact that α-helical CRF(9–41) blocks heat-induced edema at doses that do not block CRF-stimulated ACTH release.[58]

STRUCTURAL REQUIREMENTS FOR CRF
RECEPTOR BINDING—MUTAGENESIS STUDIES

One approach to assessing the structural determinants for receptor function uses mutagenesis to determine regions of the receptor that may be involved in binding and signaling. In one study, chimeric receptors were created in which domains of the GRF receptor were replaced by the corresponding domains of the CRF-R1. A chimeric receptor in which the ECD-1 of the CRF-R1 was replaced by the ECD-1 of the GRF-R, does not bind either labeled astressin or labeled urocortin. A chimera in which the ECD-1 of the GRF-R was replaced by the corresponding domain of the CRF-R, binds astressin and urocortin with a dissocuation constant K_d ~10 nM. Additional chimeras were created to explore the role of the extracellular loops, and it was found that a chimera expressing all three extracellular loops, together with the N-terminus of the CRF-R, displays nearly the same affinity as the wild-type receptor.[62]

As a further test of the role of the ECD-1 in binding CRF analogs, a chimera was created, in which the ECD of the activin type-2 receptor was replaced by the ECD-1 of CRF-R1 (CRF-R/Act-R). The activin receptor is a single transmembrane serine/threonine kinase.[63] This chimera binds astressin with nanomolar affinity (see TABLE 2). In another study, the ECD-1 was expressed as a soluble protein and it was found to display only low binding affinity for a CRF agonist.[64] These data suggest that the N-terminal domain of the CRF-R1 contains major binding determinants for CRF agonists and antagonists, but that it must be anchored to the cell membrane.

In CRF-R1, there eight conserved cysteine residues in ECD-1, -2, and -3. The role of these residues was studied by mutating them, either singly or in pairs. It was found that there is potential pairing of the Cys residues, #44 with #102, #68 with #87; and the two residues in ECD-2 and -3, #188 with #258. Mutations of C30 and C54 appear to have little effect on receptor binding. Additionally, mutations of the cysteine residues within the transmembrane and intracellular domains have no effect on either binding or signaling.[65]

Another question relates to the origin of CRF receptor selectivity as manifested by greater potency of CRF in signaling by CRF-R1 compared to CRF-R2.[25] The amino acids that differ between CRF-R1 and CRF-R2 were exchanged and it was found that substitution of Val266, Tyr267, and Thr 268 in CRF-R1 by the corresponding residues in CRF-R2 increases the EC-50 for CRF-stimulated cAMP accumulation by a factor of about ten. Other residues in ECD-2 (#175–#178, and #189) also appear to be involved in the CRF response of CRF-R1.[66,67]

At the amino acid level, the *Xenopus* CRF-R1 is about 80% homologous to the human CRF-R1, but the two receptors differ in their affinities for sauvagine, r/h CRF, and ovine CRF.[17] Whereas hCRF-R1 is not selective for these ligands, the xCRF-R1 has about one tenth the affinity for ovine CRF and sauvagine, as compared to CRF. Using mutagenesis, it was found that the five amino acids #76, #81 #83, #88, and #89 in the N-terminal domain are responsible for the observed differences.[68] These data are consistent with some published results,[62] but they contrast with others.[66,67]

The avian CRF-R1 is about 88% identical to that of the human, rat, and mouse CRF-R1, with many amino acid differences in the ECD-1, and the remainder of the differences scattered throughout the rest of the sequence.[16] In the avian receptor the relative potencies are urotensin $\cong$ sauvagine > CRF, for both binding and signaling. This pattern is more like that seen for the CRF-R2 than for CRF-R1. No mutagenesis study has yet been reported for the avian receptor, but the ECD-1 is again implicated in the ligand specificity because most of the amino acid differences appear in this domain.

Recently a series of nonpeptide CRF antagonists have been developed that bind, specifically and with high affinity, to type-1 receptors; and inhibit, both *in vitro* and

TABLE 2. Inhibitory dissociation constants, K_i (nM), for astressin and urocortin bound to COSM6 cells transfected with various chimeric and mutant receptors[a]

Receptor	Ast/Ast* K_i (nM)[b]	Ucn/Ucn* K_i (nM)[b]
rCRF-R (wt)	1.8 (1.1–2.9)	3.0 (1.6–5.7)
rGRF-R (wt)	—[c]	—[c]
E1$_g$/CRF-R	—[c]	—[c]
E1$_c$/GRF-R	13 (7.7–22)	12 (1.9–74)
E1$_c$/E2$_c$/GRF-R	10 (7.1–14)	10 (4.5–22)
E1$_c$/E3$_c$/GRF-R	7.1 (3.8–13)	—[c]
E1$_c$/E4$_c$/GRF-R	4.2 (3.0–5.8)	1.6 (0.58–4.4)
E1$_c$/E2$_c$/E3$_c$/GRF-R	5.4 (3.5–8.4)	—[c]
E1$_c$/E2$_c$/E4$_c$/GRF-R	7.9 (5.3–12)	7.0 (3.5–14)
E1$_c$/E3$_c$/E4$_c$/GRF-R	11 (5.2–23)	7.6 (2.1–27)
E1$_c$/E2$_c$/E3$_c$/E4$_c$/GRF-R	4.3 (1.9–9.6)	1.3 (0.71–2.4)
E1$_c$/ActIIB-R	3.5 (1.8–7.0)	—[c]

[a]The K_i values were determined from homologous displacement assays, assuming that the K_d values for Ast* and Ucn* were not significantly different from those for astressin and urocortin, respectively.
[b]Values in parentheses are 95% confidence limits.
[c]The specific binding was too low to measure the K_i accurately.

in vivo, CRF actions mediated by them.[69–72] One study found that the mutations H199V and M276I, two of the residues in transmembrane domains 3 and 5 that differ between CRF-R1 and CRF-R2, reduce the affinity of CRF-R1 for a nonpeptide antagonist but have no effect on the affinity for CRF.[67] In another study, a different nonpeptide antagonist, antalarmin,[72] displaced the labeled antagonist, astressin, to a much smaller degree than it displaced labeled oCRF from both the cloned CRF-R1 and the native cerebellar receptor—a tissue that predominantly expresses CRF-R1 (Perrin, unpublished). These data suggest that the binding domains of peptide and nonpeptide antagonists are different.

CONCLUSIONS

To date, four CRF receptors and one novel CRF ligand have been cloned. The type-1 receptor, widely expressed in the central nervous system and in the pituitary, is the major mediator for activation of the HPA axis. The fact that CRF-R1 is found in the reproductive and immune systems, as well as in spleen, adrenal, and skin, suggests that this receptor mediates many diverse actions. The type-2 receptor exists in different splice-variant forms that differ in their N-terminal sequences and in their tissue expression. In both the rodent and human, one variant is restricted to the central nervous system, whereas the other variants are found not only in the brain but also in peripheral sites.

A novel CRF agonist, urocortin, has been cloned and found to have characteristics that are similar, but not identical, to those of CRF. Urocortin is widely expressed in the brain, as well as in many of the peripheral tissues that express the type-2 receptor. Urocortin binds with high affinity to both types of receptors but is significantly more potent than CRF on the type-2 receptor.

Studies of mutant CRF receptors have shown that recognition of CRF peptides is governed, to a large extent, by residues in the extracellular domains, especially the N-terminus. Furthermore, the binding of nonpeptide CRF-R1–selective antagonists involves receptor domains that differ from those involved in binding of the peptide antagonists.

The future holds exciting prospects for cloning other CRF receptors and discovering novel sites of expression and action. The cloning of urocortin raises the possibility that other CRF-like molecules exist in mammals. Future studies of CRF receptor and/or urocortin knock-out mice will undoubtedly disclose expanded roles for the CRF family and increase our understanding of the roles of CRF in normal and pathological states.

ACKNOWLEDGMENTS

We gratefully acknowledge the technical assistance of D. Bain, T. Berggren, A. Blount, R. Kaiser, K. Kunitake, K. Lewis, A. McCarthy, S. Sutton, and J. Vaughan; and manuscript preparation by D. Dalton, S. Fitzpatrick, and S. Guerra.

REFERENCES

1. TORPY, D.J. & G.P. CHROUSOS. 1996. The three-way interactions between the hypothalamic-pituitary-adrenal and gonadal axes and the immune system. Baillieres Clin. Rheumatol. **10:** 181–198.

2. RICHTER, R.M. & M.J. MULVANY. 1995. Comparison of hCRF and oCRF effects on cardiovascular responses after central, peripheral, and in vitro application. Peptides **16:** 843–849.

3. FISHER, L.A. 1993. Central actions of corticotropin-releasing factor on autonomic nervous activity and cardiovascular functioning. Ciba Found. Symp. **172:** 243–253.

4. NEMEROFF, C.B., E. WIDERLOV, G. BISSETTE et al. 1984. Elevated concentrations of CSF corticotropin-releasing factor-like immunoreactivity in depressed patients. Science **226:** 1342–1344.

5. PLOTSKY, P.M., M.J. OWENS & C.B. NEMEROFF. 1998. Psychoneuroendocrinology of depression. Hypothalamic-pituitary-adrenal axis. Psychiatr. Clin. North Am. **21:** 293–307.

6. NASMAN, B., T. OLSSON, M. FAGERLUND et al. 1996. Blunted adrenocorticotropin and increased adrenal steroid response to human corticotropin-releasing hormone in Alzheimer's disease. Biol. Psychiatry. **39:** 311–318.

7. BEHAN, D.P., S.C. HEINRICHS, J.C. TRONCOSO et al. 1995. Displacement of corticotropin releasing factor from its binding protein as a possible treatment for Alzheimer's disease. Nature **378:** 284–287.

8. RAADSHEER, F.C., J.J. VAN HEERIKHUIZE, P.J. LUCASSEN et al. 1995. Corticotropin-releasing hormone mRNA levels in the paraventricular nucleus of patients with Alzheimer's disease and depression. Am. J. Psychiatry **152:** 1372–1376.

9. EAGLES, E., G. SANTILLI, A. OKOSI et al. 1998. Endogenous corticotropin releasing hormone protects neuroblastoma cells from hypoxia-induced necrosis. (Abst. # P1-420). In Endocrine Soc. Meeting, June 1988, New Orleans, Louisiana.

10. TJUVAJEV, J., Y. KOLESNIKOV, R. JOSHI et al. 1998. Anti-neoplastic properties of human corticotropin releasing factor: involvement of the nitric oxide pathway. In Vivo **12:** 1–10.

11. MOODY, T.W., F. ZIA, R. VENUGOPAL et al. 1994. Corticotropin-releasing factor stimulates cyclic AMP, arachidonic acid release, and growth of lung cancer cells. Peptides **15:** 281–285.

12. CHEN, R., K.A. LEWIS, M.H. PERRIN et al. 1993. Expression cloning of a human corticotropin-releasing factor receptor. Proc. Natl. Acad. Sci. USA **90:** 8967–8971.

13. VITA, N., P. LAURENT, S. LEFORT et al. 1993. Primary structure and functional expression of mouse pituitary and human brain corticotrophin releasing factor receptors. FEBS Lett. **335:** 1–5.

14. CHANG, C.-P., R.V. PEARSE, II, S. O'CONNELL et al. 1993. Identification of a seven transmembrane helix receptor for corticotropin-releasing factor and sauvagine in mammalian brain. Neuron **11:** 1187–1195.

15. PERRIN, M.H., C.J. DONALDSON, R. CHEN et al. 1993. Cloning and functional expression of a rat brain corticotropin releasing factor (CRF) receptor. Endocrinology **133:** 3058–3061.

16. YU, J., L.Y. XIE & A.-B. ABOU-SAMRA. 1996. Molecular cloning of a type A chicken corticotropin-releasing factor receptor with high affinity for urotensin I. Endocrinology **137:** 192–197.

17. DAUTZENBERG, F.M., K. DIETRICH, M.R. PALCHAUDHURI et al. 1997. Identification of two corticotropin-releasing factor receptors from Xenopus laevis with high ligand selectivity: unusual pharmacology of the type-1 receptor. J. Neurochem. **69:** 1640–1649.

18. ROSS, P.C., C.M. KOSTAS & T.V. RAMABHADRAN. 1994. A variant of the human corticotropin-releasing factor (CRF) receptor: cloning, expression and pharmacology. Biochem. Biophys. Res. Comm. **205:** 1836–1842.

19. KARTERIS, E., D. GRAMMATOPOULOS, Y. DAI *et al.* 1998. The human placenta and fetal membranes express the corticotropin-releasing hormone receptor 1alpha (CRH-1alpha) and the CRH-C variant receptor. J. Clin. Endocrinol. Metab. **83:** 1376–1379.

20. TSAI-MORRIS, C.H., E. BUCZKO, Y. GENG *et al.* 1996. The genomic structure of the rat corticotropin releasing factor receptor. J. Biol. Chem. **271:** 14519–14525.

21. DE SOUZA, E.B., M.H. PERRIN, T.R. INSEL *et al.* 1984. Corticotropin-releasing factor receptors in rat forebrain: autoradiographic identification. Science **224:** 1449–1451.

22. PRIMUS, R.J., W. YEVICH, C. BALTAZAR *et al.* 1997. Autoradiographic localization of CRF1 and CRF2 binding sites in adult rat brain. Neuropsychopharmacology **17:** 308–316.

23. POTTER, E., S. SUTTON, C. DONALDSON *et al.* 1994. Distribution of corticotropin-releasing factor receptor mRNA expression in the rat brain and pituitary. Proc. Natl. Acad. Sci. USA **91:** 8777–8781.

24. CHALMERS, D.T., T.W. LOVENBERG & E.B. DESOUZA. 1995. Localization of novel corticotropin-releasing factor receptor (CRF2)mRNA expression to specific subcortical nuclei in rat brain: comparison with CRF1 receptor mRNA expression. J. Neurosci. **15:** 6340–6350.

25. LOVENBERG, T.W., W.L. CHEN, D.E. GRIGORIADIS *et al.* 1995. Cloning and characterization of a functionally distinct corticotropin-releasing factor receptor subtype from rat brain. Proc. Natl. Acad. Sci. USA **92:** 836–840.

26. PERRIN, M., C. DONALDSON, R. CHEN *et al.* 1995. Identification of a second corticotropin-releasing factor receptor gene and characterization of a cDNA expressed in heart. Proc. Natl. Acad. Sci. USA **92:** 2969–2973.

27. KISHIMOTO, T., R.V. PEARSE II, C.R. LIN *et al.* 1995. A sauvagine/corticotropin-releasing factor receptor expressed in heart and skeletal muscle. Proc. Natl. Acad. Sci. USA **92:** 1108–1112.

28. STENZEL, P., R. KESTERSON, W. YEUNG *et al.* 1995. Identification of a novel murine receptor for corticotropin-releasing hormone expressed in the heart. Mol. Endocrinol. **9:** 637–645.

29. LIAW, C.W., T.W. LOVENBERG, T. OLTERSDORF *et al.* 1996. Cloning and characterization of the human corticotropin-releasing factor-2 receptor complementary deoxyribonucleic acid. Endocrinology **137:** 72–77.

30. VALDENAIRE, O., T. GILLER, V. BREU *et al.* 1997. A new functional isoform of the human CRF2 receptor for corticotropin-releasing factor. Biochim. Biophys. Acta **1352:** 129–132.

31. KOSTICH, W.A., A. CHEN, K. SPERLE *et al.* 1998. Molecular identification and analysis of a novel human corticotropin-releasing factor (CRF) receptor: the CRF2gamma receptor. Mol. Endocrinol. **12:** 1077–1085.

32. SAKAI, K., S. NAGAFUCHI, N. HORIBA *et al.* 1998. The genomic organization of the human corticotropin-releasing factor type-1 receptor. (Abst. # P3-571). *In* Endocrine Soc. Meeting, June 1988, New Orleans, Louisiana.

33. HEINRICH, N., M.R. MEYER, J. FURKERT *et al.* 1998. Corticotropin-releasing factor (CRF) agonists stimulate testosterone production in mouse leydig cells through CRF receptor-1. Endocrinology **139:** 651–658.

34. ASAKURA, H., I.H. ZWAIN & S.S. YEN. 1997. Expression of genes encoding corticotropin-releasing factor (CRF), type-1 CRF receptor, and CRF-binding protein and localization of the gene products in the human ovary. J. Clin. Endocrinol. Metab. **82:** 2720–2725.

35. SLOMINSKI, A., G. ERMAK, J. HWANG *et al.* 1995. Proopiomelanocortin, corticotropin releasing hormone and corticotropin releasing hormone receptor genes are expressed in human skin. FEBS Lett. **374:** 113–116.

36. ERMAK, G. & A. SLOMINSKI. 1997. Production of POMC, CRH-R1, MC1, and MC2 receptor mRNA and expression of tyrosinase gene in relation to hair cycle and dexamethasone treatment in the C57BL/6 mouse skin. J. Invest. Dermatol. **108:** 160–165.

37. DIBLASIO, A.M., F.P. GIRALDI, P. VIGANO et al. 1997. Expression of corticotropin-releasing hormone and its R1 receptor in human endometrial stromal cells. J. Clin. Endocrinol. Metab. **82:** 1594–1597.

38. THEOHARIDES, T.C., L.K. SINGH, W. BOUCHER et al. 1998. Corticotropin-releasing hormone induces skin mast cell degranulation and increased vascular permeability, a possible explanation for its proinflammatory effects. Endocrinololgy **139:** 403–413.

39. SLOMINSKI, A., G. ERMAK, J.E. MAZURKIEWICZ et al. 1998. Characterization of corticotropin-releasing hormone (CRH) in human skin. J. Clin. Endocrinol. Metab. **83:** 1020–1024.

40. LOVENBERG, T.W., D.T. CHALMERS, C. LIU et al. 1995. CRF2 alpha and CRF2 beta receptor mRNAs are differentially distributed between the rat central nervous system and peripheral tissues. Endocrinology **136:** 4139–4142.

41. HELDWEIN, K.A., D.L. REDICK, M.B. RITTENBERG et al. 1996. Corticotropin-releasing hormone receptor expression and functional coupling in neonatal cardiac myocytes and AT-1 cells. Endocrinology **137:** 3631–3639.

42. ROHDE, E., J. FURKERT, K. FECHNER et al. 1996. Corticotropin-releasing hormone (CRH) receptors in the mesenteric small arteries of rats resemble the (2)-subtype. Biochem. Pharmacol. **52:** 829–833.

43. OKAWARA, Y., S.D. MORLEY, L.O. BURZIO et al. 1988. Cloning and sequence analysis of cDNA for corticotropin-releasing factor precursor from the teleost fish Catostomus commersoni. Proc. Natl. Acad. Sci. USA **85:** 8439–8443.

44. STENZEL-POORE, M.P., K.A. HELDWEIN, P. STENZEL et al. 1992. Characterization of the genomic corticotropin-releasing factor (CRF) gene from Xenopus laevis: two members of the CRF family exist in amphibians. Mol. Endocrinol. **6:** 1716–1724.

45. VAUGHAN, J., C. DONALDSON, J. BITTENCOURT et al. 1995. Urocortin, a mammalian neuropeptide related to fish urotensin I and to corticotropin-releasing factor. Nature **378:** 287–292.

46. DONALDSON, C.J., S.W. SUTTON, M.H. PERRIN et al. 1996. Cloning and characterization of human urocortin. Endocrinology **137:** 2167–2170.

47. KOZICZ, T., H. YANAIHARA & A. ARIMURA. 1998. Distribution of urocortin-like immunoreactivity in the central nervous system of the rat. J. Comp. Neurol. **391:** 1–10.

48. YAMAMOTO, H., T. MAEDA, M. FUJIMURA et al. 1998. Urocortin-like immunoreactivity in the substantia nigra, ventral tegmental area and Edinger-Westphal nucleus of rat. Neurosci. Lett. **243:** 21–24.

49. OKI, Y., M. IWABUCHI, M. MASUZAWA et al. 1998. Distribution and concentration of urocortin, and effect of adrenalectomy on its content in rat hypothalamus. Life Sci. **62:** 807–812.

50. TAKAHASHI, K., K. TOTSUNE, M. SONE et al. 1998. Regional distribution of urocortin-like immunoreactivity and expression of urocortin mRNA in the human brain. Peptides **19:** 643–647.

51. WONG, M.L., A. AL-SHEKHLEE, P.B. BONGIORNO et al. 1996. Localization of urocortin messenger RNA in rat brain and pituitary. Mol. Psychiatry **1:** 307–312.

52. IINO, K., H. SASANO, Y. OKI et al. 1997. Urocortin expression in human pituitary gland and pituitary adenoma. J. Clin. Endocrinol. Metab. **82:** 3842–3850.

53. IINO, K., H. SASANO, T. SUZUKI et al. 1998. Urocortin expression in mucosal inflammatory cells of human gastrointestinal tract. (Abst. # P2-561). In Endocrine Soc. Meeting, June 1988, New Orleans, Louisiana.

54. PETRAGLIA, F., P. FLORIO, R. GALLO *et al.* 1996. Human placenta and fetal membranes express human urocortin mRNA and peptide. J. Clin. Endocrinol. Metab. **81:** 3807–3810.

55. OKOSI, A., B.K. BRAR, M. CHAN *et al.* 1998. Expression and protective effects of urocortin in cardiac myocytes. Neuropeptides **32:** 167–171.

56. BAMBERGER, C.M., M. WALD, A.M. BAMBERGER *et al.* 1998. Human lymphocytes produce urocortin, but not corticotropin-releasing hormone. J. Clin. Endocrinol. Metab. **83:** 708–711.

57. POLIAK, S., F. MOR, P. CONLON *et al.* 1997. Stress and autoimmunity: the neuropeptides corticotropin-releasing factor and urocortin suppress encephalomyelitis via effects on both the hypothalamic-pituitary-adrenal axis and the immune system. J. Immunol. **158:** 5751–5756.

58. TURNBULL, A.V., W. VALE & C. RIVIER 1996. Urocortin, a corticotropin-releasing factor-related mammalian peptide, inhibits edema due to thermal injury in rats. Eur. J. Pharmacol. **15:** 213–216.

59. SMAGIN, G.N., L.A. HOWELL, D.H. RYAN *et al.* 1998. the role of CRF2 receptors in corticotropin-releasing factor- and urocortin-induced anorexia. Neuroreport **9:** 1601–1606.

60. PERRIN, M.H., S.W. SUTTON, L. CERVINI *et al.* 1999. Comparison of an agonist, urocortin, and an antagonist, astressin, as radioligands for characterization of CRF receptors. J. Pharm. Exp. Ther. **288:** 729–734.

61. GULYAS, J., C. RIVIER, M. PERRIN *et al.* 1995. Potent, structurally constrained agonists and competitive antagonists of corticotropin-releasing factor. Proc. Natl. Acad. Sci. USA **92:** 10575–10579.

62. PERRIN, M.H., S. SUTTON, D.B. BAIN *et al.* 1998. The first extracellular domain of corticotropin releasing factor-R1 contains major binding determinants for urocortin and astressin. Endocrinology **139:** 566–570.

63. MATHEWS, L. & W. VALE. 1991. Expression cloning of an activin receptor, a predicted transmembrane serine kinase. Cell **65:** 973–982.

64. SYDOW, S., J. RADULOVIC, F.M. DAUTZENBERG *et al.* 1997. Structure-function relationship of different domains of the rat corticotropin-releasing factor receptor. Brain Res. Mol. Brain Res. **52:** 182–193.

65. QI, L.J., A.T. LEUNG, Y. XIONG *et al.* 1997. Extracellular cysteines of the corticotropin-releasing factor receptor are critical for ligand interaction. Biochemistry **36:** 12442–12448.

66. LIAW, C.W., D.E. GRIGORIADIS, T.W. LOVENBERG *et al.* 1997. Localization of ligand-binding domains of human corticotropin-releasing factor receptor: a chimeric receptor approach. Mol. Endocrinol. **11:** 980–985.

67. LIAW, C.W., D.E. GRIGORIADIS, M.T. LORANG *et al.* 1997. Localization of agonist- and antagonist-binding domains of human corticotropin-releasing factor receptors. Mol. Endocrinol. **11:** 2048–2053.

68. DAUTZENBERG, F.M., S. WILLE, R. LOHMANN *et al.* 1998. Mapping of the ligand-selective domain of the *Xenopus laevis* corticotropin-releasing factor receptor 1: Implications for the ligand-binding site. Proc. Natl. Acad. Sci. **95:** 4941–4946.

69. CHEN, C., J.R. DAGNINO, E.B. DESOUZA *et al.* 1996. Design and synthesis of a series of non-peptide high-affinity human corticotropin-releasing factor$_1$ receptor antagonists. J. Med. Chem. **39:** 4358–4360.

70. WHITTEN, J.P., Y.F. XIE, P.E. ERICKSON *et al.* 1996. Rapid microscale synthesis, a new method for lead optimization using robotics and solution phase chemistry: application to the synthesis and optimization of corticotropin-releasing factor$_1$ receptor antagonists. J. Med. Chem. **39:** 4354–4357.

71. SCHULZ, D.W., R.S. MANSBACH, J. SPROUSE *et al.* 1996. CP-154,526: A potent and selective nonpeptide antagonist of corticotropin releasing factor receptors. Proc. Natl. Acad. Sci. **93:** 10477–10482.
72. WEBSTER, W.L., D.B. LEWIS, D.J. TORPY *et al.* 1996. *In vivo* and *in vitro* characterization of antalarmin, a nonpeptide corticotropin-releasing hormone (CRH) receptor antagonist: suppression of pituitary ACTH release and peripheral inflammation. Endocrinology **137:** 5747–5750.

α-MSH Can Control the Essential Cofactor 6-Tetrahydrobiopterin in Melanogenesis

KARIN U. SCHALLREUTER,[a] JEREMY MOORE, DESMOND J. TOBIN, NICHOLAS J.P. GIBBONS, HARRIET S. MARSHALL, TRACEY JENNER, WAYNE D. BEAZLEY, AND JOHN M. WOOD

Clinical and Experimental Dermatology Department of Biomedical Sciences, University of Bradford, Bradford BD7 1DP, United Kingdom

ABSTRACT: In the human epidermis both keratinocytes and melanocytes express POMC m-RNA. Immunohistochemical studies of both cell types demonstrate significantly higher levels of α-MSH in melanocytes than in keratinocytes. Both cell types also hold the full capacity for *de novo* synthesis/recycling of the essential cofactor (6R)-L-erythro-5,6,7,8-tetrahydrobiopterin (6BH$_4$). 6BH$_4$ is critical for the hydroxylation of the aromatic amino acids L-phenylalanine, L-tyrosine, and L-tryptophan, for nitric oxide production and in various immune modulatory processes. Recently it was shown that tyrosinase activity is regulated by 6BH$_4$ through a specific allosteric inhibition. The tyrosinase/6BH$_4$ inhibition can be activated by 1:1 complex formation between 6BH$_4$ and α-MSH, but an excess of α-MSH over 6BH$_4$ can inhibit tyrosinase due to complex formation by tyr^2 in the α-MSH sequence. In both melanocytes and keratinocytes 6BH$_4$ controls the L-tyrosine supply via phenylalanine hydroxylase (PAH). Recently we were able to show that the cellular uptake of L-phenylalanine and its intracellular turnover to L-tyrosine is crucial for melanogenesis. α-MSH can promote the production of L-tyrosine via PAH due to activation of the PAH tetramer to the more active dimer by removing 6BH$_4$ from the regulatory binding domain on the enzyme. In conclusion, α-MSH can control (1) intracellular L-tyrosine formation from L-phenylalanine in both melanocytes and keratinocytes, and (2) tyrosinase activity, directly, in melanocytes.

Human skin color is the product of a concerted action involving many metabolic steps.[1] The constitutive pigment is determined by racial differences, whereas-UVB light (280–320 nm) induces facultative (*de novo*) tanning.[1,2] The factory for epidermal pigmentation resides in melanocytes, and these are surrounded by approximately 36 keratinocytes to form the epidermal unit.[2,3] In fact, melanin is formed in special organelles—the melanosomes—and it is their number and grade of maturation that determines skin color.[2] To date, it is well established that tyrosinase (monophenol dihydroxyphenylalanine oxidoreductase; EC 1.14.18.1) represents the key enzyme in melanogenesis, and that enzyme activities are significantly lower in fair skin than in dark skin, despite similar mRNA levels for both skin types.[2,4,5] The substrate for tyrosinase is L-tyrosine and its supply limits the reaction.[1] L-Tyrosine

[a]Address for correspondence: Professor K.U. Schallreuter, Clinical and Experimental Dermatology Department of Biomedical Sciences, University of Bradford, Bradford BD7 1DP, UK. +44 1274 235529 (voice); +44 1274 235290 (fax); K.Schallreuter@bradford.ac.uk (e-mail).

can either originate directly from the blood stream containing concentrations of 6×10^{-5} M, or it can be metabolized from the essential amino acid L-phenylalanine via phenylalanine hydroxylase (EC 1.14.16.1) in the presence of O_2 and the cofactor (6R)-L-erythro-5,6,7,8-tetrahydrobiopterin (6BH$_4$).[6] Recently the complete auto-crine *de novo* synthesis/recycling/regulation of 6BH$_4$ has been demonstrated in human epidermal melanocytes and keratinocytes.[7,8] It has also been realized that epidermal biopterin levels and phenylalanine hydroxylase activities correlate with photo skin types I–VI (Fitzpatrick classification) showing an almost linear increase from fair to dark skin.[7–9] Additionally, it has been shown in 12 healthy people with different photo skin types, that epidermal 6BH$_4$ *de novo* synthesis/recycling is induced 24 hours after UVB exposure with only one application of an individual minimal erythema dose (MED).[9] 6BH$_4$ downregulates tyrosinase activity by non-competitive kinetics in melanocytes ($K_i = 13 \times 10^{-3}$ M) and controls tyrosine hydroxylase (EC 1.14.16.2) activity in keratinocytes by means of an allosteric mechanism.[10] A single conserved specific binding domain for 6BH$_4$ has been identified in tyrosinases from neurospora, frogs, mice, and humans.[10] UVB can reactivate the 6BH$_4$/tyrosinase inhibitor complex in a dose-dependent manner, whereas the longer wavelengths of UVA (320–400 nm) exert no effect on this process.[11] Recently we were able to demonstrate *in vivo* epidermal hydrogen peroxide (H$_2$O$_2$) generation, resulting from UVB exposure, by using Fourier-Transform Raman spectroscopy.[12] In this context, it is noteworthy that H$_2$O$_2$ effectively oxidizes 6BH$_4$ to 6-biopterin.[12] Clearly this mechanism could be valid for reactivation of the 6BH$_4$/tyrosinase inhibitor complex.

HOW IS α-MELANOCYTE STIMULATING HORMONE (α-MSH) LINKED TO 6BH$_4$ IN MELANOGENESIS?

More than 40 years ago Lerner and McGuire demonstrated, *in vivo*, that application of α-MSH to human skin darkens skin color.[13,14] The consequence of this observation induced a plethora of pro- and contra-scientific publications on the subject (see Ref. 15 for a review). It has been shown that α-MSH upregulates tyrosinase mRNA in mouse melanoma cells.[16] Furthermore, hormone-mediated increase of tyrosinase activity was shown to occur.[17,18] α-MSH is a 13-amino-acid peptide (N-acetyl-ser^1-tyr^2-ser^3-met^4-glu^5-his^6-phe^7-arg^8-trp^9-gly^{10}-lys^{11}-pro^{12}-val^{13}-NH$_2$) cleaved from adrenocorticotropic hormone (ACTH) by prohormone convertase-2 (PC2).[19] The presence of α-MSH, as well as the presence of both convertases, PC1 and PC2, have been demonstrated in human skin biopsies.[20] FIGURE 1 shows an immunohistochemical stain of a full-skin biopsy, illustrating a much more pronounced color in melanocytes than in keratinocytes, and a close up view of melanocytes *in vitro*—where the expression of α-MSH clearly resides in granules. α-MSH was strictly located within melanosomes in melanocytes using immunoelectron microscopy (see FIGURE 2). Based on this observation, the function of α-MSH in melanocytes was further explored. The key question of interest to us was: Could α-MSH be linked to the cofactor 6BH$_4$ and consequently control 6BH$_4$-dependent processes in these cells?

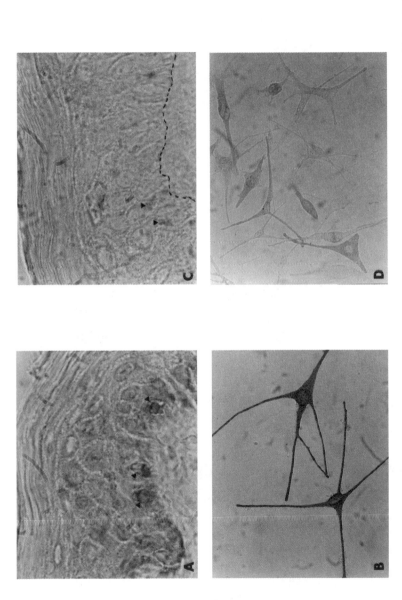

FIGURE 1. The presence of α-MSH in the human epidermis and in melanocyte granules. Sections from healthy skin (**A**, ×100) and of human cultured melanocytes (**B**, ×400) compared to negative controls (**C** and **D**). Melanocytes (▼) are stained primarily in granules with higher intensity around the nucleus. In the control (**C**), melanocytes (▼) are indicated by their pigment only. Keratinocytes show considerably less staining. Melanocytes from normal adult epidermis were established in a modified MCDB 153 medium on glass cover slips.[30]

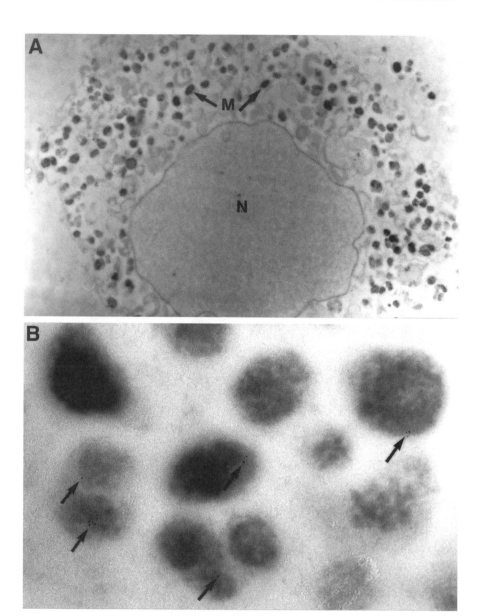

FIGURE 2. Immuno-electron microscopic evidence for α-MSH association with melanosomes. Normal adult human epidermal melanocytes were established from sun unexposed caucasian skin, as described in FIGURE 1, and processed for postembedding immunoelectron microscopy using 5 nm gold conjugate without any additional staining. Note the restriction of the gold particle to the melanosome (→) and their absence in the cytoplasm. **(A).** The melanocyte shows numerous melanosomes of different stages (magnification ×9,000; *N*, nucleus; *M*, melanosomes). **(B).** A close up view of individual melanosomes shows the α-MSH/gold conjugate as black dots (→) (magnification ×69,000).

α-MSH CAN CONTROL THE SUPPLY OF
L-TYROSINE IN HUMAN MELANOCYTES

L-Tyrosine is synthesized from L-phenylalanine in the cytosol of human melano-cytes associated with high PAH activities.[7,8] Recently a detailed study on the trans-port and metabolism of L-phenylalanine to L-tyrosine, compared with direct L-tyrosine uptake in human melanocytes cultured under *in vitro* conditions, revealed that significantly more L-tyrosine is produced via PAH.[21] $6BH_4$ controls PAH in two ways: (1) At high concentration, it binds to PAH-active dimers forming inactive tet-ramers with very little enzyme activity.[22] (2) $6BH_4$ acts as the cofactor/electron do-nor for the hydroxylation of L-phenylalanine to L-tyrosine on the catalytic site.[22] Our experiments show that α-MSH can activate PAH by removal of $6BH_4$ from inactive

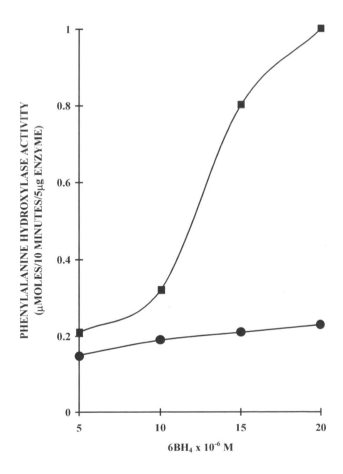

FIGURE 3. α-MSH forms active PAH dimers from inactive tetramers. The influence of $6BH_4$ on PAH activity in the presence (■) and absence of low levels of α-MSH, indicat-ing active dimer formation from inactive tetramer (●).

tetramers yielding active dimers (see FIGURE 3). As a consequence, α-MSH could effectively control the supply of L-tyrosine from L-phenylalanine in melanocytes.

THE REGULATION OF TYROSINASE BY α-MSH

Tyrosinase is subject to allosteric inhibition by $6BH_4$ by a regulatory binding domain involving 13 amino acids.[10] The tyrosinase/$6BH_4$ inhibitor complex can be fully reactivated by binding $6BH_4$ to α-MSH 1:1.[23] FIGURE 4 shows the activation of

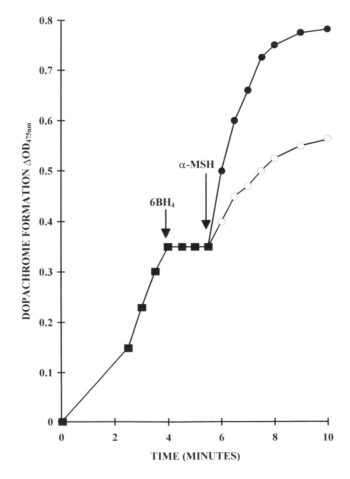

FIGURE 4. α-MSH reactivates the $6BH_4$/tyrosinase inhibitor complex. Tyrosinase activity was determined by following the formation of dopachrome at 475 nm from L-tyrosine $(10^{-3}$ M) (■). The enzyme was inhibited upon the addition of 18 μmoles $6BH_4$. After six minutes enzyme activity was fully restored with 18 μmoles α-MSH (1:1) (●). Note that enzyme activity is only partially restored using 36 μmoles α-MSH (1:2) (○).

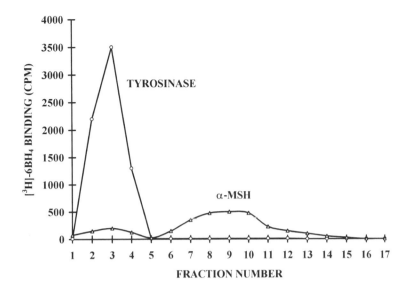

FIGURE 5. Transfer of [³H]-6BH₄ from the 6BH₄/tyrosine complex to α-MSH. Reactions contained 10 µl [³H]-6BH₄ (0.4 µCi), 100 µl tris buffer (0.05 M) pH 7.5, 200 µl human tyrosinase (63 Kd) (1.5 mg/ml) and 0.1 M DTE. The labeled inhibitor was allowed to bind for 15 minutes at 25°C followed by chromatographic separation on a Biogel P6 column (5 ml) from BioRad (540 µl/fraction). The tyrosinase [³H]-6BH₄ complex eluted in fractions 2–5 (○). The peak fractions 2 and 3 were pooled and incubated for 10 minutes with 100 µl α-MSH (4 mg/ml) and rechromatographed. Under the experimental conditions, the majority of [³H]-6BH₄/α-MSH eluted in fractions 6–12 on the same column (△).

6BH₄ inhibited tyrosinase by α-MSH. The stoichiometry for [³H]-labeled 6BH₄ transfer from human tyrosinase to α-MSH using P6 biogel chromatography is exhibited in FIGURE 5. In this context, it is noteworthy that desacetylated α-MSH cannot activate the inhibitor complex, underlining the importance of the N-acetyl group for this α-MSH activity.

THE INHIBITION OF PAH AND TYROSINASE BY α-MSH

Both PAH and tyrosinase are fully activated by the α-MSH 1:1-complex with 6BH₄. However, free α-MSH functions as a competitive inhibitor of tyrosinase activity, presumably due to the presence of tyr^2 in its sequence.[23] Based on detailed kinetic analyses it can be concluded that tyr^2 must be internalized in the structure of the complex and is, therefore, unavailable to react with its substrate binding site on the enzyme. These results suggest that the ratio of α-MSH to 6BH₄ in the melanocyte could offer a fine control mechanism for constitutive/inherited pigment in different skin types.

STRUCTURAL STUDIES OF THE α-MSH/6BH$_4$ COMPLEX

Both 500-MHz NMR and Fourier-Transform Raman spectroscopy (FT-Raman) indicate that free α-MSH has a random structure in solution.[24] The binding of [^{3}H]-labeled 6BH$_4$ to α-MSH established a 1:1 stoichiometry for the optimal α-MSH/6BH$_4$-complex formation. Stereospecificity for 6BH$_4$ binding to α-MSH was confirmed, since 7BH$_4$, dihydropterin, 6-biopterin, 7,8-dihydroxanthopterin, and substances with similar pyrimidine ring structures (such as GTP, GDP, GMP, and cyclic GMP) did not bind to the peptide.

FT-Raman spectroscopy proved the specificity of 6BH$_4$ binding to α-MSH where tyr^2, glu^5, and his^6 are strongly implicated in complex formation. The tyrosine ring stretch at 1618.9 cm^{-1} and ring breathing at 643.6 cm^{-1} decrease in intensity with complex formation, whereas, compared to the same vibrational mode for phenylalanine at 1603.1 cm^{-1}, the peak at 622.4 cm^{-1} remains unaffected. Changes in these Raman bands can be attributed to π-orbital interactions in the benzene ring of ty-

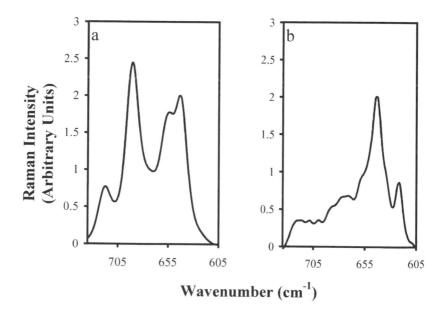

Wavenumber (cm^{-1})

FIGURE 6. FT-Raman spectrum of 6BH$_4$ and the 6BH$_4$/α-MSH complex. **(a).** The deformation modes for the pyrimidine (691.8 cm^{-1}) and pyrazine ring (635 cm^{-1}) are clearly visible. The shoulders seen at 645 and 715 cm^{-1} are due to different ring geometries found in the solid dihydrochloride salt. **(b).** After complex formation to α-MSH the pyrimidine ring deformation disappears. This is most likely to be due to steric hindrance on the pyrimidine based on three hydrogen bonds formed between glu^5 and his^6. The peak at 620 cm^{-1} is due to the tyrosine residue in position 2. FT-Raman spectra were obtained using a Bruker RFS 100/S FT-Raman spectrometer equipped with a liquid nitrogen cooled germanium detector. Solid samples were excited by using an Nd^{3+} YAG laser operating at 1064 nm with a power of 200 mW. Spectra were accumulated after 1000 scans with a resolution of 1 cm^{-1}.

rosine. These data are supported by a considerable decrease in the pyrimidine ring deformation mode at 691.8 cm^{-1}, which is one of the most intense bands of uncomplexed 6BH$_4$. There are also slightly decreased intensities of the pyrimidine ring stretch at 1578.2 cm^{-1}. The decrease in intensity of the ring stretch band is greatly perturbed, indicative of π-orbital interaction (see FIGURE 6). Therefore, we conclude that α-MSH/6BH$_4$ complex formation involves a π-π–interaction between the benzene ring of the tyrosine residue and the 6BH$_4$ molecule.[25] Glu[5] and his[6] appeared to be crucial for complex formation. In order to test the importance of glu[5], this ami-

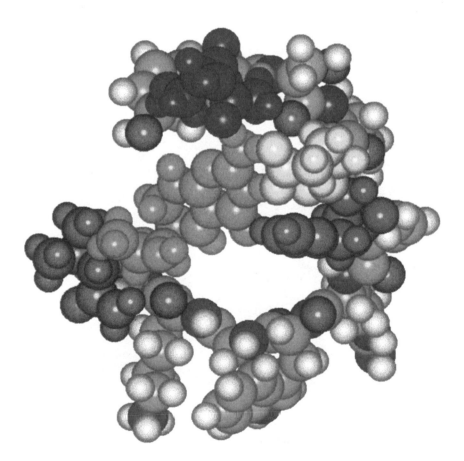

FIGURE 7. Minimized Hyperchem™ 3D-structure of the aqueous α-MSH/6BH$_4$ complex. H-bonds are confirmed from the carbonyl group of N-acetyl ser[1] to one of the H-atoms of the amino group in the pterin ring. The second H-atom of the amino group complexes to the carboxylate group of glu[5] together with a proton from N$_1$ of the pteridine ring. The N$_1$ proton of his[6] complexes to the carbonyl group of the pteridine ring. In free α-MSH his[6] is protonated on N$_3$. The amide proton of val[13] H-bonds to the OH group in position 2 of the erythro (R) side chain. After 6BH$_4$ complex formation α-MSH forms a defined cyclic 3D-structure. (Green, 6BH$_4$; purple, N-acetyl-Ser[1]; yellow, Glu[5]; pink. his[6]; red, val[13].)

no acid was replaced by ala[5]. This peptide was inactive in both $6BH_4$-binding and tyrosinase activation, emphasizing the specificity of glu[5] (data not shown).

Minimized Hyperchem™ modeling of the thermodynamically most stable form of the α-MSH/$6BH_4$ complex in water predicted H-bonds from N-acetyl-ser[1], glu[5], his[6], and val[3] with π-π–interaction between the pyrimidine ring of $6BH_4$ and tyr[2] (see FIGURE 7). This molecular model is supported by the FT-Raman data. Interestingly, this complex has a definitive 3D-structure that is cyclic and involves both the N- and C-terminal residues of α-MSH.

PROPERTIES OF THE α-MSH/$6BH_4$ STRUCTURE

Free $6BH_4$ is unstable to molecular O_2 at room temperature. A 10^{-3} M solution of $6BH_4$ at pH 7.0 is oxidized in approximately four hours. In contrast, the α-MSH/$6BH_4$ complex is stable to oxidation for three days under the same conditions. Furthermore, $6BH_4$ is photolabile to UVB-light. It is rapidly photooxidized to 7,8-dihydroxanthopterin.[11] High doses of UVB oxidize $6BH_4$ to 6-biopterin by H_2O_2 generation. In contrast, the α-MSH/$6BH_4$ complex is significantly more stable to UVB photo-oxidation.[23] Here, it is interesting that α-MSH release increases after UVB exposure.[26] The protection of $6BH_4$ by α-MSH suggests that the hormone could act as a chaperone for $6BH_4$ in the human epidermis, where pterins may play a key role in regulation of pigmentation and differentiation. The induction of both $6BH_4$ *de novo* synthesis and α-MSH synthesis by inflammatory cytokines, such as TNF-α, γ-IFN, and IL-2, indicates that the $6BH_4$/α-MSH interaction could involve a number of other biologically important processes.[27,28]

CONCLUDING REMARKS

The results presented in this report point to a novel autocrine mechanism for the regulation of melanogenesis by the concerted action of α-MSH and $6BH_4$. FIGURE 8 summarizes the proposed mechanism. The concentration of α-MSH in the melanosomes could offer a critical fine control for constitutive pigmentation; that is, inherited skin color: (1) As a consequence of lower α-MSH levels when compared to $6BH_4$ levels, low tyrosinase activity would be predicted. (2) The 1:1 complex formation of α-MSH to $6BH_4$ is presumably optimal for pigmentation activation (FIG. 4). (3) However, if α-MSH levels are higher than $6BH_4$ levels, tyrosinase should be inhibited due to tyr[2] in the peptide sequence, since this can act as a competitive substrate-inhibitor. Several questions remain to be answered.

1. Are the concentrations of α-MSH and $6BH_4$ in melanosomes isolated from photo skin types I–VI (Fitzpatrick classification) different?

2. Does the α-MSH/$6BH_4$ complex react with the MC-1 receptor?

3. Is α-MSH/$6BH_4$ interaction also involved in the control of pigmentation during the hair cycle? Recent results from our laboratory indicate that the *de novo* synthesis of $6BH_4$ follows the synchronized hair cycle in the murine C57BL/6 model, preceding the expression of tyrosinase.[29]

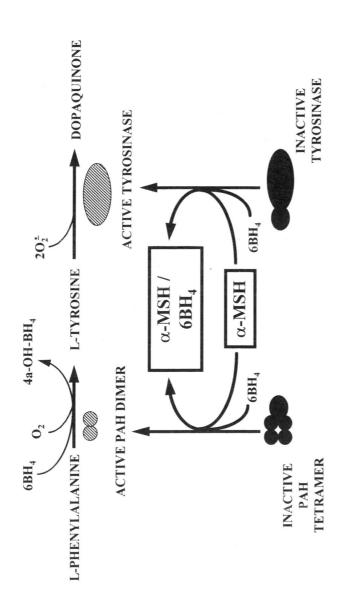

FIGURE 8. A proposed mechanism for α-MSH removal of $6BH_4$ from both regulatory domains on PAH and tyrosinase to activate melanogenesis. α-MSH converts the inactive tetramer of PAH into an active dimer, meanwhile the allosteric inhibition of tyrosinase is released due to removal of $6BH_4$ by α-MSH from the enzyme.

It has also been shown that TNF-α, γ-IFN, and IL-2 can directly upregulate 6BH$_4$ *de novo* synthesis by means of GTP-cyclohydrolase-I, the key enzyme of 6BH$_4$ *de novo* synthesis.[27,28] Future research will be directed to explore a possible link between these and other cytokines and the 6BH4/α-MSH interaction.

ACKNOWLEDGMENT

This research was generously supported by Stiefel International. The [^{3}H]-labeled 6BH$_4$ was a gift from E.R. Werner, Institute for Medical Chemistry and Biochemistry, University of Innsbruck, Austria. The α-MSH antibody was kindly provided by A.J. Thody, Department of Biomedical Sciences, University of Bradford, UK. Helen Bartle typed the manuscript.

REFERENCES

1. PROTA, G. 1976. Melanins and Melanogenesis. Academic Press, New York.
2. FITZPATRICK, T.B. *et al.* 1971. Photomedicine. *In* Dermatology in General Medicine. McGraw-Hill Book Co, New York.
3. FRENK, E. & J.P. SCHELLHORN. 1969. Morphology of the epidermal melanin unit. Dermatologica **139:** 271–277.
4. IWATA, M. *et al.* 1990. The relationship between tyrosinase activity and skin colour in human foreskins. J. Invest. Dermatol. **95:** 9–15.
5. IOZUMI, K. *et al.* 1993. Role of tyrosinase as the determinant of pigmentation in cultured human melanocytes. J. Invest. Dermatol. **100:** 806–811.
6. KAUFMAN, S. 1964. The role of pteridines in the enzymatic conversion of phenylalanine to tyrosine. Trans. N.Y. Acad. Sci. **26:** 977–983.
7. SCHALLREUTER, K.U. *et al.* 1994. Regulation of melanin biosynthesis in the human epidermis by tetrahydrobiopterin. Science. **263:** 1444–1446.
8. SCHALLREUTER, K.U. *et al.* 1994. Defective tetrahydrobiopterin and catecholamine biosynthesis in the depigmentation disorder vitiligo. Biochim. Biophys. Acta **1226:** 181–192.
9. SCHALLREUTER, K.U. *et al.* 1997. Pteridines in the control of pigmentation. J. Invest. Dermatol. **109:** 31–35.
10. WOOD, J.M. *et al.* 1995. A specific tetrahydrobiopterin binding domain on tyrosinase controls melanogenesis. Biochem. Biophys. Res. Commun. **206:** 480–485.
11. SCHALLREUTER, K.U. *et al.* 1998. 6-tetrahydrobiopterin functions as a UVB-light switch for de novo melanogenesis. Biochem. Biophys. Acta **1382:** 339–344.
12. SCHALLREUTER, K.U. *et al.* 1999. *In vivo* and *in vitro* evidence for hydrogen peroxide (H_2O_2) accumulation in the epidermis of patients with vitiligo and its successful removal by a UVB-activated pseudocatalase. J. Invest. Dermatol. Symp. Proc. In press.
13. LERNER, A.B. & J.S. MCGUIRE. 1961. Effect of alpha and beta melanocyte stimulating hormones on skin color of man. Nature **189:** 176–179.
14. LERNER, A.B. 1993. The discovery of the melanotropins. Ann. N.Y. Acad. Sci. **680:** 2–12.
15. WINTZEN, M. *et al.* 1996. Proopiomelanocortin, its derived peptides in the skin. J. Invest. Dermatol. **106:** 3–10.
16. RUNGTA, D. *et al.* 1996. Regulation of tyrosinase mRNA in mouse melanoma cells by α-melanocyte-stimulating hormone. J. Invest. Dermatol. **107:** 689–693.
17. PAWELEK, J. *et al.* 1973. Molecular biology of pigment cells. Molecular controls in mammalian pigmentation. Yale. J. Biol. Med. **46:** 430–443.

18. FULLER, B.B. *et al.* 1987. Alpha-melanocyte stimulating hormone regulation of tyrosinase in Cloudman S-91 mouse melanoma cell cultures. J. Biol. Chem. **262:** 4024–4033.

19. STRYER, L. 1988. Biochemistry, 3rd ed. 993–994. W.H. Freeman. New York.

20. WAKAMATSU, K. *et al.* 1997. Characterisation of ACTH peptides in human skin and their activation of the melanocortin-1 receptor. Pigment. Cell. Res. **10:** 288–297.

21. SCHALLREUTER, K.U. *et al.* 1998. Perturbed epidermal pterin metabolism in Hermansky-Pudlak syndrome. J. Invest. Dermatol. **111:** 511–516.

22. DAVIS, M.D. *et al.* 1996. Structure-function relationships of phenylalanine hydroxylase revealed by radiation target analysis. Arch. Biochem. Biophys. **325:** 235–241.

23. SCHALLREUTER, K.U. *et al.* 1997. Pterins and α-MSH in the control of pigmentation in the human epidermis. *In* Chemistry and Biology of Pteridines and Folates. W. Pfleiderer & H. Rokos, Eds.: 791–795. Blackwell Science, Berlin.

24. MOORE, J. *et al.* 1997. Studies in the structure of the tetrahydrobiopterin/α-MSH complex formation using Fourier-Transform Raman spectroscopy. *In* Chemistry and Biology of Pteridines and Folates. W. Pfleiderer & H. Rokos, Eds.: 831–835. Blackwell Science, Berlin.

25. SIAMWIZA, M.N. *et al.* 1975. Interpretation of the doublet at 850 and 830 cm^{-1} in the Raman spectra of tyrosyl residues in proteins and certain model compounds. Biochem. **4:** 4870–4876.

26. CHAKRABORTY, A.K. *et al.* 1996. Production and release of proopiomelanocortin (POMC) derived peptides by human melanocytes and keratinocytes in culture: regulation by ultraviolet B. Biochim. Biophys. Acta **1313:** 130–138.

27. WERNER, E.R. *et al.* 1990. Impact of tumour necrosis factor-α and interferon-γ on tetrahydrobiopterin synthesis in murine fibroblasts and macrophages. Biochem. J. **280:** 709–714.

28. ZIEGLER, I. *et al.* 1990. Control of tetrahydrobiopterin synthesis in T-lymphocytes by synergistic action of interferon-γ and interleukin-2. J. Biol. Chem. **265:** 17026–17030.

29. SCHALLREUTER, K.U. *et al.* 1998. Pterins in human hair follicle cells and the synchronized murine hair cycle. J. Invest. Dermatol. **111:** 545–550.

30. PITTELKOW, M.R. & SHIPLEY, G.D. 1989. Serum free culture of normal human melanocytes: growth kinetics and growth factor requirements. J. Cell. Physiol. **140:** 565–576.

Melanocortins and the Treatment of Nervous System Disease

Potential Relevance to the Skin?

WILLEM HENDRIK GISPEN AND ROGER A.H. ADAN

Rudolf Magnus Institute for Neurosciences, Department of Medical Pharmacology, Utrecht University, Universiteitsweg 100, 3584 CG Utrecht, The Netherlands

ABSTRACT: For several decades melanocortins have been implicated in the modulation of brain function. More recently, this idea has been supported by the identification and cloning of melanocortin (MC) receptors in the nervous system. MCs stimulate axonal growth in fetal neural tissue or in neural cell lines in culture. This feature was utilized in screening their neurotrophic or neuroprotection potential in animal studies of nervous system disease (peripheral nerve and spinal cord trauma, toxic and metabolic neuropathies, EAN, EAE, etc.). Some of these effects may be mediated by MC4 receptor activation, although as yet unknown receptors may also be involved (for instance, protection by Org 2766). To what extent MC-nervous system effects are related to known effects of MCs in skin- and neuro-immune systems, remains to be discovered. Nevertheless, it is of interest to note that activation of brain MC4 receptors profoundly affects care behavior for the body surface (skin and fur). The excessive grooming response in rodents exhibits a remarkable functional correlation with MSH activity in a brain–skin axis.

INTRODUCTION

Historically, our interest in the role that peptides related to ACTH and MSH play in nervous system function originates from the pioneering research by David de Wied.[1] In 1969, he formulated his neuropeptide concept, which was based on his findings that peptides derived from the pituitary directly influence brain function and behavior, in addition to their hormonal activity. Thus, well before the demonstration of a melanocortin peptidergic network, and the discovery of brain melanocortin (MC) receptors, neural cells were already thought to be targets for MC related peptides. By analogy with peptide hormone-peripheral target cell interactions, it was hypothesized that the effects of MCs on the nervous system could be described in terms of a modulatory and a trophic nature. The former concerns the effects on neurotransmission and a variety of behaviors, whereas for some 25 no evidence was available for the latter. In line with the trophic effect of ACTH on adrenal cortical RNA and protein synthesis, early studies by us and others revealed that MC related peptides were able to stimulate brain RNA and protein synthesis, especially in the brains of hypophysectomized rats.[2,3] Much later this trophic response was better documented in studies employing fetal neural tissue or neurons in culture.[4] Parallel *in vivo* studies, mainly using animal models of peripheral nerve neuropathy, demonstrated that

MC peptides displayed neurotrophic or neuroprotective effects that could be of significance in the quest for new and effective therapy of peripheral nervous disorders.[5]

MELANOCORTINS AND TROPHIC
EFFECTS IN NEURAL DEVELOPMENT

Early studies by the group of Swaab,[6] pointed to a fetal growth-promoting factor of hypothalamic origin. Injection of α-MSH antibodies directly into the foetus inhibited fetal and brain growth, suggesting that there was a physiological role played by α-MSH in fetal brain development, among other processes. Another example relates to the effect of neonatal administration of peptides derived from ACTH and α-MSH on brain maturation, as evidenced by a peptide-enhanced eye opening.[7] Furthermore, early postnatal treatment with these peptides also accelerated the development of the neuromuscular junction.[8] Since the latter data were interpreted to stem from both neurotrophic and myotrophic origins, they underscore the conclusion that neurotrophic effects may be seen in the CNS, as well as in the PNS.[9]

Subsequently, a variety of studies documented the effects of melanocortin peptides derived from this family on the differentiation, survival, and outgrowth of neurites in embryonal neuronal cultures. These studies employed E10-12 rat cerebral cells, E14 rat raphe neurones, E8 chick cerebral neurons, E6 quail dorsal root ganglia (DRG), E15 rat DRG, E15 rat spinal cord slices, and spinal cord cells.[4] The data collectively and unequivocally demonstrated that melanocortins exert a direct effect on CNS- and PNS-neurones in culture, and open the possibility that they may play a similar role in adults for the protection or repair of neuronal networks following noxious influences.

MELANOCORTINS AND PNS REPAIR

Although several research groups studied the effect of peptide treatment on functional parameters following brain lesions, the first systematic approach in the search for neurotrophic activity of MCs *in vivo* concerned their beneficial role in the functional recovery from injury to the peripheral nervous system. Both the group of Strand and our own group used the peripheral nerve as model for its well-documented morphology and accessibility for neurophysiologic and functional techniques. Strand and Kung,[10] and Bijlsma et al.,[11] independently reported that systemic treatment of rats with ACTH or nonhormonally active fragments resulted in an earlier return of sensori (motor) function following a crush lesion of the sciatic nerve. Importantly, it was argued that this functional effect originated from a direct neurotrophic effect of the peptides on the injured nerve and its corresponding neuronal cell bodies. The pharmacology of the peptide treatment in this animal model was extensively studied: (1) The route of administration; effective treatment following subcutaneous and local administration; ineffective following i.p., oral, or nasal application. (2) The dose-response relationship; inverted U-shaped. (3) The treatment schedule; only effective immediately following the nerve trauma. (4) The structure-activity relationships; $ACTH_{1-24}$, α-MSH, Org 2766, $ACTH_{4-10}$, and NDP-α-MSH were active.[11,12]

Peptide treatment did not increase axonal outgrowth but shortened the delay of new sprout formation and increased the number of newly formed sprouts.[13] Under proper experimental conditions the peptide treatment improved the recovery of both sensori and motor function and shortened the delay in recovery of motor and sensori nerve conduction.

This neurotrophic activity *in vivo* was further substantiated by studies using trauma of the facial nerve, oculomotor nerve and the caudal nerve in the rat. These and other data prompted us to investigate whether peptide treatment might be of significance to protection or repair in nontrauma afflictions of the peripheral nerve, such as in metabolic-, toxic-, or immune-mediated neuropathies.

MELANOCORTIN AND PERIPHERAL NEUROPATHIES

The first series of experiments addressed the putative protection by Org 2766 of cisplatin-induced neurotoxicity in the rat sciatic nerve. At that time no information on the MC receptor subtypes was available, and since Org 2766 shares many neurotrophic properties with α-MSH, this was the peptide most studied. The peptide had a somewhat longer biological half-life and could eventually be used in humans based on its safe toxicological profile. In a rat model of cisplatin-mediated neuropathy it was observed that Org 2766 treatment markedly protected the peripheral nerve.[14] As observed in the human clinic, the chemotherapeutic drug selectively lowered sensory, H-reflex-related nerve-conduction velocity, leaving motor nerve conduction velocity intact. Peptide treatment in rats of all ages almost completely blocked this effect of the drug on sciatic nerve conduction velocity without affecting the antitumor activity of the drug. After adequate animal experimentation, a multicenter randomized double-blind clinical trial was performed, involving 54 women that received cisplatin based therapy of ovarian carcinoma. The end-point parameter was the possible amelioration of treatment with Org 2766 on the cisplatin-induced increase in vibration perception threshold. In addition, clinical signs and symptoms were scored. In the group of women that received high doses of Org 2766 before and after each infusion with chemotherapy, the vibration perception threshold was not altered—as observed in the placebo cisplatin treatment patients. Likewise, the sum score of clinical signs and symptoms of their neuropathy was reduced. In a follow up of a subgroup of patients, during the period that no peptide treatment was given, a rebound effect on the vibration perception threshold was evident. In a few subsequent clinical studies by other groups involving patients with testicular or ovarian cancer and different regimens of chemotherapy, peptide treatment was less helpful and showed no effect. The only other positive clinical trial reported was a protective effect in patients treated with vincristin.[15]

One of the most common neuropathies is the symmetric peripheral diabetic neuropathy. Although the exact pathogenetic mechanism remains unclear, it seems that, despite rigid metabolic control, this diabetic complication is a severe risk for patients suffering from type-I diabetus mellitus for a long period. In the commonly used experimental model of this complication; that is, the streptozotocin treated rat or the BB-war rat; treatment with Org 2766 prevented or interfered with the neuropathy, as evidenced by a gain in sensory- and motor-nerve conduction-velocity.[16] Similar treatment also reduced the expression of autonomic neuropathy in streptozotocin rats.

The question of whether this peptide treatment affected the *vasa nervorum* or the *nervi vasorum* remains unresolved. Either way, enhanced blood supply would counteract the development of the ischemic conditions leading to the neuropathy. Only one study is available in the literature that describes some small beneficial effects from chronic treatment with Org 2766 in patients suffering from neuropathy associated with type-I diabetes mellitus.[17]

The last model of a common neuropathy is that of experimental allergic neuritis in Lewis rats. In various forms, this model is often used in the study of the human Guillain-Barré syndrome. Treatment with Org 2766 during the development, or following the first signs of the neuritis, markedly reduced the clinical signs and improved sensori-motor function—paralleled by the saving or appearance of small myelinated fibres in the tibial nerve. Although there are experimental data that argue against an immunosuppressive effect of the peptide treatment, an immune mediated mechanism in addition to a direct neuroprotective effect cannot be excluded.[18,19]

Collectively, the data on the protective effect of Org 2766 on neuropathic conditions caused by different pathogenic stimuli (trauma, toxicity, altered metabolism, or immune-related) suggest that peptides derived from MCs affect a common denominator in the process of nerve protection or repair. One hypothesis is that neurons, irrespective of the nature of the noxious stimulus, counterfight their compromised function by activating a general trophic repair program in which peptides play a pathophysiologic role. Indeed there is circumstantial evidence to suggest that endogenous POMC-derived peptides may play such role. Such a general role could be deduced from the effects of the peptides on developing neuronal cells of different origin. Peptide pharmacotherapy would then mimic or amplify that function of endogenous peptides. On the other hand, it may well be that the notion that these peptides exert profound effects on the sympathetic nervous system, and thus indirectly on nerves that receive sympathetic input on their vessels, is sufficient to explain the protective or trophic moiety of these peptides under a variety of experimentally induced neuropathies.

MOLECULAR MECHANISM OF ACTION

As is common knowledge in pharmacology, activity of a given compound *in vivo* predicts the existence of a receptor. Recognition and activation being the key principles underlying biological effects. The identification of MC receptors took a major effort of many research groups.[20–26] Once established, it became clear that there is a family of five MC-receptor subtypes, of which at least two can be found in the nervous system. In view of the heterogeneity in place, time, and function of neural tissue and the localized distribution of MC-receptor subtypes in the nervous system, it is not surprising that so many different effects of MC had been observed over the years preceding the discovery of these receptors.

There is only limited information on the MC-receptor subtype that is responsible for the neurotrophic activity of MCs as outlined above. Since Org 2766 has no affinity for MC-receptors,[27] the effects of MCs on nerve regeneration are mediated by an unidentified Org 2766 receptor that also binds MCs; or there are two distinct receptor types involved—an Org-receptor and a MC-receptor. Two lines of evidence support the latter. The potent MC-receptor agonist NDP-α-MSH stimulates nerve regeneration, and the MC4 receptor is located in brain and spinal cord (as demonstrated by RNAse protection and *in situ* binding assays). The brain and spinal cord are putative target tissues for the beneficial effect of MCs on nerve regeneration (Van der Kraan *et al.*, Mol. Brain Res., submitted for publication). We rule out involvement of the MC3 receptor since the MC3 receptor-selective agonist, γ-MSH, does not stimulate nerve regeneration.[28] Although insufficient immunocytochemical data are available to be able to precisely localize the MC-receptor subtype in the population of neurons in the spinal cord, its presence in areas involved in nociception suggests a modulatory role on the spinal neuronal network. This may influence the function of neurites communicating with, or originating from, the spinal cord (peripheral nerve). In a direct molecular approach to try to delineate the neurotrophic moiety at the receptor level, neuro-2A cells that themselves express MC4 receptors were stimulated with α-MSH.[29] Activation of these receptors by α-MSH led to pronounced neurite outgrowth. Blockade of these receptors with an MC4-specific antagonist in a dose-dependent manner, completely blocked the MSH induced outgrowth. When the receptor was bypassed using forskolin as a stimulator of the second messenger cAMP, a similar trophic response was observed in Neuro 2A cells after α-MSH. Thus, the neurotrophic influence of α-MSH *in vitro* most likely originated from MC4-receptor activation, resulting in the elevation of intracellular cAMP.

NEUROECTODERM: NERVOUS SYSTEM AND SKIN

Within the context of this volume one is forced to consider common roles that α-MSH may play in the physiology of brain and skin. Functionally, a common role of this type is nicely presented by the MSH-mediated effects on the skin melanocytes of amphibia that control their adaptation to the environment. In many higher species of vertebrates, where α-MSH–mediated effects on melanocytes are of less significance to the organism as a whole, MSH is thought to play an adaptive modulating role in brain function. There are several other examples that support a brain-skin axis based on the common ontogenetic origin of certain neurons and melanocytes. In our own research we have studied the brain–skin axis from yet another interesting functional perspective.

MC PEPTIDES AND CARE OF THE BODY SURFACE BEHAVIOR

In the search for neuroactive moieties in ACTH- and MSH-like peptides, Ferrari[30] was the first to report that in a variety of species, notably in the dog, cat, rabbit, and rat, intracisternal injection of ACTH and that of fragments related to ACTH and MSH induced a so-called stretching and yawning syndrome, which in the rat was paralleled by excessive grooming and stretching. Years later, we became interested in the latter as a potential rapid assay for CNS effectivity of MC receptors.

In mammals grooming is part of a care-of-the-body-surface (COBS) repertoire that also consists of stretching, nibbling, rubbing, wallowing, and bathing. These behaviors serve to remove ectoparasites, dirt, or aversive substances; and they may act in thermoregulation, chemocommunication, and wound healing. From studies in rodents and primates, both allo- and autogrooming may serve various other functions such as dearousal, regulation of social tension, and reconciliation.[31]

Using specific agonists and antagonists it was demonstrated that MC-receptor–mediated grooming originates from activation of the MC4-receptor subtype.[27,32] Likewise, novelty induced grooming in the rat, which is thought to reflect a dearousal mechanism, can be blocked by pretreatment with SHU 9119—a potent MC receptor antagonist (Adan *et al.*, Eur. J. Pharmacol, in press). This latter observation suggests that natural grooming, occurring during or after mild stressful stimuli, is governed by a neural substrate involving MC4 receptors. It has long been recognized that grooming consists of a fixed motor program that is centrally activated and to which peripheral inputs are of lesser significance. Classically, peptide-mediated grooming is only elicited following central application of the peptides. Recently, we were able to demonstrate that systemic injection of the potent MC4-agonist, MT-II, elicits a similar display of grooming, implying that this MSH-analog effectively penetrates the blood-brain barrier and reaches the responsible grooming induction sites in the brain.

There is little information on the significance of central MC4 receptors in humans. Intracisternally, an ACTH preparation in doses up to 0.02 μg/kg in men caused nausea and vomiting, but no grooming or stretching was observed.[33] A recent report on MT-II suggests that men with psychogenic erectile dysfunction responded favorable to the peptide treatment.[34] Side effects that were reported from MT-II treatment were nausea, decreased appetite; and, interestingly, stretching and yawning. Such observations would be in line with older animal literature on the effects of MC-peptides on penile erections in rodents, seen in parallel with the stretching and yawning syndrome, and excessive grooming.

CONCLUDING REMARKS

The identification of MC receptors has now provided us with the pharmacologic and genetic tools to identify the mechanism underlying the effects of MCs on the nervous system, the skin, and other systems (e.g. obesity). For instance, in mice with disruption of the MC5 receptor gene, a defect in subaceous gland function results in defects in thermoregulation.[35] The central effects of MCs on thermoregulation, as well as in grooming behavior (which functions to spread lipids over the skin), suggest a coordinating role played by MCs at different levels in order to control skin function. The application of stable, potent, and selective MC receptor ligands in models for nerve degeneration, obesity, and malignances of the skin, has yet to reveal whether MC receptors form a drug target in these disorders.

REFERENCES

1. DE WIED, D. 1969. Effects of peptide hormones on behavior. *In* Frontiers in Neuroendocrinology. W.F. Ganong & L. Martini, Eds.: 97–140.

2. DUNN, A.J. & P. SCHOTMAN. 1986. Effects of ACTH and related peptides on cerebral RNA and protein synthesis. In Neuropeptides and Behavior, vol. 1, CNS Effects of ACTH, MSH and Opioid Peptides. D. De Wied, W.H. Gispen & T.B. Van Wimersma Greidanus, Eds.: 165–187. Pergamon Press, Oxford.

3. DE GRAAN, P.N.E., P. SCHOTMAN & D.H.G. VERSTEEG. 1990. Neural mechanisms of action of neuropeptides: macromolecules and neurotransmitters. In Neuropeptides: Basics and Perspectives. D. De Wied, Ed.: 139–172. Elsevier Science Publishers B.V. Amsterdam.

4. HOL, E.M., W.H. GISPEN & P.R. BAR. 1995. ACTH-related peptides: receptors and signal transduction systems involved in their neurotrophic and neuroprotective actions. Peptides 16: 979–993.

5. GISPEN, W.H., J. VERHAAGEN & D. BAR. 1994. ACTH/MSH-derived peptides and peripheral nerve plasticity: neuropathies, neuroprotection and repair. Prog. Brain Res. 100: 223–229.

6. SWAAB, D.F., M. VISSER & F.J. TILDERS. 1976. Stimulation of intra-uterine growth in rat by alpha-melanocyte-stimulating hormone. J. Endocrinol. 70: 445–455.

7. VAN DER HELM-HYLKEMA, H. & D. DE WIED. 1976. Effect of neonatally injected ACTH and ACTH analogues on eye-opening of the rat. Life Sci. 18: 1099–1104.

8. STRAND, F.L., K.A. WILLIAMS, S.E. ALVES, F.J. ANTONAWICH, T.S. LEE, S.J. LEE, J. KUME & L.A. ZUCCARELLI. 1994. Melanocortins as factors in somatic neuromuscular growth and regrowth. Pharmacol. Ther. 62: 1–27.

9. STRAND, F.L., C. SAINT-COME, T.S. LEE, S.J. LEE, J. KUME & L.A. ZUCCARELLI. 1993. ACTH/MSH(4-10) analog BIM 22015 aids regeneration via neurotrophic and myotrophic attributes. Peptides 14: 287–296.

10. STRAND, F.L. & T.T. KUNG. 1980. ACTH accelerates recovery of neuromuscular function following crushing of peripheral nerve. Peptides 1: 135–138.

11. BIJLSMA, W.A., F.G.I. JENNEKENS, P. SCHOTMAN & W.H. GISPEN. 1981. Effects of corticotropin (ACTH) on recovery of sensorimotor function in the rat: structure-activity study. Eur. J. Pharmacol. 76: 73–79.

12. VAN DER ZEE, C.E.E.M., J.H. BRAKKEE & W.H. GISPEN. 1991. Putative neurotrophic factors and functional recovery from peripheral nerve damage in the rat. Br. J. Pharmacol. 103: 1041–1046.

13. VERHAAGEN, J., P.M. EDWARDS, F.G.I. JENNEKENS, P. SCHOTMAN & W.H. GISPEN. 1986. α-Melanocyte stimulating hormone stimulates the outgrowth of myelinated nerve fibers after peripheral nerve crush. Exp. Neurol. 92: 451–454.

14. HAMERS, F.P.T., C. PETTE, B. BRAVENBOER, C.J. VECHT, J.P. NEIJT & W.H. GISPEN. 1993. Cisplatin-induced neuropathy in mature rats. Effects of the melanocortin-derived peptide ORG 2766. Cancer Chemo. Pharmacol. 32: 162–166.

15. VAN KOOTEN, B., H.A. VAN DIEMEN, K.M. GROENHOUT, P.C. HUIJGENS, G.J. OSSEN-KOPPELE, J.J. NAUTA & J.J. HEIMANS. 1992. A pilot study on the influence of a corticotropin (4–9) analogue on Vinca alkaloid-induced neuropathy. Arch. Neurol. 49: 1027–1031.

16. BRAVENBOER, B., A.C. KAPELLE, T. VAN BUREN, D.W. ERKELENS & W.H. GISPEN. 1993. $ACTH_{4-9}$ analogue ORG 2766 can improve existing neuropathy in streptozocin-induced diabetic rats. Acta Diabetol. 30: 21–24.

17. BRAVENBOER, B., P.H. HENDRIKSE, P.L. OEY, A.C. VAN HUFFELEN, C. GROENHOUT, W.H. GISPEN & D.W. ERKELENS. 1994. Randomized double-blind placebo-controlled trial to evaluate the effect of the ACTH4-9 analogue ORG 2766 in IDDM patients with neuropathy. Diabetologia 37: 408–413.

18. DUCKERS, H.J., J. VERHAAGEN & W.H. GISPEN. 1993. The neurotrophic analogue of ACTH(4-9), Org 2766, protects against experimental allergic neuritis. Brain 116: 1059–1075.

19. DUCKERS, H.J.D., J. VERHAAGEN & W.H. GISPEN. 1993. A neurotrophic analogue of $ACTH_{4-9}$ protects against experimental allergic neuritis. Ann. N.Y. Acad. Sci. 680: 493–495.

20. CHHAJLANI, V. & J.E.S. WIKBERG. 1992. Molecular cloning and expression of the human melanocyte stimulating hormone receptor cDNA. FEBS Lett. **309:** 417–420.
21. CONE, R.D., D. LU, S. KOPPULA, D.I. VAGE, H. KLUNGLAND, B. BOSTON, W. CHEN, D.N. ORTH, C. POUTON & R.A. KESTERSON. 1996. The melanocortin receptors: agonists, antagonists, and the hormonal control of pigmentation. Recent. Prog. Horm. Res. **51:** 287–317; discussion 318.
22. GANTZ, I., H. MIWA, Y. KONDA, Y. SHIMOTO, T. TASHIRO, S.J. WATSON, J. DELVALLE & T. YAMADA. 1993. Molecular cloning, expression, and gene localization of a fourth melanocortin receptor. J. Biol. Chem. **268:** 15174–15179.
23. MOUNTJOY, K.G., L.S. ROBBINS, M.T. MORTRUD & R.D. CONE. 1992. The cloning of a family of genes that encode the melanocortin receptors. Science **257:** 1248–1251.
24. GANTZ, I., Y. SHIMOTO, Y. KONDA, H. MIWA, C.J. DICKINSON & T. YAMADA. 1994. Molecular cloning, expression, and characterization of a fifth melanocortin receptor. Biochem. Biophys. Res. Commun. **200:** 1214–1220.
25. GANTZ, I., T. KONDA, T. TASHIRO, Y. SHIMOTO, H. MIWA, G. MUNZERT, S.J. WATSON, J. DELVALLE & T. YAMADA. 1993. Molecular cloning of a novel melanocortin receptor. J. Biol. Chem. **268:** 8246–8250.
26. ROSELLI-REHFUSS, L., K.G. MOUNTJOY, L.S. ROBBINS, M.T. MORTRUD, M.J. LOW, J.B. TATRO, M.L. ENTWISTLE, R.B. SIMERLY & R.D. CONE. 1993. Identification of a receptor for gamma melanotropin and other proopiomelanocortin peptides in the hypothalamus and limbic system. Proc. Natl. Acad. Sci. USA **90:** 8856–8860.
27. ADAN, R.A.H., R.D. CONE, J.P. BURBACH & W.H. GISPEN. 1994. Differential effects of melanocortin peptides on neural melanocortin receptors. Mol. Pharmacol. **46:** 1182–1190.
28. VAN DER ZEE, C.E.E.M., J.H. BRAKKEE & W.H. GISPEN. 1988. αMSH and Org2766 in peripheral nerve regeneration: different routes of delivery. Eur. J. Pharmacol. **147:** 351–357.
29. ADAN, R.A.H., M. VAN DER KRAAN, R.P. DOORNBOS, P.R. BAR, J.P. BURBACH & W.H. GISPEN. 1996. Melanocortin receptors mediate alpha-MSH-induced stimulation of neurite outgrowth in neuro 2A cells. Brain Res. Mol. Brain Res. **36:** 37–44.
30. FERRARI, W. 1958. Behavioural changes in animals after intracisternal injection with adrenocoticotrophic hormone and melanocyte stimulating hormone. Nature (Lond.) **181:** 925–926.
31. SPRUIJT, B.M., J.A.R.A.M. VAN HOOFF & W.H. GISPEN. 1992. Ethology and neurobiology of grooming behavior. Physiol. Rev. **72:** 825–852.
32. ADAN, R.A.H., J. OOSTEROM, G. LUDVIGSDOTTIR, J.H. BRAKKEE, J.P. BURBACH & W.H. GISPEN. 1994. Identification of antagonists for melanocortin MC3, MC4, and MC5 receptors. Eur. J. Pharmacol. **269:** 331–337.
33. FLORIS, E. 1963. Effect delliniezone endorachnidea nell'uoma di ACTH. Boll. Soc. Ital. Viol. Sper. 558–560.
34. WESSELLS, H., K. FUCIARELLI, J. HANSEN, M.E. HADLEY, V.J. HRUBY, R. DORR & N. LEVINE. 1998. Synthetic melanotropic peptide initiates erections in men with psychogenic erectile dysfunction: double-blind, placebo controlled crossover study. J. Urol. **160:** 389–393.
35. CHEN, W., M.A. KELLY, X. OPITZ-ARAYA, R.E. THOMAS, M.J. LOW & R.D. CONE. 1997. Exocrine gland dysfunction in MC5-R-deficient mice: evidence for coordinated regulation of exocrine gland function by melanocortin peptides. Cell **91:** 789–798.

The Skin POMC System (SPS)

Leads and Lessons from the Hair Follicle

RALF PAUS,[a,b] VLADIMIR A. BOTCHKAREV,[b] NATALIA V. BOTCHKAREVA,[b] LARS MECKLENBURG,[c] THOMAS LUGER,[d] AND ANDRZEJ SLOMINSKI[e]

[b]Department of Dermatology, Charité, Humboldt-University, Berlin, Germany

[c]Department of Pathology, School of Veterinary Medicine, Hannover, Germany

[d]Department of Dermatology, University of Muenster, Muenster, Germany

[e]Department of Pathology, Loyola University Medical Center, Maywood, Illinois, USA

ABSTRACT: Human and murine skin are prominent extrapituitary sources and targets for POMC products. The expression of, for example, ACTH, α-MSH, β-endorphin, and MC-1–receptors fluctuates during synchronized hair follicle cycling in C57BL/6 mice. Since hair growth can be induced by ACTH injections in mice and mink, and since high doses of MSH peptides modulate epidermal and/or follicle keratinocyte proliferation in murine skin organ culture, some POMC products may operate as locally generated growth modulators, in addition to their roles in cutaneous pigment and immunobiology. Intrafollicularly generated ACTH and α-MSH as well as their cognate receptors may assist in the maintenance of the peculiar immune privilege of the anagen hair bulb. Possibly, they are also involved in the development of the follicle pigmentary unit, with whose generation their expression coincides. Given that murine skin also expresses (in a hair-cycle-dependent way) CRH and CRH-R, which control pituitary POMC expression and in view of the fact that CRH arrests follicles in telogen, this suggests the existence of a local *skin POMC system* (SPS). This may be an integral component of cutaneous stress response-systems, and may most instructively be studied using the murine hair cycle as a model.

INTRODUCTION TO THE MURINE HAIR FOLLICLE AS A MODEL FOR EXPLORING NEUROPEPTIDE FUNCTIONS

It is still not yet widely enough appreciated that the hair follicle (HF) can serve as an excellent model system for exploring the functional activities of neuropeptides. There is hardly another tissue system in the mammalian body that rivals the HF in its exquisite sensitivity toward a very wide range of locally or systemically administered steroid and peptide hormones, not to mention numerous growth factors and cytokines[1–5] as well as the long-appreciated, paramount influence of gonadal and thyroid hormones on hair growth.[1] For example, glucocorticosteroids are powerful inhibitors of hair growth[6,7] and melatonin administration alters the molting cycle in

[a]Address for correspondence: Ralf Paus, M.D., Department of Dermatology, University Hospital Eppendorf, University of Hamburg, Martinistr. 52, D-20246 Hamburg, Germany.
paus@uke.uni-hamburg.de (e-mail).

mink.[1] Furthermore, neurotrophins act as modulators of murine HF morphogenesis and/or cycling,[8–10] and local administration of the neuropeptide substance-P induces hair growth (anagen) in mice.[11]

It is particularly interesting to study the effects of neuropeptides on hair growth when one wishes to explore non-neuronal neuropeptide functions, such as growth-modulatory effects on epithelial cells that grow in their natural tissue architecture and in the presence of their natural mesenchymal environment. The HF represents a neuroectodermal-mesenchymal tissue interaction system, whose proper development, growth, production of pigmented fibers, and remodelling requires the stringently coordinated interaction of neuroectodermal (keratinocytes and melanocytes) and mesenchymal cells (dermal papilla fibroblasts). Furthermore, neuropeptides, neurotransmitters, and neurotrophins released from perifollicular nerve fibers, glia cells, and mast cells may all exert a modulatory effect on hair growth.[2,12,13]

Under the influence of inductive and morphogenic signals exchanged between selected, directly adjacent, epidermal and dermal cell populations, the HF develops from an epidermal invagination, followed by massive keratinocyte proliferation, until a bulbous hair shaft factory has been generated—the epithelial hair bulb[14] (see FIGURE 1A). HF morphogenesis, as well as the subsequent cyclic growth and regression activity of the HF, are controlled by specialized fibroblasts (dermal papilla) that retain inductive and morphogenic properties throughout the lifetime of the organism. This mesenchymal "command center" of the HF drives the latter through perpetual cyclic transformations between a state of rapid, apoptosis-driven organ involution (catagen), active production of a pigmented hair shaft (anagen), and relative resting (telogen) (FIG. 1A).[2,4,13,15,16]

In black mice, such as C57BL/6, HF cycling can be easily followed by assessing changes in the skin color (see FIGURE 1B). Melanin-producing melanocytes in truncal mouse skin are exclusively located in the hair bulb, and generate melanin only during the anagen stages III–VI, i.e., when a pigmented hair shaft is actively produced.[18–20] HF cycling in young mice is relatively well-synchronized. This synchrony of murine HF cycling also allows one to assess the hair cycle stage by measuring changes in skin thickness, since the entire architecture, and the patterns of epithelial cell proliferation and apoptosis dramatically change when thousands of HF simultaneously enter from the telogen stage into anagen (FIG. 1B).[5–7,16,21]

These features render the murine hair cycle ideally suited to exploring the non-neuronal functions of neuropeptides on interacting neuroectodermal and mesenchymal cells under *physiologically relevant* conditions. This applies particularly to POMC-derived neuropeptides.

POINTERS TO A ROLE FOR POMC PRODUCTS
IN HAIR GROWTH CONTROL

That the pituitary gland influences hair growth has been appreciated at least since Houssay noted[23] in 1918 that the hair coat of hypophysectomized dogs remained that of the "puppy" type. For example, in mink or weasels, hypophysectomy prevents the

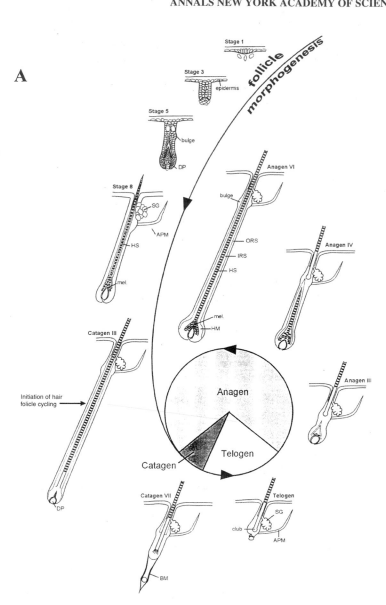

FIGURE 1A. The figure provides an overview of the major stages of hair follicle morphogenesis and cycling (adapted from Stenn *et al.*[3,4]) Note that, in all mammalian species,
hair follicle cycling commences with spontaneous and rather well-synchronized entry into
the first stage of hair follicle involution (catagen), followed by a stage of relative resting
(telogen). Entry of the hair follicle into its first genuine growth phase, during which a pigmented hair shaft is generated (anagen), again occurs spontaneously. The anagen phase is
synchronized in mice and rats, but it occurs asynchronously in man (mosaic hair cycle).
Anagen is terminated, and catagen induced spontaneously. By means of this catagen transformation the entire hair shaft "factory", the anagen hair bulb, is deconstructed and follicular melanogenesis is switched-off in a process of massive keratinocyte apoptosis,
accompanied by some melanocyte apoptosis.[2,4,5,13,17]

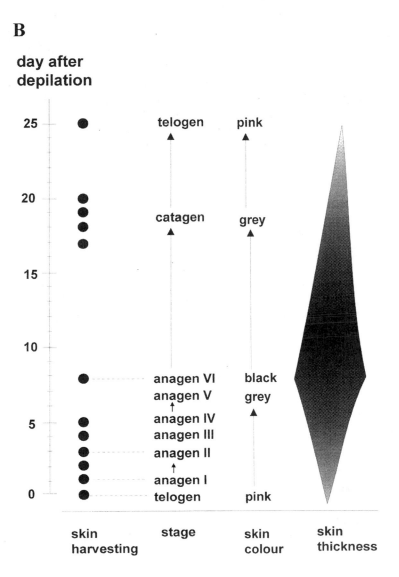

FIGURE 1B. Representation of hair cycle–associated changes in skin pigmentation and thickness after anagen induction by depilation in murine back skin. During each hair cycle, the hair follicle runs from the resting stage (telogen) through the growth stage (anagen), and via a short regression stage (catagen), back to telogen. All telogen follicles can be forced to immediately enter into anagen by plucking their hair shafts (depilation). The figure shows the highly synchronized and highly reproducible sequence of events that accompanies depilation-induced hair follicle cycling in mice. Black dots represent standardized times of skin harvesting, which were used for the neuropeptide determinations shown in FIGURES 2 and 3, and in TABLE 1. This is correlated with the corresponding stages in hair follicle cycling and the associated changes in skin pigmentation and relative skin thickness.[7,21,22]

spontaneous onset of molting, which can be corrected by the administration of α-MSH or ACTH to hypophysectomized animals.[24,25]

In man, overproduction of ACTH (by malignant epithelial tumors, for example) or therapeutic ACTH administration are well-recognized causes of acquired hypertrichosis.[26–28] Hypertrichosis is a process in which a minute, nonpigmented vellus HF is converted into a large terminal HF that produces strong, pigmented hair shafts. To at least some extent this also reflects a change in HF cycling, since hypertrichotic HF have a substantially longer anagen phase than the original vellus HF.[2,5,26,29] Thus, the induction of hypertrichosis by ACTH provides circumstantial evidence that this neuropeptide may stimulate and/or prolong anagen.

Interestingly, bilateral adrenalectomy in mink, which causes a sharp rise in pituitary ACTH release, induces a premature onset of anagen when performed during the period when most back skin HF are in telogen.[30] In mink, anagen can indeed be induced directly by the intracutaneous injection of ACTH, but not by injection of α-MSH.[31] Previously, we had already noted a similar anagen-inducing effect of intracutaneously injected ACTH in murine telogen skin,[32] and had found that ACTH can also induce the premature onset of catagen in murine anagen skin.[34] This strongly suggests that at least this POMC product is involved in hair growth control.

However, the exact underlying mechanisms remain largely obscure, and only quite recently have melanocortin receptors been discovered in mammalian skin on cells other than melanocytes,[35,36] and even in the HF (see below).

THE HAIR FOLLICLE AS A SOURCE AND TARGET OF POMC PRODUCTS

Many skin-derived cell populations, including melanocytes, endothelial cells, fibroblasts, adipocytes, and keratinocytes express POMC-derived peptides *in vitro*.[35] In 1992, we reported the first evidence that the POMC gene is also transcribed, translated, and processed in mammalian skin *in vivo;* and that very prominent β-endorphin immunoreactivity (IR) is localized in the sebaceous gland, which forms one functional unit with the HF[37] (see TABLE 1).

Subsequently, we also detected ACTH-IR in the hair bulb of human anagen HF (but only on the capillitium)[38] and in the outer root sheath of murine anagen HF.[36] Later, we found ACTH-R (MC-2R) transcripts by RT-PCR in skin.[39] Most recently, we have also detected α-MSH-IR, as well as specific IR for the corresponding receptor (MC-1R), in murine HF[45] (see FIGURE 2). The constitutive presence of ACTH and β-endorphin in unmanipulated mouse skin was confirmed by RP-HPLC and radioimmunoassay.[36,41]

Moreover, POMC expression in normal murine skin is not only strikingly restricted to defined regions of the HF epithelium, but is also surprisingly hair cycle dependent (TABLE 1 and FIG. 2).[37,42] This is also true for the POMC products β-endorphin[41] (Table 1), ACTH,[36] α-MSH, and MC-1R[40] (FIG. 2). Taken together, this makes the HF both a prominent source and a potential target for the bioactivity of POMC products.

TABLE 1. Hair cycle-dependent expression of proopiomelanocortin

	Proopiomelanocortin		
Hair cycle stages	mRNA[a]	Protein detectable by Western blot[b]	Protein detectable by immunohistochemistry[c]
Telogen	—	—	(+)
Very early anagen	(±)	—	(±)
Early anagen	+	—	+
Mid anagen	+	+	+++

NOTE: The table depicts hair-cycle-associated changes in the expression of POMC transcripts and of POMC-related protein in murine back skin during the depilation-induced hair cycle of adolescent C57BL/6 mice (modified from Slominski *et al.*[37]).

[a] 0.9-Kb transcript.

[b] 30–33 KD protein detected by anti-β-endorphin antiserum.

[c] POMC-related immunoreactivity as detected by anti-β-endorphin antiserum.

Very early anagen, day one after anagen induction by depilation in the back skin of mice with all hair follicles in the resting phase of the hair cycle (telogen); early anagen, days three and four after depilation; mid anagen, days five to eight after depilation.

POTENTIAL FUNCTIONS OF LOCALLY GENERATED POMC PRODUCTS IN HAIR FOLLICLE BIOLOGY

The dependence of the respective expression patterns of POMC, its products and of melanocortin receptors on the stage of HF cycling (TABLE 1 and FIG. 2); that is, on the rhythmic transformation of a neuroectodermal-mesenchymal tissue interaction unit; raises the intriguing possibility that selected POMC products are involved in more than just control of HF pigmentation—where their role is well-established.[20,43] Radioimmunoassay-controlled RP-HPLC analysis has recently shown the α-MSH peptide to be present in murine anagen skin, and that prominent intrafollicular α-MSH-IR is detected only in murine anagen IV skin.[40]

This is consistent with a role of intrafollicularly generated α-MSH in HF melanogenesis, as we had previously speculated,[20] and is in line with the well-established roles of α-MSH and ACTH in the control of melanogenesis,[43] which has dominated interest in the cutaneous effects of POMC products for so many years.

However, the currently available pharmacologic evidence (cited above) is quite suggestive for the assumption that ACTH, at least, also plays an active role in hair growth control, possibly both during anagen,[31,32] and during catagen development.[34] Interestingly, administration of high doses of ACTH to organ-cultured full-thickness mouse skin with all hair follicles in spontaneous, unmanipulated telogen, discretely, but significantly, inhibits follicular DNA synthesis[36] (see FIGURE 4). Although it has not yet been determined whether murine HF express functional MC-2R, even an indirect mode of action of ACTH on murine hair growth can be envisioned.

For example, ACTH is a potent secretagogue for murine skin mast cells, and the degranulation of mast cells seems to play a functionally important, though nonessen-

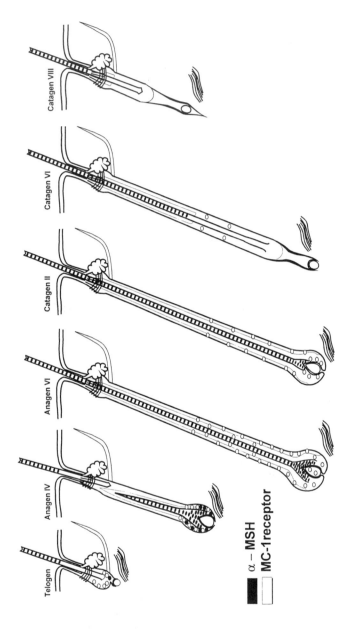

FIGURE 2A. See legend on opposite page.

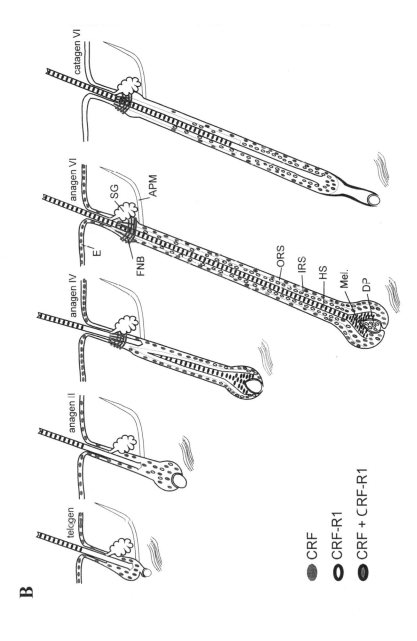

FIGURE 2B. Hair cycle-dependent expression of α-MSH-, MC-1R-, CRH-, and CRH-R-immunoreactivity in murine back skin. **A.** Patterns of α-MSH- and MC-1R-IR. **B.** Patterns of CRH- and CRH-R-IR.

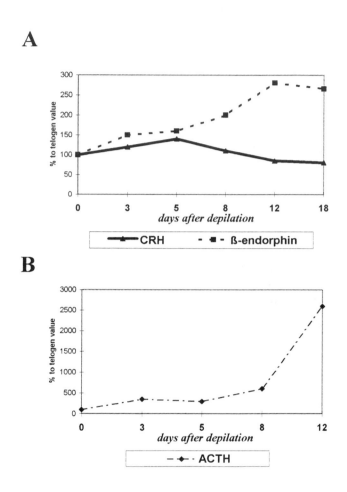

FIGURE 3. Hair cycle-dependent changes in the content of ACTH, β-endorphin, and CRH in murine skin. The figure summarizes our previously published results on hair cycle associated changes in the relative skin content of ACTH,[36] β-endorphin,[41] and CRH,[44] after anagen induction by depilation. (For absolute values, please consult the cited references.)

tial, role in the regulation of both anagen and catagen development in mice.[32,34,45] Thus, even in the absence of functional MC-2R, locally generated and secreted ACTH might still be able to exert indirect, paracrine effects on hair growth control.

The nonpigmentary roles of β-endorphin, MSH-peptides, and LPH in the biology of the pilosebaceous unit await systematic exploration. For example, high-dose (1 μM) γ_1-MSH and γ_2-MSH significantly stimulate epidermal DNA synthesis in organ-cultured telogen mouse skin,[19] whereas α-MSH inhibits it.[40,45] If sufficiently high concentrations are reached in the HF, selected melanocortins may have para- or autocrine growth-modulatory effects on HF keratinocytes.

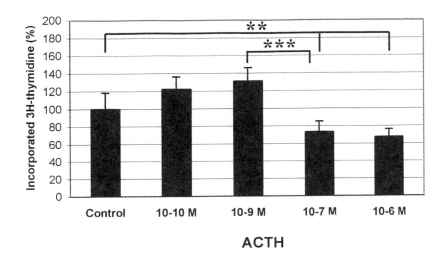

FIGURE 4. Manipulation of follicular keratinocyte proliferation by ACTH in murine skin organ culture. The graph depicts the effects of ACTH on ^{3}H-thymidine incorporation into the dermal fragment of full-thickness murine skin with all hair follicles in telogen, organ-cultured at the air-liquid-interphase.[21] Dermal ^{3}H-thymidine incorporation, in this assay, predominantly reflects the proliferative activity of keratinocytes in the proximal hair follicle epithelium. Data shown as published in Slominski *et al.*[36]

Keratinocytes, fibroblasts, endothelial cells, and adipocytes, as well, have recently been found to express functional melanocortin receptors[35] (see also elsewhere in this volume). In the light of findings indicating that the anagen hair bulb, which is located deep in the subcutis, is a prominent source of melanocortins, it is conceivable that HF-derived melanocortins stimulate cognate receptors on fibroblasts of the proximal perifollicular connective tissue sheath, as well as on adipocytes and endothelial cells of the perifollicular subcutis. Perhaps, such signalling exchanges are even related to the, as yet entirely unexplained, but very striking, hair cycle-dependent changes in skin thickness (FIG. 1B) and vascularization.[2,21]

Another intriguing area of possible functional relevance for immunosuppressive POMC products like ACTH and α-MSH is that of hair follicle immunology. The anagen hair bulb is unusual in that it has established an area of immune privilege that may serve to sequester melanogenesis-related autoantigens from immune recognition.[48,49] The proximal anagen hair bulb meets all key criteria of an immunoprivileged tissue site. For example, in mice hair matrix and inner root sheath of anagen, HF appear to be devoid of MHC class-Ia expression and antigen presenting Langerhans cells; the intraepithelial T-cells (DETC) lie behind a special protective extracellular matrix barrier and are immunoreactive for potent immunosuppressants, like TGFβ.[46-49] The proximal ORS of anagen HF displays IR for the immunosuppressant ACTH,[36] whereas α-MSH is found in the proximal outer root sheath and in the hair matrix of anagen IV HF (FIG. 2).[40]

Thus, two questions deserve to be examined. First, do locally generated immuno-suppressive POMC products like ACTH and α-MSH contribute to the establishment and maintenance of the immune privilege of the anagen hair bulb? Second, is insufficient production of these neuropeptides in any way related to the collapse of the immune privilege that may underlie the pathogenesis of a common, immunologically-mediated form of hair loss, alopecia areata?[33,47]

IS THERE A *SKIN POMC SYSTEM* (SPS)?

Certainly, it is timely to look beyond HF pigmentation when it comes to dissecting the functional activities of POMC products in HF biology. As discussed elsewhere in this volume,[36] this includes cutaneous responses to various external stressors like UV irradiation, infection, and physicochemical trauma. Even the hormone that largely controls pituitary POMC expression, CRH, is found in murine and human skin, including the murine HF, along with the corresponding receptors (FIG. 2).[44]

Most notably, the cutaneous CRH levels in murine skin peak in anagen skin extracts,[44] yet before the stage when maximal skin levels of ACTH or β-endorphin are detectable (FIG. 3).[36,41] Therefore, it is reasonable to ask whether intracutaneous CRH exerts a comparable effect on the intrafollicular expression of POMC as is seen on the hypothalamic-pituitary axis;[27] and whether mammalian skin has established an analogous signalling system to the HPA axis, of which follicular POMC products may form an integral component. Since CRH and the POMC products, ACTH and β-endorphin, are all classical stress hormones,[27] we have proposed that CRH and POMC-derived neuropeptides are integrated into a peripheral, cutaneous stress-response-system, the *skin stress system* (SSS) (for details and discussion see Ref. 36).

EXPLOITING THE HF TO CHARACTERIZE THE SPS

Since hair shaft removal by depilation constitutes a mild wounding of the HF, depilation-induced anagen is likely to be associated with follicular stress-responses. Obviously, this model lends itself to further exploration. Does an external stressor (e.g., wounding by depilation) trigger a classical stress-response cascade in this peripheral tissue? That is, CRH release → stimulation of follicular CRH-R (that are either constitutively expressed or upregulated as a result of wounding) → stimulation of follicular POMC transcription, translation, and processing → generation of defined subsets of POMC-derived neuropeptides → auto- and/or paracrine stimulation of cognate melanocortin receptors.

This easily accessible and manipulable, as well as inexpensive, physiologically and clinically relevant model offers a research arena in which to explore the fascinating question of whether peripheral tissues really are capable of executing complex response cascades similar to those that exist between hypothalamus and pituitary during systemic stress responses. Moreover, this model also allows one to dissect, with comparative ease, how the local tissue milieu (e.g., perifollicular fibroblasts, mast cells, macrophages, and endothelial cells—all of which express melanocortin receptors[35]) reacts to the secretion of melanocortins by the HF epithelium. Therefore, the less exclusive term *skin POMC system* (SPS) may be preferable, since this helps to promote the concept that POMC expression, translation, and processing in the skin is part of an entire signalling network; one that may recapitulate key aspects of comparable networks established in the HPA axis.[35,36]

The epithelial expression of CRH-R in the murine HF[44] (FIG. 2) invites one to ask whether locally generated CRH also affects the proliferation, differentiation, and/or apoptosis of HF keratinocytes. Preliminary data from our laboratory suggest that subcutaneously implanted slow-release capsules that release high concentrations of CRH in the direct vicinity of murine telogen HF, effectively arrest these in an extended telogen state (Paus, Fechner, and Mecklenburg, unpublished data). Naturally, it now needs to be asked whether this is not simply due to the high systemic CRH levels in this experiment, since this would be expected to substantially raise systemic corticosterone levels via stimulation of the HPA axis.[27] High systemic glucocorticosteroid levels would clearly suffice to explain a profound anagen-inhibitory effect of CRH implants.[1,6,7]

The C57BL/6 mouse model, advocated here as an ideal study system for exploring the non-neuronal functions of neuropeptides in the context of the putative skin POMC system (SPS), is well suited to clarify this issue. By studying the hair cycle-modulatory effects of CRH implants in adrenalectomized mice, this mouse model will also allow us to distinguish direct from indirect effects of POMC products on the HF; by studying the hair cycle-modulatory effects of ACTH (see above) in mast cell-deficient mice, mast cell-mediated indirect effects on hair growth can be excluded. Finally, the relative ease with which skin penetration and HF targeting of topically administered neuropeptides can be achieved in murine skin by using appropriate vehicle formulations (e.g., liposomes), makes the murine HF an optimal model system for studying the growth-, pigmentation-, and immunomodulatory effects of the new generations of synthetic melanocortin receptor agonists and antagonists that are now available or are being developed.

The corresponding leads and lessons that can be learnt from the HF should greatly assist us in revealing the full range of functions that POMC-derived neuropeptides display in complex neuroectodermal-mesenchymal interaction systems. We predict that the HF will enable us to do so more quickly, and under physiologically and clinically more relevant conditions than occur in most other experimental models routinely employed today in mainstream POMC research.

ACKNOWLEDGMENTS

The experimental contributions of our colleagues and collaborators are gratefully acknowledged. In particular we thank Drs. B. Roloff, J. Furkert, and K. Fechner for use of their published data—summarized in this article. Preparation of this paper was supported by grants from DFG (Pa 345/6-2) and Wella AG, Darmstadt, to R.P.

REFERENCES

1. EBLING, F.J.G., P.A. HALE & V.A. RANDALL. 1991. Hormones and hair growth. *In* Physiology, Biochemistr and Molecular Biology of the Skin. L.A. Goldsmith, Ed.: 660–696. Oxford University Press, New York.

2. PAUS, R. 1996. Curr. Opin. Dermatol. **3:** 248–258.
3. STENN, K.S., N.J. COMBATES, K.J. EILERTSEN, J.S. GORDON, J.R. PARDINAS, S. PARIMO & S.M. PROUTY. 1996. Dermatol. Clinics **14:** 543–558.
4. STENN, K., S. PARIMOO & S. PROUTY. 1998. Growth of the hair follicle: A cycling and regenerating biological system. *In* Molecular Basis of Epithelial Appendage Morphogenesis. C.M. Chuong, Ed.: 111–124. Landes Bioscience Publ., Austin.
5. PAUS, R. 1998. J. Dermatol. Sci. **25:** 793–802.
6. STENN, K.S., R. PAUS, T. DUTTON & B. SARBA. 1993. Skin Pharmacol. **6:** 125–134.
7. PAUS, R., B. HANDJISKI, B.M. CZARNETZKI & S. EICHMÜLLER. 1994. J. Invest. Dermatol. **103**(2): 143–147.
8. BOTCHKAREV, V.A., N.V. BOTCHKAREVA, K.M. ALBERS, G.R. LEWIN, C. VAN DER VEEN & R. PAUS. 1998. J. Invest. Dermatol. **111:** 279–285.
9. BOTCHKAREV, V.A., P. WELKER, K.M. ALBERS, N.V. BOTCHKAREVA, M. METZ, G.R. LEWIN, S. BULFONE-PAUS, E.M.J. PETERS, G. LINDNER & R. PAUS. 1998. Am. J. Path. **153:** 785–799.
10. BOTCHKAREV, V.A., N.V. BOTCHKAREVA, P. WELKER, M. METZ, G.R. LEWIN, A. SUBRAMANIAM, S. BULFONE-PAUS, E. HAGEN, A. BRAUN, M. LOMMATZSCH, H. RENZ & R. PAUS. 1999. FASEB J. **13:** 395–410.
11. PAUS, R., T. HEINZELMANN, K.D. SCHULTZ, J. FURKERT, K. FECHNER & B.M. CZARNETZKI. 1994. Lab. Invest. **71:** 134–140.
12. PAUS, R., E.M.J. PETERS, S. EICHMÜLLER & V.A. BOTCHKAREV. 1997. J. Invest. Dermatol. Symp. Proc. **2:** 6168.
13. PAUS, R. & G. COTSARELIS. 1999. New Engl. J. Med. **341:** 491–497.
14. PHILPOTT, M. & R. PAUS. 1998. Principles of hair follicle morphogenesis. *In* Molecular Basis of Epithelial Appendage Morphogenesis. C.M. Chuong, Ed.: 75–109. Landes Bioscience Publ., Austin.
15. JAHODA, C.A.B. & A.J. REYNOLDS. 1996. Dermatol. Clinics **14:** 573–584.
16. LINDNER, G., V.A. BOTCHKAREV, N.V. BOTCHKAREVA, G. LING, C. VAN DER VEEN & R. PAUS. 1997. Amer. J. Pathol. **151:** 1601–1617.
17. TOBIN, D.J., E. HAGEN, V.A. BOTCHKAREV & R. PAUS. 1998. J. Invest. Dermatol. **111**(6): 941–947.
18. SLOMINSKI, A., R. PAUS & R. COSTANTINO. 1991. J. Invest. Dermatol. **96:** 172–179.
19. SLOMINSKI, A., R. PAUS & J. WORTSMAN. 1991. J. Invest. Dermatol. **97**(4): 747.
20. SLOMINSKI, A. & R. PAUS. 1993. J. Invest. Dermatol. **101:** 90S–97S.
21. PAUS, R., K.S. STENN & R.E. LINK. 1990. Br. J. Dermatol. **122:** 777–784.
22. SLOMINSKI, A., R. PAUS, P. PLONKA, A. CHAKRABORTY, M. MAURER, D. PRUSKI & S. LUKIEWICZ, 1994. J. Invest. Dermatol. **102:** 862–869.
23. HOUSSAY, B.A. 1918. Endocrinology **2:** 497–498.
24. RUST, C.C. 1965. Gen. Comp. Endocrinol. **5:** 222–231.
25. RUST, C.C., R.M. SHACKELFORD & R.K. MEYER. 1965. J. Mammal. **46:** 549–565.
26. DAWBER, R. Ed. 1997. Diseases of the Hair and Scalp. Blackwell Science, Oxford.
27. WILSON, J.D., D.W. FOSTER, H.M. KRONENBERG & P.R. LARSEN, Eds. 1998. Williams Textbook of Endocrinology, 9th ed. Saunders, Philadelphia.
28. STERRY, W., R. PAUS. 1999. Checkliste Dermatologie. Thieme, Stuttgart.
29. JAHODA, C.A.B. 1998. Exp. Dermatol. **7:** 235–248.
30. ROSE, J. & M. STERNER. 1992. J. Exp. Zool. **262:** 469–473.
31. ROSE, J. 1998. J. Invest. Dermatol. **110:** 456–457.
32. PAUS, R., M. MAURER, A. SLOMINSKI & B.M. CZARNETZKI. 1994. Dev. Biol. **163:** 230–240.
33. PAUS, R., A. SLOMINSKI & B.M. CZARNETZKI. 1994. Yale J. Biol. Med. **66:** 541–545.
34. MAURER, M., E. FISCHER, B. HANDJISKI, A. BARANDI, J. MEINGASSER & R. PAUS. 1997. Lab. Invest. **77:** 319–332.
35. LUGER, T.A., T. SCHOLZEN, T. BRZOSKA, E. BECHER, A. SLOMINSKI & R. PAUS. 1998. Ann. N.Y. Acad. Sci. **840:** 381–394.

36. SLOMINSKI, A., N.V. BOTCHKAREVA, V.A. BOTCHKAREVA, A. CHAKRABORTY, T. LUGER, M. UENALAN & R. PAUS. 1998. Biochem. Biophys. Acta Mol. Cell Res. **1448:** 147–152.
37. SLOMINSKI, A., R. PAUS & J. MAZURKIEWICZ. 1992. Experientia **48:** 50–54.
38. SLOMINSKI, A., J. WORTSMAN, J.E. MAZURKIEWICZ, L. MATSUOKA, J. DIETRICH, K. LAWRENCE, A. GORBANI & R. PAUS. 1993. J. Lab. Clin. Med. **122:** 658–666.
39. SLOMINSKI, A., G. ERMAK & M. MIHM. 1996. J. Clin. Endocrinol. Metab. **81:** 2746–2749.
40. BOTCHKAREV, V.A., N.V. BOTCHKAREVA, A. SLOMINSKI, B. ROLOFF, T. LUGER & R. PAUS. 1999. Ann. N.Y. Acad. Sci. **885:** this issue.
41. FURKERT, J., U. KLUG, A. SLOMINSKI, S. EICHMÜLLER, B. MEHLIS, U. KERTSCHER & R. PAUS. 1997. Biochim. Biophys. Acta **1336:** 315–322.
42. SLOMINSKI, A., G. ERMAK, J. HWANG, J. MAZURKIEWICZ, D. CORLISS & A. EASTMAN. 1996. Biochim. Biophys. Acta **1289:** 247–251.
43. NORDLUND, J.J., R.E. BOISSY, V.J. HEARING, R.A. KING & J.P. ORTONNE, EDS. 1998. The Pigmentary System: Physiology and Pathophysiology. Oxford University Press.
44. ROLOFF, B., K. FECHNER, A. SLOMINSKI, J. FURKERT, V.A. BOTCHKAREV, S. BULFONE-PAUS, J. ZIPPER, E. KRAUSE & R. PAUS. 1998. FASEB J. **12:** 287–297.
45. MAURER, M., R. PAUS & B.M. CZARNETZKI. 1995. Exp. Dermatol. **4:** 266–271.
46. PAUS, R. 1997. Immunology of the hair follicle. *In* The Skin Immune System. J.D. Bos, Ed.: 377–398. CRC Press, Boca Raton.
47. PAUS, R., T. CHRISTOPH & S. MUELLER-ROVER. 1999. J. Invest Dermatol. Symp. Proc. In press.
48. PAUS, R., C. VAN DER VEEN, S. EICHMÜLLER, T. KOPP, E. HAGEN, S. MÜLLER-RÖVER & U. HOFMANN. 1998. J. Invest. Dermatol. **111:** 7–18.
49. RÜCKERT, R., U. HOFMANN, C. VAN DER VEEN, S. BULFONE-PAUS & R. PAUS. 1998. J. Invest. Dermatol. **111:** 25–30.

Expression of MC1- and MC5-Receptors on the Human Mast Cell Line HMC-1

M. ARTUC,[a,b] A. GRÜTZKAU,[b] TH. LUGER,[c] AND B.M. HENZ[b]

[b]Department of Dermatology, Charité, Humboldt University, Berlin, Germany

[c]Department of Dermatology, University of Münster, Münster, Germany

INTRODUCTION

Stimulation of mast cells leads to degranulation, release of mediators (histamine and LTC4, for example), and subsequent clinical symptoms such as urticaria. Stimulation can be caused either by IgE-immunoglobulins crosslinking on the cell membrane, or by IgE-independent mechanisms that are only partly understood.[1] Candidate stimuli for IgE-independent mast cell activation include substance P, SCF, and the complement peptides, C3a and C5a.[2] Although these stimuli have been well studied, many of the IgE-independent reactions remain unexplained—especially in humans.

ACTH is a neurohormone that has been shown to stimulate *rodent* mast cells via cAMP generation,[3] but until now neither its activity nor that of other related neuropeptides, such as α-MSH, has been demonstrated on *human* mast cells. Five specific receptors for α-MSH (MC1–MC5) have so far been characterized on human cells of different types, but not on human mast cells, two of them (MC1 and MC5) on human skin cells.[4,5] In this work we have studied human mast cells for MC-receptor expression and for associated cAMP generation, as a possible second messenger of neuropeptide action, using the mast cell line HMC-1 as target cells.

MATERIALS AND METHODS

Cell Culture

HMC-1 cells were grown in a basal ISCOVE medium supplemented with 10% FCS and monothioglycerol.

Total RNA was isolated from HMC-1 cells using a RNeasy total RNA isolation kit (Qiagen, Hilden, FRG). The isolated total RNA was treated with RNase-free DNase I at 37°C for 30 min and heated to 75°C for another 5 min. The quantity of total RNA was estimated photometrically at 260/280 nm. 1 μg of the total RNA was reverse transcribed using a first-strand cDNA synthesis kit for RT-PCR (Boehringer, Mannheim, FRG). The resulting cDNA was amplified using a PCR master kit (Boehringer). PCR primers sequences for detection of MC1- and MC5-receptor mRNA were published previously.[6]

[a]Address for correspondence: Dr. M. Artuc, Department of Dermatology, Charité, Campus Virchow Klinikum, Augustenburgerplatz 1, 13344 Berlin, Germany. 49-30 45065113 (voice); 49-30 45065900 (fax).

FACS-Analysis

For flow cytometric detection of MC5-receptor expression in HMC-1 cells, an affinity-purified goat serum (Santa Cruz Biotechnology, Santa Cruz, USA) was used. This enables recognition of an epitope corresponding to an amino acid sequence that maps to the carboxy terminus of the receptor. Briefly, prefixed cells (4% paraformaldehyde and 0.1% glutaraldehyde) were permeated with 0.03% saponin and were then stained with the primary antiserum at an IgG concentration of 7 µg/ml. A phycoerythrin-conjugated antibody (Jackson Immunotech, West Grove, USA) was used to fluorescence label the primary antibody. The specificity of binding was checked by preincubating the primary antiserum with an antigen-specific blocking peptide (Santa Cruz Biotechnology, Santa Cruz, USA).

Measurement of cAMP-Generation

HMC-1 cells were stimulated in flat-bottomed 96-well microtitre plates with increasing concentrations of α-MSH or ACTH, over a range from 0.1 nM to 1 µM, for 15 min at 37°C. Thereafter, the cells were lysed and the total cellular cAMP content was determined by a cAMP-specific enzyme-immunoassay, according to the protocol for nonacetylated specimens, provided by the manufacturer (Amersham, Braunschweig, Germany).

RESULTS AND DISCUSSION

RT-PCR

RT-PCR was performed on HMC-1-derived, total RNA generated fragments of 416- and 361-bp, that represent positive signals for MC1- and MC5-mRNA (see FIGURE 1). In all experiments, the MC5-receptor mRNA signal was much stronger than that for the MC1-receptor. Although signals were not normalized against an internal standard, the strength and continuity of the observed difference may be taken as an indication that MC5-receptors dominate on HMC-1 cells in comparison with MC1-receptors.

FACS-Analysis

As is shown in FIGURE 2, nearly 80% of cells stained positively for the MC5-receptor. This signal was almost completely abolished in the presence of an excess of antigen-specific blocking peptide.

c-AMP-Generation

α-MSH did not alter cAMP-generation, whereas ACTH—also known to bind specifically to MC5-receptors—activated the adenylate system to 30% above basal levels of unstimulated HMC-1 cells (975 pmol compared to 750 pmol). Due to the spontaneous activity of the adenylate system in HMC-1 cells, a weak stimulating effect of α-MSH may have been disguised.

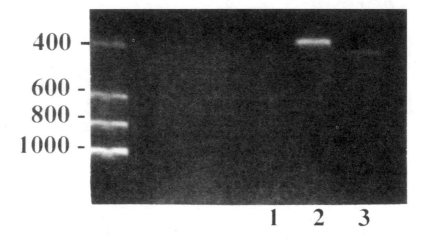

FIGURE 1. RT-PCR analysis of total RNA derived from HMC-1 cells. *Lane 1.* control (H$_2$O); *lane 2,* MC5-receptor; *lane 3*, MC1-receptor.

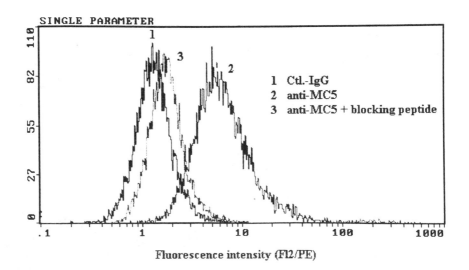

FIGURE 2. FACE-analysis of HMC-1 cells after labelling with an antibody specific for the MC5-receptor. 1, control-IgG; 2, anti-MC5; 3, anti-MC5 + blocking peptide.

Taken together, these data demonstrate that HMC-1 cells are able to express MC1- and MC5-receptors, thus providing the prerequisite for neuropeptide action on human mast cells. The precise nature of the mechanism and of the corresponding second messengers, remain to be further clarified.

REFERENCES

1. METCALFE, D.D., D. BARAM & Y.A. MEKORI. 1997. Mast cells. Physiol. Rev. **77:** 1033–1079.
2. COLOMBO, M. *et al.* 1992. The human recombinant c-kit receptor ligand, rhSCF, induces mediator release from the human mast cells and enhances IgE-dependent mediator release from both human skin mast cells and peripheral basophils. J. Immunol. **149:** 599–608.
3. BURT, D.S. & D.R. STANWORTH. 1983. Changes in cellular levels of cyclic AMP in rat mast cells during secretion of histamine induced by immunglobuline E decapeptide and ACTH peptide. Biochem Biophys. Act. **762:** 458–465.
4. MOUNTJOY, K. *et al.* 1992. The cloning of a family of genes that encode the melanocortin receptors. Science **257:** 1248.
5. BHARDWAJ, R.S. *et al.* 1997. Evidence for the differential expression of the functional α-melanocyte-stimulating hormone MC-1 on human monocytes. J. Immunol. **158:** 3378–3384.
6. BHARDWAJ, R.S. *et al.* 1996. Evidence of the expression of a functional melanocortin receptor 1 by human keratinocytes. J. Invest. Dermatol. **106:** 817.

Characterization of μ-Opiate Receptor in Human Epidermis and Keratinocytes

M. BIGLIARDI-QI,[a] P.L. BIGLIARDI, S. BÜCHNER, AND T. RUFLI

Department of Dermatology, Kantonsspital Basel, 4031 Basel, Switzerland

Recent studies suggest that the nervous system and the skin interact directly through neuropeptides.[1] Neuropeptides are able to interact with multiple types of cells in the skin in order to mediate actions that are important in skin inflammation. Thus, there is possibly, not only a neuroimmunologic axis, but also a neuroimmune–dermatologic axis. There is increasing evidence that neurotransmitters play a crucial role in skin physiology and pathology. The expression and production of proopiomelanocortin (POMC) molecules, such as β-endorphin, in the human epidermis[2] suggest that an opiate receptor is present in keratinocytes. In this paper we show that human epidermal keratinocytes do indeed express a μ-opiate receptor in the human epidermis, by using Western blot analysis and a differential display by basal cell carcinoma skin biopsy.

As we previously proved, the μ-opiate receptor is expressed in skin epidermis both at the RNA and protein levels. The staining is generally dispersed in the epidermis and confined to the cytoplasmic region, but increased immunostaining of the μ-opiate receptor was observed on the basal layer.[3] RT-PCR, amplification of cDNA, and sequencing, revealed a 433-nt DNA fragment identical to a μ-opiate receptor from human brain (MOR-1). Southern blot analysis confirmed both PCR products. *In situ* hybridization showed expression of the receptor in human epidermis, especially in the suprabasal layers.

Western blot analysis of the μ-opiate receptor was carried out after immunoprecipitation. To perform immunoprecipitation, the antibodies were linked to CNBr-activated Sepharose 4B. The membranes were isolated from human skin and cultured human foreskin keratinocytes. The receptor was precipitated by binding at antibody-coated sepharose beads. Rat brain membranes were used as a positive control, and antibody-coated sepharose beads—unexposed to membrane proteins—were used as a negative control. The Western blot analysis was performed on a Pharmacia PhastSystem™ and a specific band between 50 and 60 kD was observed with rat brain membrane proteins (see FIGURE 1) and with membranes isolated from human skin and human foreskin keratinocytes. From the literature, the expected size for μ-opiate receptor is 55 kD. We also reported that the receptor can be downregulated by ligands of the μ-opiate system and suggested that indeed a functional active receptor exists in the human epidermis.[3]

In basal-cell carcinoma skin-biopsy, tumor cells do not express the μ-opiate receptor, whereas normal epidermal cells in the surrounding epidermis express the re-

[a]Address for correspondence: Bigliardi-Qi M., Department of Dermatology, Kantonsspital Basel, 4031 Basel, Switzerland. bigliardiqi@ubaclu.unibas.ch (e-mail).

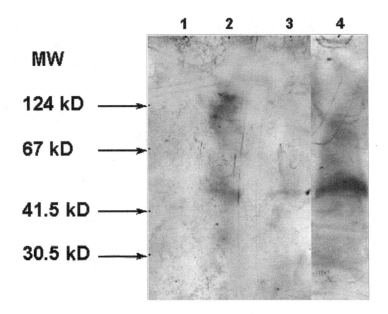

FIGURE 1. Western blot analysis of isolated skin membranes. Human μ-opiate receptor is present in human skin membrane. *Lane1:* Antibody bound CNBr-activated sepharose 4B beads alone as negative control, no band is visible; *Lane 2:* Immunoprecipitation with rat brain membrane as positive control, a positive band can be seen at 55 kD. *Lane 3:* Immunoprecipitation with isolated skin membranes, there is a positive band at 55 kD. *Lane 4:* Isolated skin membranes without immunoprecipitation, a strong band is visible at 55 kD. Immunoprecipitation and Western blot analysis used a μ-opiate receptor specific antibody (Pharmingen).

ceptor normally (see FIGURE 2). Therefore, we were able to show a differential expression of opiate receptor in one single biopsy.

The μ-opiate-receptor agonist β-endorphin is significantly elevated in sera of patients with severe atopic dermatitis[4] and psoriasis.[5] The expression of μ-opiate receptor in human epidermal skin and human keratinocytes suggests an important role of the opioids in the pathology of skin diseases, wound healing, perception of itch,[6,7] and possibly also in skin tumor cells. Further studies will open new prospects for skin physiology and pathology; and will lead to better understanding of the mechanism of the interaction between immune system, neural system, and skin.

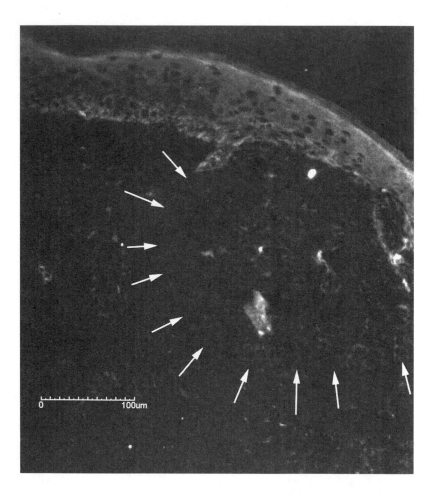

FIGURE 2. Immunostaining of the μ-opiate receptor in human carcinoma skin. Cryosections of human basal cell carcinoma were stained with μ-opiate receptor-specific antibody, and a secondary antibody labeled with Cy 2. A positive immunohistochemical signal can be seen in the membrane of epithelial cells from neighboring and overlaying epidermis, but is completely absent from the epidermal tumor cells. The *arrows* show the border of the basal cell carcinoma.

ACKNOWLEDGMENTS

This work was supported by Swiss National Foundation Grant No. 32-45991.95.

REFERENCES

1. ANSEL, J.C. *et al.* 1996. Skin-nervous system interactions. J. Invest. Dermatol. **106:** 198–204.
2. WINTZEN, M., M. YAAR, J.P.H. BURBACH & B.A. GILCHREST. 1996. Proopiomelano-cortin gene product regulation in keratinocytes. J. Invest. Dermatol. **106:** 673–678.
3. BIGLIARDI, P.L., M. BIGLIARDI-QI, S. BÜCHNER & T. RUFLI. 1998. Expression of μ-opiate receptor in human epidermis and keratinocytes. J. Invest. Dermatol. **111:** 101–105.
4. GLINSKI, W., H. BRODECKA, M. GLINSKA-FERENZ & D. KOWALSK. 1995. Increased concentration of beta-endorphin in the sera of patients with severe atopic dermatitis. Acta Derm. Venereol. **75:** 9–11.
5. GLINSKI, W., H. BRODECKA, M. GLINSKA-FERENZ & D. KOWALSK. 1994. Neuropep-tides in psoriasis: possible role of beta-endorphin in the pathomechanism of the dis-ease. Int. J. Dermatol. **33:** 356–360.
6. BERNSTEIN, J.E. & R. SWIFT. 1979. Relief of intractable pruritus with naloxone. Arch Dermatol. **115:** 1366–1367.
7. PFER, G. *et al.* 1996. Randomised crossover trial of naltrexone in uraemic pruritus. Lancet **348:** 1552–1554.

Characterization of a Polyclonal Antibody Raised Against the Human Melanocortin-1 Receptor

MARKUS BÖHM,[a] THOMAS BRZOSKA,[a] URSULA SCHULTE,[a]
MEINHARD SCHILLER,[a] ULRICH KUBITSCHECK,[b] AND THOMAS A. LUGER[a,c]

[a]Department of Dermatology and Ludwig Boltzmann Institute for Cell Biology and
Immunobiology of the Skin, University of Münster, Münster, Germany

[b]Institute for Biophysics and Physiology, University of Münster, Münster, Germany

ABSTRACT: We have generated a polyclonal antibody raised against a synthetic peptide corresponding to the amino acids 2–18 of the extracellular, N-terminal domain of the human melanocortin-1 receptor (MC-1R). Specificity of the affinity-purified anti-MC-1R antibody was confirmed by dot blot analysis with the antigenic peptide. The antibody detected MC-1R antigenicity on the surface of normal human melanocytes and WM35 melanoma cells, as shown by FACS and immunofluorescence analysis. The antibody was suitable for immunoperoxidase staining of deparaffinized skin sections, revealing prominent MC-1R staining of a cutaneous melanoma as opposed to undiseased skin in which normal melanocytes were only occasionally immunoreactive. Distinct adnexal structures in normal skin also displayed MC-1R immunostaining. Specificity of the MC-1R immunoreactivity in each technique was confirmed by preabsorption with the immunogenic peptide, omission, or substitution of the primary antibody with preimmune serum. Our results provide a baseline for future studies on MC-1R expression in diseased human skin.

INTRODUCTION

The multitude of biological activities of the proopiomelanocortin (POMC)-derived peptides, α-melanocyte-stimulating hormone (α-MSH) and adrenocorticotropin (ACTH), are mediated by binding to specific receptors located on the cell surface of target cells. These receptors are known as melanocortin receptors (MC-Rs) and have emerged from cloning the well-characterized melanocyte-stimulating hormone receptor (MSH-R) and adrenocorticotropin receptor (ACTH-R).[1] To date, five MC-R subtypes, MC-1R to MC-5R, have been discriminated.[2] They are 39–61% identical to one another at the amino acid level, and bind α-MSH, β-MSH, ACTH, and NDP-α-MSH with different affinities. Based on Northern blot analysis, expression of the five MC-R subtypes appeared to be tissue- and cell-specific. MC-1Rs and MC-2Rs were primarily expressed in melanocytes and adrenocortical cells, MC-3Rs in brain and placenta, MC-4Rs exclusively in the cen-

[c]Address for correspondence: T.A. Luger, M.D., Department of Dermatology, Westfälische Wilhelms Universität, Von Esmarch-Str. 56, D-48149 Münster, Germany. + 49-251-835 8604 (voice); + 49-251-835 6522 (fax); Luger@uni-muenster.de (e-mail).

tral nervous system, and MC-5Rs appeared to be more ubiquitously expressed.[2] With respect to MC-1R expression, this picture has been challenged, since independent studies have revealed MC-1R-specific transcripts in a number of nonmelanocytic cell types. Consequently, expression of MC-1R on the RNA level has been detected by reverse transcription-polymerase chain reaction (RT-PCR) in human dermal microvascular endothelial cells, keratinocytes, and dermal fibroblasts.[3–5] It was also reported that monocytes express MC-1Rs, as shown by RT-PCR and by binding studies using biotinylated α-MSH.[6,7] Treatment of each of these cell types with α-MSH resulted in distinct biological responses, such as modulation of cytokine secretion, downregulation of adhesion molecule expression, or modulation of cytokine-induced DNA-protein complex formation of distinct transcription factors known to regulate inflammatory responses.[7–10] In the light of these and additional activities of α-MSH,[11–13] it is important to know the actual protein expression of MC-1Rs in a given tissue and cell type, under normal and diseased conditions. Previous, studies on the MC-1R protein expression in cells in culture and *in situ* have been scarce, due to the lack of generally available antibodies. Recently, a polyclonal antibody that stained a cutaneous melanoma *in situ*, as well as COS-7 cells transfected with the human MC-1R gene, has been described.[14] MC-1R antigenicity was also detected in human testis, ovary, and placenta using a monoclonal anti-MC-1R antibody.[15] We generated a polyclonal antibody raised against a synthetic peptide corresponding to the amino acids 2–18 of the human MC-1R. Specificity and properties of the antibody for detection of MC-1Rs *in vitro* and *in situ* in human skin are described.

MATERIAL AND METHODS

Generation of an Anti-hMC-1R Polyclonal Antibody

The MC-1R immunogen was a synthetic peptide corresponding to the amino acids 2–18 (AVQGSQRRLLGSLNSTP) of the N-terminal, extracellular domain of the human MC-1R. Prior to immunization, 2 mg of the peptide was conjugated with 2 mg of hemocyanin derived from horseshoe crab (*Limulus polyphemus*) hemolymph. After purifying the conjugate by means of a Sephadex-G-25 column, 0.5 mg of conjugate was used to immunize three-month-old female ZIKA-rabbits weighing 2.0 to 2.5 Kg. 1 mL of adjuvant consisting of 95% paraffin oil, 2.4% Tween 40, 0.1% cholesterol, and 0.01% lipopolysaccharide derived from Phormidium were coinjected. Two subsequent boosts with 0.5 mg and 0.25 mg conjugate, respectively, were performed at weekly intervals. After four weeks, the animals were bled and serum was obtained by coagulation and subsequent centrifugation. Serum was stabilized by thiomersal at a final concentration of 0.02% and purified against an anti-IgG column. Total IgG fractions were tested for their specificity by dot-blot analysis. Positive fractions were affinity-purified on a CNBr-activated sepharose 4B column (Pharmacia, Piscataway, NJ) with the immunogen coupled directly to the column material. Preimmune serum was obtained prior to immunization, and did not exhibit any immunoreactivity toward the immunogenic peptide as shown by dot-blot analysis.

Cell Culture

Normal human melanocytes derived from neonatal foreskin were purchased from BioWhittaker (Walkersville, MD) and maintained with all supplements as recommended by the manufacturer. The human melanoma cell line, WM35, was a gift from Dr. M. Herlyn (The Wistar Institute, Philadelphia). They were derived from the radial growth phase of an early melanoma (16), and maintained in RPMI 1640 (Boehringer, Ingelheim, Germany) supplemented with 10% fetal calf serum (FCS), 1% glutamine, and 1% penicillin/streptomycin (all from Boehringer) in a humidified atmosphere of 5% CO_2.

Immunofluorescence Studies

Cells seeded into polystyrene tissue chambers were fixed with 4% paraformaldehyde for 30 min followed by aldehyde quenching with 50 mM NH_4CL, and permeated by methanol for 10 min at $-20°C$. Unspecific binding was blocked with 5% donkey serum for 1 h at room temperature. Cells were next incubated for 1 h at room temperature with the primary antibody (1:15). After three washes with TRIS-buffered saline containing 0,04% Tween 20, cells were incubated with secondary donkey anti-rabbit antibodies conjugated to Cy3™ (1:100, Dianova) for 1 h at room temperature. After 3 final washes, slides were mounted and examined by confocal scanning-laser microscopy. For negative controls, preimmune serum was used instead of the primary antibody. Alternatively, the primary antibody was omitted. For blocking experiments, the antigenic peptide was preincubated at a 5- to 100-fold weight excess with the primary antibody in a small volume of phosphate-buffered saline (PBS) for 1 h at 37°.

FACS Analysis

Cells were scraped into ice-cold PBS and centrifuged at 1200 rpm followed by two washes. The pellets were preincubated in PBS with 1% bovine serum albumin (BSA) at 4°C for 1 h to reduce unspecific binding. After two washes with PBS, cells were incubated with the anti-MC-1R antibody (1:10) at 4°C for 1 h. Unbound antibody was washed off and cells were incubated with a FITC-conjugated anti-rabbit antibody (Dianova) for 30 min. After one final washing step, cells were resuspended in PBS and analyzed in the presence of propidiumjodide in a coulter fluorescence cytometer (Coulter, Miami, FL). Negative controls were used as described above.

Immunohistochemistry

Samples of normal human adult skin were obtained from various body sites including face, extremities, and trunk. In one case, the specimen was derived from a patient with cutaneous melanoma undergoing routine surgery. The specimens were fixed in 7% buffered paraformaldehyde, dehydrated, embedded in parablast, and mounted on Tissue-Tek (Mikrom, Walldorf, Germany). Parablast-embedded sections were deparaffinized with xylol and ethanol at decreasing concentrations, followed by thorough washing with water. For epitope unmasking, sections were immersed in an aqueous solution containing 0.1 M citric acid/0.1M sodium citrate, and treated in a microwave for 15 min. Sections were quenched for endogenous peroxidase by incubating with 1% methanolic hydrogen peroxide for 20 min. After rinsing with PBS, unspecific binding sites were blocked with 2% BSA for 30 minutes at room temperature. Then, sections were incubated with the anti-MC-1R antibody (1:14, diluted in 1% BSA) for 45 min at room temperature. After washing with PBS, they were developed by the indirect immunoperoxidase technique using peroxidase-conjugated goat-anti-rabbit antibodies (1:250, Dianova) 0.01% hydrogen peroxide, and 3-amino-9-ethylcarbazole (Sigma, St. Louis, MO). Negative controls were used as described above.

RESULTS AND DISCUSSION

First, the ability of the affinity-purified antibody to detect MC-1Rs in human pigment cells in culture was examined. For this purpose, we performed immunofluorescence and FACS analysis on normal human foreskin melanocytes and WM35 melanoma cells derived from an early primary cutaneous melanoma. Normal human melanocytes and transformed melanocytes have been previously shown to express the MSH-R and to possess functional binding sites.[1,17,18] Immunofluorescence of WM35 melanoma cells caused the anti-MC-1R antibody to produce a characteristic granular staining of the cell membrane and the cytoplasm, while mostly sparing the nuclei (see FIGURE 1A). No specific immunostaining was observed in cells treated with the fluorochrome-conjugated secondary antibody alone (FIG. 1B) or, in cells treated with preimmune serum (FIG. 1C). Preabsorption of the anti-MC-1R antibody with the antigenic peptide resulted in subtotal abrogation of the immunostaining (FIG. 1D). Examining the human melanoma cell line, WM266-4, others have detected prominent MC-1R immunostaining mainly on the cell surface.[19] In contrast, most of the immunoreactivity in genetically engineered stable MC-1R expressing COS-7 was found within the cytoplasm and the perinuclear region.[14] It is possible that these discrepancies are due to cell-specific differences, or that they reflect the differential mode of MC-1R expression; that is, ectopic MC-1R expression in COS-7 cells with cytoplasmic sequestration of newly synthesized receptors, as opposed to melanoma cells that naturally express MC-1Rs. Internal binding sites for MSH have also been described in wild-type and variant Cloudman melanoma cells.[20]

In order to confirm the surface expression of MC-1R, we next performed FACS analysis of normal human melanocytes and WM35 melanoma cells. In these experiments, detachment of the cells from the culture flasks by trypsin was avoided since the extracellular portion of the MC-1R, to which our antibody was directed, contains cleavage sites for trypsin. Thus, the adherent cells were gently scraped into PBS. Unspecific binding of the anti-MC-R1 antibody to the cell surface of the cells was assessed by incubating the cells with preimmune serum at the same concentration as the anti-MC-R1 antibody. Normal melanocytes and WM35 melanoma cells displayed significant MC-1R antigenicity on their cell surface although the mean fluorescence intensity—and thus the number of MC-1Rs expressed—was higher in melanocytes than in the tumor cell line (see FIGURE 2A and B). Omission of the primary antibody or preabsorption with the immunogenic peptide, abolished the antibody binding (data not shown). Increasing concentrations of the anti-MC-1R

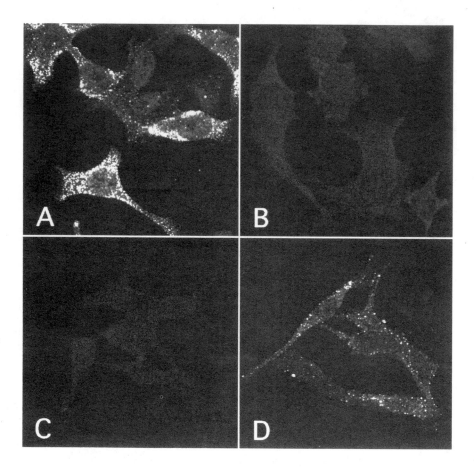

FIGURE 1. Immunofluorescence staining of WM35 melanoma cells. Cells were incubated with the anti-human MC-1R antibody. Bound antibodies were detected by a secondary donkey anti-rabbit antibody conjugated to Cy3™ followed by confocal scanning-laser microscopy; all magnifications 1:630. **A.** Specific immunostaining of the cell membrane and cytoplasmic region after incubation with the anti-MC-1R antibody, 1:15. **B.** Negative control with the secondary antibody alone. **C.** Negative control using preimmune serum. **D.** Subtotal abrogation of specific immunostaining after preabsorption of the anti-MC-1R antibody with the immunogenic peptide at a weight excess of 1:10.

antibody resulted in a dose-dependent increase in the mean fluorescence intensity (FIG. 2C).

We next examined the ability of the antibody to detect MC-1Rs *in situ*. Deparaffinized skin sections from various body sites derived from healthy donors, as well as from one patient with a cutaneous melanoma, were evaluated histochemically for *in situ* MC-1R expression using the immunoperoxidase technique. MC-1R antigenicity in normal skin was mainly expressed in hair follicle epithelia, sebocytes, and secre-

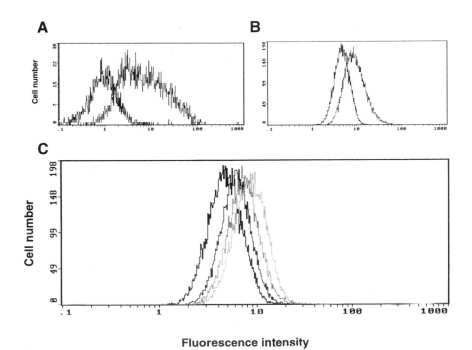

FIGURE 2. FACS analysis of MC-1R expression in WM35 melanoma cells and normal human melanocytes. Cells were scraped into PBS, incubated with the anti-MC-1R antibody (1:10), followed by incubation with an anti-rabbit FITC-conjugated secondary antibody and propidiumiodide staining. Preimmune serum was used as a control to monitor unspecific antibody binding (*left curve*). **A.** Surface expression of MC-1R on normal human melanocytes. **B.** Surface expression of MC-1R on WM35 melanoma cells. **C.** Detection of MC-1R antigenicity on the surface of WM35 melanoma cells using different dilutions of the anti-MC-1R antibody (from *left* to *right*; preimmune serum, anti-MC-1R antibody, 1:20; 1:10; 1:5).

tory and ductal epithelia of sweat glands (see FIGURE 3A). Normal melanocytes were occasionally immunoreactive (FIG. 3E). The unexpected staining pattern in adnexal structures was consistently present in more than 10 samples of normal skin, and independent from the body site. Omission or substitution of the primary antibody with preimmune serum did not produce any staining (FIG. 3B and C). Blocking experiments with the antigenic peptide completely neutralized immunostaining in the adnexal structures (FIG. 3D) confirming the specificity of the MC-1R immunostaining. Moreover, similar results were obtained in cryostat sections of normal skin, indicating that the observed MC-1R antigenicity is not an artifact due to fixation with paraformaldehyde and parablast embedding. Our findings on the observed MC-1R antigenicity of normal skin are in contrast to reports from others who could not detect any MC-1R immunoreactivity in normal skin.[14] However, the synthetic peptide,

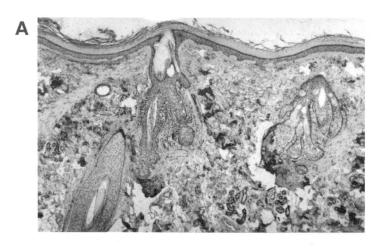

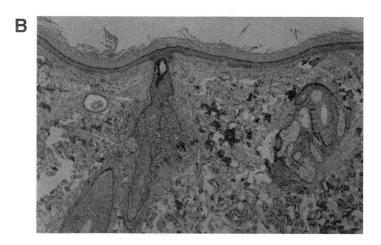

FIGURE 3. Immunohistochemical detection of MC-1R antigenicity in normal human skin and a cutaneous melanoma. Deparaffinized skin sections were incubated with the anti-MC-1R antibody (1:14), followed by the immunoperoxidase technique. **A.** MC-1R antigenicity of normal skin; note immunoreactivity of secretory cells of the sweat glands, hair follicle keratinocytes of the outer root sheath and sebocytes. **B.** Negative control with the secondary antibody alone. (Figure continued on next page).

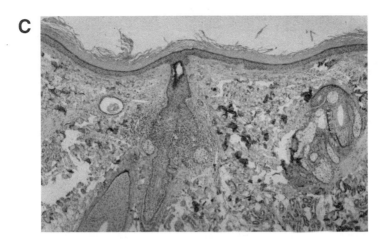

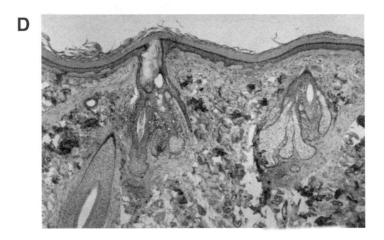

FIGURE 3/continued.   C. Negative control using preimmune serum. **D.** Blocking experiment with the antigenic peptide (10-fold weight excess) and the primary antibody. (Figure continued on next page).

E

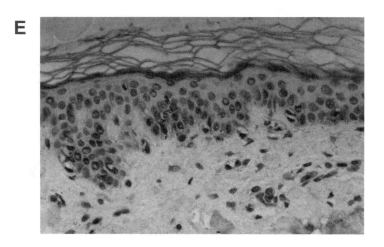

F

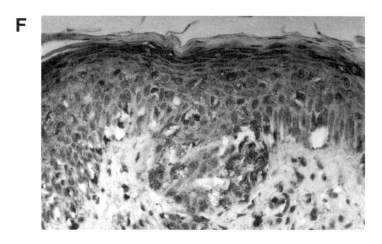

FIGURE 3/continued. **E.** MC-1R immunoreactivity of scattered melanocytes in normal skin. **F.** MC-1R immunoreactivity in a cutaneous melanoma from the back of a 40-year-old male caucasian, Clark level I–II, tumor thickness 0.3 mm. Note also immunoreactivity of epidermal cells adjacent to the tumor.

those authors used for generation of their polyclonal antiserum was somewhat different from that we used. The pilosebaceous unit has been known for some time to represent a target site for POMC-derived peptides. Accordingly, α-MSH has been shown to induce sebum secretion.[21] Moreover, binding sites for α-MSH have been found on human scalp hair follicles.[22] Thus, the observed MC-1R antigenicity in adnexal structures may represent hitherto undetected binding sites *in situ* for POMC-derived peptides. In contrast, the weak and irregular MC-1R antigenicity of melanocytes *in situ* may be due to the overall low expression of the receptor under normal conditions. In contrast to melanocytes in normal skin, melanoma cells *in situ* displayed prominent MC-1R antigenicity (FIG. 3F). Preimmune serum, on the other hand, did not produce any immunostaining (data not shown). It remains to be determined if overexpression of MC-1R *in situ* is a consistent feature of cutaneous melanomas. Preliminary data indicate that the detectable *in situ* MC-1R expression in melanomas is heterogeneous, and that a significant proportion of common nevi also display prominent MC-1R antigenicity (our own unpublished work). As reported previously, MC-1R immunoreactivity was also detected in the epidermis in the vicinity of the melanoma (FIG. 3F), suggesting that melanoma cells may secrete soluble factors that actually promote the expression of MC-1R in neighboring keratinocytes.

Taken together, these data indicate that this antibody, which is directed against the human MC-1R, may serve a useful tool for *in vitro* and *in situ* studies and thus will help to shed light into the biology of melanocortins and their respective receptors in the skin.

REFERENCES

1. MOUNTJOY, K.G. *et al.* 1992. The cloning of a family of genes that encode the melanocortin receptors. Science **257:** 1247–1251.
2. CONE, R.D. *et al.* 1996. The melanocortin receptors: agonists, antagonists and the hormonal control of pigmentation. Rec. Prog. Horm. Res. **51:** 287–318.
3. HARTMEYER, M. *et al.* 1997. Human microvascular endothelial cells (HMEC-1) express the melanocortin receptor type 1 and produce increased levels of IL-8 upon stimulation with α-MSH. J. Immunol. **159:** 1930–1937.
4. BRZOSKA, T. *et al.* 1997. UVB irradiation regulates the expression of proopiomelanocortin, prohormone convertase 1 and melanocortin receptor 1 by human keratinocytes. (Abstract). J. Invest. Dermatol. **108:** 622.
5. BÖHM, M. *et al.* 1997. Human fibroblasts express melanocortin-1 receptors and respond to alpha-melanocyte stimulating hormone with increased secretion of interleukin-6 and interleukin 8. (Abstract). J. Invest. Dermatol. **108:** 593.
6. BHARDWAJ, R. *et al.* 1997. Evidence for the differential expression of the functional α-melanocyte-stimulating hormone receptor MC-1 on human monocytes. J. Immunol. **158:** 3378–3384.
7. STAR, R.A. *et al.* 1995. Evidence of autocrine modulation of macrophage nitric oxide synthase by α-melanocyte-stimulating hormone. Proc. Natl. Acad. Sci. USA **92:** 8016–8020.
8. BÖHM, M. *et al.* Alpha-melanocyte-stimulating hormone modulates the activation of NF-κB and AP-1 and the secretion of interleukin-8 in human dermal fibroblasts. Ann. N.Y. Acad. Sci. **885:** this volume.
9. KALDEN, D.-H. *et al.* α-MSH modulates LPS-induced adhesion molecules. Ann. N.Y. Acad. Sci. **885:** this volume.

10. BRZOSKA, T. *et al.* Molecular basis of the α-MSH/IL-1 antagonism. Ann. N.Y. Acad. Sci. **885:** this volume.
11. KISS, M. *et al.* 1995. α-Melanocyte stimulating hormone induces collagenase/metallomatrix proteinase-1 in human dermal fibroblasts. Biol. Chem. Hoppe-Seyler **376:** 425–430.
12. SIMON, M.M. *et al.* 1994. POMC-derived peptide hormones alpha-MSH and ACTH affect proliferation and differentiation of cultured human keratinocytes. J. Invest. Dermatol. **103:** 419–425.
13. OREL, L. *et al.* 1997. α-Melanocyte-stimulating hormone downregulates differentiation/driven heat shock protein 70 expression in keratinocytes. J. Invest. Dermatol. **108:** 401–408.
14. XIA, Y. *et al.* 1995. Polyclonal antibodies against human melanocortin MC_1 receptor: preliminary immunohistochemical localization of melanocortin MC_1 receptors to malignant melanoma cells. Eur. J. Pharmacol. **288:** 277–283.
15. THÖRNWALL, M. *et al.* 1996. Immunohistochemical detection of the melanocortin 1 receptor in human testis, ovary and placenta using specific monoclonal antibodies. Horm. Res. **48:** 215–218.
16. HERLYN, M. *et al.* 1989. Growth regulatory factors for normal, premalignant, and malignant human melanoma cells *in vitro.* Adv. Cancer Res. **54:** 213–220.
17. CHHALJANI, V. *et al.* 1992. Molecular cloning and expression of the human melanocyte-stimulating hormone receptor cDNA. FEBS Lett. **309:** 417–420.
18. DONATIEN, P.D. *et al.* 1992. The expression of functional MSH receptors on cultured human melanocytes. Arch. Dermatol. Res. **284:** 424–426.
19. XIA, Y. *et al.* 1996. Immunological localization of melanocortin 1 receptor on the cell surface of WM266-4 human melanoma cells. Cancer Lett. **98:** 157–163.
20. ORLOW, S.J. *et al.* 1990. Internal binding sites for MSH: analysis in wild-type and variant Cloudman melanoma cells. **142:** 129–136.
21. BÖHM, M. *et al.* 1998. The pilosebaceous unit is part of the skin immune system. Dermatology **196:** 75–79.
22. NANNINGA, P.B. *et al.* 1991. Evidence for alpha-MSH binding sites on human scalp hair follicles: preliminary results. Pigm. Cell Res. **4:** 193–198.

Effects of Ethanol Consumption on β-Endorphin Levels and Natural Killer Cell Activity in Rats

NADKA BOYADJIEVA, GARY MEADOWS, AND DIPAK SARKAR[a]

Department of VCAPP, Department of Pharmaceutical Science,
Washington State University, Pullman, Washington, USA

INTRODUCTION

Natural killer (NK) cells have been implicated in immune surveillance against tumors, bacterial, and viral infections.[1] The NK cell cytotoxic activity appears to be responsive to a variety of stresses. It is markedly reduced during chronic stress and in opiate addicts. Limited work has been done on the effect of ethanol on NK cells in mice.[2] Work that is available has demonstrated alcohol action on NK cells, although variable effects have been reported.[3] There is evidence that central opioid neurons may control NK cell function[4] and alcohol abuse. Opioid peptides, particularly β-endorphin (β-EP), regulates ethanol self-administration, behavioral, and neuroendocrine abnormalities in alcohol abuse.[5] Ethanol alters β-EP by modulating the release and synthesis of the peptide *in vivo* and *in vitro.*[6] We showed previously that in primary cultures of fetal hypothalamic cells, low concentrations of ethanol rapidly stimulated β-EP release, whereas constant exposure to ethanol desensitized these cultured neurons.[7] Since the β-EP is involved in the control of alcohol abuse, and since alcohol may alter NK cell activity, a question arises as to whether alcohol intake affects NK cell function due to altered β-EP activity. To better understand the neuroendocrine-immune interactions in alcohol abuse, we determined the effects of acute and chronic intake of ethanol on hypothalamic and plasma levels of β-EP and splenic NK cell cytolytic activity in rats.

MATERIALS AND METHODS

Rats and Feeding Design

Male Sprague-Dawley rats were used throughout the experiments on a 12 h light/dark cycle at 22 to 24°C. The ethanol-treated animals received 5.5 g of ethanol/Kg body weight (b.w.), i.p., 20% w/v saline; the control animals received a corresponding volume of saline. The rats were decapitated 3 h after injection, and the spleen, hypothalamus, and blood were removed for subsequent analysis of NK cell cytolytic activity, plasma, and hypothalamic β-EP, as described below. Chronic administration

[a]Address for correspondence: Dr. Dipak K. Sarkar, Professor and Chairman, Department of Animal Sciences, Rutgers, The State University of New Jersey, New Brunswick, NJ 08901-8525, USA. 732-932-1529 (voice); 732-932-6996 (fax); sarkar@aesop.rutgers.edu (e-mail).

of ethanol involved liquid diet procedures as previously described.[10] The rats were separated in to three experimental groups: (1) an *ad libitum*–fed rodent chow meal; (2) a pair-fed group with isocaloric liquid diet; and (3) an ethanol group with liquid diet identical to group (2) except that the sucrose was replaced with 8.7% (v/v) ethanol. The liquid diet was administered for 15 days. At the conclusion of the experiments, animals were decapitated, the spleen, hypothalamus, and blood were removed for analyses of NK cell cytolytic activity and β-EP.

Natural Killer Cell Activity

NK cell cytolytic activity against YAC-1 lymphoma cells was determined from NK spleen cells by a standard 4-h 51-Cr release cytolytic assay, as described previously.[2]

Radioimmunoassay of Immunoreactive β-ET

The immunoreactive β-EP levels in plasma and hypothalamus were measured by a RIA system, as described by us previously.[7]

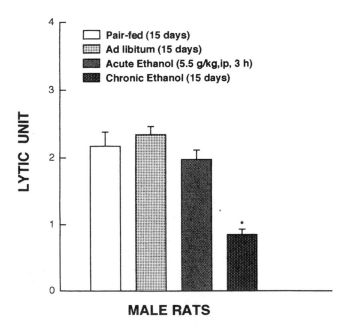

FIGURE 1. Effect of acute ethanol (5.5 g/Kg, i.p.) for 3 h and chronic consumption of ethanol for 15 days on splenic NK cell activity in male rats. Data shown are Mean + SEM of lytic unit. * $p < 0.05$.

Statistics

The mean and standard error of the data were determined and are presented in the text and figures. Data were analyzed using one-way ANOVA. The post-hoc test involved the Student-Newmann-Keuls test. A value of $p < 0.05$ was considered significant.

RESULTS

The cytolytic activity of splenic NK cells from rats after consuming ethanol for 15 days as a function of YAC-1 lymphoma targets, was significantly inhibited compared with the pair-fed and *ad libitum* groups. The acute treatment with ethanol for 3 h did not change the NK cell cytolytic activity (see FIGURE 1). In order to measure whether the ethanol administration altered the *in vivo* β-EP in rats, we determined the hypothalamic and plasma β-EP content after ethanol administration for 3 h and consumption for 15 days.The hypothalamic content of rat β-EP was significantly increased 3 h after ethanol administration, but decreased after 15 days of ethanol treatment (see FIGURE 2). Similarly, the plasma levels of β-EP were significantly increased after 3 h, but decreased following chronic consumption of ethanol for 15 days.

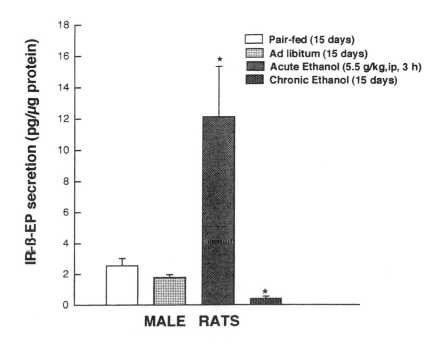

FIGURE 2. Effect of acute ethanol (5.5 g/Kg, i.p.) for 3 h and chronic consumption of ethanol for 15 days on hypothalamic IR-β-EP content in male rats. Data shown are Mean + SEM of pg of IR-β-EP/μg protein. * $p < 0.05$

DISCUSSION

The data presented here demonstrate that ethanol consumption for 15 days suppressed NK cell activity, and decreased plasma and hypothalamic content of β-EP in male rats. Acute treatment with ethanol for 3 h did not alter NK cell activity, but increased both plasma and hypothalamic β-EP levels in rats. The data presented in this study are in agreement with the majority of *in vivo* studies[6] on rats in that acute treatment with ethanol increased hypothalamic β-EP content whereas chronic consumption of ethanol decreased β-EP content. We also found that ethanol alters plasma β-EP content—similar to its effects on hypothalamic β-EP. The plasma levels of β-EP may reflect from the pituitary gland as well as from other sources, such as adrenal gland and ovary.

The results presented demonstrate that the reduction of hypothalamic and plasma β-EP levels following chronic ethanol intake correlates with the reduction of splenic NK cell activity. It has been reported that chronic ethanol consumption inhibits the NK cell activity in mice.[2] The data presented here provide the first evidence that chronic ethanol intake decreased splenic NK cell cytolytic activity in rats. The positive association between the changes of NK cell function and β-EP levels in alcohol-treated animals provides corroboration for a positive involvement of the opioid peptides in controlling NK cell function. Further studies to determine the effect of opioid agonists and antagonists on ethanol and nonethanol treated animals may establish the role played by β-EP in regulating NK cell function.

ACKNOWLEDGMENTS

This work was supported by National Institutes of Health Grants AA00220 and AA07293.

REFERENCES

1. HERBERMAN, R.B & J.R. ORTALDO. 1981. Natural-killer cells: Their role in defense against disease. Science (Wash DC) **214:** 24–30.
2. MEADOWS, G.G. *et al.* 1989. Influence of ethanol consumption on natural killer cell activity in mice. Alcoholism: Clin. Exp. Res. **13:** 476–479.
3. LI, F. *et al.* 1997. Ethanol and natural killer cells: II. Stimulation of NK activity by ethanol *in vitro.* Alcoholism: Clin. Exp. Res. **6:** 981–987.
4. SOHN, J.H. *et al.* 1986. Brain μ-opioid receptors are involved in morphine-induced suppression of immune function. Soc. Neurosci. **12:** 339.
5. ZAGON, I.S., & P.J. MCLAUGHLIN. 1983. Behavioral effects of prenatal exposure to opiates. Monog. Neural Sci. **9:** 159–168.
6. GIANOULAKIS, C. *et al.* 1987. Effect of acute ethanol *in vivo* and *in vitro* on the β-endorphin system in rat. Life Sci. **40:** 19–28.
7. BOYADJIEVA, N.I. & D.K. SARKAR. Effects of chronic alcohol on β-endorphin secretion from hypothalamic neurons in primary cultures: evidence for alcohol tolerance, withdrawal and sensitization responses. Alcoholism: Clin. Exp. Res. **18:** 1497–1501.

Murine Dendritic Cells Express Functional Delta-Type Opioid Receptors

CLEMENS ESCHE,[a] VALERIA P. MAKARENKOVA,[b] NATALIA V. KOST,[b]
MICHAEL T. LOTZE,[a] ANDREY A. ZOZULYA,[b] AND MICHAEL R. SHURIN[a,c]

[a]University of Pittsburgh Cancer Institute, Biologic Therapeutics Program,
300 Kaufmann Building, 3471 Fifth Avenue, Pittsburgh, Pennsylvania 15213, USA

[b]National Mental Health Research Center, Academy of Medical Sciences, Moscow, Russia

INTRODUCTION

Dendritic cells (DC) are the most potent antigen-presenting cells (APC), and the only APC capable of presenting novel antigens to naïve T-cells.[1] Following their departure from the bone marrow, DC migrate to nonlymphoid tissues where they reside in an immature stage. The classical example is the epidermal Langerhans cell (LC) that recognizes and processes antigens in the skin. After migration to the secondary lymphoid organs, DC mature into cells that are capable of presenting antigens and stimulating T-cell proliferation. TNF-α promotes DC maturation *in vitro* by upregulation of adhesion and costimulatory molecules, and downregulation of antigen-capturing and antigen-processing molecules. DC are involved in the pathogenesis of numerous skin diseases including psoriasis, allergic contact eczema, atopic eczema, oral hairy leukoplakia, mycosis fungoides, and melanoma. The function of epidermal LC and dermal DC is likely to be regulated by neuropeptides released from nerves ending in the skin. In fact, receptors for calcitonin gene-related peptide,[2] pituitary adenylate cyclase activating polypeptide,[3] gastrin-releasing peptide,[3] and substance P[4] have been identified on epidermal LC. The aim of this work was to evaluate presence and function of δ-type opioid receptors (DOR) on DC.

METHODS

Femur and tibia marrow cells from male C57BL/6 mice were depleted of CD4+, CD8+, and B220+ lymphocytes and adherent macrophages, and cultured with 1000 U/ml *rm*GM-CSF and *rm*IL-4. One-week-old cultures revealed a purity exceeding 90% DC by FACScan analysis. Mature DC were generated by additional supplementation with 10 ng/ml TNF-α. Extracted DNA samples from both immature and mature DC were amplified using the primers 5´-ATCTTCACCCTCACCATGATG-3´ and 5´-CGGTCCTCCTCCTTGGAACC-3´ to cDNA, encoding the third transmembrane domain and the third extracellular loop of the binding site of the murine DOR. These primers identify the second and third exon of the DOR gene, and produce a

[c]Address for correspondence: Michael R. Shurin, University of Pittsburgh Cancer Institute, Biologic Therapeutics Program, 300 Kaufmann Building, 3471 Fifth Avenue, Pittsburgh, PA 15213, USA. mshurin+@pitt.edu (e-mail).

PCR product approximately 365 base pairs in length. Mixed leukocyte reaction (MLR) was performed using cultured DC preincubated with 10^{-9}–10^{-5} M DOR ligand DADLE, [D-Ala^2, D-Leu^5]-enkephalin, for 24 hours. Then, 2.5×10^4 to 2×10^5 irradiated DC were added in triplicates to 3×10^5 purified allogeneic Balb/c T-cells isolated from the spleen. Proliferation was determined 72 hours later by incorporation of [^{3}H]thymidine and expressed as counts per minute (cpm) ± standard error of the mean (SEM). Dose dependent effects were analyzed by two-way ANOVA.

RESULTS

Electrophoresis of RT-PCR products on a 1.5% agarose gel revealed a specific band with the expected molecular size (see FIGURE 1). Mature DC (lane 3) expressed higher levels of DOR mRNA than immature DC (lane 2). MLR results showed that DADLE induced bidirectional modulation of DC function in a dose-dependent fashion (see FIGURE 2). Doses of 10^{-7} and 10^{-8} M enhanced the stimulatory capacity of immature DC by as much as 140% ($p < 0.01$); lower (10^{-9} M) or higher (10^{-5} M) doses, reduced the ability of DC to stimulate T-cell proliferation down to 10% ($p < 0.001$).

DISCUSSION

Vaccination using DC pulsed with tumor-associated antigens initiates protective and therapeutic, tumor-specific, humoral, and cellular immune responses.[1] However, the most efficient combination of cytokines and growth factors required for the development of high numbers of active DC remains to be identified.[1] Opioid agonists selective for the DOR are capable of regulating the activity of immune cells and, with the exception of DC, DOR have been identified in all major immune cell pop-

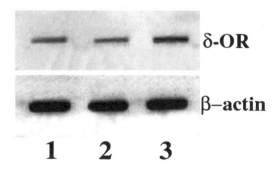

FIGURE 1. RT-PCR amplification of DOR mRNA from murine DC. Mature DC (*lane 3*) expressed higher levels of DOR than immature DC (*lane 2*). *Lane 1,* positive control using rat bulbus olfactorius cells. These data suggest a maturation-dependent expression of DOR mRNA in murine DC.

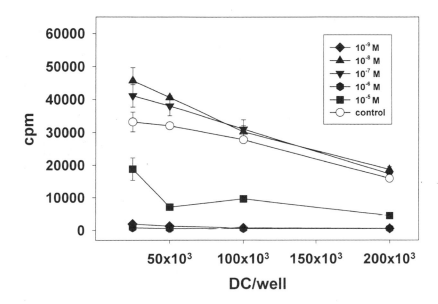

FIGURE 2. Regulation of functional activity of cultured DC by DADLE *in vitro*. Cultured murine DC were pre-incubated with 10^{-9}–10^{-5} M DADLE for 24 hours and their ability to stimulate proliferation of allogeneic T-cells was determined by MLR. These data suggest that stimulation of DOR on DC results in dose-dependent activation or inhibition of DC function *in vitro*.

ulations so far. Therefore, we evaluated the presence and function of DOR on these cells and found the functional expression of DOR on murine DC. The higher level of DOR expression on mature DC most likely reflects the involvement of opioid agonists in the regulation of DC-induced T-cell proliferation. This report provides the first evidence for opioid-receptor expression on DC and suggests a new neuroendocrine mechanism for the regulation of DC function and, thus, the development of specific immune responses.

ACKNOWLEDGMENTS

This work was supported in part by Grants Es 132/1-1 from the Deutsche Forschungsgemeinschaft (DFG) to C.E., and RO1 CA80126-01 from the National Institutes of Health (NIH) to M.R.S.

REFERENCES

1. ESCHE, C., M.R.SHURIN & M.T. LOTZE. 1999. The use of dendritic cells for cancer vaccination. Curr. Opin. Mol. Ther. **1:** 72–81.

2. HOSOI, J., G.F. MURPHY, C.L. EGAN, E.A. LERNER, S. GRABBE, A. ASAHINA & R.D. GRANSTEIN. 1993. Regulation of Langerhans cell function by nerves containing calcitonin gene-related peptide. Nature **363:** 159–163.
3. TORII, H., Z. YAN, J. HOSOI & R.D. GRANSTEIN. 1997. Expression of neurotrophic factors and neuropeptide receptors by Langerhans cells and the Langerhans cell-like cell line XS52: Further support for a functional relationship between Langerhans cells and epidermal nerves. J. Invest. Dermatol. **109:** 586–591.
4. STANIEK, V., L. MISERY, J. PEGUET-NAVARRO, J. ABELLO, J.D. DOUTREMEPUICH, A. CLAUDY & D. SCHMITT. 1997. Binding and *in vitro* modulation of human epidermal Langerhans cell functions by substance P. Arch. Dermatol. Res. **289:** 285–291.
5. CARR, D.J.J., C.H. KIM, B. DeCOSTA, A.E. JACOBSON, K.C. RICE & J.E. BLALOCK. 1988. Evidence for a δ-class opioid receptor on cells of the immune system. Cell. Immunol. **116:** 44–51.

Expression of Corticotropin Releasing Hormone in Malignant Melanoma

YOKO FUNASAKA,[a] HIROFUMI SATO, AND MASAMITSU ICHIHASHI

Department of Dermatology, Kobe University School of Medicine,
Kobe, 650-0017, Japan

Corticotropin releasing hormone (CRH), a 41-amino-acid peptide, is synthesized not only in the hypothalamus,[1] but also in several extrahypothalamic sites. These include most peripheral reproductive tissues, such as adrenals, gonads, placenta, gastrointestinal system, pancreas, and immune cells.[2–6] Higher expression of CRH in malignant cells has been detected in thyroid carcinomas[7] and breast cancers[8] without accompanying clinical manifestations of hyperadrenocorticism, as in ectopic CRH-adrenocorticotropic hormone (ACTH) tumors such as small cell lung carcinoma, bronchial and thymic carcinoids, pheochromocytoma, and thyroid carcinoma.[9] The expression of CRH and CRH-receptor (CRH-R) type-1 mRNAs has been detected in cultured human melanocytes and melanoma cells, as well as in nevus tissues.[10] We have recently shown that cultured melanoma cells express CRH mRNA at higher levels than nevus cells and epidermal melanocytes.[11] To characterize the localization of CRH expression in melanoma tissues, an immunohistochemical study was performed on surgically removed specimens. As is shown in FIGURE 1, some vertically growing melanoma cells exhibited strong expression of immunoreactive CRH peptides, in contrast with the negative staining seen for normal epidermal melanocytes. This tendency to higher CRH expression was much more clearly observed in advanced melanoma cells such as nodular melanoma, vertically growing superficial spreading melanoma, acral lentiginous melanoma, and in metastatic melanoma, than in horizontally growing melanoma cells and nevus cells (Sato *et al.*, manuscript in preparation).

α-Melanocyte stimulating hormone (MSH) has been reported to stimulate proliferation of melanoma cells and to enhance their metastatic behavior in an autocrine or paracrine manner in mouse models.[12–14] Our recent study showed that more malignant melanoma cells might produce higher level of POMC peptides that correlate with tumor progression, although the mechanism of this upregulation was unclear.[15] Upregulation of proopiomelanocortin (POMC) peptides and their receptors has been reported in cultured keratinocytes and melanocytes treated with interleukin-1 (IL-1), dibutyryl cyclic AMP (dbcAMP), 12-O-tetradecanoylphorbol-13-acetate (TPA), or ultraviolet B (UVB).[16–18] High levels of CRH peptide expression might stimulate expression of POMC peptides, thus endowing melanoma cells with enhanced growth and metastatic abilities. CRH and POMC expression coincided in about 50% of advanced melanoma cells. However, in other cells, POMC was highly expressed with-

[a]Address for correspondence: Yoko Funasaka, M.D., Ph.D., Department of Dermatology, Kobe University School of Medicine, 5-1 Kusunoki-cho 7-chome, Chuo-ku, Kobe 650-0017, Japan. +81-78-382-6132 (voice); +81-78-382-6149 (fax); funasaka@med.kobe-u.ac.jp (e-mail).

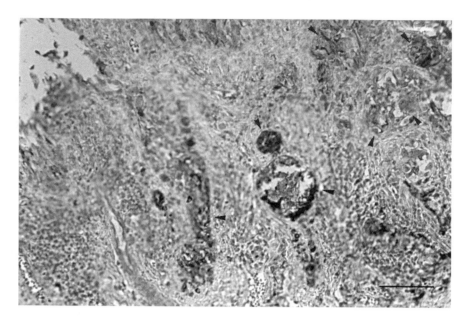

FIGURE 1. Expression of CRH in melanoma tissues. Melanoma tissues were obtained from surgical specimens, fixed in paraformaldehyde, embedded in paraffin, and sectioned. Deparaffinized sections were incubated with rabbit antiserum against r/hCRH (a gift from Dr. GP Chrousos, NIH), followed by the avidin-biotin-peroxidase detection system, with 3-amino-9-ethyl-carbazole as chromogen. Some vertically growing, invading melanoma cells in acral lentiginous melanoma showed strong positive immunostaining. *Arrows* indicate the localization of positive melanoma cells. *Bar* = 100 µm.

out concomitant high CRH expression, or vice versa (data not shown). As well as inducing POMC gene expression, CRH exerts multiple other effects on various cell types, such as stimulating endothelial chemotaxis[19] and enhancing inflammatory reactions.[20] Human tumor cells transfected with CRH have a growth advantage when transfected to nude mice, due to stimulated angiogenesis. Studies to examine the effects of CRH antagonists and CRH peptides on growth and metastasis of melanoma tumors transplanted in mice are currently underway in our laboratory.

REFERENCES

1. VALE, W., C. RIVIER et al. 1983. Chemical and biological characterization of corticotropin-releasing factor. Recent Prog. Horm. Res. **39:** 245–267.
2. THOMPSON, R.C., A.F. SEASHOLTZ et al. 1987. Rat corticotropin-releasing hormone gene: sequence and tissue-specific expression. Mol. Endocrinol. **1:** 363–370.
3. OWENS, M.J. & C.B. NEMEROFF. 1991. Physiology and pharmacology of corticotropin-releasing factor. Pharmacol. Rev. **43:** 425–473.
4. ORTH, D. 1992. Corticotropin-releasing hormone in humans. Endocr. Rev. **13:** 164–191.

5. VAMVAKOPOULOS, N.C. & G.P. CHROUSOS. 1994. Hormonal regulation of human corticotropin-releasing hormone gene expression: implications for the stress response and immune/inflamatory reaction. Endocr. Rev. **15:** 409–420.
6. ZOUMAKIS, E., A.N. MARGIORIS *et al.* 1997. Human endometrium as a neuroendocrine tissue: expression, regulation and biological roles of endometrial corticotropin-releasing hormone (CRH) and opioid peptides. J. Endocrinol. Invest. **20:** 159–167.
7. SCOPA, C.D., G. MASTORAKOS *et al.* 1994. Presence of immunoreactive corticotropin releasing hormone in thyroid lesions. Am. J. Pathol. **145:** 1159–1167.
8. CIOCCA, D.R., L.A. PUY *et al.* 1990. Corticotropin-releasing hormone, luteinizing hormone-releasing hormone, growth hormone-releasing hormone, and somatostatin-like immunoreactivities in biopsies from breast cancer patients. Breast Cancer Res. Treat. **15:** 175–184.
9. WAJCHENBERG, B.L., B.B. MENDONCA *et al.* 1995. Ectopic ACTH syndrome. J. Steroid Biochem. Molec. Biol. **53:** 1–6.
10. SLOMINISKI, A, G. ERMAK *et al.* 1995. Proopiomelanocortin, corticotropin releasing hormone and corticotropin releasing hormone receptor genes are expressed in human skin. FEBS Lett. **374:** 113–116.
11. FUNASAKA, Y., H. SATO *et al.* 1998. Expression of proopiomelanocortin, corticotropin releasing hormone (CRH), CRH receptor in malignant melanoma cells, nevus cells, and normal human melanocytes. J. Invest. Dermatol. In press.
12. BREGMAN, M.D., Z.A. ABDEL-MALEK *et al.* 1985. Anchorage-independent growth of murine melanoma in serum-less media is dependent on insulin or melanocyte-stimulating hormone. Exp. Cell Res. **157:** 419–428.
13. SHEPPARD, J.R., T.P. KOESTLER *et al.* 1984. Experimental metastasis correlates with cyclic AMP accumulation in B16 melanoma clones. Nature **308:** 544–547.
14. BENNETT, D.C., T.J. DEXTER *et al.* 1986. Increased experimental metastatic capacity of a murine melanoma following induction of differentiation. Cancer Res. **46:** 3239–3244.
15. NAGAHAMA, M., Y. FUNASAKA *et al.* 1998. Immunoreactivity of α-melanocyte stimulating hormone, adrenocorticotropic hormone, and β-endorphin in cutaneous malignant melanoma and benign melanocytic naevi. Br. J. Dermatol. **138:** 981–985.
16. SCHAUER, E., F. TRAUTINGER *et al.* 1994. Proopiomelanocortin-derived peptides are synthesized and released by human keratinocytes. J. Clin. Invest. **93:** 2258–2262.
17. CHAKRABORTY, A.K., Y. FUNASAKA *et al.* 1996. Production and release of proopiomelanocortin (POMC) derived peptides by human melanocytes and keratinocytes in culture: regulation by UVB. Biochim. Biophys. Acta **1313:** 130–138.
18. FUNASAKA, Y., A.K. CHAKRABORTY *et al.* 1998. Modulation of melanocyte stimulating hormone receptor expression on normal human melanocytes: evidence for a regulatory role of UVB, IL-1α, IL-1β, ET-1, and TNF-α. Br. J. Dermatol. **139:** 216–224.
19. KARALIS, K., H. SANO *et al.* 1991. Autocrine or paracrine inflammatory actions of corticotropin-releasing hormone *in vivo*. Science **254:** 421–423.
20. ARBISER, J.L., K. KARALIS *et al.* 1998. Corticotropin releasing hormone is a proangiogenic cytokine. (Abstract). J. Dermatol. Sci. **16:** S46.

Depression Modulates Pruritus Perception

A Study of Pruritus in Psoriasis, Atopic Dermatitis and Chronic Idiopathic Urticaria[a]

MADHULIKA A. GUPTA[b,c] AND ADITYA K. GUPTA[d]

[c]Department of Psychiatry, University of Western Ontario, 490 Wonderland Road South, Suite 6, London, Ontario, Canada N6K 1L6

[d]Division of Dermatology, Department of Medicine, University of Toronto, Toronto, Ontario, Canada

BACKGROUND

Pruritus is defined as a sensation that provokes the desire to scratch and it is reported to be the most common symptom of dermatologic disease. Pruritus has been associated with a wide range of psychopathology, including depression and suicide. We examined the relation between pruritus and depression among pruritic skin disorders—psoriasis, atopic dermatitis, and chronic idiopathic urticaria—that are also known to have a psychosomatic component. That is, psychological stress has been known to exacerbate the course of these disorders. Furthermore, "psychoneuroimmunologic" factors have also been implicated in the mediation of the psychosomatic response.

METHODS

296 consecutive consenting dermatology outpatients (97 men and 155 women; 77 with psoriasis, 143 with atopic dermatitis, 32 with chronic idiopathic urticaria; mean age ± SD, 49.1 ± 14.6 years) consented to participate in the study. Since pruritus is primarily a subjective symptom, the patients self-rated the severity of their pruritus on a 10-point scale (a rating of '0' denoted *not at all* and a rating of '9' denoted *very marked*) by responding to the following question: "How much is your rash itching at the present time?" Depression was measured using the Carroll rating scale for depression (CRSD) (Carroll *et al.*, 1981)—a 52-item self-rated instrument that is used to screen for the clinical depressive syndrome. A score of 10 on the CRSD is considered to be the cutoff-point in screening for clinical depression.

[a]Presentation abstracted from Gupta, M.A., A.K. Gupta, N.J. Schork, and C.N. Ellis. *Psychosomatic Medicine,* **56:** 36–40, 1994.

[b]Address for correspondence: 519-657-4222 (voice); 519-657-9238 (fax); magupta@julian.uwo.ca (e-mail).

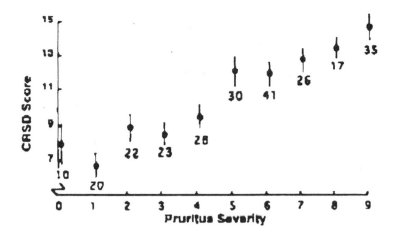

FIGURE 1. Relation between pruritus and depression.

Statistical Analysis

Because of the ordinal nature of our measure for pruritus severity, both Pearson product-moment correlations and Spearman rank-order correlations were used to examine the relation between pruritus severity and CRSD scores among all subjects.

RESULTS

The correlations obtained between pruritus severity, rated on the 10-point scale, and the depression (CRSD) score were as follows: Pearson $r = 0.34$, $p = 0.0006$, and Spearmans $\rho = 0.32$, $r < 0.005$. FIGURE 1 shows the relation between pruritus and depression (CRSD) scores over the three diagnostic groups. The plot shows the mean and standard error of the CRSD score for each level of pruritus observed with our data. The number above each pruritus severity rating indicates the number of subjects with that pruritus rating value.

COMMENT

We have observed a direct correlation between pruritus severity and depression (CRSD) scores among a range of pruritic skin disorders. The depressive state may be a primary feature of the skin disorder, or it may be secondary to the disorder. It is possible that the depressed clinical state, which has been associated with elevated levels of corticotropin-releasing factor, amplifies itch perception by increasing central nervous opiate levels.

α-MSH Immunomodulation Acts via Rel/NF-κB in Cutaneous and Ocular Melanocytes and in Melanoma Cells

J.W. HAYCOCK,[a] M. WAGNER,[a] R. MORANDINI,[b] G. GHANEM,[b]
I.G. RENNIE,[c] AND S. MACNEIL[a]

[a]University Division of Clinical Sciences, Section of Medicine, Clinical Sciences Centre, Northern General Hospital, Sheffield, S5 7AU, United Kingdom

[b]Laboratory of Oncology and Experimental Surgery (LOCE), Institut Bordet, Université Libre de Bruxelles, Rue Heger Bordet-1, B-1000 Brussels, Belgium.

[c]University Department of Ophthalmology and Orthoptics, Royal Hallamshire Hospital, Sheffield, S10 2JF, United Kingdom

INTRODUCTION

Alpha-melanocyte stimulating hormone (α-MSH) is a 13-amino-acid peptide that has a recognized role in pigmentation. However, recent reports also suggest roles in the modulation of host fever, inflammation, and immune system responses, that proceed by inhibiting the production/action of proinflammatory cytokines, or by increasing the synthesis of antiinflammatory cytokines.[1] α-MSH production is widespread and includes the pituitary gland, melanocytes, keratinocytes, and melanoma tumors. Levels are also known to increase locally when skin is exposed to UV (a stimulus that also increases local cytokine production). We previously reported on work from our own group, to show that α-MSH inhibits cytokine upregulation of intercellular adhesion molecule-1 (ICAM-1) in melanocytes and melanoma cells.[2] Cytokines mediate inflammatory responses largely through activation of transcription factors, in particular NF-κB (present in a wide range of cell types). In turn, NF-κB controls expression of many genes related to inflammation. We therefore investigated the ability of α-MSH to prevent cytokine activation of NF-κB in melanocytes and melanoma cells.

METHODS

Human uveal melanocytes[3] and melanoma tumor cells,[3] A-375SM,[4] and HBL[2] human-cutaneous melanoma cell-lines were obtained and cultured as described previously. Cells were grown to 60% confluence and the medium was changed 18 hours prior to experimentation. Effectors were added at appropriate dosages/times (α-MSH, tumor necrosis factor-α [TNF-α]) and terminated by medium removal and washing (PBS × 2). Cells were processed for nuclear extraction, and extracts mea-

[a]Address for correspondence: + 44 114 2714007 (voice); + 44 114 2560458 (fax); J.W.Haycock@Sheffield.ac.uk (e-mail).

sured for NF-κB by electrophoretic mobility shift assay (EMSA). Scanning densitometry of the resulting autoradiographs under comparative conditions allowed the measurement of relative NF-κB activity.

RESULTS

No constitutive NF-κB activity was detected for any cell types studied, as determined by EMSA. However, acute addition of the proinflammatory cytokine, TNF-α (200 U/ml), showed acute increases in DNA-binding activity. A maximum relative increase in activity was observed after two hours incubation for all cell types. Coincubation of cells with TNF-α (200 U/ml) and α-MSH (10^{-9} M) decreased the level of NF-κB binding activity, when compared with cytokine (alone)-stimulated values under identical conditions. TABLE I shows relative activity changes and FIGURE 1 shows typical results obtained by EMSA analysis. The largest inhibitory effect of α-MSH was after two hours incubation for all cell types. However, HBL cells displayed a particularly large decrease in relative binding activity after only one hour incubation. It was of note that the level of NF-κB activity was not affected by incubating the cells with α-MSH alone for between one and three hours.

DISCUSSION

A number of studies demonstrate α-MSH to have potent antipyretic and antiinflammatory activities. Although it is known that these properties are mediated by a

TABLE 1. Inhibitory action of α-MSH on TNF-α stimulated NF-κB activity[a]

| | Relative NF-κB activity in presence of α-MSH (compared with cytokine-alone stimulation) | | |
| | Cells treated with TNF-α (200 U/ml) + α-MSH (1×10^{-9} M) | | |
Cell type	1 hour	2 hours	3 hours
Ocular melanocytes	0.53 ± 0.05* (*n* = 3)	0.53 ± 0.05* (*n* = 3)	nd
Ocular melanoma tumor cells	0.63 ± 0.06* (*n* = 4)	0.53 ± 0.10* (*n* = 4)	0.87 ± 0.18* (*n* = 3)
A-375SM (cutaneous melanoma cell line)	0.56 ± 0.07* (*n* = 9)	0.28 ± 0.04** (*n* = 3)	0.60 ± 0.14 (*n* = 3)
HBL (cutaneous melanoma cell line)	0.19 ± 0.07*** (*n* = 7)	nd	nd

[a]Values shown are relative NF-κB activity (mean values ± SEM) seen in the presence of α-MSH plus TNF-α, compared to that seen with TNF-α alone.

* $p < 0.05$; ** $p < 0.01$; *** $p < 0.001$; as determined by Wilcoxon nonparametric analysis.

Number of experimental repetitions indicated in parentheses below each data entry; nd, not determined.

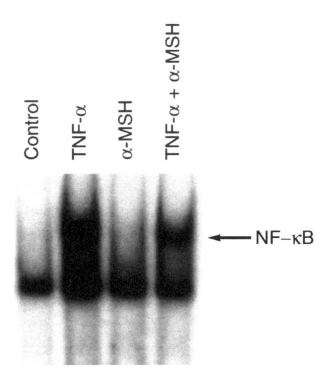

FIGURE 1. Typical results showing A375-SM (passage 30) cutaneous melanoma cells stimulated with TNF-α (200 U/ml) alone or in combination with α-MSH (1×10^{-9} M) or untreated (*control*) for one hour. Nuclear extracts were incubated with labelled oligonucleotide probe containing the NF-κB binding site. Autoradiograph obtained following electrophoretic mobility shift assay (4% acrylamide) is shown. *Arrow* indicates position of NF-κB p50/p65 specific band.

decrease in the production/action of proinflammatory cytokines or an elevation of antiinflammatory cytokines, the intracellular mechanism of action is not known.[1] α-MSH is known to be produced by melanocytes and keratinocytes, but also by melanoma tumors. UV-irradiation of skin causes local α-MSH production, together with cytokine release. One consequence of cytokine action is an increased expression of cell surface ICAM-1 necessary for T-lymphocyte interaction. Our previous work demonstrated that in melanocytes and melanoma cells α-MSH can reduce the level of TNF-α stimulated ICAM-1 expression.[2] We demonstrate, for the first time in melanocytes, ocular melanoma cells, and in two cutaneous melanoma cell lines that α-MSH can oppose the action of TNF-α stimulated NF-κB activity. Changes in activity of this transcription factor would be expected to lead to alterations in expression of several genes, but in particular those concerned with inflammation, cell migration, cellular repair, and activation of immune cells.[5] We suggest that the presence of an α-MSH–mediated paracrine/autocrine mechanism in melanocytes may assist these cells to resist a local inflammatory reaction. For melanoma cells, such a mechanism may facilitate successful transformation/metastasis by preventing immune cell recognition.

REFERENCES

1. LIPTON, J.M. & A. CATANIA. 1997. Anti-inflammatory actions of the neuroimmuno-modulator α-MSH. Immunol. Today **18:** 140–145.
2. MORANDIDI, R., J.M. BOEYNAMS *et al.* 1998. Modulation of ICAM-1 expression by α-MSH in human melanoma cells and melanocytes. J. Cell Physiol. **175:** 276–282.
3. GOODALL, T., J.A. BUFFEY *et al.* 1994. Effect of melanocyte stimulating hormone on human cultured choroidal melanocytes, uveal melanoma cells and retinal epithelial cells. Invest. Ophth. Vis. Sci. **35:** 826–837.
4. DEWHURST, L.O., J.W. GEE *et al.* 1997. Tamoxifen, 17β-oestradiol and the calmodulin antagonist J8 inhibit human melanoma cell invasion through fibronectin. Br. J. Cancer **75:** 860–868.
5. GHOSH, S., M.J. MAY *et al.* 1998. NF-κB and Rel proteins: Evolutionary conserved mediators of immune response. Annu. Rev. Immunol. **16:** 225–260.

Microinjection of Alpha-MSH Followed by UV-Irradiation Blocks HSP 72 in Human Keratinocytes

BJÖRN HELD,[a] SUSANNE AMATO, ERNST G. JUNG, AND CHRISTIANE BAYERL

Department of Dermatology, Klinikum Mannheim gGmbH, University Clinic, Faculty for Clinical Medicine Mannheim of the University of Heidelberg, Mannheim, Germany

INTRODUCTION

The aim of this study was to investigate the interaction of alpha-melanocyte-stimulating hormone (α-MSH) and heat shock protein 72 (HSP 72) in human keratinocytes in order to learn about the link between the neuroimmunocutaneus system and UV-induced immunomodulation.[1–3] α-MSH, a proopiomelanocortin (POMC) derived neuropeptide,[4] is produced in human keratinocytes[5,6] as well as in normal and pathologic human skin.[7] It is upregulated by UV-irradiation,[8] and it is a potent mediator of inflammation[9,10] and immune response.[3,11] HSP 72, a chaperoning protein that has protective properties on cells,[12,13] is upregulated by environmental stresses such as heat, UV-irradiation, drugs, and chemicals.[12,14] Orel *et al.,*[13] showed that there are inverse interactions between α-MSH and HSP 72 in the HaCat cell line. Therefore, we microinjected α-MSH into primary human keratinocytes in culture so as to study changes in HSP 72 at the protein level.

METHODS

Primary human keratinocytes were seeded on eight coverslips with an alphabetic micro-raster in Petri dishes, and were grown to 70% confluency. Using a semiautomatic micromanipulator/injector (Eppendorf, Hamburg, Germany), defined areas on the coverslips were microinjected either with PBS or with a secondary irrelevant antibody (donkey anti goat IgG, nr. 28223, Jackson ImmunoResearch, West Grove, USA) or α-MSH (Research Biochemicals Int., Natick, USA). Ninety minutes after incubation, UV-irradiation was performed with a solar simulator (300W, UVA = 0.0012 W/cm^2, UVB = 0.00135 W/cm^2, Oriel instruments, USA) for 60 sec. Controls were similarly injected, but not irradiated. Cell survival was estimated by a keratinocyte count before and six hours after microinjection/irradiation. Cell growth was stopped six hours after microinjection/irradiation in 50:50 ethanol/acetone. Qualitative immunohistochemical characterization of HSP 72 was performed by im-

[a]Address for correspondence: Björn Held, Klinikum Mannheim gGmbH, Hautklinik, Theodor-Kutzer-Ufer 3, 68135 Mannheim, Germany. 0621-383-2280 (voice); 0621-383-3815 (fax); christiane.bayerl@haut.ma.uni-heidelberg.de (e-mail).

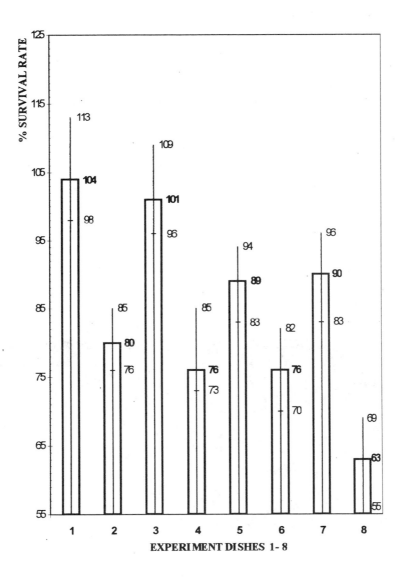

FIGURE 1. Cell survival rate of keratinocytes by morphological aspects six hours after UV-irradiation. The experiments were performed in eight groups: **1.** Control, not injected and not irradiated. **2.** Not injected, UV-irradiated. **3.** Control, injected with PBS, not irradiated. **4.** Injected with PBS, UV-irradiated. **5.** Control, injected with donkey antigoat IgG, not irradiated. **6.** Injected with donkey antigoat IgG, UV-irradiated. **7.** Control, injected with α-MSH, not irradiated. **8.** Injected with α-MSH, UV-irradiated. Cell survival rate shows the relation of cells before and 6 h after microinjection/irradiation. Each experiment was performed three times. The results are expressed as highest, average, and lowest values.

munofluorescence (IF) and immunoperoxidase (IP) staining, using a monoclonal antibody to HSP 72 (clone W27, Oncogen research products, Oxford, England).

RESULTS

FIGURE 1 shows the cell survival rates of keratinocytes. The cell survival rate in nonirradiated samples was: (1) 104% for uninjected and (3) 101% for cells injected with PBS. Cells injected with donkey anti-goat IgG (5) reached a survival rate of 89%. UV-irradiated samples showed (2) 80% for noninjected cells, (4) 76% for keratinocytes, injected with PBS, and (6) 76% for cells injected with donkey anti-goat IgG. Keratinocytes injected with α-MSH, (7) without irradiation reached a survival rate of 90%, whereas cells injected with 'α-MSH and additional irradiation (8) reached only 63%, indicating an evident decrease in cell survival. Immunohistochemical labeling for HSP 72 showed cytoplasmic staining in few cells (FIG. 1.1), accentuated for keratinocytes in mitosis. Strong labeling was achieved in irradiated controls (FIG. 1.2) indicating a UV-induced increase of HSP 72. In keratinocytes injected with PBS (FIG. 1.3 and 1.4) and donkey anti-goat IgG (FIG. 1.5 and 1.6), and in cells injected with α-MSH without irradiation (FIG. 1.7), the immunohistochem-

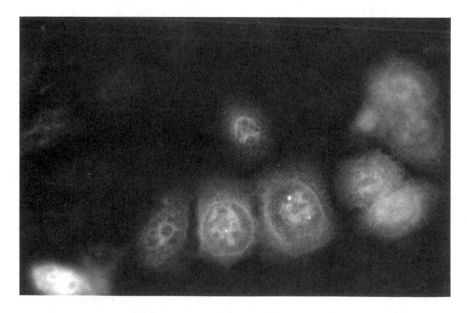

FIGURE 2. Immunofluorescence of human keratinocytes in culture, microinjection of α-MSH and UV irradiation, labeling with an antibody against HSP 72 (630x). Cells injected with α-MSH and UV-irradiation showed no labeling (*left* and *upper side*), whereas uninjected cells adjacent to the defined injection area (*right side* and *bottom*) showed bright cytoplasmic and nuclear fluorescence for HSP 72.

ical labeling for HSP 72 was not increased. In contrast, cells injected with α-MSH and additional UV-irradiation showed no IF for HSP 72 (see FIGURE 2), and only in some cells IP labeling for HSP 72 (FIG. 1.8).

DISCUSSION

Differentiation-driven HSP 72 expression in HaCat cells is downregulated by α-MSH.[12] On the protein level we were able to show that UV-induced upregulation of HSP 72 in human keratinocytes is antagonized by microinjection of α-MSH, whereas injection of PBS or donkey anti-goat IgG did not influence the expression of HSP 72. This protein is well known to be UV-protective.[12,13] Our data indicate that cells injected with α-MSH exhibit decreased survival after UV damage. Thus, after UV-irradiation, microinjected α-MSH weakens the UV-protective properties of human keratinocytes. This data may provide additional evidence for a link between α-MSH and HSP 72.

REFERENCES

1. MISERY, L. 1997. Skin, immunity and the nervous system. Br. J. Dermatol. **137:** 843–850.

2. SCHOLZEN, T., C.A. ARMSTRONG, N.W. BUNNETT, T.A. LUGER, J.E. OLERUD & J.C. ANSEL. 1998. Neuropeptides in the skin: interactions between the neuroendocrine and the skin immune system. Exp. Dermatol. **7:** 81–96.

3. LUGER, T.A., R.S. BHARDWAJ, S. GRABBE & T. SCHWARZ. 1996. Regulation of the immune response by epidermal cytokines and neurohormones. J. Dermatol. Sci. **13:** 5–10.

4. LOTTI, T., G. HAUTMANN & E. PANCONESI. 1995. Neuropeptides in skin. J. Am. Acad. Dermatol. **33:** 482–496.

5. KIPPENBERGER, S., A. BERND, S. RAMIREZ-LOITSCH, A. BOSCA, J. BREITER-HAHN & H. HOLZMANN. 1995. Alpha-MSH is expressed in cultured human melanocytes and keratinocytes. Eur. J. Dermatol. **5:** 395–397.

6. BHARDWAJ, R.S. & T.A. LUGER. 1994. Proopiomelanocortin production by epidermal cells: evidence for an immune neuroendocrine network in the epidermis. Arch. Dermatol. Res. **287:** 85–90.

7. SLOMINSKI, A., J. WORTSMAN, J.E. MAZURKIEWICZ, L. MATSUOKA, J. DIETRICH, K. LAWRENCE, A. GORBANI & R. PAUS. 1993. Detection of proopiomelanocortin-derived antigens in normal and pathologic human skin. J. Lab. Clin. Med. **122:** 658–666.

8. CHAKRABORTY, A.K., Y. FUNASAKA, A. SLOMINSKI, G. ERMAK, J. HWANG, J.M. PAWELEK & M. ICHIHASHI. 1996. Production and release of proopiomelanocortin (POMC) derived peptides by human melanocytes and keratinocytes in culture: regulation by ultraviolet B. Biochem. Biophys. Acta **1313:** 130–138.

9. LIPTON, J.M. & A. CATANIA. 1997. Anti-inflammatory actions of the neuroimmunomodulator alpha-MSH. Immunol. Today **18:** 140–145.

10. LUGER, T.A., T. SCHOLZEN & S. GRABBE. 1997. The role of alpha-melanocyte-stimulating hormone in cutaneous biology. J. Inv. Dermatol. Symp. Proc. **2:** 87–93.

11. LUGER, T.A. 1998. Immunomodulation by UV light: role of neuropeptides. Eur. J. Dermatol. **8:** 198–199.

12. OREL, L., M.M. SIMON, J. KARLSEDER, R. BHARDWAJ, F. TRAUTINGER, T. SCHWARZ & T.A. LUGER. 1997. Alpha-melanocyte stimulating hormone downregulates differentiation-driven heat shock protein 70 expression in keratinocytes. J. Inv. Dermatol. **108:** 401–405.

13. TRAUTINGER, F., I. KINDAS-MÜGGE, B. BARLAN, P. NEUNER & R.M. KNOBLER. 1995. 72-kD heat shock protein is a mediator of resistance to ultraviolet B light. J. Inv. Dermatol. **105:** 160–162.

14. BAYERL, C., J. LAUK, I. MOLL & E.G. JUNG. 1997. Immunohistochemical characterization of HSP, alpha-MSH, Merkel cells and neuronal markers in acute UV dermatitis and acute contact dermatitis *in vivo*. Inflamm. Res. **46:** 409–411.

β-Endorphin Binding and Regulation of Cytokine Expression in Langerhans Cells

JUNICHI HOSOI,[a] HIROAKI OZAWA,[b] AND RICHARD D. GRANSTEIN[b]

[a]*Shiseido Life Science Research Center, Fukuura, Kanazawa, Yokohama, Japan*

[b]*Department of Dermatology, Cornell University Medical College, New York, USA*

INTRODUCTION

The human body responds to environmental and psychological stressors. Nervous system, immune system, and endocrine system all mediate the reaction. Several immune functions of the body, including NK cell activity and CD4/CD8 ratio, are regulated by stress (see Ref. 1 for a review). Skin is one of the target organs of the stress reaction. Regulation of skin functions by stress was found in our laboratory by using animal models. Proliferation of epidermal keratinocytes was suppressed and epidermis became thinner,[2] recovery of the barrier function was delayed,[3] and activity of sebaceous gland was downregulated.[4] Phenotypic change of epidermal Langerhans cells (LC) and suppression of contact hypersensitivity were also induced.[5] These results suggest a connection between CNS and skin.

The anatomical and functional association found between nervous system and immune system provided evidence for the connection between CNS and skin. Intimate association of nerve fibers with epidermal LC was observed by confocal laser scanning microscopy and electron microscopy.[6] The antigen-presenting activity of LC was suppressed by the neuropeptide, calcitonin gene-related peptide, *in vitro*[6] and *in vivo*.[7] On the other hand, dendrite formation of PC12 cells were induced by factors secreted from LC.[8] These findings demonstrate the bidirectional interaction between the nervous and immune systems in skin.

Various hormones are secreted after exposure to stress, including ACTH, cortisol, and adrenaline. β-Endorphin (β-end) is also induced by stress in animals[9,10] and humans.[11,12] β-End is a 31-amino-acid opioid synthesized in the arcuate nucleus that inhibits several central nervous system functions. In the periphery, endorphin is synthesized in the intermediate pituitary or its vestigia.

Immunocytes also synthesize β-end,[1] and regulation of immune system by β-end has been also reported. Natural cytotoxicity was stimulated by β-end.[13] In patients with organ-specific autoimmune diseases β-end concentration is decreased[1] and the cytokine pattern of T-helper cells is shifted to Th1-type in these patients.

In this article the effects of β-end on epidermal LC are examined. We report binding of β-end and its regulation of cytokine expression in LC.

[a]Address for correspondence: Junichi Hosoi, Shiseido Research Center, 2-12-1 Fukuura, Kanazawa, Yokohama 236-8643, Japan. 81-45-788-7291 (voice); 81-45-788-7277 (fax); hosoi_junichi@po.shiseido.co.jp (e-mail).

MATERIALS AND METHODS

Cell Culture

A dendritic cell line (XS52)[14] established from newborn BALB/c epidermis was propagated in a RPMI medium containing 10% FCS, 10 U/ml recombinant murine GM-CSF (Biosource Intl, Camerrillo, CA), and NS cell supernatants.[14] This cell line is dendritic, presents antigen, and has many phenotypic characteristics of freshly-harvested LC.[15] These cells were cultured in RPMI, without any supplement, for one day before experiments were performed.

Isolation of Fresh Epidermal LC

Epidermal LC were purified from BALB/c epidermis as described previously.[16] Briefly, epidermal cells were prepared and Thy-1$^+$ cells were deleted. These cells were incubated with mouse anti-I-A^d (PharMingen) for 30 min on ice, followed by incubation with goat antimouse IgG conjugated to magnetic microspheres (Dynabeads M-450; Dynal, Oslo) for 30 min on ice with continuous gentle shaking. I-A positive cells were collected after washing out cells unbound to the beads, by holding the beads with magnetic spheres. Flow cytometry demonstrated that more than 90% of the cells obtained were I-A positive.

Binding Assay

XS52 cells were cultured for 24 hours in serum free RPMI with a combination of 50 U/ml GM-CSF and 1 µg/ml LPS. Cells were harvested with a scraper and washed once with cold PBS. 500,000 cells were resuspended in 200 µl of RPMI/1% BSA. After addition of biotin-labeled β-end (Penninsula Lab., Belmont, CA) at final concentration of 10 nM, the cells were incubated for 1 h at 4°C, washed twice with PBS, and incubated in RPMI/1% BSA containing 40 µg/ml FITC-labeled streptavidin for 30 min at 4°C, followed by washing with PBS. Cells were then resuspended in PBS and analyzed with a flow cytometer (FACScan; Becton Dickinson). Dead cells were excluded by positivity of propidium iodide. Cells for negative control were incubated without biotin-labeled β-end, but with FITC-labeled streptavidin. For competition assays, 1 µM unlabeled β-end, or 1 µM unlabeled substance P, was added to the incubation with biotinylated β-end.

ELISA

XS52 cells (2×10^5/120 µl) were cultured for 24 hours in RPMI without any supplement, and for the next 24 hours in RPMI containing 10 nM β-end and/or a combination of 50 U/ml GM-CSF and 1 µg/ml LPS, or diluent alone. Culture supernatants were collected and subjected to ELISA (IL-1β and TNFα; Endogen, Boston, MA, IL-10; Biosource, Camarillo, CA).

RT-PCR

Freshly isolated epidermal LC (1×10^5 cells) were cultured for 24 hours in RPMI containing 10 nM β-end and/or a combination of 50 U/ml GM CSF and 1 µg/ml LPS, or in diluent alone. Then poly-A$^+$ RNA was extracted from these cells (Micro-FastTrack kit; Invitrogen, Carlsbad, CA) following the procedure of Bost et al.,[17] with slight modification. Briefly, cDNA was synthesized with random primers (RT-

PCR kit; Perkin Elmer Cetus) and amplified for glyceraldehyde-3-dehydrogenase (GAPDH), IL-1β, IL-10, and TNFα (26 cycles for GAPDH and 35 cycles for cytokine of denature for 60 sec at 95°C, annealing for 60 sec at 60°C, and extension for 60 sec at 72°C). Primers for GAPDH and IL-1β were synthesized as published previously,[18] and according to Bost *et al.,* for IL-10 and TNFα.[17]

Flow Cytometry for I-A

XS52 cells ($2 \times 10^5/120$ µl) were cultured for 24 hours in RPMI without any supplement, and for the next 24 hours in RPMI containing 10 nM β-end or in diluent alone. Cells were harvested and incubated in FITC-labeled antiI-A^d antibody (1:50; Pharmingen) for one hour on ice in the dark. After washing, cells were analyzed by FACScan. Dead cells were excluded by positivity of propidium iodide.

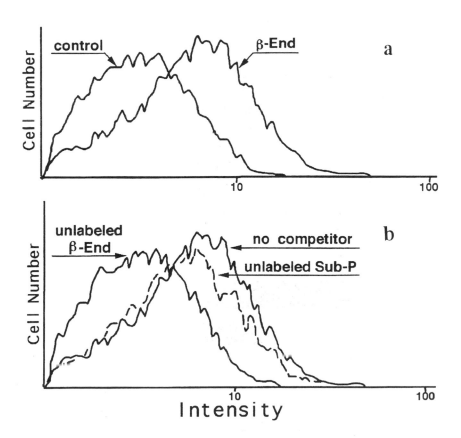

FIGURE 1. Specific binding of biotinylated β-end. **a.** XS52 cells were incubated with or without biotinylated β-end, washed, and then incubated with streptavidine-FITC. The cells were analyzed by flow cytometry. **b.** XS52 cells were incubated with 10 nM biotinylated β–end in the presence or absence of 1 µM intact β–end or substance P. The cells were washed, incubated with streptavidine-FITC, and were then subjected to flow cytometry.

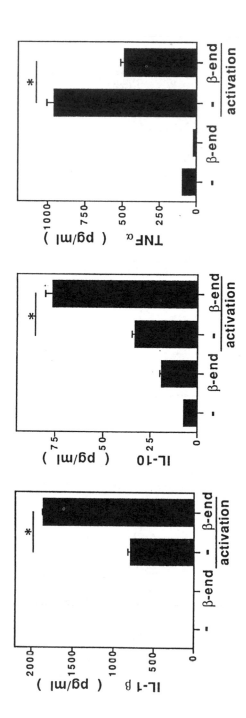

FIGURE 2. Regulation of cytokine secretion by β–end. After culturing XS52 cells for 24 h in the presence of 10 nM β–end and/or combination of 1 μg/ml LPS and 50 U/ml GM-CSF, the culture supernatants were collected and assayed for cytokines. *Bars*, SD; * $p < 0.01$.

RESULTS

Receptors for β-End

To detect the receptor for β-end on XS52 cells, a binding assay was performed by analysis with FACScan. Biotinylated β-end bound to stimulated XS52 cells by combination of LPS and GM-CSF (see FIGURE 1a). The peak was significantly shifted from the peak of control cells that were incubated with only avidine-FITC. The specificity was examined by competition assay. When cells were incubated with biotinylated β-end in the presence of unlabeled β-end, the binding was abrogated (FIG. 1b). However, there was only slight change in the presence of unlabeled substance P—a control peptide. These results suggest that LC have specific receptors for β-end on their surface.

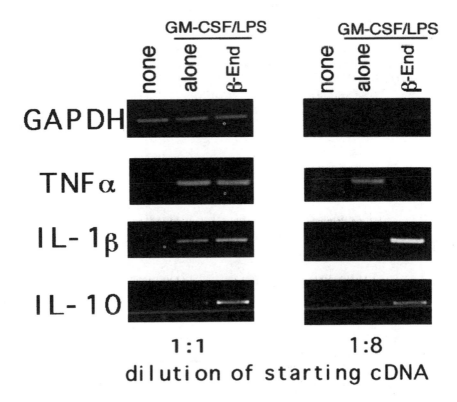

FIGURE 3. Regulation of cytokine expression in fresh LC. Freshly prepared murine epidermal LC were cultured for 24 h in the presence of 10 nM β–end and/or combination of 1 μg/ml LPS and 50 U/ml GM-CSF. Poly-A$^+$ RNA was extracted from those cells and subjected to RT-PCR.

Regulation of Cytokine Expression

Response of LC to β-end was examined by assays for cytokine expression. Culture supernatant of XS52 cells were collected and assayed for IL-1β, IL-10, and TNFα (see FIGURE 2). When XS52 cells were activated with a combination of GM-CSF and LPS, these cells were induced to secrete the cytokines into culture medium. The induction of IL-1β and IL-10 was augmented and the induction of TNFα was inhibited by β-end.

The regulation of cytokine expression in LC by β-end was confirmed in freshly purified LC by RT-PCR. When the initial RNA was diluted, the amount of amplified GAPDH products decreased (see FIGURE 3), demonstrating that the amount of the product depends on the amount of the message. After activation of LC with GM-CSF/LPS, expression of IL-1β, IL-10, and TNFα was induced. The induction of IL-1β and IL-10 was enhanced in the presence of β-end, whereas the induction of TNFα was suppressed in fresh LC. These results suggest that LC in the epidermis may be regulated by β-end.

Enhancement of Expression of I-A Molecules on XS52 Cells

The effect of β-end on expression of I-A was examined by flow cytometry. The results are shown in FIGURE 4. The fluorescence intensity derived from FITC conjugated antiI-A antibodies was stronger on XS52 cells cultured with β-end for 24 hours, suggesting that β-end enhances the expression of I-A molecules in LC.

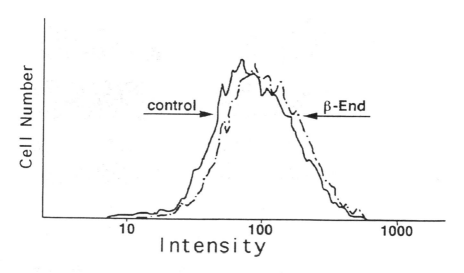

FIGURE 4. Enhancement of I-A expression by β–end. XS52 cells were cultured in the presence or absence of 10 nM β–end for 24 h and analyzed for I-A expression by flow cytometry.

DISCUSSION

β-End receptors on murine peritoneal macrophages were characterized by Woods et al.[19] Functional regulation of macrophages by β-end was also reported. β-End stimulates production of super oxide[20] and enhances phagocytosis.[21] LPS-induced release of IL-1 was potentiated by β-end.[22]

β-End bound to LC, and the binding was replaced by excess of cold β-end. These results suggest functional regulation by β-end. LPS-induced cytokine expression in LC, examined by ELISA and by RT-PCR, was regulated by β-end. IL-1β, IL-10, and TNFα are immunomodulators. IL-1β stimulates and IL-10 inhibits LC functions.[23,24] β-end may possibly regulate LC function by modulation of expression of these cytokines. Slight enhancement of expression of MHC class-II I-A molecule suggests that there is stimulatory activity of β-end.

Furthermore, regulation of proliferation of epidermal keratinocytes was also reported. IL-1β enhanced secretion of plasminogen activator, which is one of the keratinocyte proliferation cascades.[25] On the other hand, Maurer et al., reported inhibition of proliferation of mouse keratinocytes by TNFα.[26] A model implicating LC in keratinocyte proliferation control was hypothesized by Potten and Allen.[27] Epidermal keratinocytes may be regulated by β-end–induced modification of cytokine expression.

Higher concentration of β-end in serum was determined in patients with atopic dermatitis[28,29] and psoriasis[29] in comparison with healthy subjects. Glinski et al., suggested that the source of β-end is inflammatory cells at the lesion.[29] Secreted β-end may possibly regulate functions of immune cells, including LC and keratinocytes.

We have found a connection between nervous system and immune system in skin. Anatomical analysis revealed intimate association of nerve fibers with LC.[6] By functional analyses, regulation of antigen presenting function of LC by neuropeptides was found in vitro[6] and in vivo.[7] Regulation of nerve cell dendrite formation by LC-derived factors was also found.[8] Recently production of proopiomelanocortin in skin and regulation of melanocytes and LC by its product, especially αMSH, have been studied (see Ref. 30 for a review). Our work has demonstrated that β-end, either from central or local sources, modulates skin immune function.

Skin functions are regulated by nervous system, immune system, and endocrine system, which interact with each other. The importance of studying the regulatory system was advocated by O'Sullivan et al.[31] They call the regulatory system the "NICE" system, named for neuro-immuno-cutaneous endocrine system.

SUMMARY

Neuropeptides and neurohormones have been shown to be able to regulate cutaneous immune reactions. Binding of β-endorphin (β-end) on epidermal Langerhans cells (LC) and effects of β-end on cytokine expression were examined. Biotinylated β-end bound to the mouse LC-like cell line, XS52, and the binding was replaced with intact β-end but not with substance P. β-End augmented secretion of IL-1β and IL-10 from XS52 cells were induced by a combination of LPS and GM-CSF. Induction of TNFα was suppressed by β-end. The regulation of cytokine expression was confirmed in fresh LC by RT-PCR. These results suggest that β-end is a regulator of skin immune function.

REFERENCES

1. PENERAI, A.E. & P. SACERDOTE. 1997. β-endorphin in the immune system: a role at last? Immunol. Today **18:** 317–319.
2. TSUCHIYA, T. & I. HORII. 1996. Epidermal cell proliferating activity assessed by proliferating cell unclear antigen (PCNA) decreases following immobilization-induced stress in male syrian hamsters. Psychoneuroendocrinology **21:** 111–117.
3. DENDA, M., T. TSUCHIYA, J. HOSOI & J. KOYAMA. 1998. Immobilization-induced and crowded environment-induced stress delay barrier recovery in murine skin. Br. J. Dermatol. **138:** 780–785.
4. TSUCHIYA, T. & I. HORII. 1995. Immobilization-induced stress decreases lipogenesis in sebaceous gland as well as plasma testosterone levels in male Syrian hamsters. Psychoneuroendocrinology **20:** 221–230.
5. HOSOI, J., T. TSUCHIYA, M. DENDA, Y. ASHIDA, A. TAKASHIMA, R.D. GRANSTEIN & J. KOYAMA. 1998. Modification of LC phenotype and suppression of contact hypersensitivity response by stress. J. Cutaneous Med. Surgery **3:** 79–84.
6. HOSOI, J., G.F. MURPHY, C.L. EGAN, E.A. LERNER, S. GRABBE, A. ASAHINA & R.D. GRANSTEIN. 1993. Regulation of Langerhans cell function by nerves containing calcitonin gene-related peptide. Nature **363:** 159–163.
7. ASAHINA, A., J. HOSOI, S. BEISSRET, A. STRATIGOS & R.D. GRANSTEIN. 1995. Inhibition of the induction of delayed-type and CH by calcitonin gene-related peptide. J. Immunol. **154:** 3056–3061.
8. TORII, H., Z. YAN, J. HOSOI & R.D. GRANSTEIN. 1997. Expression of neurotrophic factors and neuropeptide receptors by Langerhans cell-like cell line XS52: further support for a functional relationship between Langerhans cells and epidermal nerves. J. Inv. Dermatol. **109:** 586–591.
9. SHUTT, D.A., L.R. FELL, R. CONNELL, A.K. BELL, C.A. WALLACE & A.I. SMITH. 1987. Stress-induced changes in plasma concentrations of immunoreactive β-endorphin and cortisol in response to routine surgical procedures in lambs. (1987) Aust. J. Biol. Sci. **40:** 97–103.
10. ROSSIER, J., E.D. FRENCH, C. RIVER, N. LING, R. GUILLEMIN & F.E. BLOOM. 1977. Foot-shock induced increases β-endorphin levels in blood but not brain. Nature **270:** 618–620.
11. MUTTI, A., C. FERRONI, P.P. VESCOVI, R. BOTTAZZI, L. SELIS, G. GERRA & I. FRANCHINI. 1989. Endocrine effects of psychological stress associated with neurobehavioral performance testing. Life Sci. **44:** 1831–1836.
12. KELSO, T.B., W.G. HERBERT, F.C. GWAZDAUSKAS, F.L. GOSS & J.L. HESS. 1984. Exercise-thermoregulatory stress and increased plasma β–endorphin/β-lipotropin in humans. J. Appl. Physiol. **57:** 444–449.
13. MATHEWS, P.M., C.J. FROELICH, W.L. SIBBITT, JR. & A.D. BANKHURST. 1983. Enhancement of natural cytotoxicity by β–endorphin. J. Immunol. **130:** 1658–1662.
14. XU, S., K. ARIIZUMI, G. CACERES-DITTMAR, D. EDELBAUM, K. HASHIMOTO, P.R. BERGSTRESSER & A. TAKASHIMA. 1995. Successive generation of antigen-presenting, dendritic cell line from murine epidermis. J. Immunol. **154:** 2697–2705.
15. XU, S., P.R. BERGSTRESSER & A. TAKASHIMA. 1995. Phenotypic and functional heterogeneity among murine epidermal derived dendritic cell clones. J. Inv. Dermatol. **105:** 831–836.

16. GRABBE, S., S, BRUVERS, A.M. LINDGREN, J. HOSOI, K.C. TAN & R.D. GRANSTEIN. 1992. Tumor antigen presentation by epidermal antigen-presenting cells in the mouse: modulation by granulocyte-macrophage colony stimulating factor α, and ultraviolet radiation. J. Leukocyte Biol. **52:** 209–217.

17. BOST, K.L., S.C. BIELIGK & B.M. JEFFE. 1995. Lymphokine mRNA expression by transplantable murine B lymphocytic malignancies. Tumor-derived IL-10 as a possible mechanism for modulating the anti-tumor response. J. Immunol. **154:** 718–729.

18. TORII, H., J. HOSOI, S. BEISSERT, S. XU, F.E. FOX, A. ASAHINA, A. TAKASHIMA, A.H. ROOK & R.D. GRANSTEIN. 1997. Regulation of cytokine expression in macrophages and the Langerhans cell-like XS52 by calcitonin gene-related peptide. J. Leukocyte Biol. **61:** 216–223.

19. WOODS, J.A., N.A. SHAHABI & B.M. SHARP. 1997. Characterization of a naloxone-insensitive β–endorphin receptor on murine peritoneal macrophages. Life Sci. **60:** 573–586.

20. SHARP, B.M., W.F. KEANE, H.J. SUH, G. GEKKER, D. TSUKAYAMA & P.K. PETERSON. 1985. Opioid peptides rapidly stimulate superoxide production by human polymorphonuclear leukocytes and macrophages. Endocrinology **117:** 793–795.

21. ICHINOSE, M., M. ASAI & M. SAWADA. 1995. β–endorphin enhances phagocytosis of latex particles in mouse peritoneal macrophages. Scand. J. Immunol. **42:** 311–316.

22. APTE, R.N., S.K. DURUM & J.J. OPPENHEIM. 1990. Opioids modulate interleukin-1 production and secretion by bone marrow macrophages. Immuno. Lett. **42**(2): 141–148.

23. ENK, A.H. & S.I. KATZ. 1995. Contact sensitivity as a model for T-cell activation in skin. J. Invest. Dermatol. **105:** 80S–83S.

24. ARAGANE, Y., H. RIMANN, R.S. BHARDWAJ, A. SCHWARZ, Y. SAWADA, H. YAMADA, T.A. LUGER, M. KUBIN, G. TRINCHIERI & T. SCHWARZ. 1994. IL-12 is expressed and released by human keratinocytes and epidermoid carcinoma cell lines. J. Immunol. **153:** 5366–5372.

25. ROX, J.M., J. REINARTZ & M.D. KRAMER. 1996. Interleukin-1 beta upregulates tissue-type plasminogen activator in a keratinocyte cell line (HaCat). Arch. Dermatol. Res. **288**(9): 554–558.

26. DELVENNE, P., W. AL-SALEH, C. GILLES, A. THIRY & J. BONIVER. 1995. Inhibition of growth of normal and human papillomaviirus-transformed keratinocytes in monolayer and organotypic cultures by interferon-gamma and tumor necrosis factor-alpha. Am. J. Pathol. **146**(3): 589–598.

27. POTTEN, C.S. & T.D. ALLEN. 1976. A model implication the Langerhans cell keratinocyte proliferation control. Differentiation **135**(1): 43–47.

28. GLINSKI, W., H. BRODECKA, M. GLINSKA-FERENZ & D. KOWALSKI. 1995. Increased concentration of beta-endorphin in the sera of patients with severe atopic dermatitis. Acta. Derm. Venereol. **75**(1): 9–11.

29. GLINSKI, W., H. BRODECKA, M, GLINSKA-FERENZ & D, KOWALSKI. 1994. Increased concentration of beta-endorphin in sera of patients with psoriasis and other inflammatory dermatoses. Br. J. Dermatol. **131**(2): 260–264.

30. LUGER, T.A., R.S. BHARDWAJ, S. GRABBE & T. SCHWARZ. 1996. Regulation of the immune response by epidermal cytokines and neurohormones. J. Dermatol. Sci. **13**(1): 5–10.

31. O'SULLIVAN, R.L., G. LIPPER & E.A. LERNER. 1998. The neuro-immuno-cutaneous-endocrine network: relationship of mind and skin. Arch. Dermatol. **134:** 1431–1435.

α-MSH Reduces Vasculitis in the Local Shwartzman Reaction

CORD SUNDERKÖTTER,[a,b,c] H. KALDEN,[b,d] T. BRZOSKA,[d]
CLEMENS SORG,[c] AND THOMAS A. LUGER[b,d]

[b]Department of Dermatology, University of Münster, Münster, Germany

[c]Institute of Experimental Dermatology, University of Münster, Münster, Germany

[d]Ludwig Boltzmann Institute of Cell Biology and Immunobiology of the Skin,
University of Münster, Münster, Germany

INTRODUCTION

Vasculitis denotes an inflammation whose primary event is the destruction of the wall of blood vessels by leukocytes. Inflammation of small blood vessels is characterized histologically by granulocytic infiltration and damage to the vessel wall, coupled with extravasation of erythrocytes. The infiltrating granulocytes often reveal karyorrhexis, which has led to the term leukocytoclastic vasculitis (see Refs. 1 and 2 for reviews). Although in most cases small vessel vasculitis is caused by precipitated immune complexes, it is also one prominent feature in the course of the LPS-induced local Shwartzman reaction (Shw-r).[3,4] A local Shw-r consists of a local preparatory phase, initiated by local, subcutaneous injection of low-dose LPS, followed after 24 h by a challenge phase elicited by systemic application of LPS. Clinically the subsequent local reaction reveals hemorrhage and histologically it is consistent with leukocytoclastic vasculitis. The Shwartzman reaction serves as a model for the pathogenesis of septic shock. Using different mouse models, we have shown that one characteristic finding in the preparatory phase of the Shw-r is the sustained expression (>24h) of the adhesion molecules VCAM and, especially, E-selectin. These molecules were downregulated after 6 to 24 h in other acute inflammations, such as the Arthus reaction or irritant contact dermatitis. In the Shw-r, they persisted until the systemic application of LPS was given.[4] Local, as well as systemic, injection of LPS was in both cases associated with an increase of serum TNF-α.[4] Since we have also revealed that α-melanocyte-stimulating hormone (α-MSH) reduces the LPS-induced expression of adhesion molecules *in vitro*,[5] we wondered whether α-MSH would be able to reduce the local Shw-r *in vivo*.

MATERIALS AND METHODS

For the preparatory phase of the local Shw-r, 7.5 μg LPS (Sigma, Deisenhofen) were injected sc into the left ear (preparatory dose) of 12 male BALB/c mice

[a]Address for correspondence: Cord Sunderkötter, Department of Dermatology and Institute of Experimental Dermatology, University of Münster, von Esmarch Str. 56, D-48149 Münster, Germany. sunderk@uni-muenster.de (e-mail).

(Charles River, Sulzberg). For challenge 150 µg LPS were injected intraperitoneally (i.p.) 24 h later. For treatment, mice were injected with 25 µg MSH (Bachem, Heidelberg) in 100 µl PBS i.p. 3 h after eliciting the preparatory phase in the ear. Control mice received 100 µl PBS i.p. The vasculitic response of the local Shw-r was evaluated by a semiquantitative score for vascular hemorrhage (number and size of petechiae), and histologically by analysis of the infiltrate during the challenge phase. To evaluate whether α-MSH affects expression or adhesion molecules in the preparatory phase, six mice were sacrificed after 24 h, at the end of the preparatory phase. Ears were excised and one half of each ear was prepared for cryostat and paraffin sections. Immunohistochemical staining was performed according to the indirect immunoperoxidase assay (see Ref. 6 for details), using monoclonal antibodies 10E9.6 (rat IgG2a) against murine E-selectin (kindly provided by D. Vestweber, Münster), and M/K-1.9 (rat IgG1) against murine VCAM-1 (ATCC, Rockville, MD) as well as goat F(ab′)$_2$ anti-rat IgG, conjugated with peroxidase (Dianova, Hamburg) as secondary antibody. Antibodies and, for control, isotypes of rat IgG were diluted in PBS with 1% BSA (maximum concentration 1.5 µg IgG/ml). To evaluate positive vessels, sections were examined using an ocular endowed with an eyepiece graticule (×160). To compare areas of equal size, ten graticule fields were evaluated for each section. Results were presented in terms of the absolute number of positive endothelial cells (E-selectin, VCAM-1) in the defined areas. The results were expressed as arithmetic means together with standard deviation. The U-test according to Mann and Whitney was performed in order to determine significant differences. Values of $p < 0.05$ were considered to be significant.

RESULTS

After injection of LPS s.c. for the preparatory phase, ear swelling and the infiltrate were not significantly reduced in mice injected with α-MSH compared to mice injected with PBS alone. However, in the challenge phase—after systemic application of LPS—untreated mice showed several petechiae after 3 to 6 h, whereas mice treated with α-MSH in the preparatory phase revealed a marked reduction or even abolishment of vascular hemorrhage (see FIGURE 1). When we analyzed the expression of endothelial adhesion molecules at the end of the preparatory phase—prior to LPS i.p.—we found that in mice injected with α-MSH there was a significantly lower number of E-selectin-positive vessels than in control mice (see FIGURE 2). There was also a lower number of VCAM-1-positive vessels (data not shown). Thus, inhibition of the hemorrhagic response in α-MSH-treated mice was preceded by an abrogated expression of E-selectin and VCAM-1 in the preparatory phase of the local Shw-r.

DISCUSSION

Our study has shown that α-MSH is able to markedly reduce the vasculitic reaction in the local Shw-r. A single dose 3 h after initiating the preparatory phase was sufficient to modify the effects of LPS s.c., in such a way that the systemic dose of

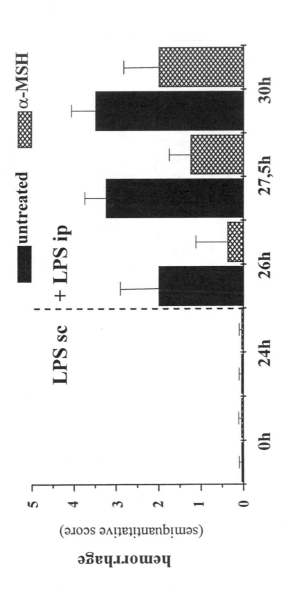

FIGURE 1. Extent of hemorrhage, given as semiquantitative score (0–5) for the number and size of hemorrhagic lesions. In ears prepared by local injection of LPS s.c., hemorrhagic lesions were induced 2 h after injecting the systemic dose of LPS i.p. The graph shows that hemorrhage is significantly reduced in mice treated with α-MSH.

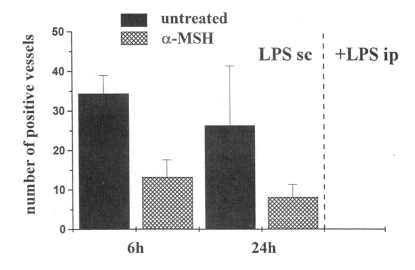

FIGURE 2. Number of vessels expressing E-selectin during the preparatory phase in ears of mice treated with α-MSH and in control mice. Mice treated with α-MSH revealed significantly fewer positive vessels than control mice, prior to eliciting the hemorrhagic reaction by LPS i.p.

LPS was curtailed in its capacity to elicit the hemorrhagic events. α-MSH exhibited similar effects when injected at the same time as the local LPS dose (data not shown). Since the inhibition was more marked when α-MSH was injected after the local administration of LPS, α-MSH appears to unfold strong activity on events already induced by LPS.

To date, the picture concerning cellular events which in the preparatory phase are responsible for the devastating effects of the succeeding systemic dose, is not complete. Our previous studies demonstrated that the sustained expression of VCAM-1 and E-selectin is one essential requirement. In rabbits ICAM-1 is another adhesion molecule involved in the pathogenesis of the Shw-r;[7] however, in the mouse ICAM-1 is expressed constitutively and, thus, its sustained expression is not unique to the Shw-r. We have suggested that the increased adhesive properties of the vascular endothelium, at the end of the preparatory phase, leads to the increased accumulation of leukocytes at the vessel wall, and perhaps to their partial activation that then assumes vessel-damaging dimensions by the systemic application of LPS.

LPS is a potent inductor of E-selectin and VCAM-1. We found that *in vitro* α-MSH was capable of inhibiting this effect, probably because it also suppressed activation of NF-κB.[5] Correspondingly, α-MSH was able to reduce adhesion of leukocytes to activated endothelial cells. Recently, the receptor specific for α-MSH (MC-1R) was found on human dermal microvascular endothelial cells and, therefore, endothelial cells may serve as a target for this peptide.[8]

This study showed that *in vivo* the application of α-MSH also resulted in a reduced expression of E-selectin and VCAM-1. We conclude, therefore, that α-MSH is able to inhibit the vasculitic response of the local Shw-r by reducing the sustained expression of endothelial adhesion molecules; thus leaving the tissue less well prepared for the challenge phase of the local Shw-r.

ACKNOWLEDGMENTS

This work was supported by Deutsche Forschungsgemeinschaft Grants DFG SO 87/11-3 Projects E and F.

REFERENCES

1. JENNETTE, J.C. & R.F. FALK. 1997. Small vessel vasculitis. N. Engl. J. Med. **337:** 1512–1523.
2. SUNDERKÖTTER, C. & G. KOLDE. 1997. Cutaneous vasculitis. *In* The Skin Immune System (SIS) Basic and Clinical Immunodermatology, 2nd ed. J. Bos, Ed.: 479–488. CRC Press, Boca Raton.
3. SHWARTZMAN, G. 1928. A new phenomenon of local skin reactivity to B. typhosus culture filtrate. Proc. Soc. Exp. Biol. Med. **25:** 560–561.
4. SUNDERKÖTTER, C., F. SCHÖNLAU, A. SCHWARZ, T. LUGER, C. SORG & G. KOLDE. 1997. Mechanisms of leukocytoclastic vasculitis. (Abstract). J. Invest. Dermatol. **108:** 332.
5. KALDEN. D.-H., M. FASTRICH, T. BRZOSKA, T. SCHOLZEN, M. HARTMEYER, T. SCHWARZ & T. LUGER. 1998. Alpha-melanocyte-stimulating hormone reduces endotoxin-induced activation of nuclear factor-kB in endothelial cells. (Abstract). J. Invest. Dermatol. **110:** 495.
6. SUNDERKÖTTER, C., W. BEIL, J. ROTH & C. SORG. 1991. Cellular events associated with inflammatory angiogenesis in the mouse cornea. Am. J. Pathol. **138:** 931–939.
7. ARGENBRIGHT, L.W. & R.W. BARTON. 1992. Interactions of leukocyte integrins with intercellular adhesion molecule 1 in the production of inflammatory vascular injury *in vivo*. The Shwartzman reaction revisited. J. Clin. Invest. **89:** 259–272.
8. HARTMEYER, M., T. SCHOLZEN, E. BECHER, R.S. BHARDWAJ, T. SCHWARZ & T. LUGER. 1997. Human microvascular endothelial cells (HMEC-1) express the melanocortin receptor type 1 and produce increased levels of IL-8 upon stimulation with αMSH. J. Immunol. **159:** 1930–1937.

Implications of the Phenotype of POMC Deficiency for the Role of POMC-Derived Peptides in Skin Physiology

HEIKO KRUDE, DIRK SCHNABEL, WERNER LUCK, AND ANNETTE GRÜTERS

Kinderpoliklinik, Charite, Campus-Virchow, Humboldtuniversität zu Berlin, Germany

INTRODUCTION

After the isolation of the POMC-derived peptide, α-MSH, from pituitary extracts in 1955, and its synthesis in 1957, several *in vivo* studies clearly demonstrated the darkening effect of α-MSH on human skin.[1] Cloning the melanocortin receptor gene family, including the MC1 receptor, revealed a molecular basis for α-MSH function on pigmentation.[2] Moreover, the observation of receptor crosstalk within the MC-receptor–POMC-peptide network, which enables binding and activation of MC1R by ACTH in addition to α-MSH, explained the phenomena of skin and hair darkening that occur during pathological situations with ACTH excess, as in Addison disease[3] and ACTH-R deficiency.[4] More recently additional functions of POMC-derived peptides have been proposed as a result of the demonstration of skin expression by the POMC gene itself, as well as the other components of the entire hypothalamus–pituitary–adrenal axis; for example, CRH, CRH-R, and ACTH-R.[5,6] An impact on skin immune responses has been especially implicated. However, the final proof of the physiological significance of POMC function, besides skin pigmentation, awaits the establishment of an animal model for POMC deficiency. Therefore, we present our preliminary and short-term observations on two patients in whom we have demonstrated a genetic defect of the POMC gene.[7]

RESULTS

The combined symptoms of isolated ACTH deficiency, severe early onset of obesity and red-hair pigmentation, cause us to hypothesize a POMC gene defect in two children affected by these symptoms and followed by us for several years. PCR amplification and subsequent direct sequencing of the coding region of the POMC gene revealed a homozygous exon-2 mutation in a seven-year-old male patient and two compound heterozygous exon-3 mutations in a four-year-old female. The mutation located in exon-2 (C3804A) creates an additional out-of-frame start codon which, according to the current scanning model of eucaryotic translation, abolishes translation of the wild-type protein. Both unaffected parents have been shown to be heterozygous for this mutation. Restriction-endonuclease digestion analysis with Sphl indicated that this mutation is not a common polymorphism. The mutations found in exon-3 truncate the POMC protein of the female patient by introduction of a stop codon (G7013T, paternal allele) and by a frame shift generated by deletion of nt

7133 in the maternal allele. Endocrine studies revealed an absence of POMC derived peptides (ACTH and α-MSH) in the serum of the female patient, and only trace amounts in that of the male patient. This suggests residual translation in the case of the homozygous C3804A mutation, and complete interruption of POMC processing downstream of γ-MSH in the female patient.

The clinical observations and the medical histories are impressive concerning the weight gain of both patients after age three months. According to both parents this is the result of an extremely stimulated eating behavior. In contrast, the mental and emotional development seems to be otherwise completely normal.

The hair color in both children is red with an orange appearance. The skin type of both children is very light, and both parents reported experiences with severe sunburns. However, if protected the skin is in general not more vulnerable to alterations than that of normal children. On palpation, the skin seems to be normal in strength and tension. The parents of the girl reported problems with skin-dryness from birth. No other alterations have been observed in both children; in particular, no infections or allergic reactions. There was not one episode of dermal abscess, phlegmona, otitis externa, mucocutaneous candidiasis, or conjunctivitis.

DISCUSSION

The functional relevance of POMC derived peptides for the pigmentation of skin and hair has remained undisputed since the *in vivo* demonstration of skin darkening after application of purified or synthesized α-MSH to human volunteers.[1] These changes in pigmentation resemble the darkening of the skin in Addison patients, and those in ACTH-R deficiency—where extreme elevation of ACTH due to adrenal insufficiency leads to dark pigmentation of skin and hair.[3,4] This darkening effect is mediated by the MC1-R expressed in skin, which can be activated by α-MSH as well as by ACTH. In contrast, patients affected by panhypopituitarism caused by defects of pituitary development, or secondary to tumors such as craniopharyngioma, and who are deficient for pituitary derived POMC peptides, do not develop changes in their skin or hair pigmentation. The same lack of cutaneous changes has been observed in mice after hypophysectomy. These discrepancies resulted in the hypothesis that ligands at the skin MC1-R are not derived from pituitary but may act in a paracrine manner; suggesting a local expression and processing of POMC within the skin. This concept has been supported by the demonstration of POMC gene expression within human skin biopsies and cell cultures using RT-PCR techniques.[5] According to the paracrine view of α-MSH function on skin pigmentation, a lightening effect could only be expected if the local action of α-MSH is blocked, or if a general POMC defect results in ubiquitous lack of MC1-R ligands. The former constellation has ben described recently in the red-orange agouti mice model, in which an overexpressed MC-R antagonist, the Agouti protein, inhibits the function of α-MSH at the keratinocyte and hair follicle MC1-R.[8] In addition, loss-of-function mutations of the MC1-R gene in Norwegian and Holstein cattle results in red-coat phenotypes.[9] The red hair and light skin observed in the two patients presented in this paper seem to reflect a lack of ligands at the MC1-R. Due to the general defect of an inherited POMC gene mutation, POMC-derived peptides are not processed in any tissue, including the skin, leading to a paracrine α-MSH deficiency, lightening of the skin, and red pigmentation of the hair. The same effect, unmasking proposed paracrine functions of POMC-derived peptides, could have been demonstrated by finding severe early onset obesity in the POMC-deficient patients described here. As demonstrated in several mouse models α-MSH plays a critical role in hypothalamic food intake regulation.[10] Thus, the POMC peptide defect in the children under investigation seems to increase food intake and induce obesity, most likely by virtue of the lack of α-MSH as a paracrine hypothalamic MC4-R ligand. Therefore, the genetic POMC defect described in these two children seems to demonstrate cryptic paracrine POMC functions, not only in the skin, but also in other tissues.

In this context, the lack of further cutaneous symptoms in both children indicates that the proposed additional roles of POMC-derived peptides in skin growth and skin immune function may not be as important as expected. However, our experience is limited to two children that we have observed for only a few years, without significant skin alterations. If more patients affected by POMC defects can be identified and diagnosed later in life, a more significant estimate of the relevance of POMC function for skin physiology, other than pigmentation, will be possible.

REFERENCES

1. LERNER, A.B. 1993. Ann. N.Y. Acad. Sci. **680:** 1–12.
2. CONE, R.D. 1996. Rec. Prog. Horm. Res. **51:** 287–318.
3. ADDISON, T. 1868. Collection of the Published Writings of the late Thomas Addison. New Syndeham Society, London.
4. MIGEON, C.J., F.M. KENNY, A.A. SNIPES, J.S. SPAULING, J.W. FINKELSTEIN & R.M. BLIZZARD. 1968. Pediatr. Res. **2:** 501–513.
5. SLOMINSKI, A., J. ERMAK, A. HWANG, J.E. CHAKROBORTY, A. MAZURKIEWICZ & M. MIHM. 1995. FEBS Lett. **374:** 113–116.
6. SLOMINSKI, A., G. ERMARK & M. MIHM. 1996. JCEM **81:** 2746–2749.
7. KRUDE, H., H. BIEBERMANN, W. LUCK, R. HORN, G. BRABANT & A. GRÖTERS. 1998. Nat. Genet. **19:** 155–157.
8. LU, D., D. WILLARD, I.R. PATEL, S. KADWELL, L. OVERTON, T. KOST, M. LUTHER, W. CHEN, R. WOYCHIK, W.O. WILKINS & R. CONE. 1994. Nature **371:** 799–802.
9. JOERG, H., H.R. FRIES, E. MEIJERNIK & G.F. STRANZINGER. 1996. Mamm. Genome **7:** 317–318.
10. FLIER, J.S. & E. MARATOS-FLIER. 1998. Cell **92:** 437–440.

Serotonin in Human Allergic Contact Dermatitis

L. LUNDEBERG,[a] E. SUNDSTRÖM,[b] K. NORDLIND,[c] A. VERHOFSTAD,[d]
AND O. JOHANSSON[e]

[a]Department of Dermatology, Karolinska Hospital,
P.O. Box 120, S-171 76, Stockholm, Sweden

[b]Division of Geriatric Medicine, Neurodeg. Res. Grp, KFC, Novum, Huddinge, Sweden

[c]Department of Dermatology, University Hospital, Uppsala, Sweden

[d]Department of Pathology, Academisch Ziekenhuis Nijmegen, Nijmegen, the Netherlands

[e]Experimental Dermatology Unit, Department of Neuroscience
Karolinska Institute, Stockholm, Sweden

INTRODUCTION

Allergic contact dermatitis (ACD) is a common clinical condition leading to considerable morbidity. Both neuropeptides and monoamines may contribute to the expression of contact hypersensitivity. Serotonin, or 5-hydroxytryptamine (5-HT), is a monoamine that acts as a neuromediator in the central and peripheral nervous systems. Serotonin is also a vasoactive amine that is stored in the blood by platelets and released at sites of inflammation. It has a wide range of actions on T-cells and other effector cells *in vitro* and *in vivo*.[1,2] *In vivo* treatment of skin-sensitized mice with ketanserin, a serotonin antagonist, inhibited their capacity to elicit a delayed-type hypersensitivity reaction, and also the ability of their lymphoid cells to transfer delayed-type hypersensitivity.[3] In a recent investigation ketanserin was found to have an inhibitory effect on established allergic contact dermatitis in humans, suggesting that serotonin contributes to the hypersensitivity response.[4]

The aim of the work described here was to further elucidate the role of serotonin in cutaneous contact hypersensitivity by comparing involved and uninvolved skin from patients with ACD with normal skin from healthy volunteers for the presence of serotonin-like immunoreactive (IR) cells; and also by comparing the concentrations of serotonin in ACD involved and uninvolved skin.

MATERIAL AND METHODS

Patients

A group of six female patients (age range 30–56 years) with patch test-verified allergic contact dermatitis caused by nickel sulfate, participated in this investigation. Six female, age-matched, healthy volunteers without any history of skin disease

[a]Address for correspondence: 46 8 517 778 51 (fax).

served as a control group. The study was approved by the local Medical Ethics Committee at the Karolinska Hospital, Stockholm, Sweden.

Test Procedure

Allergic contact dermatitis was induced by 48-hour patch testing with nickel sulfate, 5.0% in petrolatum, applied to the patients' backs. After 72 hours, 3 mm skin biopsy specimens were taken from the test reaction and from contralateral uninvolved skin. For the immunohistochemical studies biopsy specimens were also taken from the backs of the controls.

Immunohistochemistry

The biopsy specimens were immersed in a solution of 14% saturated picric acid and 10% formalin, and then rinsed in 0.1 M Sörensen's buffer containing 10% sucrose, 0.01% NaN_3, and 0.02% Bacitracin. Serial cryostat sections (14 um) were used for indirect immunofluorescence.[5] A rabbit polyclonal antibody to serotonin[6] was used at a dilution of 1:600, and a mouse monoclonal antibody to melanoma-associated antigen (NKI beteb, Sanbio, Uden, the Netherlands) at a dilution of 1:80. The sections were kept in a humid atmosphere with the above-mentioned antisera overnight at 4°C, rinsed in phosphate-buffered saline (PBS), incubated for 30 min at 37°C in lissamine rhodamine (LRSC)-conjugated goat antirabbit IgG (1:160) and/or fluorescein-isothiocyanate (FITC)-conjugated goat antimouse IgG (1:160) (both from Jackson ImmunoResearch, West Grove, Pennsylvania, USA). To test the specificity of the antiserum, a preadsorption experiment was conducted, in which the antiserum was preincubated with 1.0 uM serotonin (5-hydroxytryptamine creatinine sulfate, Sigma Aldrich, Stockholm, Sweden) for 48 h at 4°C.

HPLC

Frozen biopsy specimens were thawed and weighed, and 50 ul of 0.1 M perchloric acid was added. The tissue was homogenized by sonication and centrifuged at 13,000 g for 5 min, and the supernatant was injected onto a Supelco LC-18-DB (75 × 4.6 mm, 3 um) reverse-phase-chromatography column. The eluent was composed of a 50 mM acetate citrate buffer with 0.2 mM sodium octyl sulfate, 0.27 mM EDTA, and 16% methanol, pH 3.8; and delivered at 1 ml/min. Eluted serotonin was detected by amperometry (LC-4B, Bioanalytical Systems, West Lafayette, IN, USA), using a glassy carbon electrode set at +0.85 V and quantified with an external standard. The results were expressed as ng serotonin/g wet weight.

Statistics

The Mann-Whitney rank sum test was used for the statistical analyses.

RESULTS

Immunohistochemistry

In *the skin of normal healthy volunteers,* the serotonin IR cells were located predominantly in the basal layer of the epidermis, appearing irregularly. The signal was preferentially associated with the cellular cytoplasm. The cells appeared to be dendritic, with rich cytoplasm and short, thin processes. In *the uninvolved skin of ACD patients,* the histological picture resembled that in normal healthy volunteers, but the uninvolved skin of the patients contained a larger number of serotonin IR cells. Also, the immunofluorescence intensity was slightly increased. In *the involved skin of ACD patients,* the number of serotonin IR cells was decreased in comparison with that in the healthy volunteers, but the dendrites of the remaining cells were enlarged and elongated; seemingly divided and showing small dendritic spines. The cells were also found to be closer to each other, often at the rete ridges. The histochemical immunoreaction of the serotonin antibody was abolished by preadsorption with the same compound, except for some unspecific staining in the stratum corneum. By omitting the primary antibody, the fluorescence was totally abolished. NKI-beteb showed a strong and diffuse immunoreactivity, being seen exclusively in certain epidermal basal cells. They appeared dendritic; however, their cellular margins and cellular processes seemed less clear than in the serotonin IR cells. When double-labelling was used we found, in most situations, that the serotonin antiserum labelled cells were also NKI-beteb positive. By omitting the primary antibody, fluorescence was totally abolished.

HPLC

In all patients the concentration of serotonin was significantly ($p < 0.05$) higher in lesional skin (median value 24.25, quartile deviation 3.00 ng/g) than in uninvolved skin (median value 9.85, quartile deviation 3.85 ng/g).

DISCUSSION

This work has shown that there is an increased concentration of 5-HT in ACD lesions compared with intact skin. Blood platelets have been found in increased numbers in inflammatory tissue, and have been shown to release 5-HT at sites of inflammation.[7] Another source of serotonin may be the immunoreactive cells in the epidermis. We have shown that these cells may be melanocytes. It has been reported that highly dendritic melanocytes in rapidly growing seborrheic keratosis, pigmented basal cell carcinoma; and that epidermis overlying melanomas are positive for serotonin.[8] Melanocytes derive from the neural crest, and the neuropeptide αMSH (alpha-melanocyte stimulating hormone) inhibits acute inflammation and contact sensitivity.[9,10] There is also increasing evidence that the nervous system has an influence on the immune system and the delayed hypersensitivity response.[11]

Dendritic cells are important in cutaneous immunity; and the Langerhans cells present antigen and migrate to the lymph nodes.[12] Granstein and collaborators[13] have shown that epidermal Langerhans cells are associated, both anatomically and functionally, with epidermal nerves. The melanocyte is also a dendritic cell, though its importance in cutaneous immunity has not been studied previously. By possible production of serotonin, the melanocytes may be able to activate T-cells in a similar way that Langerhans cell do. However, it may also interplay with other cell types in the epidermis, such as Langerhans cells, and with epidermal nerve endings, thereby influencing antigen presentation and release of sensory neuropeptides—such as substance P and calcitonin gene-related peptide.[14,15]

SUMMARY

To elucidate the role of serotonin in cutaneous contact hypersensitivity, we compared ACD-involved skin and uninvolved skin from nickel-allergic patients with normal skin from healthy volunteers. In the skin of normal healthy volunteers serotonin IR cells were situated in the basal layer of the epidermis. In uninvolved skin the cells were also situated in the basal layer, but they were more numerous and their immunofluorescence intensity was increased. In involved skin, IR cells were fewer and they had migrated upwards in the epidermis. Furthermore, the configuration of these cells had changed—showing enlarged and elongated dendrites as well as dendritic spines. Based on the serotonin IR cell-location and morphology, it is most likely that these cells are cutaneous melanocytes. The serotonin antiserum-labeled cells in ACD-involved skin was also NKI-beteb positive, the latter is known as a reliable marker for melanocytes. The concentration of serotonin in involved skin was significantly higher than that in uninvolved skin in ACD patients ($p < 0.05$). These results indicate that serotonin plays an important role in ACD.

ACKNOWLEDGMENTS

This investigation was supported by grants from the Swedish Asthma and Allergy Association, the Cancer and Allergy Foundation, Karolinska Institutet, the Welander/Finsen Foundation, and the Swedish Foundation for Health Care Science and Allergy Research. The technical assistance of Ms. Gunilla Holmkvist is gratefully acknowledged.

REFERENCES

1. AUNE, T.M., H.W. GOLDEN & M. MCGRATH. 1994. Inhibitors of serotonin synthesis and antagonists of serotonin 1 a receptors inhibit T lymphocyte function *in vitro* and cell-mediated immunity *in vivo*. J. Immunol. **153:** 489–498.
2. YOUNG, M.R., J.L. KUT, M.P. COOGAN, M.A. WRIGHT, M.E. YOUNG & J. MATTHEWS. 1993. Stimulation of splenic T-lymphocyte function by endogenous serotonin and by low-dose exogenous serotonin. Immunology **80:** 395–400.
3. AMEISEN, J.C., R. MEADE & P.W. ASKENASE. 1989. A new interpretation of the involvement of serotonin in delayed-type hypersensitivity. J. Immunol. **142:** 3171–3179.
4. BONDESSON, L., K. NORDLIND, V. MUTT & S. LIDÉN. 1996. Inhibitory effect of vasoactive intestinal polypeptide and ketanserin on established allergic contact dermatitis in man. Acta Dermatol. Venereol. **76:** 102–106
5. LJUNGBERG, A. & O. JOHANSSON. 1993. Methodological aspects of immunohistochemistry in dermatology with special reference to neuronal markers. Histochem. J. **25:** 735–745.
6. VERHOFSTAD, A.A.J., H.W.M. STEINBUSCH, H.W.J. JOOSTEN, B. PENKE, J. VARGA & M. GOLDSTEIN. 1983. Immunocytochemical localization of noradrenaline, adrenaline and serotonin. *In* Immunocytochemistry: Practical Application in Pathology and Biology. J.M. Polak & S. Van Noorden, Eds.: 143–168. Wright, Bristol.
7. GEBA, G.P., W. PTAK, G.M. ANDERSON, V. PALIWAL, R.E. RATZLAFF, J. LEVIN & P.W. ASKENASE. 1996. Delayed-type hypersensitivity in mast cell deficient mice: dependence on platelets for expression of contact sensitivity. J. Immunol. **157:** 557–565.

8. IYENGAR, B. 1994. Indoleamines and the UV-light-sensitive photoperiodic responses of the melanocyte network: a biological calendar. Experientia **50:** 733–736.
9. HILTZ, M.E. & J.M. LIPTON. 1990. Alpha-MSH peptides inhibit acute inflammation and contact sensitivity. Peptides **11:** 979–982.
10. RHEINS, L.A., A.L. COTLEUR, R.S. KLEIER, W.B. HOPPENJANS, D.N. SAUNDER & J.J. NORDLUND. 1989. Alpha-melanocyte stimulating hormone modulates contact hypersensitivity responsiveness in C57/BL6 mice. J. Invest. Dermatol. **93:** 511–517.
11. BLALOCK, J.E. 1994. The syntax of immune-neuroendocrine communication. Immunol. Today **15:** 504–511.
12. LAPPINS, M.B., I. KIMBER & M. NORVAL. 1996. The role of dendritic cells in cutaneous immunity. Arch. Dermatol. Res. **288:** 109–121.
13. ASAHINA, A., O. MORO, J. HOSOI, E.A. LERNER, S. XU, A. TAKASHIMA & R.D. GRANSTEIN. 1995. Specific induction of cAMP in Langerhans cells by calcitonin gene-related peptide: Relevance to functional effects. Proc. Natl. Acad. Sci. USA **92:** 8323–8327.
14. HARA, M., M. TOYODA, M. YAAR, J. BHAWAN, E. AVILA, I. PENNER & B. GILCHREST. 1996. Innervation of melanocytes in human skin. J. Exp. Med. **184:** 1385–1395.
15. ROSÉN, A., J. FRANCK & E. BRODIN. 1995. Effects of acute systemic treatment with the 5HT-uptake blocker alaproclate on tissue levels and release of substance P in rat periaqueductal grey. Neuropeptides **28:** 317–324.

Differential Temporal and Spatial Expression of POMC mRNA and of the Production of POMC Peptides During the Murine Hair Cycle

J.E. MAZURKIEWICZ,[a,b] D. CORLISS,[b] AND A. SLOMINSKI[c]

[b]Department of Microbiology, Immunology, and Molecular Genetics,
Albany Medical College, Albany, New York, USA

[c]Department of Pathology, Loyola University Medical Center, Chicago, Illinois, USA

Proopiomelanocortin (POMC) is a 27-kDa precursor protein that is posttranslationally processed to yield a number of neuropeptides, including ACTH, melanocyte-stimulating hormones (α-MSH, β-MSH, and γ-MSH), β-lipotropins, and endorphin opioids (α-endorphin, β-endorphin, and γ-endorphin).[1] Originally identified as products of the pituitary gland and the hypothalamus, POMC and POMC-derived peptides have been shown to be produced by a variety of nonpituitary tissues.[1] More recently, they have also been shown to be produced by keratinocytes in culture, in skin and skin derivatives, and by melanomas and melanocytic tumors of cutaneous origin.[2–4] It has been suggested that cutaneously produced POMC-derived peptides play significant roles in skin physiology, including immune modulation and local responses to stress.[5,6]

In the pituitary and hypothalamus, posttranslational proteolysis of POMC is performed by the prohormone convertases, PC1 and PC2. Cleavage by PC1 results primarily in the production of ACTH and β-lipotropin; and, to a minor extent, β-endorphin. Cleavage by PC2 elicits β-endorphin and N-terminally extended corticotropin, containing the joining peptide and either α-MSH or desacetylated-α-MSH. Processing of β-endorphin$_{1-31}$ to yield β-endorphin$_{1-27}$ is mediated solely by PC2.[7,8]

To directly study the relationship between POMC gene transcription and the production of POMC peptides resulting from depilation-induced anagen in murine skin, we used *in situ* hybridization (ISH) to identify sites of POMC mRNA expression, and immunohistochemistry to identify the cells that contained POMC peptides (β-endorphin, ACTH, and β-MSH), and the prohormone convertases, PC1 and PC2.

At telogen, POMC message levels were below the limit of detection by ISH, but were detectable in skin extracts by RTPCR. On days three, five, and ten after induction, sebaceous units were positive for POMC mRNA, on day five scattered epidermal and follicle keratinocytes contained POMC mRNA, and on day ten all keratinocytes were positive. POMC products also displayed a differential cellular localization and temporal expression during anagen. β-Endorphin immunoreactivity (IR) was primarily limited to sebocytes. β-endorphin IR was detected throughout the

[a]Address for correspondence: Dr. Joseph E. Mazurkiewicz, Department of Microbiology, Immunology, and Molecular Genetics, Mail Code A-68, Albany Medical College, 47 New Scotland Avenue, Albany, NY 12208, USA. 518-262-5381 (voice); 518-262-5748 (fax); jmazurki@amc.edu (e-mail).

hair cycle; it was present at telogen and the concentration increased as anagen progressed. ACTH-IR was limited to epidermal and follicle keratinocytes. Although absent at telogen, ACTH-IR tested positive at anagen day three, and increased to day 15. β-MSH-IR was absent at telogen. On day three, keratinocytes, some sebocytes, and sebaceous gland duct cells were IR-positive; and on day five, the outer root-sheath cells were also positive. There was a striking increase in β-MSH-IR intensity in keratinocytes and sebocytes on day 11, and this returned to telogen levels by day 15. Cells that contained POMC peptides also expressed POMC mRNA, and as immunoreactivity increased there was a parallel increase in mRNA.

We examined the cellular localization of PC1 and PC2 at telogen and at anagen-VI. As with POMC mRNA and POMC-derived peptides, these peptidases also displayed a differential temporal and spatial pattern of expression. PC1 and PC2 were present at very low levels in epidermal keratinocytes in telogen; the PC1-IR level was greater than that of PC2-IR. Immunoreactivity for both convertases increased in anagen-VI, with PC1 showing the greater elevation. In sebaceous units in telogen, PC1-IR was present at low levels in sebocytes and in adjacent small cells, whereas PC2-IR was just at, or below, detectable levels. In anagen-VI, IR for both convertases increased, with PC1 again showing the greater increase. Both sebocytes and adjacent small cells showed the increase in PC1-IR, but only small cells exhibited the increase in PC2-IR.

In skin cells, as in cells of the anterior pituitary,[8] the differential expression of PC1 and PC2 may play a role in posttranslational processing. For example, when considering the results of the PC1 and PC2 immunolocalizations, PC1 could certainly be responsible for all of the POMC processing in keratinocytes. Likewise, PC1, which was present at low levels in sebocytes in telogen, could be responsible for processing POMC to β-endorphin. In contrast, in anagen-VI, where β-endorphin-IR was very high in sebocytes, both PC1-IR and PC2-IR were increased. This differential β-endorphin-IR could result from the differential expression of the prohormone convertases in these cells.

ACKNOWLEDGMENT

This work was supported in part by National Science Foundation Grants IBN-9405242 and IBN-9604364.

REFERENCES

1. SMITH, A.I. & J.E. FUNDER. 1988. Proopiomelanocortin processing in the pituitary, central nervous system, and peripheral tissues. Endocrine Rev. **9:** 159–179.
2. SLOMINSKI, A., R. PAUS & J.E. MAZURKIEWICZ. 1992. Proopiomelanocortin expression in the skin during induced hair growth in mice. Experentia **58:** 50–54.
3. SLOMINSKI, A., J. WORTSMAN, J.E. MAZURKIEWICZ, L. MATSUOKA, R. PAUS & K. LAWRENCE. 1993. Detection of the proopiomelanocortin-derived antigens in normal and pathologic human skin J. Lab. Clin. Med. **122:** 658–666.
4. WINTZEN, M., M. YAAR, E.M. AVILLA, B.J. VERMEER & B.A. GILCHREST. 1996. Proopiomelanocortin, its derived peptides, and the skin. J. Invest. Dermatol. **106:** 3–10.
5. SLOMINSKI, A., R. PAUS & J. WORTSMAN. 1993. On the potential role of proopiomelanocortin in skin physiology and pathology. Mol. Cell. Endocrinol. **93:** C1–C6.

6. PAUS, R., C. VAN DER VEEN, S. EICHMULLER, T. KOPP *et al.* 1998. Generation and cyclic remodeling of the hair follicle immune system in mice. J. Invest. Dermatol. **111:** 7–18.

7. SEIDAH, N.G., R. DAY, M. MARCINKIEWICZ & M. CHRÉTIEN. 1993. Mammalian paired basic amino acid convertases of prohormones and proproteins Ann. N.Y. Acad. Sci. **680:** 135–146.

8. ZHOU, A., B.T. BLOOMQUIST & R.E. MAINS. 1993. The prohormone convertases PC1 and PC2 mediate distinct endoproteolytic cleavages in a strict temporal order during proopiomelanocortin biosynthetic processing. J. Biol. Chem. **269:** 1763–1769.

Effective Treatment of Pruritus with Naltrexone, an Orally Active Opiate Antagonist

D. METZE,[a] S. REIMANN, AND T.A. LUGER

Department of Dermatology, Ludwig Boltzmann Institute for Cellbiology and Immunobiology of the Skin, University of Münster, Münster, Germany

INTRODUCTION

Clinical and experimental observations have shown that opiates can evoke or intensify itch, and to do so independently of their histamine-releasing effect.[1] The action of opiates results from specific binding to opiate receptors in the central and peripheral nervous system, thus mimicking the physiological effects of endorphins and enkephalins.[2] The role of opiate receptors in the perception of pruritus is emphasized by the observation that opiate antagonists suppress pruritus of different origin. It has been long recognized that parenteral and oral administration of opiate antagonists reverse epidural morphine-induced pruritus and effectively suppress otherwise intractable cholestatic pruritus.[3-5] Furthermore, a randomized crossover trial demonstrated amelioration of pruritus in hemodialysis patients using naltrexone, a newly developed oral opiate antagonist.[6] Only recently was it possible to show that naltrexone can significantly diminish itching and alloknesis after a histamine stimulus.[7] Transient response of itch caused by urticaria and atopic dermatitis could be observed after a single dose of nalmefene. However, other authors were not able to demonstrate any alleviation of pruritus in psoriasis and eczematous diseases using this oral opiate antagonist in a long-term study.[8,9]

The aim of our pilot study was to evaluate the efficacy and safety of naltrexone in the treatment of severe, antihistamine-resistant pruritus in dermatologic and internal diseases.

PATIENTS AND METHODS

A total of 35 patients with pruritus caused by liver cirrhosis, chronic renal failure, cutaneous lymphoma, hydroxyethyl starch (HES), atopic dermatitis, macular amyloidosis, lichen simplex chronicus, and prurigo nodularis, as well as patients with pruritus of unknown origin, were randomly selected to receive naltrexone (Nemexin®) orally in a single daily dose of 50 mg (see TABLE 1). In many cases, pruritus was refractory to regular therapeutic trials prior to administration of naltrexone. The patients did not receive any other local or systemic antipruritic therapy, such as antihistamines, steroids, and phototherapy. The pruritus intensity was rated by the

[a]Address for correspondence: Dieter Metze, M.D., Department of Dermatology, University Münster, Von-Esmarchstrasse 56, D-48149 Münster, Germany. +49-251-835-6504 (voice); +49-251-835-6522 (fax); metzed@uni-muenster.de (e-mail).

TABLE 1. Diagnoses, number of patients, and therapeutic response of pruritic symptoms to naltrexone therapy

Diagnoses	Number of patients	Therapeutic response	Antipruritic effect
Liver cirrhosis	1	1	70%
Chronic renal failure	1	1	100%
Pruritus of unknown origin	6	3	50–70%
HES-induced pruritus	4	3	50–100%
Cutaneous-lymphoma	5	3	60–100%
Atopic Dermatitis	4	2	20–100%
Macular amyloidosis	1	1	100%
Prurigo/lichen simplex	13	9	30–100%

patients before and during therapy by using a visual analogue scale ranging from 0 (no pruritus) to 10 (severe pruritus).

RESULTS

First relief of the pruritic sensations could be observed within two to eight days. Therapeutic response was achieved in 65.5%, in which 22.8% of all treated patients reported a complete elimination of pruritus, 28.5% reported a reduction of more than 50%. Tachyphylaxis was infrequent (8.5%) and occurred late. Naltrexone was of high antipruritic effect in lichen simplex and prurigo nodularis, and it contributed to healing of the skin lesions.

Adverse drug effects were transient. During the initial 1–2 weeks of treatment, 25.7% of the patients complained of nausea that could be ameliorated by metoclopramid; and 2.8% experienced fatigue and dizziness. No transient elevation of liver enzymes, no thrombocytopenic purpura, and no withdrawal reaction of opiate addiction could be observed.

CONCLUSION

The efficacy of currently available therapeutic agents for pruritus is often disappointing. Since the perception of pruritus is modified by endogenous opiates via central opiate receptors in a histamine-independent manner, opiate antagonists show a high capacity to suppress pruritus. Of further interest is the observation that opiate antagonists have a greater therapeutic effect in placebo *non*responder patients than in placebo responders.[10] The current pilot-study showed that the oral administration of naltrexone (Nemexin®) effectively suppressed pruritus in dermatologic and internal diseases. Most remarkably, naltrexone proved to be a well-tolerated therapeutic alternative in many cases that were refractory to regular antipruritic therapy. In particular, an excellent response was seen in lichen simplex chronicus and prurigo nodularis, where arrest of scratching contributed to healing of the lesions.

Adverse drug effects of naltrexone are minimal and are restricted to the initial weeks of treatment. Nausea could be ameliorated by metoclopramid; fatigue and dizziness were rare. Transient elevation of liver enzymes and reversible idiopathic thrombocytopenic purpura were not observed at the low dosage currently used. Transient symptoms of opiate withdrawal syndrome have been reported only in patients treated for cholestatic pruritus and these can be attributed to increased levels of endogenous opiates in liver diseases.[4]

In conclusion, our preliminary results suggest that oral opiate antagonists offer an exciting approach to the treatment of pruritus.

REFERENCES

1. BERNSTEIN, J.E., R.M. SWIFT, K. SOLTANI & A.L. LORINCZ. 1982. Antipruritic effect of an opiate antagonist, naloxone hydrochloride. J. Invest. Dermatol. **78:** 82–83.
2. STEIN, C. 1995. The control of pain in peripheral tissue by opioids. N. Engl. J. Med. **332:** 1685–1690.
3. BERNSTEIN, J.E. 1979. Relief of intractable pruritus with naloxone. Arch. Dermatol. **115:** 1366–1367.
4. JONES, E.A. & N.V. BERGASA. 1992. The pruritus of cholestasis and the opioid system. JAMA **268:** 3359–3362.
5. WOLFHAGEN, F.H., E. STERNIERI, W.C. HOP, G. VITALE, M. BERTOLOTTI & H.R. VAN BUUREN. 1997. Oral naltrexone treatment for cholestatic pruritus: a double-blind, placebo-controlled study. Gastroenterology **113:** 1264–1269.
6. PEER, G., S. KIVITY, O. AGAMI, E. FIREMAN, D. SILVERBERG, M. BLUM & A. LAINA. 1996. Randomised crossover trial of naltrexone in uraemic pruritus. Lancet **348:** 1552–1554.
7. HEYER, G., M. DOTZER, T.L. DIEPGEN & H.O. HANDWERKER. 1997. Opiate and H1 antagonist effects on histamine induced pruritus and alloknesis. Pain **73:** 239–243.
8. MONROE, E.W. 1989. Efficacy and safety of nalmefene in patients with severe pruritus caused by chronic urticaria and atopic dermatitis. J. Am. Acad. Derm. **21:** 135–136.
9. HARRISON, P.V.J. 1990. Nalmefene and pruritus. Am. Acad. Dermatol. **23:** 530.
10. SUMMERFIELD, J.A. 1981. Pain, itch and endorphins. Br. J. Derm. **105:** 725–726.

Developmentally Regulated Expression of α-MSH and MC-1 Receptor in C57BL/6 Mouse Skin Suggests Functions Beyond Pigmentation[a]

V.A. BOTCHKAREV,[b] N.V. BOTCHKAREVA,[b] A. SLOMINSKI,[b] B. ROLOFF,[b,c] T. LUGER,[d] AND R. PAUS[b,e]

[b]Department of Dermatology, Charité, Humboldt Universität zu Berlin, D-10117, Berlin, Germany

[c]Department of Pathology, Loyola University, Maywood, Illinois 60153, USA

[d]Department of Dermatology, University of Münster, D-48149, Münster, Germany

α-MSH is an endogenous proopiomelanocortin-derived neuropeptide that can act as hormone, neurohormone, neurotransmitter, cytokine, biological response modifier, and growth factor.[1–41] In the skin, α-MSH is understood to primarily control melanogenesis and to exert immuno-suppressive functions.[1–5] In the skin, the α-MSH receptor (MC1R) has been identified and characterized in melanocytes,[1,6] keratinocytes,[7,8] endothelial cells, and macrophages.[9,10] However, the role of α-MSH in hair growth control is still unclear. In this paper, we report our immunohistology studies of α-MSH and MC1-receptor expression during hair follicle morphogenesis and cycling in mouse skin. We have assessed the effects of α-MSH on epidermal and hair follicle keratinocyte proliferation in skin organ culture.

Back skin of neonatal C57BL/6 mice (PO-P14) was used to study hair follicle morphogenesis,[11,12] and the depilation-induced hair cycle of adolescent C57BL/6 mice was investigated to study hair follicle cycling.[13,14] α-MSH- and MC1-receptor-immunoreactivity (IR) in skin cryosections was examined by immunofluorescence[15] (using rabbit anti-α-MSH- and anti-MC1-receptor antisera.[16,17] The action of α-MSH on ^{3}H-thymidine incorporation into epidermal and hair follicle keratinocytes during different hair-cycle stages was tested in murine skin organ culture.[13,18,19]

During murine hair follicle morphogenesis, α-MSH-IR appeared in basal epidermal keratinocytes, as well as in the central outer root sheath and in the proximal hair matrix of developing hair follicles in morphogenesis stages 4–5 (see FIGURE 1A). At stages 4–5 of hair follicle development, MC-1R-IR was found in the outer and inner root sheath, and in suprabasal epidermal keratinocytes (see FIGURE 1 and 2B). With progressing hair follicle morphogenesis (stages 6–8), both α-MSH- and MC1R-IR were seen in keratinocytes (KCs) of the developing central and proximal outer root

[a]NOTE: The results reported here represent preliminary results. An extended manuscript containing specific data is in preparation.
[e]Address for correspondence: Dr. R. Paus, Department of Dermatology, University Hospital Eppendorf, University of Hamburg, D-20246 Hamburg, Germany. paus@uke.uni-hamburg.de (e-mail).

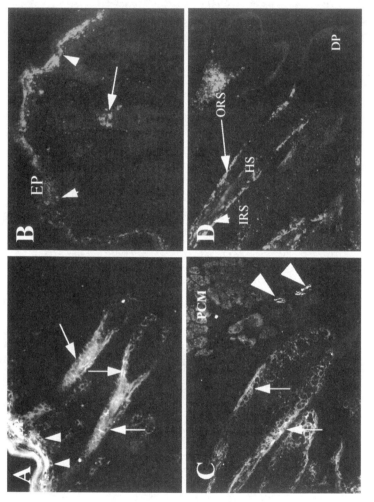

FIGURE 1. α-MSH and MC1R are expressed in keratinocytes during hair follicle morphogenesis. Cryostat sections (8 μm thick) of neonatal C57BL/6 murine back skin of the defined age were immunostained with antisera against α-MSH or MC1 receptor. Stages IV-V: **A.** α-MSH-IR in epidermal keratinocytes (*arrowheads*), central and proximal hair follicle outer root sheath (*arrows*). **B.** MC1R-IR in suprabasal layer of epidermis (*arrowheads*) and in follicular outer and inner root sheath (*arrow*). Stages VI–VIII: **C.** α-MSH-IR in hair follicle outer root sheath (*arrows*), and in subcutaneous nerve bundles (*arrowheads*). **D.** MC1R-IR in hair follicle outer (*arrow*) and inner root sheath (*arrowhead*). Abbreviations: EP, epidermis; DER, dermis; DP, dermal papilla; HM, hair matrix; HS, hair shaft; IRS and ORS, inner and outer root sheath; PCM, panniculus carnosus muscle; SC, subcutis.

sheath; α-MSH-IR was observed in the proximal hair matrix and in large subcutaneous nerve bundles (FIG. 1C and D).

In unmanipulated telogen skin α-MSH-IR was detected in nerve bundles (FIG. 1A) and in the circular fibers, located around hair follicle isthmus (follicular network B), confirmed by α-MSH-IR/PGP9.5 double immunovisualization (not shown). α-MSH-IR in adolescent skin was detected in keratinocytes of the proximal outer root sheath and the hair matrix of anagen IV hair follicles (FIG. 2B). With the assays employed, α-MSH-IR was below the level of detection in follicular keratinocytes during anagen II, V, VI, and catagen.

Low levels of MC1-R-IR were detected in the outer root sheath and hair germ of telogen hair follicles (FIG. 2D), whereas numerous MC1-R positive cells were found in the hair matrix of anagen IV–V hair follicles (FIG. 2E). In mature anagen VI hair follicles, MC1-IR was present in hair matrix, dermal papilla, and in the outer and inner root sheath (FIG. 2F). During catagen, MC1R-IR was restricted to hair bulb melanocytes and to the inner root sheath keratinocytes (FIG. 2G).

Organ culture assays of murine telogen skin revealed that pharmacological doses of αMSH inhibited DNA synthesis in both epidermal and hair follicle keratinocytes (see FIGURE 3). No proliferation effect was found in anagen II and IV skin.

This study provides further support for the notion that the biological activities of α-MSH in skin extend beyond the control of melanogenesis and skin immune responses,[4,5] and may include an involvement in hair growth control. The prominence of α-MSH and MC1-R expression in the developing hair follicle epithelium raises the possibility that α-MSH forms part of the signalling system that regulates hair follicle morphogenesis (see Refs. 11 and 20 for a review). α-MSH expression in nerve fibers around the hair-follicle isthmus and bulge might modulate hair follicle cycling by functionally altering the epithelial hair follicle stem cells located in this region.[21]

The onset of strong follicular α-MSH coincides with the onset of follicular melanogenesis, both during neonatal hair follicle morphogenesis and adolescent hair follicle cycling. This is consistent with the concept that locally generated α-MSH is a key factor in controlling hair follicle pigmentation.[4,5,22] α-MSH may also be involved in regulating the migration of immature melanocytes into the hair matrix and in stimulating their differentiation into pigment–producing hair follicle melanocytes. Expression of MC1-R in the outer and inner root sheath, and in the hair matrix during anagen, suggests a role of α-MSH in the control of hair follicle keratinocyte proliferation and/or differentiation. That α-MSH inhibits epidermal and hair follicle keratinocyte proliferation *in situ* raises the possibility that α-MSH—directly or indirectly—might be involved in the control of epithelial homeostasis in murine skin.

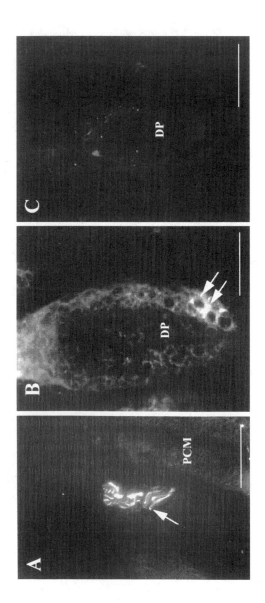

FIGURE 2. Hair follicle-associated α-MSH- and melanocortin receptor 1-immunoreactivity expression shows hair-cycle dependent changes. Cryostat sections of adolescent C57BL/6 murine back skin in the defined stages of induced hair cycle (telogen, unmanipulated skin, day 0; anagen IV and VI, respectively, 5 and 8–12 days after anagen induction) were immunostained with antisera against α-MSH and MC1 receptor. **A.** Expression of α-MSH-IR in subcutaneous nerve bundle (*arrow*). **B.** In anagen IV skin α-MSH-IR was expressed by individual hair matrix keratinocytes (*arrows*). **C.** Negative control of immunostaining with antiserum against α-MSH preincubated with 100 μg/ml cf α-MSH peptide. **D.** Relatively weak MC1R-IR expression in hair germ (*arrowhead*) and outer root sheath (*arrow*) in telogen skin. **E.** Numerous MC1R-positive cells in the developing hair bulb of anagen IV–V hair follicles (*arrows*). MC1R-IR is also visible between melanin granules (*arrowhead*). **F.** MC1R-IR in proximal outer (*arrow*) and inner (*small arrowhead*) root sheath, in hair matrix (*large arrowhead*), and among melanin (*asterisk*) in anagen VI hair follicle. **G.** In catagen-II hair follicles, MC1R-IR is seen in the inner root sheath (*small arrowhead*), in hair matrix (*large arrowhead*), and in hair bulb melanocytes (*arrow*). Abbreviations: DP, dermal papilla; HM, hair matrix; HS, hair shaft; IRS and ORS, inner and outer root sheath; Mel, melanin; PCM, panniculus camosus muscle. *Scale bars,* 50 μm. (Figure continued on opposite page.)

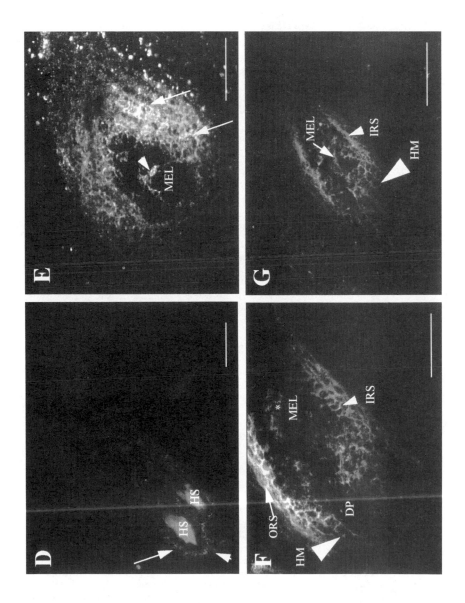

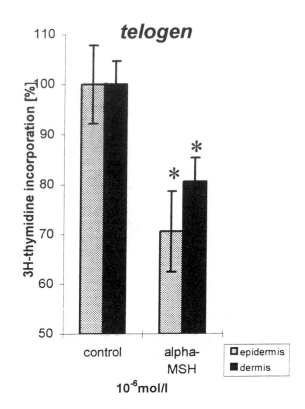

FIGURE 3. Influence of α-MSH to keratinocyte proliferation *in situ*. Ten to twelve 4 mm punch biopsies of murine skin in telogen were cultured in the presence of α-MSH and ^{3}H-thymidine during 20 hours at the air-liquid interface on gelatin gel[18,19] in Williams medium E. The epidermal and dermal fragments were then separated by 2 M NaBr. Incorporation of ^{3}H-thymidine was measured by liquid scintillation spectrometry. Dermal ^{3}H-thymidine incorporation largely reflects the proliferation of hair follicle keratinocytes.[18,19] Mean ± SEM, *$p < 0.05$.

REFERENCES

1. EBERLE, A., Ed. 1988. The Melanotropins. Karger, Basel.
2. CATANIA, A. & J. LIPTON. 1993. Alpa-melanocyte stimulating hormone in the modulation of host reactions. Endocr. Rev. **14:** 564–576.
3. LIPTON, J.M. & A. CATANIA. 1997. Anti-inflammatory actions of the neuroimmunomodulator αMSH. Immunol. Today **18:** 140–145.
4. LUGER, T.A., T. SCHOLZEN & S. GRABBE. 1997. The role of α-melanocyte-stimulating hormone in cutaneous biology. J. Invest. Dermatol. Symp. Proc. **2:** 87–93.
5. SLOMINSKI, A., R. PAUS & J. WORTSMAN. 1993. On the potential role of proopiomelanocortin in skin physiology and pathology. Mol. Cell Endocrinol. **93:** C1–C6.
6. HUNT, G. 1995. Melanocyte-stimulating hormone: a regulator of human melanocyte physiology. Pathobiol. **63:** 12–21.

7. CHAKRABORTY, A. & J. PAWELEK. 1993. MSH receptors in immortalized human epidermal keratinocytes: a potential mechanism for coordinated regulation of the epidermal melanin unit. J. Cell Physiol. **157:** 344–350.

8. OREL, L., M.M. SIMON, J. KARLSEDER, R. BHARDWAJ, F. TRAUTINGER, T. SCHWARZ & T.A. LUGER. 1997. α-Melanocyte stimulating hormone downregulates differentiation-driven heat shock protein 70 expression in keratinocytes. J. Invest. Dermatol. **108:** 401–405.

9. AUTELITANO, D.J., J.R. LUNDBLAD, M. BLUM & J.L. ROBERTS. 1989. Hormonal regulation of POMC gene expression. Annu. Rev. Physiol. **51:** 715–726.

10. SMITH, A.L. & J.E. FUNDER. 1988. Proopiomelanocortin processing in the pituitary, central nervous system, and peripheral tissues. Endocrine Rev. **9:** 159–179.

11. HARDY, M. 1992. The secret life of the hair follicle. Trends Genet. **8:** 55–61.

12. PAUS, R., K. FOITZIK, P. WELKER, S. BULFONE-PAUS & S. EICHMÜLLER. 1997. Transforming growth factor receptor type I and type II expression during murine hair follicle development and cycling. J. Invest. Dermatol. **109:** 518–526.

13. PAUS, R., K.S. STENN & R.E. LINK. 1990. Telogen skin contains an inhibitor of hair growth. Br. J. Dermatol. **122:** 777–784

14. PAUS, R. 1996. Control of the hair cycle and hair diseases as cycling disorders. Curr. Opin. Dermatol. **3:** 248–258.

15. BOTCHKAREV, V.A., S. EICHMÜLLER, O. JOHANSSON & R. PAUS. 1997. Hair cycle-dependent plasticity of skin and hair follicle innervation in normal murine skin. J. Comp. Neurol. **386:** 379–395.

16. GRAHEM, G., J. VERSTEGEN, A. LIBERT, R. ARNOULD & F. LEJEUNE. 1989. Alpha-melanocyte-stimulating hormone immunoreactivity in human melanoma metastases extracts. Pigment Cell Res. **2:** 519–523.

17. BOHM, M. *et al.* 1998. (Abstract). Exp. Dermatol. **7:** 222.

18. LI, L., R. PAUS, A. SLOMINSKI & R. HOFFMAN. 1992. Skin histoculture assay for studying the hair cycle. In Vitro Cell Dev. Biol. **28:** 695–698.

19. PAUS, R., M. LÜFTL & B.M. CZARNETZKI. 1994. Nerve growth factor modulates keratinocyte proliferation in murine skin organ culture. Br. J. Dermatol. **130:** 281–289.

20. PHILPOTT, M. & R. PAUS. 1998. Principles of hair follicle morphogenesis. *In* Molecular Biology of Epithelial Appendage Morphogenesis. 75–85. R,G. Landes, Austin.

21. COTSARELIS, G., T.T. SUN & R. LAVKER. 1990. Label-retaining cells reside in the bulge area of pilosebaceous unit: implications for follicular stem cells, hair cycle and skin cancerogenesis. Cell **61:** 1329–1337.

22. SLOMINSKI, A. & R. PAUS. 1993. Melanogenesis is coupled to murine anagen: toward new concepts for the role of melanocytes and the regulation of melanogenesis in hair growth. J. Invest. Dermatol. **101:** 90S–97S.

Plasma β-Endorphin Concentrations During Natural and Artificially Induced Winter Hair Growth in Mink (*Mustela vison*)

J. ROSE,[a,b] K. WOOD,[b] J. BILLINGSLEY,[b] J. OLBERTZ,[b]
A. LOVERING,[c] AND J. CARR[c]

[b]*Department of Biological Sciences, Idaho State University,
Pocatello, Idaho 83209, USA*

[c]*Department of Biological Sciences, Texas Tech University,
Lubbock, Texas 79409, USA*

Exogenous melatonin (MEL) or bilateral adrenalectomy (ADX) of mink when hair follicles are in the resting (telogen) stage of the hair growth cycle, initiates winter hair growth (anagen) 5–6 weeks earlier than controls.[1] The mechanism by means of which these treatments induce anagen is unknown; however, intradermal injections of adrenocorticotropin (ACTH) initiates localized anagen responses in mink[2] and rats.[3] Consistent with ADX-induced anagen is a concomitant increase in blood ACTH levels. Furthermore, exogenous MEL increases blood β-endorphin levels in rams.[4] Because β-endorphin and ACTH are secreted simultaneously in some species,[5] it is possible that MEL-induced anagen is mediated, in part, by ACTH. We measured plasma β-endorphin levels in mink to provide an indicator for ACTH secretion, in order to determine whether natural, ADX- and MEL-induced anagen are correlated with increased ACTH secretion; and whether suppression of ACTH/β-endorphin secretion with exogenous cortisol (CORT) inhibits the onset of anagen.

In control mink winter anagen commences during mid–late September and plasma β-endorphin concentrations exhibit no change during the onset of anagen (see FIGURE 1). Thus, it would appear that increased pituitary ACTH secretion is not involved in the normal initiation of winter anagen in mink. ADX + deoxycorticosterone (DOC, a mineralocorticoid supplement) treated mink exhibited winter anagen one month earlier than controls ($p < 0.05$). Supplementation of ADX-mink with CORT (ADX + DOC + CORT) delayed anagen by two weeks in comparison with ADX + DOC ($p < 0.05$), although anagen still occurred 2–3 weeks before controls ($p < 0.05$). Plasma β-endorphin levels increased threefold in response to ADX and remained elevated between July 25 and November 24 ($p < 0.05$). There was no difference in β-endorphin levels between ADX + DOC and ADX + DOC + CORT; and the resulting pelage in both groups of mink was representative of normal winter fur. Treatment with CORT, CORT + DOC, or with DOC, resulted in onset of anagen at approximately the same time as in controls. There was no difference in plasma β-endorphin levels among the three groups. However, the pelage that developed following CORT or CORT + DOC treatment, was devoid of under hair-type fibers, con-

[a]Address for correspondence: Dr. Jack Rose, Idaho State University, Department of Biological Sciences, Campus Box 8007, Pocatello, ID 83209, USA. rosewill@isu.edu (e-mail).

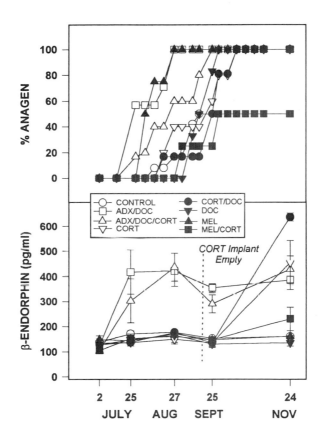

FIGURE 1. Percent of animals in the anagen stage of the hair growth cycle, and plasma β-endorphin concentrations in female mink from July 2 to November 24, 1997. Mink were treated with melatonin (MEL, $n = 6$), cortisol (CORT, $n = 5$), deoxycorticosterone (DOC, $n = 6$), MEL + CORT ($n = 4$), CORT + DOC ($n = 6$), bilateral adrenalectomized + DOC (ADX + DOC, $n = 6$), ADX + DOC + CORT ($n = 4$), or controls ($n = 6$). β-Endorphin values are expressed as the mean ± SEM, derived from duplicate determinations. MEL (25 mg/implant) and DOC (100 mg/implant) were administered in Silastic (Dow Corning, Midland, MI) tubing implants inserted subcutaneously (sc) over the interscapular region. CORT was administered in dissolvable implants (200 mg each, 60 day release; Innovative Research of America, Sarasota, Fl). Implants were administered July 2 and ADX between July 7 and 9. Onset of anagen was determined as the day on which hair growth could be measured above the skin surface.

sisting only of a thin coat of guard hairs. Following depletion of CORT from the implants in mid-September (FIG. 1), a significant increase in β-endorphin levels occurred in mink with intact adrenals (CORT or CORT + DOC) on November 24 ($p < 0.05$).

Mink that were treated with MEL alone, displayed onset of winter anagen one month before the controls ($p < 0.05$), and there was no change in plasma β-endorphin levels during the telogen to anagen transition. It would appear that the winter anagen-inducing actions of MEL are not mediated by pituitary β-endorphin/ACTH secretion. Interestingly, mink treated with MEL + CORT exhibited a one month delay in onset of anagen in comparison with MEL alone ($p < 0.05$), and 50% of the MEL + CORT mink failed to exhibit winter anagen. The MEL + CORT–treated mink also developed a pelage that was for the most part devoid of under-hair-type fibers. Because β-endorphin levels were not different in mink treated with MEL or MEL + CORT, this suggests that the anagen inhibiting effects of CORT in MEL-treated mink are not mediated by pituitary β-endorphin/ACTH secretion. Because glucocorticoids inhibit hair growth when administered systemically or topically[6] in numerous species, including the mink, it is possible that CORT inhibited anagen through direct actions on the skin and/or hair follicle.

Although increasing plasma levels of ACTH and/or β-endorphin do not appear to play a role in the induction of winter anagen in mink, we hypothesize that increased production of either, or both, of these peptides within the skin, may be a prerequisite for anagen induction. ACTH and other proopiomelanocortin (POMC) derived peptides and their receptors have been shown to be synthesized by the skin,[7] with some (POMC and β-endorphin) produced in a hair-cycle-dependent manner—highest during anagen and lowest during telogen. Slominski and colleagues[7] have proposed that the equivalent of a hypothalamic-pituitary-adrenal axis exists in the skin that may play a role in hair growth cycles. Studies are in progress in our laboratory to determine whether MEL binding sites are present in the skin of mink, and whether POMC expression increases in response to exogenous MEL prior to the onset on winter anagen.

ACKNOWLEDGMENT

This work was supported by the American Mink Farmers Research Foundation.

REFERENCES

1. ROSE, J. *et al.* 1998 Serum prolactin and dehydroepiandrosterone (DHEA) concentrations during the summer and winter hair growth cycles of mink (*Mustela vison*). Comp. Biochem. Physiol. Part A, **121:** 263–271.
2. ROSE, J. 1998. Adrenocorticotropic hormone (ACTH) but not apha-melanocyte stimulating hormone (α-MSH) as a mediator of adrenalectomy induced hair growth in mink. J. Invest. Dermatol. **110:** 456–457
3. PAUS, R. *et al.* 1994. Mast cell involvement in murine hair growth. Dev. Biol. **163:** 230–240.
4. LINCOLN, G.A. *et al.* 1992. Effects of placing micro-implants of melatonin in the mediobasal hypothalamus and preoptic area on the secretion of prolactin and β-endorphin in rams. J. Endocrinol. **134:** 437–448.

5. GUILLEMIN R. *et al.* 1977. β-Endorphin and adrenocorticotropin are secreted concomitantly by the pituitary gland. Science **197:** 1367–1369.
6. STENN, K.S. *et al.* 1993. Glucocorticoid effect on hair growth initiation: A reconsideration. Skin Pharmacol. **6:** 125–134.
7. SLOMINSKI, A.J. *et al.* 1996. Potential mechanism of skin response to stress. Int. J. Dermatol. **35:** 849–851.

Expression of Proopiomelanocortin Peptides and Prohormone Convertases by Human Dermal Microvascular Endothelial Cells

THOMAS E. SCHOLZEN,[a] THOMAS BRZOSKA,[b] DIRK-HENNER KALDEN,[b] MECHTHILD HARTMEYER,[b] THOMAS A. LUGER,[b] CHERYL A. ARMSTRONG,[a] AND JOHN C. ANSEL[c]

[a]Department of Dermatology, Emory University School of Medicine, Atlanta, Georgia 30322, USA

[b]Ludwig Boltzmann Institute for Cellbiology and Immunobiology of the Skin, Department of Dermatology, University of Münster, Germany

INTRODUCTION

Proopiomelanocortin (POMC) peptides such as α-melanocyte stimulating hormone (α-MSH) and adrenocorticotropin (ACTH) are expressed in the epidermal and dermal compartments of the skin. In epidermal cells, such as keratinocytes or melanocytes, the transcription and release of POMC-peptides *in vivo* and *in vitro* increases as a result of noxious stimuli such as UV-light or infection, either directly, or possibly by the induction of secondary mediators such as IL-1. POMC-peptides, especially α-MSH, are considered to be potent immunomodulators with antipyretic and immunosuppressive properties. The expression and regulation of cellular adhesion molecules and cytokines by dermal microvascular endothelial cells is crucial in mediating leukocyte-endothelial cell interaction and transmigration into the extravascular tissue during cutaneous inflammation.[1,2] In this paper we address the hypothesis that human dermal microvascular endothelial cells (HDMEC) are capable of expressing both the POMC and prohormone convertases (PC) that are required to generate POMC peptides.

RESULTS AND DISCUSSION

HDMEC were isolated and cultured as previously described.[3] Cells were treated with IL-1β (0.1–10.0 ng/mL) after they had been grown to 90% confluency for 1–48 h. Following total RNA isolation, semiquantitative RT-PCR studies revealed a constitutive expression of POMC mRNA by HDMEC *in vitro* that could be upregulated by IL-1β at one and five hours after stimulation. This occurred in a dose-dependent manner (data not shown). Since UV-irradiation is one of the major stimuli for POMC mRNA and peptide expression in epidermal cells *in vitro*, we tested the pos-

[c]Address for correspondence: John C. Ansel, Emory University School of Medicine, Department of Dermatology, 5313 Woodruff Memorial Building, Atlanta, GA 30322, USA. 404-727-5107 (voice); 404-727-5217 (fax); jansel@emory.edu (e-mail).

sibility that UV-irradiation may also have a direct impact on HDMEC POMC production. Exposure of HDMEC to UVA1 (30 J/cm^2, UVASUN 5000 irradiation source) or UVB-light (12.5 mJ/cm^2, FS20 Westinghouse bulbs) significantly enhanced POMC expression (data not shown). In order to investigate whether UV-induced expression of POMC mRNA is accompanied by an increased accumulation and release of POMC peptides, HDMEC lysates and supernatants were harvested after UV-irradiation as previously described,[4] and subjected to analysis using ACTH- and α-MSH-specific radioimmunoassays (see TABLE 1). UVB or UVA1 treatment of HDMEC resulted in increased intracellular ACTH 12 h after stimulation, this declined 24 h after UV, and was slightly elevated again 48 h post UV-exposure. The induction of intracellular ACTH was also dose-dependent, with maximum ACTH accumulation observed 12 h after 20 mJ/cm^2 UVB or 30 J/cm^2 UVA1 The effect of UV on released ACTH and α-MSH was also determined (TABLE 1). Our results demonstrate that ACTH and α-MSH release were also significantly increased in the supernatants of UVA1-irradiated HDMEC (30 J/cm^2) with a maximum quantity detected 24 h after irradiation for both of these POMC-derived peptides. Similar data were obtained when HDMEC were treated with UVB (data not shown).

In neuroendocrine tissues, PC-1 is required to generate ACTH and β-lipotropin, whereas PC-2 cleavage generates MSH and β-endorphins. Since both ACTH and α-MSH are released by HDMEC, we examined the expression of PC-1 and PC-2 in HDMEC by semiquantitative RT-PCR. HDMEC express low levels of PC-1

TABLE 1. ACTH and α-MSH production by HDMEC after UV exposure

		12 h	24 h	48 h
		ACTH (intracellular); pmol/mg protein^a		
control		44.32 ± 14.07	17.59 ± 10.87	20.88 ± 5.55
UVB (mJ/cm^2)	10	88.13 ± 5.05	12.77 ± 1.82	23.99 ± 6.75
	20	110.58 ± 14.07	19.00 ± 1.15	46.16 ± 7.10
	30	42.18 ± 2.85	10.63 ± 0.95	12.50 ± 0.85
UVA1 (J/cm^2)	10	72.67 ± 0.55	7.03 ± 1.33	28.93 ± 1.75
	30	142.05 ± 5.42	5.00 ± 0.35	41.97 ± 1.15
	50	86.81 ± 1.15	3.31 ± 0.05	56.28 ± 1.25
		ACTH (supernatant); pmol/mL^a		
control		n.d.	33.00 ± 8.51	11.6 ± 2.27
UVA1 (30 J/cm^2)		n.d.	100.27 ± 3.68	4.54 ± 3.02
		α-MSH (supernatant); pmol/mL^a		
control		n.d.	16.26 ± 0.23	14.46 ± 0.43
UVA1 (30 J/cm^2)		n.d.	43.28 ± 0.51	28.21 ± 1.26

^{a}HDMEC (2 × 10^6 cells) were left untreated or stimulated with UVB or UVA1. Cells or cell supernatants were harvested after the indicated time as previously described.[4] ACTH and α-MSH were determined by specific RIA. All values are given as mean ± SEM.

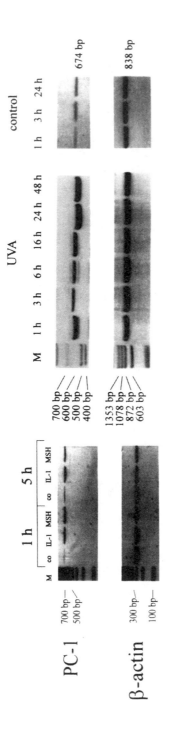

FIGURE 1. Kinetics and concentration dependence of PC-1 mRNA upregulation in relation to β-actin expression after stimulation with IL-1β and α-MSH (**left**) or UVA1-light (**right**). HDMEC (2×10^6 cells) were left untreated (**control**) or stimulated with 1 ng/ml IL-1β, 10^{-8} M α-MSH or 30 J/cm^2 UVA1. Total RNA was harvested at the indicated times and subjected to semiquantitative RT-PCR using PC-1 and β-actin-specific primer pairs. PCR-conditions allowing reliable comparison of PC-1 expression with β-actin mRNA expression in different samples were established by making serial dilutions of template cDNA at constant cycle numbers for each primer pair to verify the linearity of PCR amplification. Subsequently, cDNA-mixtures were diluted to obtain equal amounts of PCR product specific for amplified β-actin and subjected to amplification of PC-1-specific PCR products. Amplification products of PC-1 (674 bp) and β-actin cDNA (300 or 838 bp) were separated on agarose gels.

mRNA that are significantly upregulated by stimulation with IL-1β or α-MSH (see FIGURE 1). Kinetic studies on PC-1 mRNA expression after UVA1 exposure revealed a biphasic induction profile with an initial induction of PC-1 expression after 1 h, a subsequent decline at 6 and 16 h, and a second induction phase at 24 and 48 h (FIG. 1). However, the PC-2 that is required to generate MSH could not be detected in HDMEC, although a specific PC-2 PCR product could be amplified from a pituitary gland cDNA library that was used as a positive control (not shown).

These data demonstrate that in HDMEC UV-light is capable of inducing the expression of POMC and of PC-1. PC-1 is one of the major proteolytic enzymes required to process the POMC prohormone. Under certain experimental conditions the expression of neurohormone convertases and their substrates might be regulated by similar mediators. The PC-2 that cleaves the POMC precursor into α-MSH was not found to be expressed in HDMEC, suggesting that there might be an alternative pathway for the generation of α-MSH in endothelial cells. HDMEC were found to express functional MC-1R, that were also regulated by IL-1β and α-MSH.[3] Thus, UV-light, by the induction of IL-1 and α-MSH, may increase the sensitivity of HDMEC for POMC peptides by upregulating melanocortin receptor expression. This may be important for the autocrine regulation of dermal endothelial cell functions, as we have discussed in another paper in this volume. It can also be speculated that α-MSH and ACTH, released by HDMEC into the vascular lumen after UV *in vivo,* might alter functions of circulating leukocytes. Thus, due to the multiple antiinflammatory and immunosuppressive properties of endothelial cell-derived POMC peptides, these mediators may significantly contribute to UV-mediated immunosuppression.

REFERENCES

1. LUGER, T.A., T. SCHOLZEN & S. GRABBE. 1997. The role of alpha-melanocyte-stimulating hormone in cutaneous biology. J. Invest. Dermatol. Symp. Proc. **2:** 87–93.
2. SWERLICK, R.A. & T.J. LAWLEY. 1993. Role of microvascular endothelial cells in inflammation. J. Invest. Dermatol. **100:** 111 S–115S.
3. HARTMEYER, M., T. SCHOLZEN, E. BECHER, R.S. BHARDWAJ, T. SCHWARZ & T.A. LUGER. 1997. Human dermal microvascular endothelial cells express the melanocortin receptor type-1 and produce increased levels of IL-8 upon stimulation with alpha-melanocyte-stimulating hormone. J. Immunol. **159:** 1930–1937.
4. CHAKRABORTY, A., A. SLOMINSKI, G. ERMAK, J. HWANG & J. PAWELEK. 1995. Ultraviolet B and melanocyte-stimulating hormone (MSH) stimulate mRNA production for alpha MSH receptors and proopiomelanocortin-derived peptides in mouse melanoma cells and transformed keratinocytes. J. Invest. Dermatol. **105:** 655–659.

ACTH Production in C57BL/6 Mouse Skin

ANDRZEJ SLOMINSKI,[a] NATALIA V. BOTCHKAREVA,[b]
VLADIMIR A. BOTCHKAREV,[b] ASHOK CHAKRABORTY,[c]
THOMAS LUGER,[d] MURAT UENALAN,[b] AND RALF PAUS[b]

[a]Department of Pathology, Loyola University Medical Center, Maywood, Illinois, USA

[b]Department of Dermatology, Charite Hospital, Humboldt University, Berlin, Germany

[c]Department of Dermatology, Yale University School of Medicine,
New Haven, Connecticut, USA

[d]Department of Dermatology, Ludwig Boltzmann Institute of Cell Biology and
Immunobiology of the Skin, University of Münster, Münster, Germany

Skin is a recognized target for POMC-derived ACTH and MSH peptides.[1] In our previous studies we have documented hair-cycle-dependent POMC gene transcription and translation in the skin of the C57BL/6 mouse.[2,3] In addition, it was reported that intracutaneous administration of ACTH induces hair growth in C57BL/6 mice[4] and in mink.[5] To further investigate a possible role of ACTH in skin physiology we used the C57BL/6 mouse model.[6]

The presence of ACTH peptide in anagen-VI skin was demonstrated by reversed-phase (RP) HPLC analysis[7] combined with specific radioimmunoassay (RIA). The major immunoreactive (IR) peak had the same retention time (18–19 min) as the synthetic ACTH standard. No specific IR was detected at the retention time for the desacetyl-α-MSH (13 min), α-MSH (15 min), diacetyl-α-MSH (17 min), or β-endorphin (21 min). The ACTH concentration, that was low in telogen (3.06 + 3.59 pg/mg protein), increased during anagen in two steps: a rapid phase in anagen-I, and a slower rise that reached its peak in anagen-VI (107.6 + 8.4 pg/mg protein). By indirect immunofluorescence, ACTH-IR was detected in keratinocytes of basal layer of epidermis, of proximal and distal ORS of hair follicle, and in subcutaneous muscle of anagen-VI skin.

Northern hybridization techniques showed the production of 4.5- and 2.0-Kb mRNAs hybridizable to the coding region of the MC2 (receptor for ACTH) gene (see FIGURE 1). The expression of both transcripts was similar through the entire hair cycle.[8]

To study the effect of ACTH we applied a previously established skin organ culture model.[9] At physiological doses (10^{-9} M) ACTH stimulates DNA synthesis in dermal ($p < 0.01$) but not in epidermal ($p > 0.05$) compartments, and at pharmacological doses (10^{-6}–10^{-7} M) it inhibited DNA synthesis in both dermis and epidermis ($p < 0.01$ and $p < 0.001$, respectively). Previous organ culture studies have documented that ^{3}H-thymidine (Tdr) incorporation into epidermal and dermal compartments represented almost exclusively DNA synthesis by epidermal and follicular

[a]Address for correspondence: Dr. Andrzej Slominski, Department of Pathology, Loyola University Medical Center, 2160 South First Avenue, Maywood, IL 60153, USA. 708-327-2613 (voice); 708-327-2620 (fax); aslomin@wpo.it.luc.edu (e-mail).

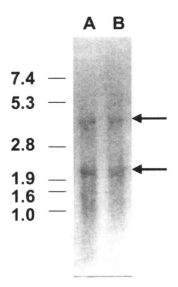

FIGURE 1. Production of ACTH receptor (MC2) mRNA in anagen-VI skin. Two micrograms of poly(A) + RNA were separated on 1% agarose gel. Samples were blotted on nylon membranes and hybridized with a cDNA probe representing the coding region of the mouse MC2 gene (see Ref. 8). Skin at early (*A*) and late (*B*) anagen-VI. MC2 hybridizable transcripts (*arrows*). *Left*, RNA size markers (Kb).

keratinocytes, respectively.[9] Therefore, we suggest that ACTH stimulates DNA synthesis in follicular keratinocytes at physiologic concentration, and inhibits it at pharmacologic doses in both epidermal and follicular keratinocytes.

In summary, we have identified, for the first time, ACTH peptide in mouse skin. We have demonstrated significant hair-cycle-associated fluctuation in its concentration and we have localized ACTH-IR in keratinocytes of epidermis and ORS, as well as in skeletal muscle. We have demonstrated that this peptide can affect keratinocyte proliferation. These findings are in agreement with detection of MC2-R mRNA (receptor for ACTH) in human skin.[10] Therefore, we propose that local production of ACTH is a part of the skin-associated regulatory system governing epidermal and follicular keratinocyte activity, and of anagen-associated melanogenesis.

ACKNOWLEDGMENT

The project was supported in part by grants from NSF (#IBN-9604364), Bane Charitable Trust (LU#9178) to A.S., by grants from Deutsche Forschungsgeimeinschaft (Pa 345/6-1) and Wella AG, Darmstadt to R.P., and Deutsche Forschungsgeimeinschaft SFB 293 to T.L.

REFERENCES

1. SLOMINSKI, A. *et al.* 1993. On the potential role of proopiomelanocortin in skin physiology and pathology. Mol. Cell. Endocrinol. **93:** C1–C6.
2. SLOMINSKI, A. *et al.* 1992. Proopiomelanocortin expression in the skin during induced hair growth in mice. Experientia **48:** 50–54.
3. SLOMINSKI, A. *et al.* 1996. The expression of proopiomelanocortin (POMC) and of corticotropin releasing hormone receptor (CRH-R) genes in mouse skin. Biochim. Biophys. Acta **1289:** 247–251.
4. PAUS, R. *et al.* 1994. Mast cell involvement in murine hair growth. Developmental Biol. **163:** 230–240.
5. ROSE, J. 1988. Adrenocorticotropic hormone (ACTH) but not alpha-melanocyte stimulating hormone (α-MSH) as mediator of adrenalectomy induced hair growth in mink. Invest. Dermatol. **110:** 456–457.
6. SLOMINSKI, A. & R. PAUS. 1993. Melanogenesis is coupled to murine anagen: Toward new concepts for the role of melanocytes and the regulation of melanogenesis in hair growth. J. Invest. Dermatol. **101:** 90S–97S.
7. SLOMINSKI, A. 1998. Identification of β-endorphin, α-MSH and ACTH peptides in cultured human melanocytes, melanoma and squamous cell carcinoma cells by RP-HPLC. Exp. Dermatol. **7:** 213–216.
8. ERMAK, G. & A. SLOMINSKI. 1997. Production of POMC-, CRH-, ACTH-, and α-MSH-receptor mRNA and expression of tyrosinase gene in relation to hair cycle and dexamethasone treatment in the C57BL6 mouse skin. J. Invest. Dermatol. **108:** 160–167.
9. PAUS, R. *et al.* 1991. The epidermal pentapeptide pyroGlu-Glu-Asp-Ser-GlyOH inhibits murine hair growth *in vivo* and *in vitro*. Dermatologica **183:** 173–178.
10. SLOMINSKI, A. *et al.* 1996. ACTH receptor, CYP11A1, CYP17 and CYP21A2 genes are expressed in skin. J. Clin. Endocrinol. Metab. **81:** 2746–2749.

Coexpression of Nitric Oxide Synthase and POMC Peptides in the Dystrophic C57BL/6J Mouse

MARGARET E. SMITH[a] AND RAVINDER K. PHUL

Department of Physiology, Medical School, University of Birmingham, Birmingham B15 2TT, United Kingdom

The C57BL/6J mouse can inherit muscular dystrophy and this is characterized by pathological changes in both the motoneuron and the muscle.[1] The genetic defect is the same as that present in Fukuyama muscular dystrophy in humans.[2] Previously, we showed that increased expression of POMC peptides accompanies this condition,[3] and also other neurodegenerative conditions in the mouse.[4] The POMC peptides have been shown to play a number of trophic roles in the neuromuscular system (for a review see Ref. 5). Excessive nitric oxide (NO) formation, which leads to free radical production, has been implicated in the pathogenesis of many neurodegenerative conditions.[6] Prolonged production of NO has also been implicated in initiating intracellular cascades involving the expression of immediate early genes,[7] and these may transactivate genes for neurotrophic peptides. Nitric oxide synthase (NOS), the enzyme that catalyses the formation of NO by oxidation of L-arginine to L-citrulline, exists as three principle isoforms: the constitutively expressed neuronal and endothelial isoenzymes, and an inducible isotype, macrophage NOS. The expression of NOS increases in the spinal cord after injury.[8] We investigated the question of whether there is a correlation between the expression of nitric oxide synthase and POMC peptides in motoneurons, in normal and dystrophic mice.

Spinal cord tissue from normal and dystrophic mice, twelve-weeks old, was used. The mice were killed by cervical dislocation and the spinal cord was rapidly dissected out. Twenty-μm transverse cryostat sections were prepared from the cervical and lumbar regions of the spinal cord. The expression of POMC peptides was studied by using histochemical *in situ* hybridization with cDNA oligoprobes for the $ACTH_{4-11}$ and β-endorphin$_{1-8}$ encoding regions of POMC mRNA, as previously described,[9] and immunocytochemistry with antibodies to β-endorphin and α-MSH.[10]

Tritiated nitro-L-arginine, a potent inhibitor of NO synthesis in the brain,[6] was used with autoradiography to quantify NOS in the ventral horn of the spinal cord as previously described.[11] Immunocytochemistry with antibodies to the three isoforms of the enzyme was used to identify the isoforms present.

FIGURE 1 shows that POMC mRNA was expressed at very few motoneurons in normal animals, but that it was expressed at a high proportion of these neurons in the dystrophic animals. There was also a higher incidence of motoneurons that were immunoreactive for β-endorphin and α-MSH. FIGURE 2 shows the B_{max} values for

[a]Address for correspondence: Prof. M.E. Smith, Department of Physiology, Medical School, University of Birmingham, Birmingham, B15 2TT UK. 0161 414 6903 (voice); 0121 414 6919 (fax); M.E.Smith@bham.ac.uk (e-mail).

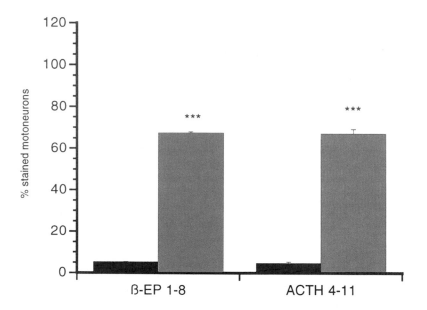

FIGURE 1. Comparison of the numbers of motoneurons that expressed POMC mRNA in normal and dystrophic mice. The values are expressed as the proportion of motoneurons that stained for each cDNA oligoprobe. Normal (*black columns*) and dystrophic (*grey columns*). The values are given as the means ± SEM (*bars*). *** $p < 0.001$.

binding of [³H]nitro-L-arginine, in cervical and lumbar spinal cord, in normal and dystrophic mice. The maximum binding density (B_{max}) was significantly higher in dystrophic mice than in normal mice, in both regions. In the normal spinal cord, the binding profiles of the ligand indicated that the ligand was binding to a single saturatable site with a K_d of approximately 60 nM. This suggests the possibility that the ligand was labelling a single isoform of the enzyme with high affinity. Immunocytochemistry indicated that this isoform was the constitutive isoenzyme normally present in neuronal cells. However, in the diseased condition, the binding profiles implied that there were two saturatable binding sites, with K_d values of approximately 40 nM and 410 nM, indicating that the ligand was labelling two different forms of NOS at sites with different ligand binding affinities. Immunocytochemistry results suggested the presence of both constitutive and inducible isoforms of the enzyme in the ventral horn cells of the dystrophic mice.

Thus, our results indicate that both POMC peptides and the inducible isoform of NOS are upregulated in motoneurons in muscular dystrophy in the C57BL/6J mouse. These results are consistent with a role played, by both POMC peptides and inducible NOS, in the regenerative response in this condition. The mechanisms whereby these molecule are induced is unclear. It is possible that impairment of the neuron-muscle relationship may bring about increased expression of NOS in motoneurons, either through loss of a retrograde signal from the muscle, which normally suppresses NOS expression, or by compensatory increases in excitatory inputs to

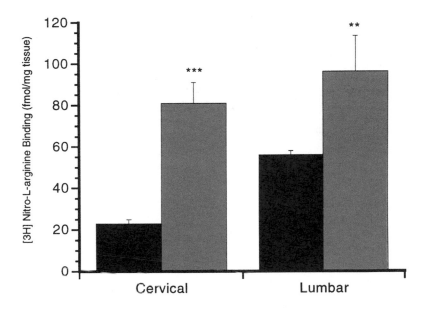

FIGURE 2. Comparison of B_{max} values for specific binding of [^{3}H]nitro-L-arginine in cervical and lumbar regions of the spinal cord. The values are expressed as means ± SEM (*bars*) for four animals in each case. **$p < 0.01$; ***$p < 0.001$.

glutamate receptors that could result in the overexpression of NOS. The increased NO production may then initiate the intracellular cascades that are responsible for both degeneration and regeneration. The latter could include upregulation of the POMC peptides.

REFERENCES

1. BRADLEY, W.G. & M. JENKINSON. 1973. Abnormalities of peripheral nerves in murine muscular dystrophy. J. Neurol. Sci. **18:** 227–247.
2. XU, H., X. WU, U.M. WEWER & E. ENGVALL. 1994. Murine muscular dystrophy caused by a mutation in the laminin α_2 (Lama 2) gene. Nature Genetics **8:** 297–301.
3. HUGHES, S. & M.E. SMITH. 1994. Upregulation of the POMC gene in spinal motoneurones in muscular dystrophy in mice. Neurosci. Lett. **163:** 205–207.
4. HUGHES, S. & M.E. SMITH. 1989. Proopiomelanocortin peptides in mice with motoneurone disease. Neurosci. Lett. **103:** 169–173.
5. STRAND, F.L., K.J. ROSE, L.A. ZUCCARELLI, J. KUME, S.E. ALVES, F.J. ANTANOWICH & L.Y. GARRETT. 1991. Neuropeptide hormones as neurotrophic factors. Physiol. Rev. **71:** 1017–1046.
6. MONCADA, S., R.M.J. PALMER & E.A. HIGGS. 1989. Biosynthesis of nitric oxide from L-arginine: a pathway for the regulation of cell function and communication. Biochem. Pharmacol. **38:** 1709–1715.
7. LEE, J-H., G.L. WILCOX & A.J. BEITZ. 1992. Nitric oxide mediates FOS expression in the spinal cord induced by mechanical noxious stimulation. Neuroreport **3:** 841–844.

8. Wu, W., F.J. Liuzzi, F.P. Schinco, A.S. Depto, Y. Li, J.A. Mong, T.M. Dawson & S.H. Snyder. 1994. Nitric oxide synthase induced in spinal motoneurones by traumatic injury. Neurosci. **61:** 719–726.
9. Hughes, S. & M.E. Smith. 1994. Upregulation of the pro-opiomelanocortin gene in motoneurones after nerve section in mice. Molec. Brain. Res. **25:** 41–49.
10. Hughes, S. & M.E. Smith. 1989. β-Endorphin and α-melanotropin immunoreactivity in transected and contralateral motoneurones in rats. J. Chem. Neuroanat. **2:** 227–237.
11. Phul, R.K., M.E. Smith, P.J. Shaw & P.G. Ince. 1998. Expression of nitric oxide synthase in the spinal cord in ALS. J. Neurol. Sci. In press.

Ligand Binding Profile and Effects of Melanin-Concentrating Hormone on Fish and Mammalian Skin Cells

T. SUPLY, B. CARDINAUD, S. KANAMORI, C. DAL FARRA,
S. RICOIS, AND J.L. NAHON[a]

*Institut de Pharmacologie Moléculaire et Cellulaire, CNRS UPR411,
660 route des Lucioles, Sophia-Antipolis, 06560 Valbonne, France*

Melanin-concentrating hormone (MCH) is a 17-amino-acid cyclic peptide in fish[1] and a 19-amino-acid peptide in mammals.[2] In teleost fish, MCH is produced by hypothalamic neurons, and it acts as a potent paling factor either by direct action on melanocytes, or by inhibition of α-MSH release at the level of the pituitary gland (for a review see Ref. 3). In mammals, MCH synthesis is confined to the lateral hypothalamus and zona incerta, whereas MCH fibers are widely distributed in the central nervous system.[4] MCH is involved as a neuromediator/neuromodulator in a broad array of functions in the brain (see Refs. 3 and 5 for reviews). In the periphery, MCH acts as a paracrine/autocrine inducer of water and electrolyte secretion in the gut. It may also regulate spermatogenesis in rodent and human testis (see Ref. 5 for a review).

PHARMACOLOGIC CHARACTERIZATION OF MCH BINDING SITES ON SVK14 CELLS

MCH interacts with putative membrane receptors that have not yet been characterized in fish or mammalian tissues. Recently, we have identified MCH binding sites expressed by cell lines of human and rodent origins. The highest values of [^{125}I]-[Phe^{13},Tyr^{19}]-MCH binding were found with human skin carcinoma cells,[6] including SVK14 keratinocytes and melanoma, and the rat pheochromocytoma PC12 cell line. This is in agreement with previous studies.[7]

The binding properties of two radiolabeled [^{125}I]-[Phe^{13},Tyr^{19}]-MCH ligands, determined by applying the chloramine T (designed ligand-I) or the lactoperoxydase (ligand-II) methods, were compared on membranes prepared from human SVK14 cells. With ligand I, scatchard analysis of saturation experiments indicated a K_d approximately 1 nM and a B_{max} about 10,000 sites/cell (see FIGURE 1A). With ligand II, scatchard analysis revealed a $K_d \cong 2$ nM and a $B_{max} \cong 170,000$ sites/cell (FIG. 1B). Competition experiments also revealed differences between ligands I and II. For instance, salmon MCH displaced [^{125}I]-[Phe^{13},Tyr^{19}]-MCH with a $K_i \cong 93$ nM when ligand I was used, whereas it did not displace ligand II (not shown). Taken together,

[a]Address for correspondence: J.L. Nahon, I.P.M.C.-CNRS UPR 411, 660 route des Lucioles, Sophia-Antipolis, 06560 Valbonne, France. 33 4 93 95 77 53 (voice); 33 4 93 95 77 08 (fax); Nahonjl@ipmc.cnrs.fr (e-mail).

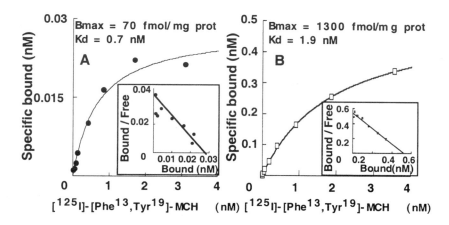

FIGURE 1. Saturation experiment on SVK 14 membranes using chloramine T (**A**) or lactoperoxydase iodination (**B**) labelled [^{125}I]-[Phe^{13},Tyr^{19}]-MCH.

the results of MCH receptor binding experiments suggest that the binding properties of the [Phe^{13},Tyr^{19}]-MCH ligand is highly dependent on the labeling process and/or membrane preparations. These important parameters should be taken into account when this [Phe^{13},Tyr^{19}]-MCH ligand is used in future studies.

EFFECTS OF MCH ON TRANSDUCING
SIGNAL PATHWAYS AND CELL GROWTH

We investigated cellular effects or pathways potentially involved in mediating the effect of MCH on SVK14 cells. It is unlikely that changes in intracellular calcium content were associated with MCH binding, as demonstrated by monitoring the Fura 2 fluorescence in SVK14 cells (our unpublished data). However, MCH might activate the cAMP pathway and inhibit cell growth under restricted cellular conditions (Cardinaud *et al.*, manuscript in preparation).

CHARACTERIZATION OF MCH RECEPTOR ON EEL SKIN CELLS

We primarily determined the physiological action of MCH on pigmentation, using fish skin models.[1] However, our knowledge of the fish MCH-receptor is at present very sparse.[8] In order to characterize the MCH-receptor in fish, we have established an eel skin bioassay and a cellular model of eel melanophores. Using these models, the synthetic salmon MCH and rat MCH were found equipotent, whereas ANF was inactive (see FIGURE 2). Furthermore, treatment with pertussis toxin did not abolish the MCH-induced melanosome aggregation in either the skin or the isolated melanophore bioassays, suggesting that G_i/G_o proteins are not involved in the effect of MCH (Cardinaud *et al.*, manuscript in preparation).

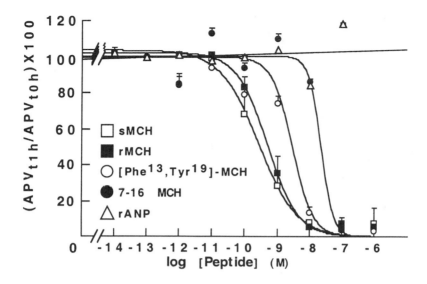

FIGURE 2. Dose-response curves for MCH-like peptides in the eel skin model.

PERSPECTIVES

Cloning the MCH-receptor is becoming a major challenge in the field. Human SVK14 cells and eel skin cells certainly represent good sources from which to prepare cDNA libraries, and to isolate MCH receptor cDNA. However, we are still missing a ligand of value for screening a library by means of an expression cloning strategy. We also need to be able to define precisely the MCH signaling pathways in mammalian and fish cells. Selection of potent agonists/antagonists (of peptidic and nonpeptidic nature) depends on very well characterized cellular models that express MCH-receptor in large amounts.

ACKNOWLEDGMENTS

This work was supported by a grant from the Institut de Recherches Servier (11392). Thomas Suply is a recipient of a Convention CIFRE-I.R.I.S./IdRS (137/97).

REFERENCES

1. KAWAUCHI, H., I. KAWAZOE, M. TSUBOKAWA, M. KISHIDA & B.I. BAKER. 1983. Characterization of melanin-concentrating hormone in chum salmon pituitaries. Nature **305:** 321–323.

2. VAUGHAN, J.M., W.H. FISCHER, C. HOEGER, J. RIVIER & W. VALE. 1989. Characterization of melanin-concentrating hormone from rat hypothalamus. Endocrinology **125:** 1660–1665.
3. BAKER, B.B. 1994. Melanin-concentrating hormone updated. Functional considerations. Trends Endocrinol. Metab. **5:** 120–126.
4. BITTENCOURT, J.C., F. PRESSE, C. ARIAS, C. PETO, J. VAUGHAN, J.L. NAHON, W. VALE & P.E. SAWCHENKO. 1992. The melanin-concentrating hormone system of the rat brain: an immuno- and hybridization histochemical characterization. J. Comp. Neurol. **319:** 218–245.
5. NAHON, J.L. 1994. The melanin-concentrating hormone: from the peptide to the gene. Crit. Rev. Neurobiol. **8:** 221–262.
6. BURGAUD, J.L., R. POOSTI, J.-A. FEHRENTZ, J. MARTINEZ & J.L. NAHON. 1997. Melanin-concentrating hormone binding sites in human SVK14 keratinocytes. Biochem. Biophys. Res. Commun. **241:** 622–629.
7. DROZDZ, R., W. SIEGRIST, B.I. BAKER, J. CHLUBA-DE TAPIA & A.N. EBERLE. 1995. Melanin-concentrating hormone binding to mouse melanoma cells *in vitro.* FEBS Lett. **359:** 199–202.
8. ABRAO, M.S., A.M. DE L. CASTRUCCI, M.E. HADLEY & V.J. HRUBY. 1991. Protein-kinase C mediates MCH signal transduction in teleost, *Synbranchus marmoratus,* melanocytes. Pigment Cell Res. **4:** 66–70.

Occurrence of Four MSHs in Dogfish POMC and Their Immunomodulating Effects

AKIYOSHI TAKAHASHI,[a] YUTAKA AMEMIYA,[a] MASAHIRO SAKAI,[b]
AKIKAZU YASUDA,[c] NOBUO SUZUKI,[d] YUICHI SASAYAMA,[d]
AND HIROSHI KAWAUCHI[a]

[a]Laboratory of Molecular Endocrinology, School of Fisheries Sciences,
Kitasato University, Sanriku, Iwate 022-0101, Japan

[b]Faculty of Agriculture, Miyazaki University, Miyazaki, 889-2192, Japan

[c]Suntory Institute of Bioorganic Research, Simamoto, Mishima, Osaka 618-9924, Japan

[d]Noto Marine Laboratory, Faculty of Science, Kanazawa University,
Uchiura, Ishikawa 927-0553, Japan.

INTRODUCTION

Primary structures of proopiomelanocortin (POMC) have been determined in two out of three taxonomic classes of fish; lamprey[1,2] of cyclostomes in the agnathans, and the sturgeon[3] of chondrosteans, gar[4] of holosteans, chum salmon,[5] rainbow trout,[6] and sockeye salmon[7] of teleosts in the osteichthyans. In contrast to the consistent occurrence of three melanotropins (MSH) in tetrapod POMC,[8] fish POMC varies in the number of MSH types it contains. POMC is, therefore, thought to have evolved in early fish by duplication, insertion, and deletion of MSH genomic segments. However, determination of POMC structure in chondrichthians, the remaining class of fish, is necessary in order to provide insight into the molecular evolution of POMC. On the other hand, it has been indicated that POMC-related peptides exhibit immunomodulating activity. The work described here was undertaken to determine the nucleotide sequence of dogfish POMC cDNA, to identify MSHs in the pituitary gland, and to evaluate the immunomodulating effects of dogfish MSHs.

MATERIALS AND METHODS

Nucleotide Sequence of POMC cDNA

The internal fragment of dogfish POMC cDNA was amplified by RT-PCR by using degenerate primers, based on dogfish $ACTH_{32-38}$[9] and β-MSH_{3-8}[10] from the pituitary of dogfish, *Squalus acanthias*. The remaining regions were amplified from double-strand cDNA that was inserted into a λZAP-II vector by PCR with primers specific to the internal sequence and to λZAP-II. The nucleotide sequence was determined for PCR-amplified cDNA inserted into plasmid.

[a]Address for correspondence: Akiyoshi Takahashi, 81-192-44-1925 (voice); 81-192-44-3934 (fax); akiyoshi@kitasato-u.ac.jp (e-mail).

Purification of MSHs

The acid-acetone extract prepared from dogfish pituitary was subjected to gel filtration, ion-exchange HPLC, and reversed-phase HPLC to purify the MSHs. In each chromatogram, chemically synthesized dogfish MSHs, based on the POMC cDNA, were used as standards. The amino acid sequences of purified dogfish MSH were determined by amino acid sequence-analysis and mass spectrophotometry.

Effect of MSH on Phagocyte

Phagocytes (10^7 cells/ml) prepared from the head kidney of carp, *Cyprinus carpio,* were incubated with chemically synthesized MSH for 24 h at 20°C. The intracellular superoxide anion in phagocytes was determined by reduction of the redox dye, nitroblue tetrazolium.

RESULTS AND DISCUSSION

POMC cDNA prepared from dogfish pituitary is 1315-bp without a poly-A tail. Northern blot analysis detected a 1.4-Kb signal of dogfish POMC mRNA. An open reading frame for the POMC cDNA encodes 320-aa sequence including a signal peptide of 26-aa. The dogfish POMC includes γ-MSH, ACTH, α-MSH, β-MSH, and β-endorphin at positions (50–61), (115–153), (115–127), (239–256), and (259–294), respectively. In addition to these classic peptides, a newly discovered MSH, which we have termed δ-MSH, is present in dogfish POMC at position (184–195), see FIGURE 1.

The four dogfish MSHs can be separated into two groups based on their sequence identities; one pair consists of α-MSH and γ-MSH; the other consists of β-MSH and δ-MSH—suggesting that γ-MSH and δ-MSH may have been duplicated during evolution from α-MSH and β-MSH, respectively. γ-MSH might have first appeared in early gnathostomes, because it is absent in the most primitive vertebrate group, the agnathans. δ-MSH, which at this time is found only in chondrichthians, might have appeared after the divergence of chondrichthians from a lineage leading to osteichthyans and tetrapods.

We identified all four MSHs that are encoded on POMC cDNA, from the dogfish pituitary extract (see FIGURE 2). The amino acid sequences of the most basic and the second most basic MSHs were identical to dogfish POMC sequences (50–61) and (184–195), respectively. Their C-termini are amide. Thus, the former and the latter were identified as γ-MSH and δ-MSH, respectively. These peptides were newly identified MSHs in this work.

The most acidic MSH was identical to dogfish $POMC_{239-254}$. This peptide is two residues shorter than that encoded on POMC cDNA and is identical to β MSH previously described.[10] Thus, this peptide was identified as $\beta\text{-MSH}_{1-16}$. The second acidic MSH showed identical sequence to dogfish $POMC_{115-127}$ and its C-terminus was amide. Thus, this peptide was identified as des-N-Ac-α-MSH, and it is identical to that reported by Bennett *et al.*[10]

Our results show that MSHs enhance the activities of carp phagocytes. Namely, the cells treated with des-N-Ac-α-MSH (1 and 10 ng/ml), $\beta\text{-MSH}_{1-16}$ (0.1 to 100 ng/

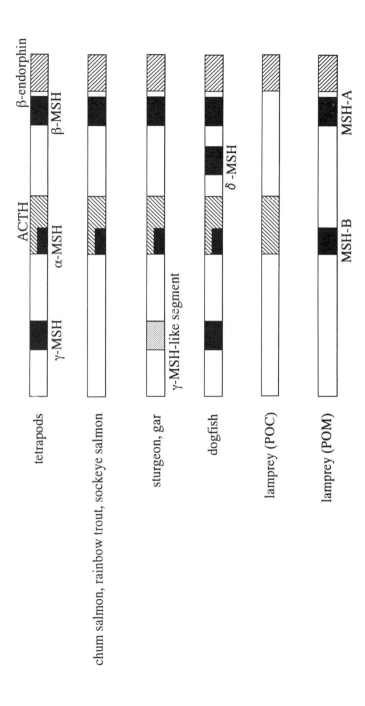

FIGURE 1. Molecular architecture of dogfish POMC compared with those of other vertebrates.

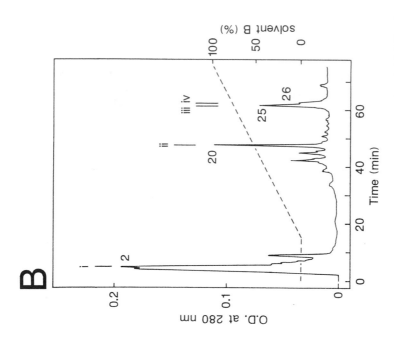

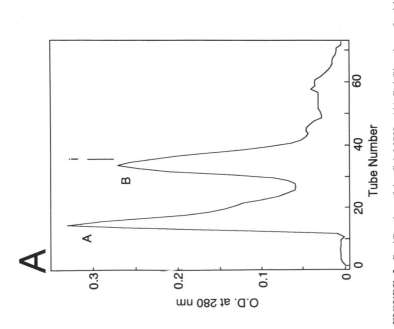

FIGURE 2. Purification of dogfish MSHs. (**A**) Gel filtration of acid-acetone extract of dogfish pituitary glands on a Sephadex G-25 (M) column (2.64 × 40 cm) in 0.1 M acetic acid. Fraction size, 4 ml/tube after forerunning of 50 ml. (**B**) Ion-exchange HPLC of fraction A obtained in (**A**) on a TSKgel CM-3SW column (0.75 × 7.5 cm) with a linear gradient of solvent A and solvent B. Solvent A: 10 mM ammonium acetate, pH 7.0/acetonitrile = 9/1 (v/v). Solvent B: 1 M ammonium acetate, pH 7.0/acetonitrile = 9/1 (v/v). Retention time of chemically synthesized MSH is shown by (*i*) for β-MSH(1–16), (*ii*) for des-N-Ac-α-MSH, (*iii*) for δ-MSH, and (*iv*) for γ-MSH.

ml), γ-MSH (0.1 to 100 ng/ml), and δ-MSH (0.1 to 100 ng/ml) showed increased production of superoxide anion. α-MSH and des-N-Ac-α-MSH with the common structure also increased the production of superoxide anion.

REFERENCES

1. TAKAHASHI, A. *et al.* 1995. Melanotropin and corticotropin are encoded on two distinct genes in the lamprey, the earliest evolved extant vertebrate. Biochem. Biophys. Res. Commun. **213**: 490–498.
2. HEINIG, J.A. *et al.* 1995. The appearance of proopiomelanocortin early in vertebrate evolution: cloning and sequencing of POMC from a lamprey pituitary cDNA library. Gen. Comp. Endocrinol. **99**: 137–144.
3. AMEMIYA, Y. *et al.* 1997. Sturgeon proopiomelanocortin has a remnant of γ-melanotropin. Biochem. Biophys. Res. Commun. **230**: 452–456.
4. DORES, R.M. *et al.* 1997. Deciphering posttranslational processing events in the pituitary of a neopterygian fish: Cloning of a gar proopiomelanocortin cDNA. Gen. Comp. Endocrinol. **107**: 401–413.
5. KITAHARA, N. *et al.* 1988. Absence of a γ-melanocyte-stimulating hormone sequence in proopiomelanocortin mRNA of chum salmon *Oncorhynchus keta*. Comp. Biochem. Physiol. **91B**: 365–370.
6. SALBERT, G. *et al.* 1992. One of the two trout proopiomelanocortin messenger RNAs potentially encodes new peptides. Mol. Endocrinol. **6**: 1605–1613.
7. OKUTA, A. *et al.* 1996. Two types of cDNAs encoding proopiomelanocortin of sockeye salmon, *Oncorhynchus nerka*. Zool. Sci. **13**: 421–427.
8. NAKANISHI, S. *et al.* 1979. Nucleotide sequence of cloned cDNA for bovine corticotropin-β-lipotropin precursor. Nature **278**: 423–427.
9. LOWRY, P.J. *et al.* 1974. The isolation and amino acid sequence of an adrenocorticotrophin from the pars distalis and a corticotrophin-like intermediate-lobe peptide from the neurointermediate lobe of the pituitary of the dogfish *Squalus acanthias*. Biochem. J. **141**: 427–437.
10. BENNETT, H.P.J. *et al.* 1974. Structural studies of α-melanocyte-stimulating hormone and a novel β-melanocyte-stimulating hormone from the neurointermediate lobe of the pituitary of the dogfish *Squalus acanthias*. Biochem. J. **141**: 439–444.

Specific Binding Sites for β-Endorphin on Keratinocytes

K. EGELING, H. MÜLLER, B. KARSCHUNKE, M. TSCHISCHKA,
V. SPENNEMANN, B. HAIN, AND H. TESCHEMACHER[a]

*Rudolf-Buchheim-Institute of Pharmacology, Justus-Liebig-University,
D-35392 Giessen, Germany*

β-Endorphin, the C-terminal fragment of proopiomelanocortin (POMC) has recently been shown to bind specifically[1] to vitronectin,[2] an extracellular matrix constituent able to enhance spreading in keratinocytes.[3] β-Endorphin might participate in this spreading process by acting through specific binding sites on vitronectin, as well as on keratinocytes. We attempted to find specific binding sites for β-endorphin in a keratinocyte model system by using an immortalized human keratinocyte cell line, HaCaT,[4] kindly provided by Dr. Fusenig, Heidelberg, Germany.

HaCaT cells were cultured at 5% CO_2 in DMEM (1.8 mM calcium) containing 10% (v/v) fetal bovine serum, penicillin (100 units/ml) and streptomycin (100 µg/ml). Binding experiments, with cell layers grown to confluency in culture dishes, were performed essentially as described by Schülein and colleagues.[5] In brief, after removing the culture medium, dishes were washed with cold (4°C) Dulbecco's PBS (D-PBS) containing 0.1% BSA. Subsequently the cell layers were incubated on ice with D-PBS containing (^{125}I) $β_H$-endorphin (1–31) in absence or in presence of $β_H$-endorphin (1–31), or fragments thereof, at various concentrations and for various periods of time. Then cells were washed with ice-cold D-PBS and lysed with 0.1 M NaOH at room temperature. The lysate was transferred to polystyrene tubes in order to measure the cell-associated radioactivity in a gamma-spectrometer. For binding experiments with cells in suspension, cells were harvested from culture dishes after incubation with Trypsin (0.05%) and EDTA (0.02%) for about 30 min at 37°C. The cells were washed by centrifugation at 280 g and 4°C, and resuspended in PBS buffer lacking calcium and magnesium. Binding experiments were performed by using a method described by Schweigerer and colleagues[6] with modifications. The cells were incubated in polypropylene vials together with (^{125}I)-$β_H$-endorphin and various concentrations of $β_H$-endorphin (1–31), as well as fragments thereof, at 4°C for two hours. Subsequently an aliquot of the cell suspension was layered over 20% (v/v) saccharose in microfuge tubes. The tubes were centrifuged in a Beckman Microfuge at 4°C, the tips of the tubes were cut off and transferred to polystyrene tubes in order to measure the cell-associated radioactivity in a gamma-spectrometer.

β-Endorphin was found to bind specifically to HaCaT cell layers grown to confluency in culture dishes. The binding showed the characteristics of a specific ligand-receptor interaction, such as time dependence, reversibility, saturability, high affini-

[a]Address for correspondence: Prof. Dr. H. Teschemacher, Rudolf-Buchheim-Institute of Pharmacology, Frankfurter Str. 107, D-35392 Giessen, Germany. +49-641-99 47640 (voice); +49-641-99 47609 (fax); Hansjoerg.Teschemacher@pharma.med.uni-giessen.de (e-mail).

ty, and structural specificity. Moreover, properties such as binding site interaction with the C-terminal β-endorphin fragment, and a K_D in the nM range, proved to be nearly identical with the characteristics previously observed for a vitronectin-β-endorphin interaction.[1]

Specific binding sites for β-endorphin were also found on keratinocytes in suspension after their detachment from culture dishes. However, the structural specificity was different in so far as the binding was mediated via the N-terminal fragment of β-endorphin.

In pilot experiments specific $β_H$-endorphin binding was also found to a human melanoma cell line, G 361 (V. Spennemann, Thesis in preparation).

It appears to be possible that β-endorphin modulates keratinocyte-spreading that is controlled by vitronectin, interacting via its N-terminal fragment with keratinocytes and via its C-terminal fragment with vitronectin bound to the culture dish. However, vitronectin might not just be associated with extracellular matrix or culture dish constituents, since there is some indication that cell association occurs, or even evidence for internalization of vitronectin into keratinocytes.[7] Thus, β-endorphin might also be bound to vitronectin on the keratinocyte surface and might subsequently be internalized to elicit intracellular effects via its N-terminal fragment.

REFERENCES

1. HILDEBRAND, A., K.T. PREISSNER, G. MÜLLER-BERGHAUS & H. TESCHEMACHER. 1989. A novel β-endorphin binding protein. Complement S protein (= vitronectin) exhibits specific non-opioid binding sites for β-endorphin upon interaction with heparin or surfaces. J. Biol. Chem. **264:** 15429–15434.
2. PREISSNER, K.T. 1991. Structure and biological role of vitronectin. Annu. Rev. Cell Biol. **7:** 275–310.
3. STENN, K.S. 1981. Epibolin: A protein of human plasma that supports epithelial cell movement. Proc. Natl. Acad. Sci. USA **78:** 6907–6911.
4. BOUKAMP, P., R.T. PETRUSSEVSKA, D. BREITKREUTZ, J. HORNUNG, A. MARKHAM & N.E. FUSENIG. 1988. Normal keratinization in a spontaneously immortalized aneuoid human keratinocyte cell line. J. Cell Biol. **106:** 761–771.
5. SCHÜLEIN, R., U. LIEBENHOFF, H. MÜLLER, M. BIRNBAUMER & W. ROSENTHAL. 1996. Properties of the human arginine vasopressin V2 receptor after site-directed mutagenesis of its putative palmitoylation site. Biochem. J. **313:** 611–616.
6. SCHWEIGERER, L., W. SCHMIDT, H. TESCHEMACHER & CH. GRAMSCH. 1985. β-Endorphin: Surface binding and internalization in thymoma cells. Proc. Natl. Acad. Sci. USA **82:** 5751–5755.
7. DAHLBÄCK, K., H.-CH. WULF & B. DAHLBÄCK. 1993. Vitronectin in mouse skin: Immunohistochemical demonstration of its association with cutaneous amyloid. J. Invest. Dermatol. **100:** 166–170.

Skin POMC Peptides

Their Binding Affinities and Activation of the Human MC1 Receptor

MARINA TSATMALIA,[a] KAZUMASA WAKAMATSU,[b] ALISON J. GRAHAM, AND ANTHONY J. THODY[a,c]

Department of Dermatology, University of Newcastle upon Tyne, Medical School, Framlington Place, Newcastle upon Tyne, NE2 4HH, United Kingdom

INTRODUCTION

Melanocyte stimulating hormone (MSH) and related peptides, such as adrenocorticotropin (ACTH), are derived from the precursor protein proopiomelanocortin (POMC) by differential enzymatic cleavage. The main site of production for these POMC peptides is the pituitary, but they are also produced in other sites, including the skin, where they have numerous effects through paracrine and/or autocrine mechanisms. α-MSH was the first POMC peptide to be found in human skin.[1] This peptide is best known for its pigmentary action through activation of the melanocortin-receptor-1 (MC1R) that is expressed on melanocytes. It is generally considered that the acetylated form of α-MSH is the most potent of the MSH peptides in regulating melanocyte function. However, ACTH also stimulates melanogenesis in human melanocytes. We have recently shown that the concentrations of ACTH peptides in the human epidermis exceed those of the α-MSH peptides.[2] In this paper we describe our measurements of the binding affinities for the different ACTH and MSH peptides that are present in human skin at the human MC1R, and our comparison of their abilities to couple to this receptor and to increase melanogenesis.

METHODS

Binding studies were carried out in human embryonic kidney (HEK 293) cells, stably transfected with the human MC1R. The K_i values of the POMC peptides that were tested were obtained from competition binding assays (see FIGURE 1a). ^{125}I-Nle^{4}DPhe^{7}α-MSH was used as the labelled ligand, as previously described.[3] Data were analyzed by a non-linear regression fitting computer program (Prism-GraphPad). The transfected HEK 293 cells were also used to measure adenylate cy-

---

[a]Present address: Department of Biomedical Sciences, University of Bradford, Bradford, West Yorkshire, BD7 1DP, United Kingdom.

[b]Present address: Fujita Health University, School of Health Sciences, Toyoake, Aichi, 470-11, Japan.

[c]Address for correspondence: +44 (0)1274 236212 (voice); +44 (0)1274 309742 (fax); A.J.Thody@bradford.ac.uk (e-mail).

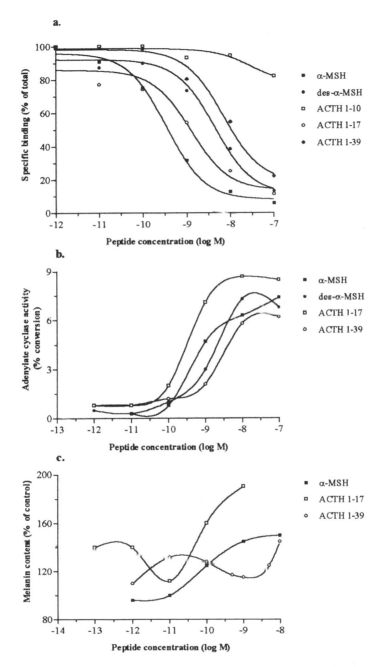

FIGURE 1. (a) Displacement curves obtained from competition binding assays. The concentration of ^{125}I-$Nle^4$$_D$$Phe^7$$\alpha$-MSH was constant (1nM), with varying concentrations of POMC peptides. **(b)** Effect of POMC peptides on adenylate cyclase activity. **(c)** Effects of α-MSH, $ACTH_{1-17}$, and $ACTH_{1-39}$ on melanin content of cultured human melanocytes.

TABLE 1. K_i and EC_{50} values at the human MC1R

POMC peptide	K_i (nM)	EC_{50}-adenylate cyclase activity (nM)	EC_{50}-melanogenesis (nM)
α-MSH	0.13 ± 0.005	1.08 ± 0.21	0.1
des α-MSH	1.12 ± 0.29	6.56 ± 0.20	nd
$ACTH_{1-10}$	40.40 ± 11.14	25.00 ± 0.55	nd
$ACTH_{1-17}$	0.21 ± 0.03	0.43 ± 0.06	0.0001, 0.08
$ACTH_{1-39}$	3.76 ± 1.22	3.02 ± 1.14	0.001, 6.3

clase activity.[2] The effect of POMC peptides on melanogenesis was examined on cultured human melanocytes, as in previous studies.[4]

RESULTS AND DISCUSSION

The K_i values for the POMC peptides are shown in TABLE 1 and displacement curves in FIGURE 1a. Acetylated α-MSH showed the highest affinity for the human MC1R. Desacetyl α-MSH, which is the major peptide in the skin, showed lower binding to the MC1R. Of the ACTH peptides, $ACTH_{1-17}$ was the most potent, with a binding affinity comparable to that of α-MSH. $ACTH_{1-10}$ and $ACTH_{1-39}$ had lower binding affinities.

All the POMC peptides tested increased adenylate cyclase activity (TABLE 1, FIG. 1b) and the EC_{50} value for $ACTH_{1-17}$ was higher than that for α-MSH.

$ACTH_{1-17}$ was also more potent than acetylated α-MSH in stimulating melanogenesis in cultured human melanocytes (TABLE 1). However, the dose response curve for $ACTH_{1-17}$ and the full length peptide, $ACTH_{1-39}$, differed from that of α-MSH in that they were biphasic (FIG. 1c). The reasons for this are not entirely clear but, as suggested previously,[4] it is possible that ACTH peptides can stimulate melanogenesis in human melanocytes by binding to a different receptor, or by coupling to an alternative signalling pathway.

These results demonstrate that ACTH peptides, as well as α-MSH, can bind the human MC1R, activate adenylate cyclase, and increase melanogenesis. These findings, together with the fact that ACTH peptides are present in the skin in greater concentrations than α-MSH, raise the possibility that ACTH peptides are natural ligands at the human MC1R, and that they regulate pigmentary and other responses mediated by this receptor.

ACKNOWLEDGMENT

We are pleased to acknowledge the support of Stiefel Laboratories.

REFERENCES

1. THODY, A.J. *et al.* 1983. MSH peptides are present in mammalian skin. Peptides **4:** 813–816.
2. WAKAMATSU, K. *et al.* 1997. Characterisation of ACTH peptides in human skin and their activation of the melanocortin-1 receptor. Pigment Cell Res. **10:** 288–297.
3. DONATIEN, P.D. *et al.* 1992. The expression of functional MSH receptors on cultured human melanocytes. Arch. Dermatol. Res. **284:** 424–426.
4. HUNT, G. *et al.* 1994. ACTH stimulates melanogenesis in cultured human melanocytes. J. Endocr. **140:** R1–R3.

The Expression of α-MSH by Melanocytes Is Reduced in Vitiligo

ALISON GRAHAM,[a] WIETE WESTERHOF,[b] AND ANTHONY J. THODY[a,c]

[a]Department of Dermatology, University of Newcastle upon Tyne, United Kingdom

[b]The Netherlands Institute for Pigmentary Disorders, Amsterdam, The Netherlands

INTRODUCTION

Vitiligo is an acquired hypopigmentary disorder of the skin that is characterized by an absence of functional melanocytes. The pathogenesis of vitiligo is poorly understood; however, recent evidence suggests that it may involve a breakdown in antioxidant defence mechanisms.[1]

Proopiomelanocortin (POMC) derived peptides such as ACTH and α-MSH are produced in the pituitary and at other sites, including the skin. In 1983, Thody *et al.*, reported that concentrations of α-MSH are reduced in the epidermis of vitiligo patients.[2] Although α-MSH is best known for its role in regulating melanogenesis, it affects other aspects of melanocyte behavior and may protect melanocytes from oxidative damage.[3] A reduction in skin α-MSH might therefore impair the mechanisms involved in the antioxidant defence of melanocytes and could contribute to the pathogenesis of vitiligo.

The aims of this work were to reexamine the expression of α-MSH in vitiligo and to investigate whether the reduction in expression is associated with melanocytes.

MATERIALS AND METHODS

Punch biopsies of lesional, perilesional, and nonlesional skin were taken from the trunk or limbs of six patients with vitiligo (age range 28–65 years) and from six control subjects (age range 9–84 years). Cryostat sections were immunostained using antibodies to α-MSH, ACTH, and the prohormone convertases, PC1 and PC2, as previously described.[4] Of these convertases the former, PC1, cleaves POMC into N-terminally extended ACTH, which is then further cleaved by PC2 into smaller peptides such as ACTH.[5] Melanocytes were identified by their positive staining with the MEL-5 antibody. Antibody reactivity was visualized using the vectorstain peroxidase kit method and nickel-enhanced diaminobenzidine (DAB). Negative controls lacking primary antibody were included in each run.

[a]Address for correspondence: A.J.Thody, Department of Biomedical Sciences, University of Bradford, Bradford, UK. +44(0)1274-236212 (voice); +44(0)1274-309742 (fax) A.J.Thody@bradford.ac.uk (e-mail).

RESULTS AND DISCUSSION

MEL-5 positive melanocytes were present in the epidermis of control skin and in nonlesional and perilesional skin from vitiligo patients (see TABLE 1). As expected the number of MEL-5 positive melanocytes was reduced in lesional skin (TABLE 1).

Immunoreactivity was observed for α-MSH throughout the epidermis of control skin and was particularly strong in melanocytes located at intervals along the basal layer (see FIGURE 1A). α-MSH positive melanocytes were also present in both non-lesional and perilesional skin of the vitiligo patients, but their numbers were significantly reduced (FIG. 1B and C, and TABLE 1). Since there were no corresponding reductions in the number of melanocytes staining positively with MEL-5, it would appear that the loss of staining for α-MSH resulted from decreased expression of the peptide rather than a reduction in melanocyte numbers. Positive staining for the pro-hormone convertases, PC1 and PC2, was also observed throughout the epidermis of control skin. Isolated basal cells, presumably melanocytes, often showed a strong reaction, especially to PC2. As found for α-MSH there was a reduction in the number of strongly PC1- and PC2-positive cells in the basal layer of the epidermis in vitiligo patients (TABLE 1). Immunostaining for ACTH differed from that of α-MSH in that, although a positive reaction was seen in keratinocytes for control skin, there was no enhanced staining of melanocytes. This confirms our earlier findings.[4] Furthermore, the pattern of staining in vitiligo skin was similar to that of the controls (results not shown).

These results confirm our earlier findings that human epidermal melanocytes express α-MSH.[4] They also demonstrate that there is a reduction in the level of this peptide in the melanocytes of vitiligo patients. The reasons for this are not clear but, since the expression of PC1 and PC2 were similarly reduced, it is possible that in vitiligo there may a defect in the ability of melanocytes to cleave POMC to α-MSH. Whether such changes are the consequence of melanocyte damage, or whether they contribute to the pathogenesis of vitiligo, is not clear. However, since α-MSH affects melanocytes in various ways[6] and appears to have a role in protecting these cells from oxidative damage,[3] it is not inconceivable that a reduction in its expression could contribute to the loss of functioning melanocytes in vitiligo.

TABLE 1. Number of MEL 5-, α-MSH-, PC1-, and PC2- positive basal cells in the epidermis of control subjects and vitiligo patients

	Control	Vitiligo		
		nonlesional	perilesional	lesional
MEL-5	33.3 ± 2.9	26.6 ± 7.2	18.7 ± 1.2	2
α-MSH	23.8 ± 2.5	7.0 ± 2.3^a	5.8 ± 0.8^b	1
PC-1	9.5 ± 1.6	< 1	0	< 1
PC-2	14.0 ± 2.3	8.3 ± 4.7	0.6 ± 0.4	< 1

Numbers are expressed as mean per 200 basal cells. Where no standard errors are given, values were obtained from only two subjects. $^a p = 0.004$ vs. control. $^b p = 0.00004$ vs. control by unpaired *t*-test.

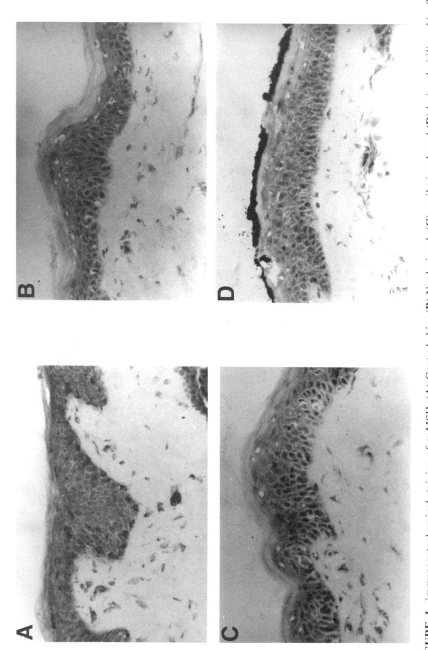

FIGURE 1. Immunocytochemical staining of α-MSH. **(A)** Control skin. **(B)** Nonlesional, **(C)** perilesional, and **(D)** lesional vitiligo skin. The *black mark* on the stratum corneum was used to delineate the lesion prior to removal of the biopsy. Note the strong staining in melanocytes from the control skin and the reduction in number of strongly positive melanocytes in all three vitiligo skin sites.

ACKNOWLEDGMENTS

We are pleased to acknowledge the support of Stiefel Laboratories.

REFERENCES

1. SCHALLREUTER, K.U. *et al.* 1991. Low catalase levels in the epidermis of patients with vitiligo. J. Invest. Dermatol. **97:** 1081–1085.
2. THODY, A.J. *et al.* 1983. MSH peptides are present in mammalian skin. Peptides **4:** 813–816.
3. VALVERDE, P. *et al.* 1996. Tyrosinase may protect human melanocytes from the cytotoxic effects of the superoxide anion. Exp. Dermatol. **5:** 247–253.
4. WAKAMATSU, K. *et al.* 1997. Characterisation of ACTH peptides in human skin and their activation of the melanocortin-1 receptor. Pigment Cell Res. **10:** 288–297.
5. SEIDAH, N.G. *et al.* 1993. Mammalian paired basic amino acid convertases of prohormones and proproteins. Ann. N.Y. Acad. Sci. **680:** 135–146.
6. THODY, A.J. 1999. α-MSH and the regulation of melanocyte function. Ann. N.Y. Acad.Sci. **885:** this volume.

α-MSH Inhibits Lipopolysaccharide Induced Nitric Oxide Production in B16 Mouse Melanoma Cells

MARINA TSATMALI,[a] PHILIP MANNING,[b] CALUM J. McNEIL,[b] AND ANTHONY J. THODY[a,c]

[a]Department of Biomedical Sciences, University of Bradford, Bradford, United Kingdom

[b]Department of Clinical Biochemistry, University of Newcastle upon Tyne, Newcastle upon Tyne, United Kingdom

INTRODUCTION

α-Melanocyte stimulating hormone (α-MSH) is produced in the skin where it functions as a local hormone to regulate melanogenesis in melanocytes. It does, however, act on other cells and there is evidence that α-MSH has a number of immunomodulatory and anti-inflammatory actions. It has been suggested that in some cells (for example, macrophages) α-MSH brings about these effects by blocking the production of nitric oxide (NO) induced in response to lipopolysaccharide (LPS) and/or pro-inflammatory cytokines.[1]

α-MSH has also been shown to affect NO production in melanocytes, but rather than having an inhibitory effect, it enhances the production of NO that occurs in response to UVR.[2] It is not clear whether the contrasting effects in melanocytes and macrophages are related to cell type, or whether they reflect the different stimuli with which α-MSH interacts. In this paper we, therefore, examine the effect of LPS on NO production by pigment cells, and how this might be affected by α-MSH.

METHODS

Cell Culture

B16 F1 mouse melanoma cells were maintained in Dulbecco's Modified Eagle Medium (DMEM) with 10% foetal calf serum, 50 IU/ml penicillin, and 50 mg/ml streptomycin.

Measurement of NO

B16 melanoma cells were seeded into petri dishes at a density of 10^6 cells per dish. After allowing them to attach overnight at 37°C in a humidified incubator, fresh medium was added. NO production was measured in real time using a commercially

[c]Address for correspondence: +44 (0)1274 236212 (voice); +44 (0)1274 309742 (fax); A.J.Thody@bradford.ac.uk (e-mail).

TABLE 1. Effect of LPS on NO production

LPS (ng/ml)	NO peak current (pA)
5	150
10	280
15	510
20	880

available ISO-NO sensor probe (ISO-NO meter, World Precision Instruments Ltd., Sarasota, USA).[3] A peak current of 350 pA at the NO electrode corresponded to 75 nM of NO. The electrode was inserted into each culture, allowed to settle prior to the addition of LPS, and measurements were continued for up to 5 min.

RESULTS AND DISCUSSION

In a preliminary experiment it was shown that the addition of LPS produced immediate, dose-related increases in the concentrations of NO (see TABLE 1). On the basis of these results 15 ng/ml of LPS were used to stimulate NO release in all sub-

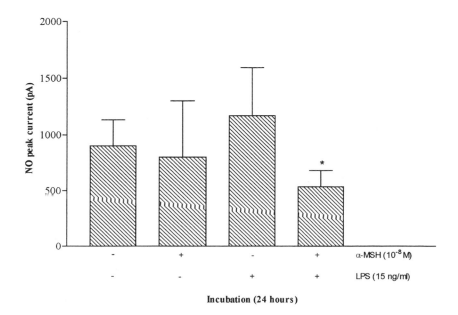

FIGURE 1. Effect of α-MSH on nitric oxide production in the presence and absence of LPS. The results are the mean ± SD of three determinations. *$p < 0.02$ compared with LPS alone.

sequent experiments. In contrast, the addition of α-MSH produced no immediate increase in NO. Preincubation of the cultures with 10^{-8} M α-MSH for 24 hours had no effect on the increase in NO that occurred in response to LPS (see FIGURE 1).

Cultures that had been preincubated with 15 ng/ml of LPS for 24 hours, showed an increase in NO concentration when stimulated acutely with LPS. This increase was inhibited by the presence of 10^{-8} M α-MSH, (FIG. 1).

These results demonstrate that α-MSH is able to inhibit LPS-induced NO production in B16 mouse melanoma cells. Therefore, it appears that in pigment cells α-MSH inhibits the induction of iNOS, as it does in macrophages. These findings, however, contrast with the NO increase in response to α-MSH in melanocytes and B16 cells following UV stimulation. It appears, therefore, that in pigment cells, α-MSH has both inhibitory and stimulatory influences on the production of NO. How α-MSH produces these opposing effects is not clear, but the fact that it exhibits these different actions suggests that the peptide may have a role as a modulator of NO production in melanocytes.

REFERENCES

1. STAR, R.A. *et al.* 1995. Evidence for autocrine modulation of macrophage nitric oxide synthase by α-melanocyte stimulating hormone. Proc. Natl. Acad. Sci. USA **92:** 8016–8020.
2. GRAHAM, A. *et al.* 1997. α-MSH induces nitric oxide production in melanocytes. (Abstract). Pigment Cell Res. **10:** 327.
3. BRODERICK, M.P. & Z. TAHA. 1995. Nitric oxide detection using a popular electrochemical sensor-recent applications and the development of a new generation of highly sensitive and selective NO-microsensors. Satell. Symp. 4th IBRO World Cong. Neurosci. Kyoto, Japan.

Index of Contributors

Abdel-Malek, Z., 117–133
Adan, R.A.H., 342–349
Airaghi, L., 183–187
Akcali, C., 117–133
Alard, P., 196–208
Amato, S., 400–404
Amemiya, Y., 459–463
Ansel, J.C., 239–253, 444–447
Armstrong, C.A., 239–253, 444–447
Artuc, M., 364–367

Barsh, G.S., 143–152, 173–182
Basak, A., 57–74
Bayerl, C., 400–404
Beazley, W.D., 329–341
Becher, E., 188–195
Benjannet, S., 57–74
Bianchi, B., 262–267
Bigliardi, P.L., 368–371
Bigliardi-Qi, M., 368–371
Billingsley, J., 440–443
Birch-Machin, M., 134–142
Blalock, J.E., 161–172
Böhm, M., 277–286, 372–382
Bolognia, J., 100–116
Boston, B.A., 75–84
Botchkarev, V.A., 287–311, 350–363, 433–439, 448–450
Botchkareva, N.V., 350–363, 433–439, 448–450
Boyadjieva, N., 383–386
Brzoska, T., 188–195, 209–216, 230–238, 239–253, 254–261, 372–382, 414–418, 444–447
Büchner, S., 368–371

Cardinaud, B., 455–458
Carlin, A., 183–187
Carr, J., 440–443
Catania, A., 173–182, 183–187

Chakraborty, A.K., 100–116, 448–450
Chartrel, N., 41–57
Choudhry, M., 287–311
Chrétien, M., 57–74
Corliss, D., 427–429
Cutuli, M., 183–187

Dal Farra, C., 455–458
De Pità, O., 268–276
Delgado, R., 183–187
Demitri, M.T., 183–187
Desrues, L., 41–57

Egeling, K., 464–465
Esche, C., 387–390

Fastrich, M., 239–253
Fazal, N., 287–311
Fechner, K., 287–311
Flanagan, N., 134–142
Frezzolini, A., 268–276
Funasaka, Y., 100–116, 391–393
Furkert, J., 287–311

Galas, L., 41–57
Garofalo, L., 183–187
Ghanem, G., 396–399
Gibbons, N.J.P., 329–341
Gispen, W.H., 342–349
Grabbe, S., 188–195
Graham, A.J., 470–473, 466–469
Granstein, R.D., 405–413
Grüters, A., 419–421
Grützkau, A., 364–367
Gunn, T.M., 143–152
Gupta, A.K., 394–395
Gupta, M.A., 394–395

Hadley, M.E., 1–21
Hain, B., 464–465
Hamelin, J., 57–74
Hartmeyer, M., 239–253, 444–447
Haskell-Luevano, C., 1–21
Haycock, J.W., 396–399
Healy, E., 134–142
Held, B., 400–404
Henz, B.M., 364–367
Holick, M.F. 85–99
Hosoi, J., 405–413

Ichihashi, M., 100–116, 391–393
Ichiyama, T., 173–182
Im, S., 117–133

Jackson, D.M., 85–99
Jenner, T., 329–341
Johansson, O., 422–426
Jung, E.G., 400–404

Kalden, D.-H., 188–195, 230–238,
    239–253, 254–261, 444–447
Kalden, H., 209–216, 277–286, 414–418
Kanamori, S., 455–458
Karschunke, B., 464–465
Kawauchi, H., 459–463
Kikuyama, S., 41–57
Kost, N.V., 387–390
Krause, E., 287–311
Krude, H., 419–421
Kubitscheck, U., 372–382

Lerner, M.R., 153–162
Lipton, J.M., xi–xiv, 173–182, 183–187
Lotti, T., 262–267, 268–276
Lotze, M.T., 387–390
Lovering, A., 440–443
Luck, W., 419–421
Luger, T.A., xi–xiv, 188–195, 209–216,
    230–238, 239–253, 254–261,
    277–286, 350–363, 364–367,
    372–382, 414–418, 430–432,
    433–439, 444–447, 448–450
Lundeberg, L., 422–426

MacNeil, S., 396–399
Mahnke, K., 188–195
Makarenkova, V.P., 387–390
Mamarbachi, A.M., 57–74
Manning, P., 474–476
Marcinkiewicz, J., 57–74
Marcinkiewicz, M., 57–74
Marshall, H.S., 329–341
Mauviel, A., 262–267, 268–276
Mazurkiewicz, J.E., 427–429
Mbikay, M., 57–74
McNeil, C.J., 474–476
Meadows, G., 383–386
Mecklenburg, L., 350–363
Metze, D., 430–432
Miller, K.A., 143–152
Moore, J., 329–341
Mor, A., 41–57
Morandini, R., 396–399
Müller, H., 464–465

Nahon, J.L., 455–458
Nicolas, P., 41–57
Niizeki, H., 196–208
Nordlind, K., 422–426

Olbertz, J., 440–443
Ollmann, M.M., 143–152
Ozawa, H., 405–413

Paus, R., xi–xiv, 287–311, 350–363,
    433–439, 448–450
Pawelek, J.M., 100–116
Perrin, M.H., 312–328
Phillips, S., 134–142
Phul, R.K., 451–454
Puddu, P., 268–276

Rees, J.L., 134–142
Reimann, S., 430–432
Rennie, I.G., 396–399
Ricois, S., 455–458
Roloff, B., 287–311, 433–439
Rose, J., 440–443
Rufli, T., 368–371

Sakai, M., 459–463
Sarkar D., 383–386
Sasayama, Y., 459–463
Sato, H., 391–393
Sayeed, M., 287–311
Schallreuter, K.U., 329–341
Schiller, M., 372–382
Schnabel, D., 419–421
Scholzen, T., 209–216, 230–238, 239–253, 254–261, 444–447
Schulte, U., 277–286, 372–382
Schwarz, A., 209–216
Schwarz, T., 209–216
Seidah, N.G., 57–74
Shurin, M.R., 387–390
Slominski, A., xi–xiv, 100–116, 287–311, 350–363, 427–429, 433–439, 448–450
Smith, M.E., 451–454
Sodi, S., 100–116
Solomon, S., 22–40
Sorg, C., 414–418
Spennemann, V., 464–465
Streilein, J.W., 196–208
Sunderkötter, C., 414–418
Sundström, E., 422–426
Suply, T., 455–458
Suzuki, I., 117–133
Suzuki, N., 459–463

Tada, A., 117–133
Takahashi, A., 459–463
Teofoli, P., 262–267, 268–276
Teschemacher, H., 464–465

Thody, A.J., 217–229, 466–469, 470–473, 474–476
Tobin, D.J., 329–341
Todd, C., 134–142
Tonon, M.C., 41–57
Tsatmali, M., 474–476
Tsatmalia, M., 466–469
Tschischka, M., 464–465

Uenalan, M., 448–450

Vale, W.W., 312–328
Vaudry, H., 41–57
Verhofstad, A., 422–426

Wagner, M., 396–399
Wakamatsu, K., 466–469
Wei, E., 287–311
Westerhof, W., 470–473
Wilson, B.D., 143–152
Wood, J.M., 329–341
Wood, K., 440–443
Wortsman, J., 287–311

Yasuda, A., 459–463

Zanello, S.B., 85–99
Zbytek, B., 287–311
Zhao, H., 173–182
Zipper, J., 287–311
Zozulya, A.A., 387–390